Diagnostic Methods in Speech Pathology

Diagnostic Methods in Speech Pathology

SECOND EDITION

Frederic L. Darley
Mayo Clinic

D. C. Spriestersbach
University of Iowa

and contributors:
Charles V. Anderson
Arnold E. Aronson
Margaret C. Byrne
Julia M. Davis
Hughlett L. Morris
Dean E. Williams

Harper & Row, Publishers
New York / Hagerstown / San Francisco / London

Sponsoring Editor: James B. Smith
Project Editor: Robert Ginsberg
Designer: Emily Harste
Production Supervisor: Marion Palen
Compositor: Port City Press, Inc.
Printer and Binder: The Maple Press Company
Art Studio: J & R Technical Services Inc.

Diagnostic
Methods
In Speech
Pathology
Second Edition

Library of Congress Cataloging in Publication Data

Darley, Frederic L.
    Diagnostic methods in speech pathology.

    Edition of 1963 by W. Johnson, F. L. Darley, and
D. C. Spriestersbach.
    Includes bibliographical references and index.
    1. Speech, Disorders of—Diagnosis.
I. Spriestersbach, D. C., joint author. II. Johnson,
Wendell, 1906–1965. Diagnostic methods in speech
pathology. III. Title.
RC423.J58   1978   616.8′55′075   77–28596
ISBN 0–06–041497–9

To Jack—
Mentor, Collaborator, Friend—
In the hope that this revision projects anew his
teaching that to know and to do effectively require
objective answers to pertinent questions.

CONTENTS

ACKNOWLEDGMENTS

We express our appreciation to the publishers and to the authors for permission to reproduce or adapt material from the following:

Academic Press, Inc.
Fraser, C., Bellugi, U., Brown, R., Control of grammar in imitation, comprehension, and production. *Journal of Verbal Learning and Verbal Behavior*, 1963, 2:121–135.

American Dental Association
Lunt, R. C., and Law, D. B., A review of the chronology of eruption of deciduous teeth. *Journal of the American Dental Association*, 1974, 89:872–879.

American Medical Association
Ziegler, F. J., and Imboden, J. B., Contemporary conversion reactions. II. A conceptual model. *Archives of General Psychiatry*, 1962, 6:279–287.
Ziegler, F. J., Imboden, J. B., and Rodgers, D. A., Contemporary conversion reactions: III. Diagnostic considerations. *Journal of the American Medical Association*, 1963, 186:307–311.

American Psychological Association
Irwin, O. C., and Chen, Han Piao, Development of speech during infancy: curve of phonemic types. *Journal of Experimental Psychology*, 1946, 36:431–436.
Irwin, O. C., Development of speech during infancy: curve of phonemic frequencies. *Journal of Experimental Psychology*, 1947, 37:187–193.

American Society of Dentistry for Children
Hurme, V. O., Ranges of normalcy in the eruption of permanent teeth. *Journal of Dentistry for Children*, 1949, 16:11–15.

American Speech and Hearing Association
Kaplan, Lucille T., A descriptive continuum of language responses in aphasia. *Journal of Speech and Hearing Disorders*, 1959, 24:410–412.

McReynolds, Leija V., and Huston, Kay, A distinctive feature analysis of children's misarticulations. *Journal of Speech and Hearing Disorders,* 1971, *36*:155–166.

Prather, Elizabeth M., Hedrick, Dona Lea, and Vane, Carolyn A., Articulation development in children aged two to four years. *Journal of Speech and Hearing Disorders,* 1975, *40*:179–191.

Rosenbek, John C., McNeil, Malcolm R., Lemme, Margaret L., Prescott, Thomas E., and Alfrey, Allen C., Speech and language findings in a chronic hemodialysis patient: a case report. *Journal of Speech and Hearing Disorders,* 1975, *40*:245–252.

Sander, Eric H., When are speech sounds learned? *Journal of Speech and Hearing Disorders,* 1972, 37:55–61.

Sax, Mary R., A longitudinal study of articulation change. *Language, Speech, and Hearing Services in Schools,* 1972, 3:41–48.

Weiner, Paul S., The standardization of tests: criteria and criticisms. *Journal of Speech and Hearing Research,* 1973, *16*:616–626.

Wepman, Joseph M., The relationship between self-correction and recovery from aphasia. *Journal of Speech and Hearing Disorders,* 1958, 23:302–305.

Wingate, M. E., A standard definition of stuttering. *Journal of Speech and Hearing Disorders,* 1964, 29:484–489.

Young, Martin A., Predicting ratings of severity of stuttering. *Journal of Speech and Hearing Disorders,* Monograph Supplement No. 7, 1961, 31–54.

Bobbs Merrill Co., Inc., Test Division

Baker, H. J., and Leland, B., *Detroit Tests of Learning Aptitude.*

College of Speech Therapists

Boller, F., Albert, M., and Denes, F., Palilalia. *British Journal of Disorders of Communication,* 1975, *10*:92–97.

Cortex

Benson, D. F., Fluency in aphasia; correlation with radioactive scan localization. *Cortex,* 1967, *3*:373–394.

Shankweiler, D., and Harris, K. S., An experimental approach to the problem of articulation in aphasia. *Cortex,* 1966, 2:277–292.

Harper & Row, Publications, Inc.

Fairbanks, Grant, *Voice and Articulation Drillbook.*

Johnson, Wendell, *People in Quandaries: The Semantics of Personal Adjustment.*

Indiana University, Institute for Sex Research

Kinsey, A. C., Pomeroy, W. B., and Martin, C. E., *Sexual Behavior in the Human Male,* Philadelphia: W. B. Saunders Co., 1948.

S. Karger, Verlag

Van Riper, C., Stuttering and cluttering: the differential diagnosis. *Folia Phoniatrica,* 1970, 22:347–353.

The MIT Press

Menyuk, Paula, *Sentences Children Use.*

National Council of Teachers of English, Committee on Research
O'Donnell, R. D., Griffin, W. J., and Norris, R. C., *Syntax of Kindergarten and Elementary School Children: A Transformational Analysis.* Research Report No. 8.

Northwestern University Press
Lee, Laura L., *Developmental Sentence Analysis.*

Prentice-Hall, Inc.
Gleason, J. B., The child's learning of English morphology. Pp. 153–157 in Bar-Adon, A., and Leopold, W. F., Eds., *Child Language: A Book of Readings.*
Van Riper, C., *The Nature of Stuttering*
Wood, Nan E., *Delayed Speech and Language Development*

The Psychological Corporation
Eisenson, J., *Examining for Aphasia*

Random House, Publishers
Williams, Roger J., *You Are Extraordinary*

W. B. Saunders Company
Darley, F. L., Aronson, A. E., and Brown, J. R., *Motor Speech Disorders.*

Charles C Thomas, Publishers
Heaver, L., Spastic dysphonia. Ch. XII, pp. 250–263 in Barbara, D. A., Ed., *Psychological and Psychiatric Aspects of Speech and Hearing.*

University of Iowa Bureau of Educational Research and Service
Templin, Mildred C., and Darley, Frederic L., *The Templin-Darley Tests of Articulation.*

University of Minnesota Press
Johnson, Wendell, Ed., *Stuttering in Children and Adults.*
Templin, Mildred C., *Certain Language Skills in Children,* Child Welfare Monograph No. XXVI.

PREFACE

This is a textbook for students who are learning to be speech and language pathologists. It is designed to give them a philosophy for clinical practice, to teach them how to be efficient observers of oral communicative behavior and of the speech mechanism, and to help them develop skills for arriving at therapy decisions based on differentiations made among the possible etiological implications of the communicative behaviors they observe.

The book is divided into three sections. Chapter 1 introduces the student to a philosophy of diagnosis and appraisal. Part One is concerned with appraisal—what to observe and how and why. Part Two is concerned with differential diagnosis—how to interpret what has been learned about the patient and how to integrate data from observations in order to make a differential diagnosis—which leads to a defensible rationale for a therapy plan.

We assume that the book will be used by students at several points during their course of study to become speech pathologists. Part One is designed for a course in clinical practice early in the student's training, whereas Part Two is for use in one or more advanced courses which deal with specific disorders of communication.

This book is the result of over 25 years of experience in working with methods and materials for teaching diagnosis and appraisal in speech and language pathology. Our first attempt to deal with the matter was *Diagnostic Manual in Speech Correction* (Harper & Row, 1952), by Wendell Johnson, Frederic L. Darley, and D. C. Spriestersbach. In that book we brought together the various materials that we were using in teaching our several courses in introduction to clinical practice, articulation and voice disorders, stuttering, and organic communication disorders. In large measure it was a workbook replete with tear-out forms introduced with minimal explanatory material. It was designed to teach the student to become a skilled and disciplined observer but it had an unintended cookbook flavor.

Eleven years later we updated our efforts (*Diagnostic Methods in Speech Pathology,* Harper & Row, 1963). In this edition the substantive material describing the speech and language behaviors to be observed was much enlarged and the tearout forms were gone, although suggested forms for recording observations were still present. The cookbook character of the material was much less evident.

The current edition represents yet another stage in our thinking about the most effective way to teach diagnosis and appraisal. The forms have largely disappeared and the substantive material has been further enlarged. The major change, however, relates to our recognition that the previous editions were concerned primarily with appraisal; little was said about diagnosis. In this edition a major section of the book concerns diagnosis. The material on language development and disorders, organic communication disorders, and voice disorders has been much enlarged. Material on auditory sensation and perception and their disorders has been added. This new material is not included to prepare students to be audiologists; rather, it is intended to prepare speech pathologists to make appropriate referrals to audiologists and to prepare them to use audiological information appropriately in the development of therapeutic plans for persons with speech, voice, and language disorders.

The most significant change in this edition comes, however, from the absence of our former senior author, Wendell Johnson. Jack died in 1965, but his impact is evident in this edition. He was our mentor and he taught us well. His stress on the imperative of understanding the processes which undergird normal and disordered speech behavior as a prerequisite to diagnosis and appraisal is still a thesis of this edition. His concern for sensitivity in the appropriate use of language in describing communication behaviors expresses itself throughout the chapters of this book.

Additional contributors, all practicing speech pathologists or audiologists, have joined us in preparing the material for this edition. They include Charles V. Anderson, Departments of Speech Pathology and Audiology and Otolaryngology and Maxillofacial Surgery, University of Iowa; Arnold E. Aronson, Consultant in Speech Pathology, Mayo Clinic; Margaret C. Byrne, Department of Speech Pathology and Audiology, University of Kansas; Julia M. Davis, Department of Speech Pathology and Audiology, University of Iowa; Hughlett L. Morris, Departments of Speech Pathology and Audiology and Otolaryngology and Maxillofacial Surgery, University of Iowa; and Dean E. Williams, Department of Speech Pathology and Audiology, University of Iowa. Their particular contributions are recognized by identification of the authors at the beginning of each chapter. Their knowledge has contributed immeasurably to the continued vitality of this effort.

FREDERIC L. DARLEY
D. C. SPRIESTERSBACH

Rochester, Minnesota
Iowa City, Iowa
October, 1977

1
A PHILOSOPHY OF APPRAISAL AND DIAGNOSIS

Frederic L. Darley

A CHALLENGE TO THE CLINICIAN

A speaker has an impairment of communication. The speech pathologist-audiologist who examines him embarks on an intricate bit of detective work: he or she must discern what this person is like, how he came to be what he is, what the specific nature of his communication problem is, how it came to be, what variables might conceivably be relevant to its maintenance and its disappearance, and what procedures might be adopted to reduce whatever makes this communication difference a difference. The clinician in charge of evaluating the problem—appraising and diagnosing it—must be aware of at least four blocks of information, must investigate and make use of them critically, and must arrive at decisions which may have significant implications for the speaker and those about him.

1. The Individual Is Unique

Alexander Pope stated that "the proper study of mankind is man." But "man" is an abstraction. There are only individual men and women, and each is unique. To neglect that individuality can immediately set us off on the wrong foot in understanding a speaker. The importance of this is dramatized in the following analogy:

> A group of people is something like a collection of colorful marbles. In the assortment of marbles all are reasonably round, but they are of different sizes; some are made of pottery, some of glass, some of agate, some of plastic and some of steel. They may be all colors of the rainbow, and individually they may be multicolored, striped, mottled,

stippled, translucent, decorated with lustrous flecks and patterned in a multitude of ways.

Try to average these marbles and one comes out with nonsense. Marbles are not made partly of pottery, partly of glass, partly of plastic, partly of agate and partly of steel. Such marbles wouldn't hold together. Try to find the average color of the marbles; mount them on a circular disk, rotate rapidly and observe. The color comes back a dirty gray. But there isn't a dirty-gray marble in the lot! People are as distinctive as marbles, but when we attempt to average them we come up with dirty-gray "man." This doesn't have anything to do with you or me, for we are colorful, interesting specimens more marvelously unique than any marbles. Averaging when applied in this careless way to people can be vicious. (21, pp. 3–4)

How do we individuals differ from one another? Let us count the ways: finger prints; acuity of peripheral vision; size and shape of our stomachs, hearts, kidneys, sinuses, blood vessels; blood groups; number, arrangement, and structure of teeth; toe prints; heart action; color vision; breathing patterns; length of fingers and toes; pattern of body hair; hair texture; stance; gait; blood chemistry; thickness of skin; ear size and shape; brain waves; heart action; size, number, and distribution of neurons in our central nervous systems; skin color; shape of semicircular canals; number of muscles; rate of blood clotting; distribution of nerve endings on the body surface; height-weight ratio; sensitivity of skin to sun; manner of attachment of muscles to ribs; voice quality; character of pain receptors; hearing sensitivity at various frequencies; the format of our faces; the profile of our intellectual abilities; and on and on to infinity (20, 21).

In short, "biologically, each member of the human family possesses inborn differences based on his brain structure and on his vast mosaic of endocrine glands—in fact, on every aspect of his physical being. . . . No one ever 'recovers' from the fact that he was born an individual" (22).

As an examiner you are confronted with an individual unlike anybody you have ever seen or will ever see again. It is this individual whose capabilities and problems you must assess. You will not understand or properly serve the speaker if you think only in terms of "the child," "the woman," "men," "the stutterer," or "a cleft palate." You will do best to envision each speaker as an individual among individuals who are unaverageable.

2. Each Environment Is Distinctive

Not only is a speaker unique with regard to his or her nature but also with regard to his or her nurture. From the moment of birth each of us has been surrounded by a unique milieu shared by no one in every excruciating detail. Here is uniqueness compounded, for as Travis (19) has stated, "Every individual is the resultant of the interaction between his original endowment and the environment into which he is thrust."

In many respects the environment serves to knock off the rough edges and to shape the rugged individual into something roughly conforming to a norm established by society. The social institutions that impinge upon you—family, peer group, community, ʻchurch, school—may in certain ways reduce your individuality and mold you into something that fits. But many personal characteristics are obviously not significantly altered by environmental influences; on the contrary, "teaching" may heighten differences and exaggerate uniqueness.

None of us "outgrows" the fact that we had our parents and not somebody else's; that we were an only child or had a twin or had 12 siblings; that food at home was abundant and nutritious or was scanty but filling; that Mrs. Utterback saw us through the second grade while Miss Miller scared us spitless in the fourth. We bear our distinctive scars and bruises and carry our personal joyful memories and bitter resentments.

If we as clinicians are to fathom what makes Johnny run, we must understand who spurs him on, who deters him, who rewards him, who punishes him, who trains him, who treats his wounds, who plans his diet, who embraces him, and who attacks him—and how all these things are done to him and how he responds.

3. Communication Is Multiphasic

Communication itself, like the individual who communicates and the environment that surrounds him or her, is complex. Oral expression involves the sequential execution and coordination of several basic functions:

1. Underlying speech is the *symbolization* process involving the formulation and comprehension of language and other symbolic forms. One must have symbols or symbol systems—languages—and sets of rules, or habits perhaps, for using them, as well as things to say, if one is to speak coherently or meaningfully, or in conventional and recognizable or acceptable ways.
2. *Respiration* provides the energy—the breath—from which speech is made.
3. In *phonation* this energy sets the vocal folds into vibration, producing tones that vary in pitch, loudness, duration, and wave composition.
4. *Resonance* results in the selective amplification of these tones which gives them certain distinctive characteristics. Nasal resonance, for example, characterizes the normal production of the consonants /m/, /n/, and /ŋ/, and occasionally an excess of nasal resonance gives a speaker's voice a distinctive quality called hypernasality. Differences in oral resonance brought about by adjustments of the shape and

size of the oral cavity and its orifice serve to differentiate the vowels from each other and have some effect on voice quality.

5. In *articulation* the breath stream is interrupted or impeded in certain ways by the articulators (tongue, teeth, and lips). Incidentally, the close relationship between resonance and articulation is pointed up by the term "vowel articulation," which refers to the speech sounds called vowels that result from changes in oral resonance effected by adjustments of jaw opening, tongue position, and lip rounding or retraction.

6. In *pronunciation* the speech sounds are arranged in prescribed sequences of syllables with applications of appropriate syllabic stress.

7. *Prosody*—or melody of speech—embraces all the variations of pitch, time, and loudness introduced by the speaker in order to emphasize words and syllables and make his or her speech interesting.

8. Finally there must be a certain communicative set—a willingness and readiness to speak, a confidence that one can speak well enough, a drive to engage in the kind of interaction we call communication.

The clinician is concerned with the speaker as a person. You may listen to a total performance and emerge with a Gestalt impression, but you must also listen analytically. One of your basic purposes is to identify the phenomena that constitute the speech impairment and to determine the basic process or processes involved. Do you hear impairment of respiration, of phonation, of resonance, of articulation, of prosody, or of all of these? Or is the problem less one of speech execution than one of language formulation? Or is the problem primarily in the speaker's attitude toward the act of speaking?

In speech and voice problems associated with cleft palate and other palatal anomalies, resonance and articulation are likely to be the processes of major concern to you. In cases of dysarthria, the respiration, phonation, resonance, articulation, and prosody all may be affected because of motor limitations; and language formulation may be disturbed too, as well as the speaker's adjustment to the speaking situation. A young boy who is brought to you as a stutterer may have moments of normal speech, while at other moments he refrains from speaking because of his anxiety about stuttering; when he does speak his avoidant behavior tends to interfere with respiration, phonation, and articulation.

Observations of speech behavior, then, must be fractionated in order to discern the nature of specific deviations and develop a properly detailed as well as comprehensive plan to remedy them.

4. The Armamentarium Is Abundant

In order to grapple with the problems facing them, clinicians draw upon a large supply of clinical tools. They may use certain personal resources—ingenuity in asking relevant questions, an ability to listen in a discriminating way, observations with trained eyes, the analyses and summations they imaginatively create. They can draw upon a large battery of tests, some perhaps intuitive and primitive, others standardized and highly sophisticated. They can extend and amplify their perceptions by using various kinds of instrumentation. They will arrive at a set of data, interpret them in terms of generalizations that have been drawn about normal and abnormal behavior, and will communicate these findings with varying degrees of precision to those who need to know them.

The clinician, then, has no small task in trying to fathom the nature of and the explanation for individual communication problems presented by unique speakers each of whom lives in a distinctive world. But fathom them one can if one sets about the task systematically and with appropriate appreciation of both one's powers and one's limitations and indeed the powers and limitations of all those other professional people upon whom one may depend. One can understand them if one carefully weighs one's information, selects one's hypotheses, tests them carefully, and without undue haste arrives at one's conclusions.

DEFINITION OF THE PROCESS

Speech-language pathologists seek to describe adequately any communication problem with which they deal in order to distinguish it from other problems that it may resemble and to determine its distinctive character. They undertake, that is, to diagnose the problem by making an appropriate examination and placing the data they gather in historical perspective. On the basis of their findings and their interpretations of them, they propose a remedial program and attempt to predict its outcome.

Five Steps

In carrying out these basic responsibilities one, as a speech-language pathologist, goes through the following steps:

1. The Background   One obtains adequate information about the speaker's past development and status. The clinician is interested in finding out how the person came to be what he or she is today. Especially interested in the onset of the speech problem, the clinician secures the desired information in a number of ways and from a variety of informants, making use especially of the case history interview (see Chapter 2).

2. The Appraisal   The clinician obtains a comprehensive and detailed description of the speaker's problem and of related aspects of his or her present status. In order to do this one makes considerable use of interview techniques, but one relies also on a variety of tests and observational procedures for identifying and measuring relevant aspects of speech and related behavior.

3. The Diagnosis   From study of the information gathered, the clinician makes a tentative identification of the problem and a determination of causes. One considers possible hypotheses regarding the conditions and circumstances that could have served to precipitate and maintain it. One tries to decide the dynamics of the problem and possibly of what "disease" entity it is a manifestation. As one weighs the data, one discards some hypotheses, and retains others for further testing.

4. The Therapy Plan   The clinician uses the facts obtained and the hypotheses drawn from them to formulate an appropriate remedial program.

5. The Prognosis   Finally, the clinician attempts a prognosis; that is, given the problem as one sees it with the causes as one understands them, one predicts as best one can the effects of the proposed remedial measures on the future course of the disorder.

You may ask, "When is a diagnosis completed?" or a related question, "Does diagnosis always precede treatment?" For obvious reasons a diagnostic workup typically precedes remedial steps, which in speech pathology are usually called "therapy." Clinicians want to know with what they are dealing and to have a rationale for doing what they do about it. Nevertheless, it should be understood that there is no absolute division between diagnosis and therapy. Just as the diagnostic procedures employed may have therapeutic effects, so the treatment itself can be diagnostic. In a given case the descriptions of the past and present status may not adequately clarify the causes. Therefore, the clinician prescribes a tentative course of treatment and withholds a diagnosis pending further observation. In speech pathology, as in other "helping professions," it may be necessary for the clinician to embark upon some well-structured experiments in order to arrive at a clear understanding of the nature and scope of the problem at hand. Furthermore, the clinician may continue to do much of what is called appraisal and diagnosis, at least at intervals, throughout the period of the activities ordinarily called therapy. Diagnosis is seldom, if ever, completed at one sitting, never to be reviewed. The clinician should continue the critical thinking implied by the term so long as he or she has any responsibility for the problem.

Although the terms *appraisal* and *diagnosis* are often used together, they are not synonymous. When a clinician specifies the presenting aspects of a problem and says something about their relative severity, he is appraising the problem. This appraisal may be an integral part of a diagnostic workup, or it may be something done by the clinician from time to time in order to chart progress or perhaps to form a basis for prognostic judgments. Appraisal is represented in the second of the five steps presented above. It is not to be thought of as the complete diagnostic process, for in diagnosis the clinician evaluates the description of present status—the appraisal—in the light of what the case history reveals about the past status. The goal is to reach a conclusion about the characteristics of the person or of his or her environment that may be responsible for the occurrence and continuation of the disorder. Having reached a conclusion regarding etiology, the clinician proceeds to formulate therapy and to make a prognosis thereby fulfilling—at least for the first round—the responsibility undertaken.

The activities involved in appraisal and diagnosis demand critical thinking on the part of clinicians. They are committed to the thoughtful—not perfunctory—application of well-understood and well-practiced methods. They are dedicated to the gathering of all the pertinent facts that they can collect, and they value the fact above a guess. They depend more on what they can hear and see and verify than on their intuitions. In trying to piece together a coherent picture, they are committed to a thoughtful analysis of the data which can lead to a resolution of apparent contradictions. As they develop and test hypotheses, they do not proliferate them but in appreciation of the principle of parsimony pursue what appear to be the simplest and the most reasonable. Knowing that there is simplicity in nature, they recognize that "the simplest explanation consistent with pertinent observations is most probably correct" (2, p. 117). As an understanding of the problem congeals, they are committed to the thoughtful planning of therapy. In short, they make use of the method of science no less than their fellow worker in the laboratory. They use the methodology of science to secure dependable answers to questions about the problem at hand.

Who Needs a Label?

If one were to view the process of diagnosis narrowly, one might conceive it to be no more than simply "hanging a label on a person." What more is there to this process than simply stuffing a person into a pigeon-hole?

There are, to be sure, dangers implicit in applying diagnostic procedures too superficially and coming up with only a name or label that may serve to delimit an individual's problem too narrowly, or to refer to it too vaguely or ambiguously—or even to contribute needlessly to the aggravation, indeed the very creation, of the problem. There is always a danger in lumping together things which appear to be similar but which are by no means identical. It is hazardous to conclude that a person displays behavior which warrants assignment of a certain label and to assume, then, that certain other things must be true of that person because of the fact that he or she now bears that given label.

A crucial consideration is that we all tend to think of other persons and to react to them according to the ways we classify them and the names or labels we give them. Our future perceptions and judgments are influenced by the words we have used in reporting—most fatefully to ourselves as our own most affected listeners—the perceptions and judgments we have already made. In medical dictionaries there is a dramatic word for the grave consequence of this sort of interaction between what we say and what we do. The word is "iatrogenic." An iatrogenic disorder is one that is caused by the physician—or the clinician of any sort—by a certain way of talking about or to the patient and by ways of dealing with the patient generally.

Consider, for example, some of the problems involved in using the term *cerebral palsy*. What this term stands for generally is not a readily defined entity with a given set of characteristics invariably distinguishing it. In fact, it encompasses such dissimilar things as spasticity, athetosis, ataxia, rigidity, and tremor. These dissimilar characteristics are lumped together by the pediatric neurologist because of an understanding of certain common aspects of the neuropathologies involved: all affect the central nervous system, all occasion motor dysfunctions, all involve lesions above a certain point in the central nervous system. But we cannot assume that the term cerebral palsy implies anything in particular about the speech and language behavior of a given child. It is not appropriate, therefore, to speak of cerebral palsied speech.

"Stuttering" is another blanket term often imprecisely employed. It is commonly used to refer ambiguously to many kinds of behavior, to many degrees and varieties of personal adjustment, to many different attitudes about one's self, one's listeners, and the speaking situation, to various patterns of interaction between speaker and listeners, and to the problem into which all these components are woven.

There is, of course, a proper use to be made of classification in clinical speech work. Certain understandings and implications follow from an accurate delimitation and naming of a problem. Appropriate classification can be useful in helping to decide what to do and to predict the outcome of one's efforts. For example, we may take five children severely retarded in speech. One, we shall say, is cerebral palsied with severe involvement of the speech mechanism; one has a severe bilateral hearing loss; one is mentally retarded to a marked degree; one gives evidence of profound emotional disturbance; the fifth we find to be an emotionally disturbed, mentally retarded, cerebral palsied child with a profound bilateral hearing loss. What we do with each of these children and how far we expect each to go in a program of remediation depends importantly upon the conclusions reached in our diagnostic workup. If we have been thorough and discriminating we have not merely labeled each child. We have arrived at a kind of classification which will be useful to us in sorting the children and assigning them to appropriate sections of our remedial program. Because the diagnostic classification is to be followed in each case by constructive management, an accurate and importantly distinctive classification is essential.

METHODS OF COMPILING CASE STUDY DATA

In order to do the detective work clinicians must master techniques for gathering information about a patient. They must become expert at examining people and must learn how to conduct case history interviews. Once mastered, these procedures provide the instruments or levers or handles by which clinicians can get "inside" the patient, analyze his or her problems, and set into motion appropriate management.

1. The Case History

By means of interviewing the patient and other individuals who affect him or her critically, the clinician learns about the nature of the communication impairment, the conditions which preceded it, aspects of his or her life and situation which conceivably set the stage for it, and features of the present situation which may be maintaining, reducing, or exacerbating the problem. The communication problem will be the focus of the investigation, but the clinician may explore rather widely in trying to clarify its onset, its development, its alterations in course, and its importance to the patient and others.

The goal of a case history is a detailed description of a unique individual with a personal problem. If this description is to be helpful, it must be comprehensive. Furthermore, the description should make clear the relationships that exist between the various facts which the historian has ascertained. The several groups of clinically relevant data and their interrelationships may be formulated diagrammatically as shown in Figure 1.1.

> In this diagram four general groups of factors are represented, and each is shown as interrelated with all the others. . . . We may regard the four factors as four general kinds of observations that can be made of "Henry"—that is, of any individual. Or for certain purposes we may regard them as four ways of talking about "Henry"—four special languages, as it were. The point of including "Henry" in the diagram is to emphasize that any one factor or point of view represented is partial and incomplete, and that all four, at least, are required for anything resembling a relatively full account. . . .
>
> By *semantic environment* is meant the individual's environment of attitudes, beliefs, assumptions, values, ideals, standards, customs, knowledge, interests, conventions, institutions, etc. . . . It is to be understood that beyond a person's immediate semantic environment is that more extensive environment that we call his culture, the larger

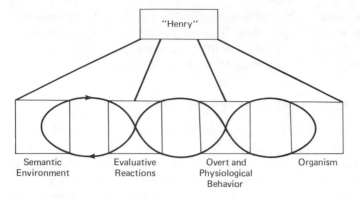

FIGURE 1.1
Diagram of interrelationships among groups of factors to be
taken into account. (Reprinted by permission from Wendell
Johnson, *People in Quandaries: The Semantics of Personal
Adjustment,* New York: Harper & Row, 1946.)

social order in which he lives, and in which his parents and teachers
live too. . . .
    Evaluative reactions include the individual's own attitudes, beliefs,
assumptions, values, ideals, etc. Taken all together, they may be regarded as that part of his semantic environment which the individual
has interiorized, or adopted. . . .
    Under the heading of *overt and physiological behavior* we include
generally what the person does—his predominantly nonverbal behavior. . . .
    By *organism* is meant not a static unchanging organic structure, but
the relatively invariant relationships involved in the processes of growth
and deterioration. In the living organism there is no fine line between
"physiology" and "anatomy." Roughly speaking, by physiological behavior we mean those bodily changes that can be observed from
moment to moment; by the organism we mean those bodily characteristics which change so slowly that from one day, or week, or month,
to the next they seem to remain constant. (*11,* pp. 411–413)

The clinician scrutinizes all of these matters as far as necessary for
clear understanding and orders the facts chronologically, using such
groupings as will clarify relationships. The report ultimately prepared
will reflect as much detail as the reader or the listener can use effectively.
Specific procedures to be followed in case history interviewing are presented in Chapter 2, along with suggestions for the preparation of the
consequent report.

2. The Test

Everyone, professional or nonprofessional, who is getting to know another
human being does it by eliciting a sample of behavior which is interest-

ing and apparently relevant. By means of a handshake, exchange of greetings, asking questions, watching someone's general behavior, and other techniques, we "feel out" and get to know a person.

The physician gathers special kinds of needed information by having a patient cough, breathe with his mouth open, say "ah," squat and rise several times, provide a urine specimen or a blood sample for analysis. The physician also fingers his pulse, takes his blood pressure, puts a thermometer in his mouth, feels his glands and his joints, and has his chest x-rayed.

The neurologist elicits even more special information: He taps the patient's patellar tendon with a reflex hammer, scratches the bottoms of his feet and watches his toes move, touches him with the dull and the sharp ends of a pin. He has the patient alternately touch his finger to his nose and to the examiner's finger, walk a straight line, walk on his toes and his heels, identify odors, move his eyes in all directions. He has him hooked up to a set of electrodes so that his brain waves can be studied by electroencephalography; by inserting needles into his muscles he studies speed of conduction of nerve impulses through electromyography; through the help of a neurosurgeon he may secure radiographic views of portions of the central nervous system when air or dye is injected; or he may observe alterations in behavior when sodium amytal is injected into his internal carotid arteries.

The clinical psychologist in appraising an individual's intellectual capacity may ask him to build structures or duplicate designs with blocks, draw a picture of a man, assemble puzzles, identify absurdities in pictures, answer questions of general information, report similarities between pairs of things, define words, or do some calculation. If he is more interested in his personality, he may ask him to answer a wide spectrum of true-false questions, tell what he sees in ink blots, complete unfinished sentences, or play with dolls.

The speech-language pathologist and the audiologist present other kinds of stimuli to elicit other samples of behavior. The speech-language pathologist may ask his subject to name some pictures using words containing specific phonemes, prolong vowels in order to assess quality of phonation, repeat syllables rapidly to determine oral diadochokinetic rate, repeat sentences to test articulation or to appraise auditory retention span, talk about a picture in order to get a sample of his syntactic structures and vocabulary, complete sentences in order to discern his mastery of syntactic transformations, follow instructions or answer questions about a story in order to assess auditory comprehension, recite the days of the week or some other automatic series, name pictures and objects, define words, explain proverbs, write to dictation, spell aloud, talk in unison with the examiner, read a passage repeatedly, speak to the accompaniment of delayed feedback, read and execute commands, blow into an oral manometer or respirometer, speak in front of cinefluorographic equipment, or talk about his problem. The audiologist presents a pure tone, a word, a warble, a succession of tones, sometimes through earphones, sometimes in a sound field, and he asks the subject to drop a marble, jot down a number, push a button, repeat what he heard, point to a picture, raise his hand, or just sit there and look around.

Anybody can make up a test. A test becomes a useful instrument for appraisal when one can be quite certain what it tests and what the range of responses is for a group of people judged to be normal or in some respect abnormal. The more precise the data it provides, the more useful the test. The more highly trained the examiner is in the use of the test, the more likely it will be that the expenditure of time required by the procedure will be profitable.

For certain determinations clinicians have no better tool than their own unaided eyes and ears. For other information they must obviously resort to some kind of instrumentation. They may need to wield a flashlight and tongue depressor, depend upon a tape recorder to listen repeatedly to a response, resort to gauges for measuring air pressure and airflow, or analyze the intricacies of vocal energy distribution via the sound spectrograph. They have available a wide range of electronic and mechanical equipment which can extend the range of observation and critical analysis. Your power as a clinician, then, depends upon your sophistication in the use of your own senses and the range of your intimate familiarity with instrumentation.

Our power as clinicians is also tempered by the degree to which we comprehend the limits of our own observation and appreciate the infinite sources of error which creep into our work because of the fact that we all, subjects and clinicians, are human. The possibility exists that the samples of behavior one thought one should elicit were not the crucial samples in the case at hand. The very fact that one was the examiner may have importantly influenced the behavior samples that one obtained. Peculiar circumstances of the subject's life on the particular day on which he or she was tested may have resulted in some distortion of behavior which made the responses more artifactual than typical.

The clinician must be particularly cautious in evaluating the results of testing young children, and in predicting the future course of their problem. Paraphrasing the words of Anderson (1): (a) the earlier your observations, the less reliance you can place upon a single observation in predicting subsequent development; (b) the earlier your observations, the greater care you should take to observe accurately and to record carefully what you see and hear; (c) the earlier your observations, the more weight you should give to the possibility of disturbing factors— negativism, refusals, distractions, fatigue—that operate to introduce error into your conclusions.

3. A Special Technique

Sometimes the refusal or inability of the patient to cooperate in an examination prevents our eliciting adequate samples of behavior for appraisal. The clinician may need to resort to a sort of pseudo test, a procedure which makes use of case history procedures to secure descriptions of samples of behavior which may be scaled just as we scale samples of behavior themselves. The Vineland Social Maturity Scale (8), for example, is not, technically speaking, a test since it does not involve the clinician's interacting with the patient and observing directly samples of behavior. Instead the clinician interviews a parent who can report firsthand observation of the child's behavior; he or she then abstracts from the information a positive or a negative rating with regard to specific items in the scale, and a measure of social age is calculated. Similarly Mecham's Verbal Language Development Scale (13) is designed to quantify information obtained from a parent about the child's acquisition of communication skills. Prevented from personally observing enough of the child's performance, the clinician utilizes a substitute observer, hoping that he or she can report objectively, without too much wishful hearing and seeing, what the child does.

Questionnaires can similarly be used in place of personal interview or to supplement face-to-face interview or to supplement direct interaction with the patient.

THE CLINICIAN AS OBSERVER AND REPORTER

Speech clinicians must become a special kind of observer. As they gather data by taking case histories and administering tests, they must interact efficiently with informants and clients—or patients, as they may prefer to refer to them, in accordance with the kind of setting in which they work. The ear must be attuned to detect clinically significant aspects of voice, speech, and language behavior. They must be sensitive to the feelings of those whom they seek to help and be alert to their subtle as well as obvious expressions of puzzlement, concern, hostility, inquiry, superstition, trust, misgiving, guilt, and anxiety. Having made and used their own observations, they are responsible for communicating what they have learned to others—judiciously, ethically, in good time, and as required. They are frequently called upon in staffings, clinical conferences, reports, and in other ways to share their knowledge and opinions through writing or speaking.

In doing your job and meeting your obligations, you as clinician may profitably be reminded of certain practices:

1. Observe and Report Enough

If you are to be "the compleat diagnostician," you must not arrive at the conclusion too soon that you understand all about the speaker whom you are examining and his or her problem. You will attempt to make your observations of the speaker and the speech and the surroundings as comprehensive and in as much detail as possible. The more complex the problem the greater your need for information about the speaker's past and present status—and no speech disorders can be called simple after thorough scrutiny. In even the simplest case, no one-to-one relationship is found between the speech problem in its entirety and any single causal factor. We have long known, for example, that a description of dentition is by no means adequate in all cases to account for a distorted /s/, or that the severity of a client's voice or articulation problem does not parallel exactly the degree to which cerebral palsy has impaired his or her motor system, or that the height of the palatal vault may have little or nothing to do with how he or she speaks.

More than superficial observation is necessary. The clinician has not completed the task by noting merely that a tooth is missing, that a parent is thoughtless and impatient, that a home is broken, that a child has a bilateral hearing loss, or that he or she cannot get a word in edgewise at home. We are enamored of drawing arrows relating cause to effect, but often we draw too few of them and thereby oversimplify the relationships.

In considering how comprehensive our observations about individuals should be, let us consider an analogy. Do you recall the fable about the six blind men confronted by an elephant for the first time? The one who felt only the trunk visualized the elephant as a snake; the one who felt only a tusk imagined the animal to be shaped like a spear; the one who grasped the ear identified the elephant with a palm leaf; the one who felt of his side pictured him as a stone wall; the massive hind leg suggested to one the dimensions of a tree trunk; and the sixth, upon grasping the tail, identified the elephant as a rope.

In clinical practice, you need to beware of making the mistake of the six blind men. From fragmentary information, considered out of context and without proper perspective, you are likely to draw faulty inferences and reach wrong conclusions.

An elementalistic view—the isolating of a single element in a complex situation and regarding it as sole cause—will not suffice. The speech-language pathologist, as Cable (4) reminds us, must be nonelementalistic and "see the relationships and connections among all things." To oversimplify is to lose something that is needed.

Consider a child who is brought to the clinic for examination. He is 3¼ years of age, but on the Vineland Social Maturity Scale he earns a social age of only 1 year, 9 months. He wears a brace on one leg, and although he moves about fairly well, he is somewhat restricted by his parents in his explorations and in his attempts to show off his physical prowess. He does a great deal of gesturing, but he is using few understandable words. His parents spend some time romping with him, but they have spent little time reading to him or playing games with him, have not encouraged association with other children, and have done little to foster self-help. Instead they have provided a governess who looks after his every need and who protects him from all possible harm. He has never had to pull off his own socks or brush his own teeth, and he has little need to ask for anything because every wish is anticipated.

In considering the cause of the speech problem, one would certainly be mistaken in referring only to impairment in the pyramidal and extrapyramidal tracts of the child's central nervous system. The adequacy of the child's speech mechanism is of interest, but so are the adequacy of the speech stimulation he has received, the need for speech which he has experienced, the reward he has received for his speech efforts, the breadth of experiences to which he has been exposed in the world around him, and the role communication plays in it. His language retardation does not have *a cause* but numerous *causes*.

It is just this point which Brown and Oliver (3) made in their report of a study of 33 cases of cleft palate. It was their purpose to look beyond the function of the palate and to consider the role of other factors in relation to the adequacy of each subject's speech. They made thorough examinations of the oral speech structures of the 33 subjects, rating each of more than 25 different activities or conditions of various structures on a 3-point scale. A rating of 1 indicated that the particular condition being rated was judged to have no adverse effect on speech; a rating of 2 suggested a possible adverse effect; a rating of 3 indicated that the particular condition would almost certainly have an adverse effect on speech.

They found no subject who did not have some abnormality of the speech mechanism in addition to an abnormality of palatal function itself. Eighty-two percent of the subjects had one or more of the structures rated 3. The median subject had 2 structures rated 3 and 12 rated 2. Even within the mouths, then, of persons with cleft palates we find multiple possible causes for any speech deviation we might observe, and we have also to look beyond the speakers' mouths to consider the attitudes of their families and associates, the attitudes of the speakers themselves and their intelligence, the adequacy of their hearing, the amount of speech stimulation they have had, the adequacy of their speech models, their need for speech and their reward for speech attempts.

The further you go in the study of communication disorders, the more likely you are to agree that "the cause of anything is everything." You must be interested not only in the persons who have speech problems but also in the persons and institutions which help make them what they are and possibly keep them from becoming what they otherwise might be.

All of us do well to remind ourselves that sometimes it is difficult to distinguish between cause and effect. In our search for the causes of problems, we may be tempted to consider as causal something that is really symptomatic of some more remote cause, and we may consider as "simply a symptom" something that can have tremendous significance as a cause of other clinically significant conditions or behavior. Consider, for example, a child with an articulatory problem who is reported to have done little babbling as an infant. Does the commonly held view that mastery of speech sounds grows from the matrix of vocal play or babbling point to the cause of this child's articulation difficulty? Or is the lack of babbling a symptom of some other more important cause—perhaps a hearing loss, or parental neglect, or parental lack of understanding of how speech develops and of the importance of the child's pleasure and reward in making sounds like those of some loving and responsive person?

As another example, suppose that a child with a cleft palate has poor articulation and marked hypernasality with speech almost unintelligible at times and a voice scarcely audible. What is the cause here? Have the misarticulations and the possible facial disfigurement themselves brought about personality changes which, in turn, have affected the child's speech behavior? Are the weakness of voice and unintelligibility of speech caused solely or primarily by structural deformities or physio-logical inadequacies, or is it possible that they result at least in part from the fact that the child has never found talking to be fun and rewarding, has found it instead to be a punishing experience which she wishes to avoid as much as possible? Does she in consequence shrink from speaking out so that she holds her head down, keeps her lips almost closed, and swallows her words? To what extent, that is, have such reactions become causal as well as symptomatic?

As a further illustration of the interaction and blending of cause and consequence, consider the case of a young stutterer who appears to be apprehensive about his speech disfluencies and seeks to avoid them at any cost. He has developed various mannerisms, grimaces, and contor-tions in his struggle to avoid the stuttering he dreads and, as he puts it, to "help the words come out." His way of speaking has become in-creasingly tense and his anxieties have mounted instead of subsided. Are we confronted with symptoms here? If they are symptoms, they are obviously also causes. They are ways of reacting which, in turn, make the child's behavior increasingly avoidant and disruptive of the activities essential in speaking. They magnify his unease and discourage him from speaking so that he tends to speak less. In trying to help him, therefore, you would be just as interested in attacking these symptoms as anything else you might regard as causes. Actually you would be dealing with causes in trying to manipulate what you might think of as symptoms. The word "reaction" or "response" is in many ways a better term than "symptom" in referring to whatever a speaker does that you regard as stuttering, simply because what the speaker does is behavior. Just as the terms "response" and "reaction" are particularly suitable for talking about *behavior,* so "symptom" is peculiarly appropriate for describing *disease.* And we use the word "stuttering" to refer to something that seems more validly classified as a form of behavior than as a type of disease.

2. Observe and Report Objectively

As a clinician one is not to ride one's hobbyhorse and see in every patient only what one wants to see, or to explain every behavior in terms of some favorite rationale. "The scientific method abhors such slanting; it insists, rather, that one observe dispassionately, hypothesize coldly, test hypotheses disinterestedly, and accept inevitable conclusions unreservedly" (6, p. 9).

It is important that clinicians distinguish between what they observe and what they conclude from their observations. They must distinguish, in other words, between fact and inference. It is not easy to make this kind of distinction and to communicate the results of observation with appropriate objectivity. Without our even recognizing what is happening our own interests, biases, and convictions distort our perceptions, our conclusions, and our reports. We filter all of our sensations through personal filters; and as we report, the filtering process goes on.

It should be the clinician's constant goal to be as objective as possible and to acknowledge and reduce as much as possible the distorting elements in observations and reports. One of the purposes of this book is to help the clinician and the clinician-in-training to minimize distorting personal projections by learning to use certain diagnostic tools designed for detailed, objective, reliable observation.

How can a clinician reduce the undesirable effects of subjectivity in his observations? One helpful way is to recognize the difference between two-valued systems (dichotomies) and multi-valued systems (continua). He can learn early, for example, that children are not either clean or dirty, either bright or backward, either attractive or homely. After he has become acquainted with a number of children, he finds that they vary along the continuum of cleanliness—or of brightness or attractiveness—from "not so very" to "rather" to "quite." As he extends his observations, he discovers that the members of a species practically never can be satisfactorily locked into categories but are dealt with most appropriately by recognizing the differences among them and appreciating that they are distributed over an infinite number of degrees of variation.

It is also helpful to clinicians to carry this practice one step further and make use of scaling procedures in comparing individuals with regard to specified characteristics. They find it useful to get into the habit of assigning numerical values to the extremes of the continua, or graduated scales, that they are dealing with and of thinking about the points along the continua as being equally spaced in the degrees of variation they represent. They also find it useful to think of a 5-point scale of hypernasality, for example, or a 9-point scale of severity of stuttering, or other kinds of scales such as "much more than average," "somewhat more than average," "about average," "somewhat less than average," and "much less than average."

3. Observe and Report Precisely

Clinicians should, insofar as possible, adopt practices in questioning and observing which will permit them to communicate exactly what they did and precisely what they saw and heard. Even when you must make judgments, you should be sensitive to the need to check your observations and ratings against your own repeated judgment and against the judgment of others. In other words, a clinician becomes concerned with the reliability and the validity of personal observations and judgments. You want to know the degree of your consistency on repeated applications of the same test or on repeated judgments of the same behavior (intra-observer reliability). The clinician must also be concerned with how well these judgments agree with those of other equally or more competent observers (interobserver reliability). And the clinician should ask whether the yardstick in use really measures what it purports to measure. You cast about for outside criteria against which you can measure the validity of your observations and of the tools you are using.

Increasingly the clinician becomes impressed with the need for compiling empirical data, that is, facts derived from experience or experiment, facts that arise from observation. And he or she learns the necessity of keeping the interpretation of these empirical data quite distinct from the data themselves. More and more the clinician learns to distrust hunches and intuitive procedures which, because they cannot be communicated to others effectively, cannot, therefore, be adequately subjected to checking and rechecking. Although at times clinicians necessarily rely upon a clinical hunch or a clinical impression, they should feel duly restrained in drawing conclusions until they are able to check them against the observations of someone else or against further data.

The clinician is a kind of detective, and Sherlock Holmes reminds us that "detection is, or ought to be, an exact science." The clinician as a practicing scientist seeks ultimately to reduce observations to quantitative terms. You should join with Sir Thomas Browne (*Religio Medici*) in his admiration of "the secret magic of numbers." For it is through the precision of numbers that you can best summarize your observations, grasp them yourself, communicate them to others, and allow replication of your procedures and conclusions. Lord Kelvin summed it up: "When you can measure what you are speaking about and express it in numbers, you know something about it; and when you cannot measure it, when you cannot express it in numbers, your knowledge is of a meager and unsatisfactory kind. It may be the beginning of knowledge, but you have scarcely in your thought advanced to the stage of a science" (12, p. 73).

By exercising ingenuity clinicians can develop for their tests numerical scoring systems in order to make their measures quantitative. They can scale the performance of a child on a series of volitional oral tasks in order to arrive at an overall score that represents his or her performance in comparison with that of other children. The aphasic patient's anomia can be summed up as 10 successes out of 20 trials on a naming task with pictures and objects. The child's equivocal response to a watch tick can be replaced by a precise description of a sensorineural hearing loss as measured by pure-tone audiometry. Degree of nasal air leakage can be translated into the ratio between the number of ounces of intra-oral pressure impounded by a child with nostrils open divided by the number of ounces impounded with nostrils occluded. The clinician can learn to use something as sophisticated as a 16-point multidimensional scale in the Porch Index of Communicative Ability (15): it captures and communicates to another clinician the accuracy of a patient's response on each of 180 items in an aphasia battery, its completeness, the facility and promptness with which he made it, and the amount of information he needed before he could make an appropriate response.

As a clinician, one may view onself as a kind of artist, sensitive to the feelings of the clients, adapting one's procedures intuitively to the nature of each examination situation. But we would better view ourselves as artist-scientists who can supplement qualitative richness with quantitative exactness; who can not only inspire admiration for skilled personal interactions and acute perception of the dynamics of our patients' problems but can also with precise detail elucidate what we have observed and inferred in a manner that makes our work repeatable and our contribution fully interpretable.

INTERPRETATION OF CASE STUDY DATA

One of the values of exact quantitative information derived in a standardized way is that such information can then be related to what we know about the behavior of other individuals. Our goal is to decide whether the behavior at hand falls within normal limits or whether it represents a point on the spectrum of human behavior sufficiently extreme to constitute a problem.

We know that *people* are not averageable, but it is perfectly reasonable to average *information* about them with respect to certain specific features. As Williams has said:

> Such words as *average, typical,* or *normal* have meaning only when one can answer the question: *average, typical or normal with respect to what?* If we were asked to pick out a book average or typical with respect to thickness, or print size, or paper thickness, or number of words, or number of chapters, or number of paragraphs, or size of index, we would have relatively little difficulty. But if we were required to pick out a book that was typical in *all* these respects, as well as having typical subject matter treated with typical literary skill, we would be really stumped. Such a book doesn't exist, and if it did it would be a most extraordinary book (in a most uninteresting way) and not a typical book at all. (*21*, pp. 170–171)

Our goal in clinical work is not to arrive at a conclusion that a given speaker is as a total being average or typical or normal, or deviant or atypical or abnormal. No useful purpose would be served in any such generalization about anyone. But to be helpful to persons with a disorder of communication it is reasonable to ask whether they fall within normal limits with regard to the size of their vocabulary, their mastery of syntactic structures, their ability to impound intraoral breath pressure or sustain a prolonged vowel, their repertoire of phonemes, their rate of speech, their fluency, and their reactions to their perceptions of their own status in all of these dimensions. We do not sacrifice the individual or exalt the mediocre by scrutinizing his or her relative status with regard to some discrete measure, whether it be a physical measure such as height, weight, pulse rate, or blood pressure; or an intellectual measure such as degree of orientation in time and space or ability to calculate mentally; or "personality" measures such as happy-go-luckiness or level of aspiration or depression; or a measure of communicative behavior such as voice quality, articulatory precision, or fluency of speech. The individual is unique in his or her pattern of excellences and weaknesses. The full import of these emerges only as we place the individual in the perspective of the performance of other individuals who display the entire spectrum of variations of the traits and skills we are interested in.

As a clinician you are, or will be, concerned with the practical evaluation of the persons whom you try to serve to the best of your ability. When engaged in diagnostic work, for example, you will find yourself continually making comparisons between the speaker at hand and other people you know about. You will ask questions such as: "Is this boy's behavior to be reasonably expected from a person of his age and sex and circumstances, or is it in some significant way deviant? Is this boy somewhat accelerated in his acquisition of this particular skill, or does he appear to be somewhat retarded?" You will view a given child in the perspective of all the children you have known; and since your experience is always necessarily limited, you must go beyond it and build into your perspective data compiled by those who have studied many children, whom they have regarded as normal and abnormal. Without establishing mediocrity as an ideal, you must keep in mind statistical information about the average performance in groups of children, and be conscious also of ways in which individual children deviate from the central tendency of an appropriately defined group.

All of this means that as a practicing clinician you need to build into your evaluative system a set of norms, compiled carefully and objectively, to which you can refer in sizing up any given speaker. Only by means of such norms, properly evaluated, can you understand adequately the behavior you observe and decide whether it indicates a need for remedial treatment. You enrich your understanding of an individual by referring to what we can expect from the study of a number of people, even while we freely realize that nobody duplicates anybody else and nobody wants to have this duplication.

In several of the following chapters, you will find relevant norms. You will want to become familiar with these and other norms and learn to use them with due discrimination. Several important questions are to be asked about any set of norms and among these are the following:

1. What Is the Purpose of These Norms?

As Meredith (14) has indicated, norms are established in different ways and serve various purposes. Some norms are simply *descriptive*, indicating the characteristics or behavior of the groups tested. The data reported tell what the groups were like but present no implicit or explicit value judgments. Most norms for height and weight, development of physical skills, development of phoneme articulation, vocabulary size, age of acquisition of bowel and bladder control, and number of hours of sleep per night tell only what the mean or median performance or characteristic is and the pattern in which subjects are distributed according to the measure applied to them. (See, for example, Table 8.2, p. 238, and Table 11.2, p. 327). In themselves, such norms do not tell whether a given child is "tall enough," "too heavy," "abnormal," "satisfactory," or "just right."

In the field of speech pathology and audiology we have a few norms of a second type—norms designed *for evaluation*. In these instances the descriptive norms are related to some value such as freedom from disorder, intelligibility, or some other criterion essential to the indicated classification. Only when we take the additional step of relating a statistical value to an appropriate value system can we express such judgments as "too," "abnormal," "satisfactory," or "fit." For an example of norms for evaluation, refer to the Social Adequacy Index described by Davis and Silverman (7, pp. 193–194).

When norms for evaluation are wanting, we may make use of a third type, *screening norms.* These constitute an approach to norms for evaluation and help in the selection of individuals for further scrutiny. They combine descriptions of characteristics in more than one dimension, utilizing jointly two or more sets of descriptive norms in ways suggested by clinical experience. For example, Templin (*18*) used norms on a 176-item diagnostic test of articulation together with scores on a 50-item screening test of articulation in order to arrive at a set of cut-off scores which she proposed as scores separating adequate and inadequate articulation in children (see Table 8.3, p. 238). Technically, these cutoff scores do not constitute norms for evaluation, as they do not relate descriptive norms to such values as "intelligibility" and "speaker acceptability." She simply used two sets of descriptive norms in a way suggested by clinical experience to derive a clinically useful screening instrument. In public school hearing surveys use is commonly made of screening tests of hearing acuity (see Chapter 12).

2. Is the Population Adequately Defined?

The compiler of each set of norms has chosen a population for study, out of which he has selected a sample for specific scrutiny (see Section 3 below). On the basis of his study of the subjects in his sample he makes certain generalizations about the population. It is important to know just how—and especially how precisely—this population is defined. Has the compiler kept in mind all of the important variables that have some bearing upon the measurement being made?

3. Is the Population Sample Large Enough?

How large is the sample of the population studied? Is it large enough to minimize sampling error sufficiently? Is it sufficiently representative of the population as defined?

4. What Is the Nature of the Data?

Are the data cross-sectional or longitudinal? In longitudinal normative studies the investigator follows a given group over a period of time, taking readings at intervals. He may study a group of children with regard to height and weight when they are 2 years old, and the same children when they are 3 years old, then 4, and again at 5. On the other hand, he may choose to study these four age levels all at once by selecting different groups of children, one group at each of the four age levels. In the latter case the data derived are cross-sectional. Both kinds of norms serve important purposes, and they are especially useful when available to supplement each other.

5. Are the Measures Adequately Defined?

Having selected this population sample, the investigator elicits a sample of each subject's behavior and analyzes it, using certain specified measures. How precise is each of the measures which he has applied? What steps has the investigator taken to define each measure distinctively? Was the definition adhered to as the data were compiled? What is known about the reliability and validity of each measure?

6. Is the Behavior Sample Adequate?

How substantial a sample of each subject's behavior was elicited and evaluated? Was the sample large enough to allow for the deriving of stable values?

7. In what Terms Are the Data Presented?

Are the normative data presented in units that indicate status or in units that indicate progress (increments)?

8. How Comprehensive Are the Data?

Are measures of dispersion (ranges, standard deviations, Q-values, quartiles, or deciles) presented as well as measures of central tendency (means, medians, modes)? Are separate norms provided where variables are judged to warrant such a breakdown—for example, norms for both sexes or norms for various socioeconomic levels? Are observer reliabilities and test-retest reliabilities reported?

9. How Applicable Are the Data?

How recently were the data collected? The passage of time can make a great difference in the interpretation and usefulness of normative information; in general, other things being equal, the more recent the norms, the better. Is extrapolation or interpolation necessary in using the norms? There are dangers in trying to extend the shapes of distributions beyond the data at hand. We prefer not to have to estimate values intermediate between known values (interpolation), and we should exercise due alertness and caution in guessing—if we feel we must guess —at values beyond those that are presented (extrapolation). Finally, we may ask whether the norms appear to be applicable to our own particular subjects and purposes.

A FEW WARNINGS

1. Exalt the Patient, Not the Clinical Procedure

Just as the platform speaker must give careful consideration to the nature of an audience and must adapt his or her remarks and delivery style to it, so, as a clinician, you must begin with your patients where they are, not where you would like them to be. Although you must be ready to use sophisticated measures in prescribed standardized ways and pose a planned series of questions in a logical sequence, you may find it necessary to abandon these choices and resort to less ideal procedures, although admittedly you will lose precision and detail thereby. An interview technique or a test procedure is not sacred. It should be replaced by alternative procedures that work better in a particular situation. To persist rigidly in testing that turns off the patient or in questioning that heightens resistance is only to ask for failure.

One should view the procedures described in Part One of this book, then, as a sort of idealized structure calculated to provide desired information under optimal conditions. Application of the procedures should be kept flexible, subject to the exigencies of the situation, to be trimmed down or replaced as necessary. The clinician will use creatively every tool that contributes to an understanding of the patient and the communication problem, and will use them judiciously, with discretion, and in a spirit of total willingness to sacrifice them in order to preserve and learn from the relationship with the patient. One must not let the tail wag the dog.

2. Adhere to Terminology that Clarifies

Especially in an earlier day the terminology relating to communication disorders proliferated, as a glance at a dictionary of speech pathology and audiology will show (16). Some of this overlapping and confusing terminology remains as a vestigial organ of the profession.

People who become specialized in certain disorders tend to develop personal classification systems. It is not always evident how one moves from one classification system to another, how a patient who seems to fit into a given slot in one system can be fitted into a slot in another system. Creators of classification systems often reflect individual interests in the terminology they select. After a few years of proliferation of such special vocabularies, a clinician may find himself in a quandary as to what label best designates the problem and communicates to another clinician what he has in mind.

An example of terminological confusion is to be found in the distinctive articulatory disorder, first described by Broca in 1861, which may be observed in the speech of patients who incur a lesion of the anterior left cerebral hemisphere. The disorder is characterized by variable off-target approximations of phonemes despite the absence of significant weakness, slowness, incoordination, or alteration of tone of the speech musculature. Broca called the problem aphemia and attributed it to impairment of a specific faculty, "the faculty of articulated language," which he considered to be quite separate from a "general faculty of language," impairment of which he called "verbal amnesia." Subsequently Trousseau criticized the term "aphemia" and replaced it with the term "aphasia" and developed around it an armchair classification of language disorders which ignored the specific phenomenologic distinction that Broca had emphasized. A few years later Wernicke described what came to be called "sensory aphasia" and acknowledged the existence of a motor equivalent, represented by Broca's aphemia. Subsequently the terms "Broca's aphasia," "motor aphasia," and "subcortical motor aphasia" came to be substituted for what Broca had described. Marie later tried to straighten out the terminological confusion by redescribing the disorder and renaming it "anarthria," meaning by this the loss of control of all those mechanical abilities employed in the exteriorization of language. But Dejerine argued that anarthria denoted simply a paralysis and Dejerine's interpretation of the term persists to this day, so that in current usage the terms "anarthria" and "dysarthria" usually refer to speech problems caused by weakness, slowness, incoordination, or alteration of tone of the speech musculature. Liepmann grouped this type of speech problem with a large family of inabilities to perform volitional acts despite intactness of muscle strength and coordination and gave a new name to these manifestations: "apraxia." In later years Henry Head classified the problem within his designation "verbal aphasia." Kleist divided it into two variants which he renamed "speech sound muteness" and "word muteness." Weisenberg and McBride obscured its distinctness by burying it within their classification "predominantly expressive aphasia." Alajouanine, Ombredane, and Durand renamed it "the syndrome of phonetic disintegration in aphasia." Nathan called it "apraxic dysarthria." Goldstein called it "peripheral motor aphasia." Other people have called it "cortical dysarthria," "articulatory dyspraxia," "apraxia of vocal expression," "literal paraphasia," and "phonemic paraphasia."

A review of the literature suggested by the above list (10) reveals that essentially the same phenomena appeared in the descriptions of the behavior presented by all of the authors; they were probably talking about the same disorder. The designations used, however, revealed the authors' different conceptualizations of the dynamics of the problem. If one calls it a form of aphasia, one implies an impairment of the patient's ability to handle the symbolic code by which we communicate; it becomes a linguistic problem. If one refers to it as a kind of dysarthria, one implies that there is some degree of weakness, slowness, incoordination, or alteration of tone of the speech apparatus directly responsible. If one calls it apraxia, one implies that the source of the problem is impairment of the programming of the movements of oral speech in spite of intact strength and independent of any problem in dealing with meaning-bearing units of language.

Another example of terminological unclearness is the use of the term "functional." Some people, among them many speech-language pathologists, use the term to describe articulatory problems for which there is no apparent organic basis. In such usage the term is a generous wastebasket term, including errors due to lags in development, faulty learning, dialectal influences, inadequate stimulation, and others. But other kinds of clinicians, among them many physicians, use the term "functional" to mean "psychogenic." There is a clear implication in their usage that the patient is displaying psychoneurotic behavior and that the given behavior represents some sort of conversion symptom.

The clinician should prefer terminology which is as unambiguous as possible and which communicates his or her intent as directly as possible. The terms used to represent parts of a classification should (1) be mutually exclusive, (2) indicate the dynamics of the problem, and (3) eliminate the need for intervening steps of explanation. With reference to the above examples, one can use the terms "aphasia," "dysarthria," and "apraxia of speech" to represent three separate entities, each of them denoting a distinctive pathophysiologic process, and each capable of communicating the clinician's intent without elaboration. It is preferable to designate the brain-injured patient's trial-and-error searching behavior in attempting to produce phonemes and sequences of them as "apraxia of speech" rather than to adopt more traditional terminology and announce that he has a "motor aphasia," finding it necessary immediately thereafter to say, "But I don't really mean that he is aphasic; what I mean is that he gropes for the right position, tries and tries again to get his lips and tongue in the right place, produces variable off-target errors, all in the absence of any weakness, slowness, incoordination, or alteration of tone of the speech apparatus at the same time that he is in total command of the word he is trying to say." Similarly the clinician will do well to avoid the vague designation of a "functional" articulatory defect and rather designate it as an "articulatory disorder of undetermined origin," an "articulatory problem due to faulty habit of tongue carriage," or something else unambiguous.

In a somewhat different vein, it may be pointed out that as a clinician you will find your effectiveness as a reporter increased if you will keep reports simple and direct. You will probably communicate more effectively with others, including your fellow clinicians, if you talk about a child's delayed speech rather than his or her "paralalia prolongata." A few of your professional colleagues may understand what is meant by a child's "rhinolalia aperta" but none will understand less if you record it as "hypernasality" or "excessively nasal voice quality."

Witness this report furnished by one speech clinic to another: "His speech was severely retarded with all the consonants incorrect or missing completely. There was a mild lingua-labial agnosia and apraxia with some lingua-alveolar apraxia." One cannot tell from this report how the determination of speech retardation was arrived at, since only the status of articulation is reported. And one becomes dubious about the report of articulation when one reads that *all* of the consonants were either incorrect or missing, since testing that is exhaustive enough nearly always shows that a child can make some of the consonant phonemes in some position or in some phonetic context or other. Similarly, it is difficult to know what the child was asked to do or in what way he performed that led to the conclusion that he presented "a lingua-labial agnosia and apraxia," much less one that was only "mild." You should avoid jargon and obscure technical terminology and use descriptive language when your purpose is to communicate effectively about problems involving clinical procedures and classification systems that may differ from clinician to clinician.

3. Beware of Dichotomies That Do Not Dichotomize

It is easy to group some disorders under the general heading "organic" and other disorders under the general heading "nonorganic." You will do well to remind yourself periodically that although this dichotomy has a certain usefulness, there is a no-man's-land—a range rather than a line—between the two. Of course you will encounter certain speech problems that stem primarily from anatomical or physiological conditions, and other speech problems which clearly result mainly from faulty learning, perseveration of infantile habits, or possibly lack of adequate stimulation or motivation. But you will also find essentially normal speech where substantial organic deviations would seem to militate against it. Occasionally you may see a person who can talk without a tongue, or an individual with an open cleft of the palate speaking with a high degree of intelligibility. You will see speakers with significant anatomical and physiological deviations who compensate for them and produce good speech, whereas others with similar or lesser deviations are apparently unable to compensate for them and as a result produce faulty speech. You will find cerebral palsied children with involvement of certain speech muscles displaying speech errors unrelated to their neuromuscular involvement (23), and you will see aphasic patients with demonstrated neurologic deficits varying in the adequacy of their performance as different kinds of motivating instructions are given to them (17)—evidence of nonorganic components in clearly organic disorders.

In short, a so-called nonorganic problem may have a heretofore unrecognized organic component, whereas an allegedly organic disorder may have a large nonorganic component. The fact that we can use the words "organic" and "nonorganic" separately does not mean that the processes of speech production and the various speech disorders can be effectively fragmented and classified in terms of these two words. Structure and function interact—so far, that is, as we can determine which is which. Just as matter and energy, or wave and particle, are no longer sharply distinct from one another for the modern physicist, so for the modern clinician structure and function, or, for example, muscle and tension, are by no means always to be clearly differentiated.

Another trap into which you could fall if not forewarned is in the words "simple" and "complex" (or "complicated"). Avoid the tendency to think that developmental disorders of articulation comprise simpler problems, with which clinicians having minimal training can deal adequately, whereas problems such as are found in aphasia, dysarthria, and cleft palate are more involved, or complicated. Obviously there is nothing simple about the problem of a child who has perfect hearing acuity, superior phoneme discrimination ability, excellent motor control of the speech mechanism, and splendid ability to produce phonemes in isolation following stimulation, but who, week after week and month after month, fails to incorporate these correct phonemes into conversational speech.

Thorough consideration of the language process does not lead to the conclusion that it is to be appropriately called simple. It might seem that it would be easier for a patient with traumatically incurred aphasia to recall and speak a single noun such as the word "leaf," a single number such as "four," a single verb such as "look," or another noun such as "clover" than it would be to put all of these together into some sort of meaningful sentence. But interestingly enough, although a patient cannot speak any of these words individually, he or she may very well put them all together and sing them with perfect rhythm and melody in the song "I'm Looking Over a Four-Leaf Clover." *Calling* a process or a problem simple does not *make* it so. All it does is to make it harder to deal with the problem intelligently.

4. Beware of Instant Diagnosis

Nearly everyone seems to admire the clinician who appears to be able to take a quick look at a child and come up with the right answer. But cursory examination can lead easily, of course, to erroneous conclusions and decisions. No law requires us to arrive at a firm conclusion about the nature of any given child's problem before next Tuesday afternoon. A medical dictionary (9) suggests that there is such a thing as a "tentative diagnosis, a diagnosis based upon the available sources of information but subject to change." We may and should defer the diagnosis if we feel none is warranted at the moment. We serve better those whom we seek to help if we refuse to be defensive, are willing to acknowledge the limits of our knowledge and understanding, and take the time we need to do all we can to insure in each case the best understanding of the problem that we can achieve.

Sometimes we find that the best way to arrive at or to confirm a diagnosis, to map out a meaningful remedial course, and to estimate prognosis is to embark upon a period of experimental therapy. As pointed out earlier, treatment itself can be diagnostic. The clinician should be willing to capitalize upon it to arrive at correct decisions rather than to arrive earlier at more absolute conclusions which later turn out to have been premature.

5. Function Ethically

In diagnostic work as well as in therapy we are bound by the principles embraced in the Code of Ethics of the American Speech and Hearing Association (5). We are reminded by the Code of Ethics that the welfare of those we serve must be paramount; therefore we must become as highly skilled as possible in the use of diagnostic tools and we must refrain from undertaking without adequate supervision diagnostic work for which we are not properly qualified.

The Code of Ethics reminds us that we must use every resource available, including referral to other specialists as needed. We do not depend upon our own skills alone but readily call upon others to counsel and guide us and in fact to take over where we cannot perform effectively.

The Code of Ethics further reminds us that we should "establish harmonious relationships with members of other professions" and should "endeavor to inform others concerning the services that can be rendered by members of the speech and hearing profession and in turn should seek information from members of related professions." The pattern is becoming increasingly well established for the speech-language pathologist and the audiologist to function as integral parts of diagnostic teams. They join the plastic surgeon, orthodontist, prosthodontist, pediatrician, psychologist, and social worker on the cleft palate team. They identify neurologists, pediatric neurologists, neurosurgeons, psycholinguists, psychologists, and rehabilitation personnel as fellow aphasiologists. Other rehabilitation enterprises involve cooperation of speech-language pathologists and audiologists with physiatrists, orthopedic surgeons, physical therapists, occupational therapists, nursing personnel, psychiatrists, psychologists, and social workers. Effective understanding and management of psychogenic voice disorders requires cooperation of speech pathologists with laryngologists, neurologists, psychiatrists, and psychologists.

To function side by side with other professional specialists in comprehensive appraisal and cooperative diagnosis is not simply an ideal about which we may dream. It is a necessity which must be implemented and made a daily reality by the ethical speech-language pathologist and audiologist.

ASSIGNMENTS

1. Distinguish between the terms "diagnosis" and "appraisal."
2. What is meant by the diagnostic uses of therapy? Suggest some hypothetical cases in connection with which you might wish to make diagnostic use of therapy.
3. Distinguish between the terms "reliability" and "validity." How might you in a specific instance choose the outside criteria for determining the validity of a testing procedure?
4. Distinguish between the terms "empiricism" and "intuition."
5. Give examples to illustrate how important it may be to understand a person's society and culture in trying to understand him or her. How might your evaluation of an individual's behavior depend upon the cultural norms to which you are accustomed?
6. What is meant by one's "philosophy of life"? One's "professional philosophy"? Make a list of the principles which might comprise your personal professional philosophy.
7. What is meant by a nonelementalistic approach? Why should you be nonelementalistic in your approach to a person with a communication problem?
8. Suppose that a child severely retarded in speech is brought to you for a diagnosis of her problem and your recommendations for helping her. What does the nonelementalistic approach imply in terms of the testing procedures you will use and the questions you will ask in the case history interview?
9. Describe some situations in which the administration of tests and interpretation of the results obtained might produce more artifacts than facts.
10. Distinguish between the terms "extrapolation" and "intrapolation." Think of some situations in which extrapolation from data available might be risky.
11. To what individuals and groups do you as a person specializing in speech pathology and audiology have responsibilities?
12. If you contemplate specializing in speech pathology and audiology, how should you ready yourself to do an adequate job? What kinds of courses would you consider relevant? What kinds of professional training experiences would best fit you to emerge from a trainee status into the status of an efficient professional worker? If you were tailoring your own curriculum with an eye to how you would want to feel on first being interviewed for a job or on first being confronted with the need for making decisions about policies and

practices in a job situation, what would you include in your program of study?

13. With what other professional and nonprofessional groups or agencies or individuals will you be expected to cooperate as a practicing speech clinician? What principles will guide you in your professional relations with them? What boundaries will delimit your areas of responsibility from theirs? To what extent is there likely to be overlapping of responsibility?

14. Secure a copy of the official curriculum or program of the speech pathology and audiology program of your own college or university. What basic philosophy appears to underlie the choice of courses prescribed? What appears to be the rationale for the inclusion of each course? How do the graduate-course requirements differ from the undergraduate? What, in your opinion, are the reasons for these differences?

15. Write out your own general definition of "speech problem." How do we know when a speech problem has been eliminated?

16. Suppose that as a practicing speech clinician you read about a new remedial technique that someone has suggested for use with stutterers. How do you decide whether you will adopt the technique in your own work?

17. Secure copies of the *Journal of Speech and Hearing Disorders,* the *Journal of Speech and Hearing Research, Language, Speech, and Hearing Services in Schools,* and *Asha.* Who are the individuals and what is the organization responsible for the publication of these journals? What kinds of articles and features are included in each?

18. Secure a copy of *dsh Abstracts* ("dsh" stands for Deafness, Speech and Hearing), published quarterly by Deafness, Speech and Hearing Publications, Inc., sponsored jointly by the American Speech and Hearing Association and Gallaudet College, the national college for the deaf, in Washington, D.C. Note the general character of the abstracts and the system of classification used in the *dsh Abstracts.* Who are the persons responsible for writing, editing, and publishing *dsh Abstracts?* What professional purposes does it serve? What uses can you make of it personally?

19. Make a list of journals other than those listed in assignment 17 which have some bearing on the work you will do as a speech clinician. What kinds of materials do they include which will be of use to you?

20. Secure a recent *Directory of the American Speech and Hearing Association* and study the introductory portions.

    a. What are the purposes of the Association and of the American Speech and Hearing Foundation as given in the bylaws of the American Speech and Hearing Association?

      b. What are the qualifications for membership in the association? What are the requirements for clinical certification?

      c. Read the Code of Ethics of the association.

        (1) What practices are specifically listed as unethical? Why?

        (2) What are the limits to which the obligation of secrecy can be carried so far as the revelation of confidential information about specific cases is concerned? For what purposes might information in clinic case files be revealed?

        (3) Is critical scrutiny and discussion of the research of other members of the profession unethical?

21. Do you have a state speech and hearing association? Who are its officers? What is the purpose of the organization? When does it meet? Does it publish a journal or newsletter? Can you belong? How can you join? How can you personally contribute to the greater effectiveness of the organization?

REFERENCES

1. Anderson, J. E., The limitations of infant and preschool tests in the measurement of intelligence. *Journal of Psychology,* 1939, 8:351–379.

2. Beck, S. D., *The Simplicity of Science.* New York: Doubleday, 1959.

3. Brown, S. F., and Oliver, D., A qualitative study of the organic speech mechanism abnormalities associated with cleft palate. *Speech Monographs,* 1939, 6:127–146.

4. Cable, W. A., A speech correctionist's professional code. *Journal of Speech Disorders,* 1946, 11:225–231.

5. *Code of Ethics of the American Speech and Hearing Association,* published in the *Annual Directory.* Washington, D.C.: American Speech and Hearing Association.

6. Darley, F. L., *Diagnosis and Appraisal of Communication Disorders.* Englewood Cliffs, N.J.: Prentice-Hall, 1964.

7. Davis, H., and Silverman, S. R., *Hearing and Deafness.* Rev. ed. New York: Holt, Rinehart and Winston, 1960.

8. Doll, E. A., *The Vineland Social Maturity Scale.* Philadelphia: Educational Test Bureau, 1946.

9. *Dorland's Illustrated Medical Dictionary.* 24th ed. Philadelphia: Saunders, 1965.

10. Johns, D. F., and Darley, F. L., Phonemic variability in apraxia of speech. *Journal of Speech and Hearing Research,* 1970, 13:556–583.

11. Johnson, W., *People in Quandaries: the Semantics of Personal Adjustment.* New York: Harper & Row, 1946.

12. Kelvin, Lord, *Popular Lectures and Addresses.* I, 1883.

13. Mecham, M. J., *Verbal Language Development Scale.* Minneapolis, Minn.: American Guidance Service, 1959.

14. Meredith, H. V., Measuring the growth characteristics of school children. *The Journal of School Health,* 1955, 25:267–273.

15. Porch, B. E., *Porch Index of Communicative Ability.* 2 vols. Palo Alto, Calif.: Consulting Psychologists Press, 1967.
16. Robbins, S. D., *A Dictionary of Speech Pathology and Therapy.* Cambridge, Mass.: Sci-Art Publishers, 1951.
17. Stoicheff, M. L., Motivating instructions and language performance of dysphasic subjects. *Journal of Speech and Hearing Research,* 1960, *3:* 75–85.
18. Templin, M. C., Norms on a screening test of articulation for ages three through eight. *Journal of Speech and Hearing Disorders,* 1953, *18:*323–331.
19. Travis, L. E., A point of view in speech correction. *Quarterly Journal of Speech,* 1936, *22:*57–61.
20. Williams, R. J., *Free and Unequal.* Austin: University of Texas Press, 1953.
21. Williams, R. J., *You Are Extraordinary.* New York: Random House, 1967.
22. Williams, R. J., The biology of behavior. *Saturday Review,* January 30, 1971, *54:*17–19, 61.
23. Wolfe, W. G., A comprehensive evaluation of 50 cases of cerebral palsy. *Journal of Speech and Hearing Disorders,* 1950, *15:*234–251.

PART ONE

Appraisal

2
THE CASE HISTORY

Frederic L. Darley

BUILDING A PROBLEM PROFILE

In order to help people with speech problems effectively, the clinician needs to see them clearly as they are now and describe fully their present problems. The majority of the procedures in this book are designed as parts of a systematic plan for securing the profile of a person as he or she presently is. The meaning of such a profile can be fully appreciated, however, only when it is viewed in context—that is, within a background of antecedent conditions and a framework of maintaining circumstances. In order to plan appropriate management, we want to learn about the origin and development of his or her present problem and to estimate its future course with and without remedial attention. So as clinicians we need to answer in any given case this basic question: "How did this person come to be what now appears in his profile?"

Several procedures are useful in gathering the information necessary for completing the problem profile and its background:

1. The Questionnaire

The questionnaire can be used for gathering a good deal of information from one person or from many in a brief time, and indeed will serve to collect data from several informants simultaneously. The procedure is economical in providing a record of the answers in usable form without further write-up. We can make a questionnaire as comprehensive or as brief as we wish, and by using it we can cover the same ground in each of a series of cases.

There are also several disadvantages in the use of the questionnaire. Although uniform coverage of the relevant areas is provided for, we cannot be sure that all respondents have interpreted the questions in the same way or even that they have understood the main point of each question. Well do we know that words can mean different things to different people, and that some words mean nothing to some people. Furthermore, the questionnaire method gives only limited guidance in ascertaining the areas to be explored further. Structured as it is, it carries the implication that the areas covered are *the* important ones. Actually some of the areas covered may be almost irrelevant in certain cases.

2. The Autobiography

If the individual under study is old enough and has the necessary ability, we may ask him or her to write a personal life history. It is enlightening to see how individuals size up themselves as well as their associates and their past and present environments. We may obtain insight into how they perceive the world and their roles in it. Also, it may be enlightening to see how they emphasize or undervalue certain points in their histories. We may get a comprehensive and helpful report, for in writing the document an individual may dredge up facts and attitudes that he or she might not reveal during an oral review. A particularly important consideration is that the autobiography, properly used, tends to have remedial as well as diagnostic value.

Unless due precautions are taken, this procedure can sometimes be unduly time consuming. It should be noted also that persons vary in ability to reconstruct the past, to remember events, and to relate what they remember. In the preparation of such a personal document there is also bound to be conscious and unconscious selection of items. Inevitably topics will be omitted which we might want to know about.

3. Spectator Observation

By observing a child or adult in a clinic room through a one-way window, or by watching a group of children at play, or by observing the interactions of parents and children in the clinic or at home, we are able to gain the kind of firsthand knowledge of behavior that is not dependent upon a written report or upon observation by some other person. Through firsthand observation we can obviate some of the biases which enter into any written abstract of what presumably went on in a given situation. We can observe details which are usually lost in verbal reports of observations. We can observe behavior in a specific context with regard to time, space, and participants and thus interpret the meaning of the behavior more readily.

We need to be sensitive, of course, to the fact that if we are seen by those whom we are observing, even though we do not interact with them, we influence their behavior. Furthermore, the range of behavior and the types of social interaction that can be observed are obviously limited in this type of procedure.

4. Participant Observation

We can carry our observations a step further by injecting ourselves into the activity of the person whom we are observing. We can structure the situation in certain ways so as to make specific observations. Of course, our presence in the activity makes it different from what it would be if someone else were participating or if no one were present to observe. It might be said that all of the procedures of standardized testing, including those outlined in this book for making systematic observation of behavior of persons with speech, voice, and language problems, are special types of participant observation techniques, involving particular kinds of structuring of the situation.

5. The Oral Interview

When we interview an informant, we operate in a special kind of interpersonal relationship which involves a two-way conversation and a mutual viewing. What the informant sees will determine in large part whether and to what degree rapport develops between the two participants. With rapport, the situation tends to be one of maximum cooperation, confidence, trust, and lack of constriction on the part of the informant. Out of this relationship we can derive at least some of the information needed in order to understand the client and his or her problems and to bring about desirable changes in behavior or situation.

This type of interview is one designed to secure information. Its goal is to ascertain important elements of the client's problem profile and relevant antecedent and maintaining conditions. It is conducted so as to determine certain facts and, in addition, a body of attitudes, value judgments, emotions, and reactions related to those facts. It is not an "uncovering" interview in the psychiatric sense, designed to unearth material in the informant's unconscious. It is not a therapeutic interview designed primarily to help or to change the informant, although in some respects the interview may incidentally provide some release for the informant. It is not primarily an information-giving interview, designed to answer the informant's questions and guide him or her to a course of action. It is a two-way conversation, but with a difference: the interviewer provides a structure to the exchange and he or she provides the probes which elicit the desired information; the interviewee does most of the talking in response to the probes, confident that there is cordial interest, sympathy, and respect on the part of the interviewer, purpose in the questions, and profit in the answering of them.

THE INTERVIEW OUTLINE

In order to secure an adequate problem profile one should explore many areas of information, as listed in the case history outline on pp.   – . One may ask, "How long should the case history be?" Wallin (5) stated that as he saw it, case study data must satisfy four conditions: relevancy, sufficiency, representativeness, and reliability. Apparently the question of how long the history should be can be answered in any specific instance only by another question: "How long *must* it be to accomplish its purpose adequately, with reference to Wallin's four conditions, *in this particular case*?" It seems that no single set of questions, such as are listed in case history questionnaires with blanks to be filled in, can be adequate for every case, although indeed some are admirably detailed and extremely useful to study. (For example, see that of Van Riper, 4, pp. 491–502.) The reason is that a question irrelevant in some cases may only begin to delve into matters of crucial importance in other cases. And what of the myriad questions not included in the questionnaire simply because there had to be a stopping place somewhere? Every person with a problem is unique. No inflexible case history questionnaire will do the job; and even though the questionnaire may be intended to be flexible, "fill-in-the-blanks" thinking tends to inflexible.

The interview outline included here has been developed through many years of clinical work in several speech and hearing clinics. The headings and questions are suggestive rather than exhaustive. Since the outline cannot be complete, it has been made brief intentionally; it represents a skeleton outline and it is up to the user of it to put the flesh on the bones. In the mutual exchange of words that characterizes the particular type of interpersonal relationship which we call a case history interview, you as interviewer need to be alert to hints of fruitful areas for exploration, interesting cues to follow up, unsuspected relationships to scrutinize. You will not be able as a rule to follow the outline carefully as you pursue the conversation, but it will help to look at it from time to time, and your prior study of it will go far to guarantee adequate coverage.

You will find the outline particularly useful in organizing your information in order to make a written record of the completed interview. It provides a way to systematize and order a mass of data. In preparing your report you can assign to each part the weight you think it should be given in pointing up the particular problems of the individual. You are sure to find sometimes that sections of the interview overlap and need to be combined. Properly employed, the outline makes it possible to arrive at a balanced account of a given problem in which many interacting variables are to be seen in perspective.

Before attempting to use such an outline, you should understand clearly why such questions are to be asked. You should understand not only what the words themselves mean but how each question relates to other questions and to the presenting problem. For example, ask yourself, "Why am I questioning the mother of this stuttering boy about his childhood diseases?" Is it because a direct causal relationship is known to exist between a reported illness and the problem of stuttering? Or is it rather because a *supposed* causal relationship in the thinking of the parents is likely to affect their evaluation of the child and his problem? Or is it because of psychological factors associated with the specific illness, such as the concern and solicitousness of the parents shown at the time of the illness, and their consequent effects? Or is it for some other reason?

You may wonder particularly about the use you are expected to make of certain kinds of medical information which we suggest you ask questions about. We are, of course, not suggesting that you independently diagnose medical conditions to which some of the suggested questions relate. The basic point is that you need to be aware of the kinds of information which are necessary in arriving at certain diagnoses, which serve to clarify the nature of specific disorders of communication and to indicate the needs and possibilities for particular kinds of improvement in speech, language, or hearing. You have a responsibility to be sensitive to the possible significance of these kinds of information in relation to the communication problems with which you are professionally concerned.

Just to be sure that you do not mistake this outline for a complete list of questions (as a case history questionnaire too often is mistakenly supposed to contain blanks about *all* the important questions), it would be well for you to take time to ask yourself about the implications of some of the listed questions. For example, if you were to try to obtain a picture of the home relationships as suggested under social history, what specific questions would you like to ask in order to obtain the details needed to clarify the rather general answers most informants give to such questions? When you have filled several pages, you can remind yourself, "This list is only a beginning. And even when I've supplemented these questions with scores of others, the data I might obtain could not be more than an abstract of all that conceivably could be secured."

Following the basic case history outline presented at the close of this chapter are several supplementary case history outlines. These present additional topics of inquiry and specific questions that you may use in order to obtain more nearly adequate special information that is needed regarding certain problems. In order to make the relevance of these additional questions clear, we have included certain information about each of the disorders. Not all of the questions one might ask have been listed. The questions that are presented will indicate which areas deserve particular scrutiny, but it will be up to you to explore each such area in sufficient detail for your specific purposes.

You may sometimes be at a loss to interpret some of the data you obtain from your informants. The normative information presented in some of these chapters will help you to understand whether the individual whose history you are securing is generally average or accelerated or retarded in certain aspects of development.

To derive maximum usefulness from these and other tables of normative data, you should become familiar with the studies upon which they are based. Definitions and procedures used by investigators in compiling specific sets of normative data are crucial in interpreting them for specific purposes.

THE HOW OF INTERVIEWING

A subject that many books cannot exhaust is impossible to cover fully in these pages. Here are a few suggestions offered as practical guides in conducting most information-getting interviews, together with a list of some useful references on the techniques of effective interviewing.

1. Set the Right Tone

Experienced interviewers have learned and repeatedly confirmed that the atmosphere most conducive to successful gathering of information is one of mutual respect. You and the informant are by no means on equal grounds, for he or she has come for help which you are in a position to give. It is to be expected that most of the questions and the guidance of the interview will issue from you, while most of the information will come from the interviewee. And yet you as the interviewer cannot afford to be aloof, superior, critical, moralistic, rigid, intolerant, disdainful, or amused.

You must show an acceptance of the person and sincerely try to understand his or her behavior and problems. You must certainly refrain from ridicule or condemnation. Rapport grows only as you show the informant that you still will accept and respect him or her and do your best to help no matter what you hear. You do this largely by accepting and acknowledging (not necessarily approving outwardly) what you are told, by trying to fit together in a meaningful pattern the various bits of information provided, and by making obvious that you want, above all else, to understand and help with the problem as well as you possibly can. Some experts in interviewing people about sensitive topics have stated it this way:

> One is not likely to win the sort of rapport which brings a full and frank confession from a human subject unless he can convince the subject that he is desperately anxious to comprehend what his

experience has meant to him. . . . Histories often involve a record of things that have hurt, of frustration, of pain, of unsatisfied longings, of disappointments, of desperately tragic situations, and of complete catastrophe. The subject feels that the investigator who asks merely routine questions has no right to know about such things in another's history. The interviewer who senses what these things can mean, who at least momentarily shares something of the satisfaction, pain, or bewilderment which was the subject's, who shares something of the subject's hope that things will, somehow, work out all right, is more effective though he may not be altogether neutral. (2, p. 42)

From the opening handshake and friendly greeting your intent is to convey your cordiality toward the patient and your deep interest in the problems communicated to you. You will show that you appreciate this chance to talk together, and you will from the beginning talk *with*, not *at* or *to*, the patient. You will be your natural self, display sincere concern for both the individual and the case, and without verbalizing it persuade the interviewee not to be on the defensive.

2. Get the Interview Off to a Good Start

Do not assume that the person you are questioning understands the purpose of the interview without having it explained. When a parent comes to a speech and hearing clinic for help, he or she may be unprepared for the kind of questioning you will be doing. Structure the situation by explaining who you are and the function you serve, the purpose of the interview, the use that will be made of the information, to whom it will—and will not—be revealed, why information is needed in such detail. The informant will submit readily to a great deal of questioning if convinced that the answers are needed and will be handled responsibly.

See that the informant is comfortable. Be alert to conditions of temperature and ventilation; see that the light is not in anyone's eyes; arrange a comfortable, relaxed interviewing situation; avoid noisy environments.

It is always desirable to encourage the person who has come for help to talk as freely as possible about his or her problem or the child's problem, as the case may be. With an attitude and posture that suggest that you have all the time in the world, let the person put into his or her own words the feelings, the questions, the beliefs and curiosities, the anxiety and sense of guilt perhaps, the hope and the doubt that need to be expressed before you begin to ask questions. In some cases the person will want, and may deeply need, to talk quite a long while. In most cases, however, you will sense fairly soon that the informant rather expects to be questioned or perhaps tested and examined in some way. If an individual does not seem to have any particular need to "get talked out," at least a few minutes of friendly conversation at the

beginning without the intrusion of note taking may be helpful in establishing rapport early. Usually you can get down to business at hand
fairly soon. If the informant obviously is ready to cooperate, there is no
need to delay the questioning.

3. Learn to Listen

Generally informants find it annoying to be asked a question, provide
the answer, and then be asked the question once or perhaps even more
times subsequently. Such a sequence indicates to them that the interviewer simply did not listen the first time. You should become sufficiently
familiar with your interviewing procedures and the particular sequence
of questions you are likely to use so that as the interview progresses you
need not be worried about how you are doing or what questions you
will be asking next; rather you should be concerned about the feelings
and replies of the person you are interviewing. Although you probably
will be making notes on what you hear (see Section 15 below), you will
need to absorb the information even as you are obtaining it. Do not
let the process of questioning become automatic. Keep it vital, and
listen actively. As Long (3) has written concerning the way medical
students should take histories,

> The eager beaver who knows all the questions and gives his patients
> little opportunity to say anything but 'yes' or 'no' rarely gets a decent
> history. Once we missed a diagnosis of late syphilis from the patient
> because we talked too much, and did not let the patient give us this
> final confidence about himself. So be easy and take it easy.

You will find it easier to listen if you have allowed yourself plenty
of time for taking the case history. Quoting again from Long, "One
can't rush through a history and do anyone justice. . . . A relaxed patient
and doctor result in the most satisfactory histories" (3, p. 61). You will
want to work your way rather rapidly through the case history (see
Section 10 below), but the informant should not get the impression that
you are in a hurry.

4. Frame Questions Clearly

Although the general atmosphere you establish is more important than
the specific way you frame any question, you can learn a lesson from
the experienced public opinion pollster and word your questions clearly.
If you do, you will save yourself time and will secure more reliable
information.

First of all, make sure you understand why you are asking each
question. What is the main point of it? Now state it briefly in words
of one syllable if you can. It makes sense to use the sort of vocabulary
and style of expression your informant seems to be in the habit of

using; if you err in any direction, err in the direction of underestimating the informant's sophistication.

In clarifying the point of a question, you may need to define some terms, even fairly common ones. For example, if you want to find out how often a child is punished at home, you will need clearly to differentiate punishment from reprimands or scolding and even give some examples of each so you and the informant will mean essentially the same things by the terms you are using.

5. Frame Direct Questions

Avoid starting a question, then qualifying part of it, then going back and reframing it, ending lamely with an ambiguous set of incoherent ideas for the informant to sort out. Not this: "How old was your child when you began to teach him habits of—uh, well, letting him know that he should go to the bathroom—you know, control his bladder?" But perhaps this: "When did you begin Eddie's toilet training?"

Avoid asking double or multiple questions. Make it possible for the informant to concentrate on one item at a time. You will obtain sharper answers and you won't miss information that got left out because a part of a multiple question was forgotten.

6. Avoid Yes-No Questions

Frame your questions so that you get the information you want rather than a "yes" or "no" which will need to be supplemented with further questions for clarification. Questions requiring factual answers place more of a burden upon the informant. For example, "What illnesses has John had?" is a more efficient question than the more general "Has John been sick much?" The latter, whatever the answer, will need to be followed up with other questions framed to elicit details.

It is usually poor strategy to describe a disorder or situation and then ask the informant to agree or disagree with what you have described. Make the informant provide the description.

7. Frame Questions Neutrally

Avoid "leading" and "loaded" questions which by their wording suggest what would be an "acceptable" answer. Try to word each question so as not to bias the answer. If you ask the parent of a stuttering child, "You didn't tell Tommy to stop and start over, did you?" you will often get "Oh, no!" for a reply. A less slanted question such as "What have you done to help Tommy talk better?" or "Have you sometimes suggested that Tommy stop and start over?" is likely to elicit a more valid reply. Avoid putting answers in the informant's mouth. Avoid suggesting how answers will be received.

However, in order to expedite answers to some questions, you may find it helpful to provide the informant with a set of possible answers or a rating scale for making a judgment. For instance, it may help a parent to describe how he or she handles a child if you suggest that some parents reprimand their children by hollering at them, others by threatening. Then: "What do you mostly do in reprimanding your child?" Again, statement of the frequency of parental reprimands may be more easily secured by suggesting various possible frequencies— 25 times a day, or once a week, or once a day, or 10 times a day— avoiding any particular sequence in the suggested answers and avoiding making the last of the suggested answers seem to be the most appropriate or expected answer.

We sometimes want parents to evaluate their children with regard to particular types of behavior or personality traits. A useful tool to offer them—partially to objectify their evaluations in terms of what they know of other children (their own or somebody else's)—is the following 5-point scale: In comparison with other children of her age, would you rate the amount of talking your child does as much more than average, somewhat more than average, about average, somewhat less than average, or much less than average?

8. Ask Questions Straightforwardly

Inevitably you will get around to matters that are intimate, emotion-laden, socially involved. How shall questions about parental relations be asked—questions about sources of conflict in the home, separations, divorces—or questions about speech and other disorders in the family history, home disciplinary practices, parental estimates of the intelligence of the child, and the like?

The best practice, though it takes most beginning interviewers a while to recognize this and boldly try it out, is to be matter-of-fact. Having laid a solid foundation of rapport, mutual understanding, and respect, ask the questions in a direct manner—as Kinsey, et al. have said, "without hesitancy and without apology." They add, "If the interviewer shows any uncertainty or embarrassment, it is not to be expected that the subject will do better in his answers. . . . Evasive terms invite dishonest answers" (2, p. 53).

Sometimes the posing of a ticklish question will result in a long painful pause while the informant wrestles with the problem of deciding how best to answer or evade it. Resist the impulse to ease the tension by talking yourself, by interposing a too ready "I understand" or an equivalent expression. If you have properly laid the groundwork for a profitable discussion of some vital question, don't throw your work away by unwisely doing the thinking and deciding for the informant.

9. Provide Transitions in Questioning

As you progress in your interview from topic to topic, try to avoid abrupt shifts in questioning which may puzzle the informant. For instance, a question about a child's speech problem followed immediately and without warning by a question about the mother's pregnancy constitutes a jarring non sequitur. Help the informant understand what is going on by building in a transitional explanation: "We've covered the subject of Sue's speech pretty thoroughly. I wonder now if we might talk about some related aspects having to do with her development, even going back to her birth and early growth."

Another occasion for a transitional statement is when the informant has wandered away from the question you asked and has seemingly gotten off the track. You can get someone back on the track without being offensive: respond to what the informant is telling you, suggest that you may want to get back to that topic later, and hark back to an earlier relevant response. "I can see what you mean and perhaps we can get into that later; you were saying a moment ago that Alan seemed unaware that anything was the matter with his speech. Did he . . .?"

10. Adjust the Sequence of Topics to the Anxiety of the Informant

Some anxiety on the part of the informant is implicit in the interviewing situation. The fact that someone has come for help means that he or she is more or less concerned about something. It has been said that an informant who feels no anxiety won't talk—indeed, probably will not have come to the clinic at all. But if an individual feels too much anxiety, the course of the interview may be seriously impeded. Arrange the sequence of topics so as to allow time for gradual building of rapport without touching on emotion-laden matter too early.

Ordinarily the informant comes ready to supply factual information about a speech disorder, details of growth and development, matters of health, and routines of life and social activities. Questioning in these areas typically appears "legitimate" and nonthreatening to most informants. On being questioned about details of family relationships, the informant may feel some reluctance to reveal material not usually discussed with outsiders. And when we raise questions that relate to attitudes about people and events, feelings, and fears, defenses rise if the informant feels the intrusion is unwarranted or the material is too highly charged.

You will do well to establish your role and confirm the informant's trust in you and respect for you by concentrating early on more neutral, factual material and maximizing the informant's verbal output. As the sequence of questions moves along, you are helping him or her feel more and more accustomed to sharing information and feelings. Finally you will feel secure in focusing your probes more and more specifically on attitudinal matters, and the informant will more likely be willing to respond honestly and openly.

11. Attempt to Get Beneath Superficial Answers

An informant may not realize the importance of a question or, trying to take the easy way out and evade a crucial subject, may dismiss a question hurriedly. You may ask: "Did you ever do anything to correct your son's stuttering?" "No," is an easy but seldom accurate answer. Dig under that too ready "No." Ask additional specific questions. Ask questions that put the burden of denial on the informant, such as, "How many times a day do you ask him to slow down?"

Parents often have a hard time recalling details of events remote in time, such as the age of first steps, the kind of approval and disapproval they expressed during the child's early toilet training, the times and details of early illnesses, the nature of first so-called stuttering reactions and the specific situation in which they were first noticed. Here is a tremendous and important challenge to your ingenuity. Suggest to the informant ways of pinning down an event. Help to establish certain milestones such as family moves from one community to another, changes in employment, visits to or from relatives, entrance into school, births, deaths, marriages, memorable trips, and so on; and then relate to these markers the incidents about which you are asking. Frame a question in various ways, suggesting details you wish recalled, and don't give up too readily in your search for these details.

Unless you can establish a reasonably clear relationship in time and place between two events, you cannot conclude that they are, in fact, related. For example, parents will often say something like, "The stuttering started at the time Arthur had a ruptured appendix and had such a bad time in the hospital." Such a statement is by no means to be taken at face value. Get both events, the rupturing of the appendix and the onset of the stuttering, dated as precisely as possible by relating them to other clear family time-markers. It is impressive how often such questioning of time relationships results in the disclosure that the two events actually occurred several months apart. We all feel the need to explain to ourselves and to others the important events in our lives or in the lives of our children. Sometimes in trying to work out the needed explanations we put close together in memory events that were far apart in reality. This is such a strong and common tendency among people that as a clinical interviewer you need to cultivate a keen sensitivity to it.

Even in cases in which it is established that events did occur together, or nearly so, *in time*, it must still be established that they were related *in space*. This may seem a strange way to put it, but a moment's reflection will probably make it seem sensible. For example, having established that an appendix ruptured in an organism at about the same time that a listener first decided that stuttering was beginning to occur in that organism, you must somehow get from the appendix to the mouth, as it were. Indeed, in such a case as this one, you would first have to determine whether the child had, in fact, begun to speak in some new and different way or the parents had begun to pay attention to and wonder about something the child had been doing all along. Assuming that the child had begun to speak in some unusual way, then it has to be determined what *relevant* events inside the organism took place between the rupturing of the appendix and the uttering of, possibly, "Wh—wh—wh—where is my c—c—c—cap?" a few hours later, or even within the next minute—to saying nothing of four weeks later. Even when such questions clearly cannot be answered, you should ask them of yourself, and often of the informant. It is essential that everyone concerned understand as thoroughly as possible that a causal relationship between two events is necessarily a relationship between them not only in time but also, and necessarily, in space.

Often the answer "I don't know" is most revealing and important. A parent who comes to the clinic convinced that a child's cerebral palsy is due to the use of instruments at time of birth, or that a youngster's stuttering was caused by a bad fright, takes a basic step toward better understanding of the problem in recognizing a lack of precise and sufficient supporting information, if such recognition is in order. Usually it will enable the parent to consider, at least, other and more sound and helpful interpretations than those previously made.

One specific problem in this connection is worthy of special mention. Quite often you will find that the parents of a stuttering child, when asked how long the child has stuttered, will reply, "From the beginning," or "All her life," or "From the time she first began to talk." Of course such an answer is not to be accepted at face value. A moment's reflection can only lead to genuine questioning about what such a statment could possibly mean. On the basis of what specific standards or norms of speech development might you conclude that a child has "always" stuttered?

Moreover, you must recognize the need to visualize or imagine as vividly as possible just what, if anything, is being described when a parent says, for example, that a child *suddenly* "could not say a word," or "was blocked," presumably at some exact time by the clock such as 9:15 of a particular Tuesday forenoon—after two or three or even more years of evidently normal functioning of the speech mechanism and, on top of that, in the absence of any apparent cause, or "just after a fall," or "when he had the measles," or "when he started school," or some other circumstance under which a sudden failure of normal neuro-muscular functioning would not usually be expected and no explanation for it is apparent. The onset of any problem is a matter to be investigated with the keenest possible sensitivity to vagueness, memory fashioned to accord with "what must have happened," and confusions of fact and unexamined assumption, not only on the part of the informant but of yourself as well. In general, you should consistently take care to have the informant *describe* quite exactly what he or she allegedly has ob-served, to distinguish at all times between vague or generalized family legends and actual memories of specific events, and to relate everything as closely as possible to times, places, and persons. This kind of inter-viewing takes more time than routine questioning, of course, and often it cannot be carried as far as you would like. Even so, it is to be kept in mind as a standard, and general information obtained hurriedly and without thorough pinpointing and evaluating is to be weighed and dis-counted accordingly.[1]

12. Note Discrepancies in the Account and Check Them

The longer the interview, the greater its reliability, for the chances of your including interlocking questions are greater and there is greater likelihood that a given item will be touched on more than once by the informant. As the informant expresses more and more attitudes and adds more details, you may recognize inconsistencies. These may be accidental and unimportant or they may suggest uncertainty, evasion, ambivalence, or untruth somewhere along the line.

Do not ignore these inconsistencies as probably trivial or due to an error on your part; likewise do not simply let them stand for someone else to puzzle out and interpret. Rather, check the point concerning which the discrepancy was noted in each instance. Do it unobtrusively later in the interview, avoiding a blunt challenge to the informant's veracity.

13. Move Rapidly Through the Interview

In some areas of questioning you may choose to ask a series of questions rather rapidly. Moving along quickly probably results in greater relia-bility, for it allows the informant less time to ponder an answer and to compare it with some presumably ideal answer and therefore modify it or try to justify it. Yet some questioning must be almost exhaustingly slow if certain subtle details are to be dredged up and clarified.

[1] The sorts of problems discussed in this section are illustrated particularly well in parts of tape recorded interviews, reproduced with comments and explanations, in Johnson (*1*).

14. Maintain Appropriate Visual Relationship

It is important to look at the informant in a way that encourages free communication. It is not good to look at people constantly, of course, as though staring them down, nor should you eye them as though you were doubtful of the truth of their statements. It is not good either always to look down at your notes or to look past your informant or in other ways to seem to avoid direct eye contact. Much of the times your eyes should meet. "People understand each other when they look at each other" (2, p. 48).

15. Record Information During the Interview

Take notes as expeditiously as possible, using a shorthand system, or telegraphic English, or some system of codes to avoid either long silences after answers while you catch up in your notes or inhibition of the flow of important material from your informants by asking them to wait while you catch up. Probably less harm is done to rapport than one might suppose by note taking; some informants actually find it reassuring to have the interviewer making an accurate record as the questioning progresses. Some seem to feel more at ease if the interviewer is doing something. But note taking must be kept within reasonable limits and should be done on a clipboard or pad that can be maneuvered easily so the informant cannot read the notes.

You may want to consider tape-recording your interview. The tape recorder is being used more and more in clinical situations. It is probably used more, however, in counseling and therapy than in case history taking. If you tape-record your case study interviews, you then must transcribe each recording in order to abstract the transcription, or else work directly from the tape, taking notes as you listen to it. In either case the extra time consumed will be considerable. If you do use a tape recorder you would be well advised, in our judgment, to be open with the informant, making clear at the onset of each instance that you are going to tape-record the interview, that this will make it unnecessary for you to take notes and so you will be able to give your undivided attention to the interview. In our experience most persons accept the microphone and recorder as tools of the clinician's trade, and after the first few moments they seem to pay no attention to them and talk as freely as they would without them.

16. Obtain the Informant's Interpretation of the Events Narrated

As a clinician you are interested in what the informant and the child or other person in question have done and the things that have happened to them, but you are also interested in their own evaluations of these happenings. It may be important for you to know that the child first walked at 15 months of age; it may be equally important for you to know whether the parents considered the child retarded, average, or advanced with regard to this aspect of development. It is good to see the child's report cards and to know that her grade average is B; it is also valuable to know whether her family approves or disapproves of such a record. It is important to know not only what it is a child does in speaking that his parents classify as stuttering, but also whether the child's parents believe that he does this sort of thing because of nervousness, fatigue, a change of handedness, a serious illness, a fall, a burn, tongue-tie, being tickled, thinking faster than he can talk, talking faster than he can think, imitation, faulty school handling, or their own mismanagement of the child. It is important, moreover, to know how well they understand such explanations, how they defend them and feel about them.

Consideration of how an informant interprets the significance of the things he or she relates will often remind you that the narrative of events cannot always be taken at face value and will give you valuable insights into the whole situation with which you must grapple as a speech clinician—for we work not just with speech problems but also with the people who are caught up in them. You will see repeatedly that ignorance, motivated or even innocent forgetting, the desire to explain things simply, and a need for approval, as well as feelings of resentment, anxiety, guilt, and shame can color and even render invalid an apparently factual report.

17. Encourage Free Expression of Opinion and Emotion, but Keep in Mind the Limitations of the Interview Situation

Your primary goal in the interview is to compile the information necessary for a properly balanced understanding of the current situation. It is not primarily to foster catharsis. Informants may experience welcome relief in unburdening themselves to you as a sympathetic listener, and you should not inhibit the outpouring of feelings unless you have to. Receive with interest what someone says, keeping alert, empathic, and spontaneous in your reactions. But occasionally in this type of interviewing you may have to stem the flow in order to accomplish your task of thorough coverage in a limited time. Do it tactfully, suggesting that there are other matters you need information about which may prove equally important to both of you.

18. Handle Emotional Scenes Tactfully

You can expect some proportion of the persons you interview to become upset and weep as their feelings of anxiety find an outlet, as they recall moments of sorrow or anxiety, or as feelings of guilt or shame overwhelm them. One possible way to handle the situation is to express understanding and then present a new question that leads off in a quite different and more neutral direction. Don't, however, be too anxious to distract your informant. Such a course of action may make a person even more uncomfortable. The emotion expressed by the informant may be anger; he or she may become hostile, resentful, or aggressive. In such a case reassurance should be offered, a mistake in judgment acknowledged, and a new tack taken if possible.

19. Be Prepared for Questions from the Informant

If you have succeeded in establishing a warm relationship with your informant, it is natural for you too to be asked a question now and then—especially a question about which the informant needs reassurance. How you handle a question should depend upon your role in the clinic routine and upon whether your answer will help or hinder the progress of the interview.

If someone else is in charge of the final disposition of the case and of counseling that normally follows the clinical routine of examination and history taking, you might well refer the informant to that person. For example, a mother says to you, "I'm so worried about Jean's not talking. What do you think is the matter?" You as interviewer can avoid a long and useless, if not harmful, discussion of your ideas by telling the parent that your function is to get as full a picture as possible of the child and the many influences that have molded her, and that the clinic supervisor will review the history and the examination results later and will discuss them with her.

In some cases a truthful answer will jeopardize the relationship you have labored to build. A parent says, "Whenever Jerry stuttered, I just told him to wait until he could say it clearly and then to speak. That's all right, isn't it?" If you say "Yes" in order to get yourself off the hook, you are giving questionable advice and very possibly doing harm. If you say, "No, you shouldn't have done that," you may put the parent on the defensive and spoil to some degree the rapport already established. It is better to refer the question to the person responsible for counseling the parent, or, if it is up to you to give the answer, better to postpone it until a more appropriate time.

Some questions may be handled simply by responding to the emotion expressed in the question rather than to the question itself. An answer such as, "It certainly is hard to know what to do," or "Children surely create problems," or "I can see why you would feel that way," often satisfies the questioner. At other times a direct truthful answer should be given the informant so as to direct his or her thinking elsewhere as soon as possible.

20. Record Your Observations of the Characteristics of the Informant

The behavior, the speech, the attitudes of informants are just as much grist for your mill as are the facts they relate to you. Report these in the section on comments at the close of the history. Some of the observations you might make are these:

Development of Rapport: Was the informant friendly and open? Or indifferent or nonchalant, parrying your questions? Or overtly hostile, refusing to answer or answering only cryptically?

Language Behavior: What does his language suggest about the informant's intellectual or educational level? Is he critical, specific, clear, careful in qualifying his answers? Or does he speak in general terms, using emotionally colored words, confusing fact with opinion? Is he glib in using labels, catchwords, and cliches, rigidly either-orish in his orientation? Is there a recurrent theme song that runs through his conversation, repeated allusions to some topic?

Expressive Movements: What do the informant's handshake, gait, posture, directness or shiftiness of gaze, quality of voice, rate of speech, inflections, and facial expressions suggest to you?

Emotional Reactions: What significant reactions to specific questions and to the interview situation generally do you notice—sighing, pausing, speeding up, weeping, anger, bland indifference?

Insight: How well does the informant see into the heart of the problem, recognize the interrelationships of various aspects in the history and present situation? How clearly does he see his own role in the problem?

Rationalizing: Does the informant strive to justify his acts and behavior, explain away things that might be unfavorably interpreted, give "good" reasons instead of the real reasons?

Unconscious Projection: Does the informant blame someone or something else, or attribute to others the emotions, attitudes, or behavior he sees in himself but cannot admit? Does he talk about people and events as though they were in fact what he takes for granted they are, not seeming to be aware of the degree to which he is projecting his unexamined assumptions and preconceptions about them?

Ambivalence: Does the informant seem to harbor conflicting feelings about the child, about himself, about the speech problem, or even about you?

21. Bring the Interview to a Close Gracefully

Explain that you have asked the questions which you have considered most important and express your appreciation to the informant for cooperating in answering them. Inquire if there is anything further which might have some important bearing on the problem. Explain when there will be an opportunity to discuss the decisions and recommendations with the person responsible for case disposition. Repeat your thanks and take your leave.

22. Write a Functional Report

In writing your report of an interview, your fundamental purpose is to communicate effectively the fruits of your questioning. The following suggestions will help you do an effective job.

a. Come to the point—whatever it may be—clearly, quickly, precisely. Use the simple expression, the direct phrase. You don't have to be fancy in your writing.

b. Quote exactly (and if you are to do it *exactly*, you can't quote at length) those statements which are so unusual, questionable, or revealing that a paraphrase of them would lack something important.

c. Use a question mark in parentheses (?) to indicate that the information immediately preceding is questionable as furnished. If the reason why it is questionable is not obvious, explain.

d. List all informants in the heading of the case history report. If there are more than one, ascribe to each the information whose source it is important to know.

e. Use complete sentences, composing a readable, flowing narrative, not merely the outline for a narrative.

f. Vary sentence structure and sentence length, avoiding monotony.

g. Be factual. Distinguish fact from inference. The statement "His grades are good" is somebody's inference. What are the actual grades —A's, B's, C's? The sentence "Home discipline is strict" describes an attitude, either yours or the informant's; tell instead what disciplinary measures are used, by whom, for what offenses, with what frequency. "The child started to stutter when he was five" refers to a classification made by you or the informant of something the child did "when he was five." What exactly did the child do that was so classified?

h. Adhere to accepted usage of capitals and punctuation marks; and if you aren't sure, consult a reliable guidebook.

i Don't be reluctant to check doubtful spellings, using an ordinary or medical dictionary as necessary.

j. Be professional, serious, sincere in tone, but not pedantic or overly formal. Avoid "asides," frequent underlining for emphasis, and exclamation points.

k. Be human and informal enough to refer by name to the person the history is about rather than to refer monotonously (and depressingly) to the patient, the subject, or the client.

l. Follow a uniform format throughout the history with regard to spacing, indentation, capitalization, underlining, and punctuation of headings. The form of the outline presented at the end of this chapter is suggested as a model.

m. See that the sources of what you record are properly indicated. Use first-person reference to yourself to indicate clearly, especially in the section for comments, the evaluations or observations reported that are your own rather than the informant's. Do not use first-person reference to yourself in recording observations and opinions of the informant or someone else.

n. Form careful habits of signing and dating reports. In writing dates include day, month, *and year.* See that the names of the client, the parents, informants, siblings, physicians, and other persons involved are written in full. Include adequate addresses of parents, physicians, teachers, and others to whom you or your supervisor might want to write. Write your own name and the full date on all reports and papers bearing interview notes.

FOR FURTHER GUIDANCE

The interview is one of our fundamental tools as speech and hearing clinicians. You may find helpful the following sources of information on conducting effective interviews:

1. Basset, G. A., *Practical Interviewing.* New York: Macmillan, 1965.
2. Benjamin, A., *The Helping Interview.* Boston: Houghton Mifflin, 1969.
3. Emerick, L., *The Parent Interview: Guidelines for Student and Practicing Speech Clinicians.* Danville, Ill.: Interstate, 1969.
4. Fenlason, A. F., *Essentials of Interviewing: For the Interviewer Offering Professional Services.* Rev. ed. New York: Harper & Row, 1962.
5. Garrett, A., *Interviewing: Its Principles and Methods.* 2d ed. New York: Family Service Association of America, 1972.
6. Kahn, R. L., and Cannell, C. F., *The Dynamics of Interviewing.* New York: Wiley, 1957.
7. Lisansky, E. T., "History Taking and Interviewing," in "Symposium on Psychiatry in Medical Practice." *Modern Treatment,* 1969, 6:656–687.
8. Richardson, S. A., Dohrenwend, B., and Klein, D., *Interviewing: Its Forms and Functions.* New York: Basic Books, 1965.

ASSIGNMENTS

1. Interview another member of the class, using the case history outline at the end of this chapter. If the person you interview does not have a generally recognized type of speech problem, ask him or her to describe his or her most important shortcoming or difficulty in speech and language behavior—stage fright perhaps, or a feeling of uneasiness in conversing with certain persons or kinds of persons, or uncertainty about grammar or pronunciation, unsureness or distress in using the telephone, or some other definable problem in oral com-

munication. In most cases this will not be a speech disorder, as this term is ordinarily used, but it might well be a problem that is important to the person who is concerned with it. Prepare a case history report.

2. Interview the mother of a preschool child in order to get practice in asking questions especially pertaining to younger children. Prepare a case history report. If the child in question has no speech problem, the section in the case history on the history of the speech problem may be designated a history of speech development.

3. The point has been emphasized that the case history outline presented in this chapter does not include all the questions that might be asked. Make a list of some of the specific questions you might ask in securing adequate information about each of the following areas:
   a. Early speech stimulation and need for speech
   b. Feeding practices and problems
   c. Child's school relationships
   d. Parent-child relationships
   e. Family discipline practices
   f. Child's personality
   g. Sibling relationships

4. How is the information-getting interview different from other kinds of interviews?

5. As you practice interviewing, what obstacles to adequate information getting appear to arise—in you, in the informant, in your relationship with the informant? Try to verbalize these specifically and discuss them with your fellow participants in the interviews. What can you do to overcome these obstacles?

6. List five questions that you wish you didn't have to ask in the interview of a parent. What makes these questions difficult? Frame three alternative ways of asking each question. Evaluate their probable relative effectiveness as probes.

7. Listen to one of the public affairs television programs with an interview format—"Meet the Press," "Face the Nation," "Questions and Answers," et cetera. Evaluate the technique of the questioners. In what respects and to what degree were their questions effective? How might they have conducted the interview differently?

Basic Case History Outline

Name: _____   Date history taken: _____
Birthdate: _____   Interviewer: _____
Address: _____   Informant(s): (Full name and rela-
                                         tionship to speaker)– _____

Complaint:

State in informant's own words, if possible. Is this the only problem?

Referral:

Full name of individual or agency making referral. Indicate relationship.

History of Speech Problem:

Age of patient when first regarded as having a speech problem? Who first so
regarded him or her? Under what circumstances? What sort of treatment has
been attempted? By whom? Have parents made any effort to correct problem
at home? What have they done? What results from treatment? Has patient
made any effort to improve his or her speech ? If so, what has he or she done?
What results? What has been the general course of the problem—has it
become better or worse? Parents' estimate of present severity. Patient's own
estimate of present severity. What things have seemed to affect the severity
of the problem? Anyone else in family or among friends with similar problem
or other speech problem? Did problem cause any adverse comment from
relatives and others? Were such comments made in patient's presence?
    Patient's attitude toward speech problem. Has he or she withdrawn from
speech or other situations because of it? Attitude of parents, siblings, and other
relatives. Variations in attitude with different situations
    (If the problem has been present from the time the child would normally
have started to talk, complete the supplementary case history on language
development and its disorders. If the problem developed after language was
partially established, complete those sections of that supplementary case
history that are appropriate for the age of the patient or the general level of
functioning.)

Developmental History

Birth weight. Unusual birth circumstances? Any feeding difficulties? Ages of
sitting up, first steps, bowel and bladder control. Toilet training techniques.
Handedness, manual dexterity, bodily coordination.

Medical History

Illnesses—age of patient at each significant illness, degree of severity, duration,
amount of fever, any complications or sequelae. Care provided when ill.
Were parents overly concerned or solicitous or matter of fact? Same for all
injuries and operations. Condition of tonsils and adenoids. History of mouth

breathing? Ever worn glasses? If so, why? Parents' or patient's own estimate of hearing and vision.

School History

Age when entered school. Ever failed or skipped a grade? Present grade placement. Kind of grades child makes. Any special difficulties with school subjects? How has patient gotten along with teachers and schoolmates? Amount of education completed. If patient is a child, parents' estimate of his or her intelligence.

Social History

Estimate of family socioeconomic status, based upon parents' occupations, amount of education, source of income, house size and type. Leisure-time activities of family and of patient, community activity participation. Parental, parent-child, and sibling relationships. Discipline practices of parents when patient was a child; present relationship between patient and parents. Personality characteristics of patient. Behavior abnormalities as a child—thumb sucking, temper tantrums, destructiveness, hyperactivity, nail biting, et cetera; present adjustment problems. Age of patient's associates, especially in childhood. If patient is an adult, include work history and estimate of his or her own socioeconomic status.

Family History

Age and health of parents and siblings. Any family health problems? Speech abilities and disabilities in the family background, and family reactions to them.

Comments on Intervew

Development of rapport, nature of informant's language behavior, expressive movements, emotional reactions, insight, evidence of rationalization, of unconscious projection. Any other important observations.

REFERENCES

1. Johnson, W., *Stuttering and What You Can Do About It*. Minneapolis: University of Minnesota Press, 1961.
2. Kinsey, A. C., Pomeroy, W. B., and Martin, C. E., *Sexual Behavior in the Human Male*. Philadelphia: Saunders, 1948.
3. Long, P. H., Editor's page: On the history and physical examination of the patient. *Resident Physician*, 1961, 7:59–62.
4. Van Riper, C., *Speech Correction: Principles and Methods*. 4th ed. Englewood Cliffs, N.J.: Prentice-Hall, 1963.
5. Wallin, P., The prediction of individual behavior from case studies. In Horst, P., *The Prediction of Personal Adjustment*, pp. 183–239. New York: Social Science Research Council, 1943.

Supplementary Case History Outline

LANGUAGE DEVELOPMENT AND ITS DISORDERS

Margaret C. Byrne

GENERAL INFORMATION ABOUT THE DISORDER

In Chapter 4 we describe an oral language disorder as a level of comprehension or use of a standard linguistic system that is inappropriate to the age of the child and the community in which he or she is living. It can be viewed as a deficit in meaningful vocabulary or grammatical structures with respect to understanding or expression. Some children are deficient in all four aspects.

The capacity a child has for learning language influences the quality and quantity of his or her communication. In addition, children tend to learn to talk when someone provides a model and encourages them at home and in preschool. Many children who grow up in deprived homes have limited language skills. Children who have neurological or genetic damage may also have language deficits. Those who are not able or willing to relate to parents, siblings, and peers find little need for oral language. They may not communicate at all or do it with limited gestures or with minimal or inappropriate words and sentences.

As a child reaches school age, all of these factors can converge and then we may be able to discern the basic reason for the language delay. The status of comprehension and use of language now reflects a combination of several of these factors.

SOME POINTS TO BE EMPHASIZED

1. Your problem is threefold:
   a. To determine the child's present language proficiency, that is, what he has achieved with respect to the stages of language development. Your parent interview should provide you with

details sufficient to guide you in your observations and testing of the child.

   b. To obtain a historical report of the child's language development. From such background you may obtain cues that require follow-up conferences with and referrals to other professional specialists.

   c. To learn how the members of the family view the child's communication. This information will help you determine the amount of family education you will need to provide and how much you can expect from the parents as team members in a language program for their child.

2. Many parents have difficulty recalling when their children performed certain tasks. Therefore, ask them to bring the child's baby book if they have one filled out.

3. If the information is not already available from a social worker, you will need to determine whether the child's social maturity is appropriate for his age. He may be slow in developing and in learning in areas such as walking, dressing, eating, toilet training, group play activities, independence in managing his time, and helping with family chores in line with his age. The results of administration of the Vineland Social Maturity Scale can tell you whether the child has deficits in addition to those of communication.

4. Some children manifest a language problem after a period of normal development. If that is the case with the child you are evaluating, try to obtain information about the circumstances in which the child either stopped talking or failed to continue normal language development.

5. The following outline is developmental in nature. Therefore, you can start the questioning at whatever point seems appropriate for a specific child. Obtain an in-depth report rather than a cursory picture of his past and current competence. Use examples to illustrate the points you are asking about. For instance, parents may not understand the word *modelling*. Give them examples of both antecedent and consequential modelling. Obtain examples of the child's performance from the parents.

SUPPLEMENTARY QUESTIONS: OUTLINE OF DEVELOPMENT

1. Obtain an estimate of the daily amount and types of early language stimulation the child received from age 2 or 3 months to the present: modelling; expansion; echoing; reading.

2. What has been the child's reaction to the language stimulation from age 2 or 3 months to the present? Sound-making, as in vocal play and babbling; gesturing; listening; looking at the speaker; smiling;

laughing; imitating the model; self-correction; spontaneous speech; carrying out requests.

3. The child's vocabulary: How many single word utterances does he have? What are they? (As you list them, classify them as functors or contentives.) How does he use them? Are they intelligible to everyone in the home? How many two-word utterances does he have? What are they? (Classify them as pivot-open or open-open classes if possible.) What do they signal? What relationships do they show? Does he use them appropriately?

4. Phrase structure: What kinds of phrases is he using? List some of them. Do they follow the order of the adult arrangement of words: NP, VP? Does he omit the functors? Does he use a VP only? Does he expand either the NP or the VP? How? Are they meaningful to the parents; to other listeners? Are they intelligible?

5. Inflections: Is he using those inflections that appear during the early stages of development: plural inflections on nouns, verb tenses, possessive, comparative and superlative forms of the adjectives? Which ones does he use correctly all of the time; some of the time?

6. Transformations: Which of the early developing transformations is he using? Negatives; questions; contractions; the verbs *get, be, do*; attributes, pronouns.
Types of syntactic structures: Which structures listed in Table 4.2, p. 108, is he using regularly?

7. Concepts: How many of the following concepts does he have? How do you know? I, you, they; one and more than one; time (present, past, future); same and different; negative; attributes, including colors; place (prepositions); classifications (clothes, foods, people); and; or.

8. Sequencing of ideas: When the child tells about an event, does he talk about it in some selected order? Does he bring in extraneous ideas that seem inappropriate?

9. Comprehension: How many of the following does he understand? How do you know? Names of things; grammatical structures involving subject-verb-object; expanded noun phrases; expanded verb phrases; transformations; inflections.

10. Parent interactions with the child: What do parents do when they don't understand him? Is there a sibling or a peer who understands him better than the parents do?
What does he do when listeners don't understand him? How soon does he give up? Does he try to describe what he's saying with gestures, with drawings? What do parents do when child doesn't understand them? Repeat their utterance? Change their utterance in some way? When do they give up? What does child do when he doesn't understand parents? How do they know he doesn't understand?

Has parents' behavior toward him changed over time as a result of difficulties in communication? How has it changed?

Has his behavior changed over time as a result of his failures in communication? How has it changed?

11. Teacher interactions with the child: How does his teacher react to his speech? Does she fill in words for him; ignore him; have someone else interpret his utterances for him? How do you know?

Supplementary Case History Outline

THE STUTTERING PROBLEM

Dean E. Williams

The onset and development of stuttering is related closely to problems in interaction between the speaker and listener. In adapting the basic case history outline described in this chapter to the study of the stuttering problem, you should investigate those speaker-listener relationships that contribute to the development of—and promote the maintenance of —hesitant, cautious, fragmented speech attempts. At the same time, keep a keen ear tuned to the nature of those relationships that create positive interactions resulting in the increase of spontaneous, forward-moving speech behavior. You are interested in obtaining information that can be used not only to decrease undesirable behavior but also to increase desirable behavior.

The stuttering problem is dynamic: it is constantly changing in complexity from childhood to adulthood. Although the general structure of the case history outline remains the same for all ages, you will need to emphasize or "zero in on" different facets of the problem as the stutterer gets older. The exact point at which one facet is emphasized over another one is difficult, if not impossible, to specify. Any human problem that is constantly developing does so on a continuum and not in discrete "jumps" or "stages." An artist, for example, can blend colors to represent different shades of gray from white to black. A writer cannot do this with words. One must categorize in order to write and hence must depend upon the reader to do the blending and overlapping. With due regard to this limitation, the supplementary case history outline is divided into three sections. The first is for the preschool-age child, the second for the elementary-school-age stutterer, and the third for the high-school-age and adult stutterer.

PRESCHOOL-AGE CHILD

When the subject is between the ages of approximately 3 and 5, the informant will most likely be one or both of the parents. The most crucial aspects of the problem to pursue with the parents include (1) frequency, duration, and type of disfluencies in the child's speech to which they refer as "stuttering"; especially, attention should be directed toward the variability in them (the times and situations where they are more likely or less likely to occur); (2) the ways in which the important listeners in the child's environment react to these disfluencies; and (3) the ways in which the child evaluates and reacts to his or her own efforts at speaking generally, and particularly to both the disfluencies and the listener reactions to his or her speech efforts.

Supplementary Questions and Considerations

For the preschool child, most of the information sought in the basic case study interview is applicable and should be pursued in detail. The child is young enough so that the information requested should be relatively fresh in the parents' memory. However, while obtaining pertinent developmental, medical, and social history information, question the parents carefully about their belief and their opinions about the degree to which events mentioned in those parts of the history affected— and were affected by—the developing stuttering problem.

Special effort and sufficient time should be devoted to obtaining as much detailed information as possible about how the child was talking and the situation(s) in which the parents first considered the child to be "stuttering." What were the types, the frequency, and the duration of disfluencies at that time? What were the situations (insofar as you can determine the nature of the conversation and the persons involved in it) in which the parents concluded that he had a stuttering problem?

Question the parents about their *beliefs* as to why their child stutters. In doing this, note the language they use. Is it reflective of a belief that stuttering is a "symptom" of something wrong *within* their child? If so, what? Or does the language reflect a belief that stuttering is a "response" on the part of the child to conditions in his environment? What have the parents done to help the child talk—or to correct the stuttering? How has the child responded to their help? In what ways has the child's fluency behavior changed from the time they first considered that he had a problem until the current interview? Have the child's reactions to speaking changed? If so, how? In what ways have the parents' reactions changed toward the child and to the speaking that he does? What is the parents' outlook on the future? Do they seem to expect him to get better as he gets older, or are they inclined to worry about the future course of his problem? That is, are they especially concerned about the way the child "sounds" and his reactions *today* or are they relatively more concerned about the effects that his stuttering might have on his social and vocational life as he gets older?

Variability of Disfluency

Certain conditions in the home are likely to produce conflict in verbal interaction, increase the frequency and duration of disfluency, and increase the hesitancy of speaking, thereby decreasing spontaneity and fluency. In obtaining information about the variability of disfluency, that is, situations in which the child is more or less disfluent than average, investigate the nature of the parents' observations and evaluations concerning factors that may be contributing to the variability. Exploring these can provide valuable information for future counseling with parents as to what they can do to reduce excessive disfluency and to increase the normal talking the child does. Examples of these conditions include the following:

1. To what extent and at what times does the child attempt to explain occurrences and happenings which he doesn't understand and has had little or no experience in talking about?
2. To what extent does he speak to responsive or unresponsive listeners? How do they attend to the child when he's talking? How do they react to what he is saying? How often do they give him enough time to say what he wants to say in a faltering, groping way? Do they, by their verbal and nonverbal reactions promote on the child's part a feeling that he has the time to search for the right words and the right ways to say things without the fear that mother and dad will turn away and resume their activities.
3. To what extent does the child need to "say things in a hurry" to offset the threat or fear of being interrupted? Do the parents or other important listeners interrupt him a great deal when he is halfway through a story or when he is trying to explain something?
4. To what extent does he have to explain verbally why he did or did not do something and attempt to explain it under the pressure of threat of punishment for whatever he says?
5. To what extent is he "shushed" or told "don't talk now" at times when it is not important, merely "inconvenient" or "bothersome" to listen, for example, when the parents are watching TV?

The specific examples mentioned above can be pursued in the context of the more general atmosphere and "pace" of the home environment. To what extent does general "tension" exist in the home? Is the family on a tight time-schedule so that it's always "hurry, hurry"? Is it a talkative family where everyone is talking at once? Are there considerable conflict and arguments in the home in which the child participates either verbally or as an observant bystander?

Contrasted with the above information is a need to explore the ways in which the parents react to the child at times when he is excessively disfluent. Do they attend to what he says *only* when he is disfluent? Do they "shush" everyone else up only when he becomes disfluent? Do they excuse him for misbehaving if he becomes "excessively disfluent" in explaining? In other words, to what extent does he receive "special consideration" when he is disfluent that he does not receive at other times?

ELEMENTARY-SCHOOL-AGE CHILD

As the child moves through the elementary grades, the elapsed time since the beginning of the stuttering problem increases. Many answers by the parents to the questions discussed above for the preschooler may be affected by this time interval. Their memory becomes hazy, and more and more they report information about their *beliefs* of what must have happened rather than the factual information about what occurred. However, what the parents believe the facts were is quite as important as the facts themselves, whatever they might have been. What people believe to be true affects their attitudes, feelings, and actions. Keep this in mind as you cover the basic case history outline. However, for the elementary-school-age child, increased attention should be directed toward the ways in which the child is coping with the problem and with his success in doing it. Develop a profile of the child's problem as perceived by different members interwoven in the problem.

Problem Profile from the Parents

Generally you will want to obtain the parents' views and attitudes about the stuttering problem *now* and the effect that they perceive it has had on their child. Reflected in their attitudes will be hints about the way the child has been treated in the family. Examples of questions that may be asked include: Why do you believe that he continues to stutter? How serious a problem is it to you or to him? How do you handle it and how do you think it should be handled by other people? In what ways do you feel it has affected your child? What kind of child is he now? In what ways do you think he would be different if he had not stuttered? How does he get along with boys and girls his own age while in school or playing? To what degree has stuttering influenced his relationship with children or with adults (teacher, grandmother, others)? How has it limited what he has achieved socially or educationally? How much help does he need in meeting new situations or new problems? What special allowances do you think he should receive because of his stuttering? How independent is he in comparison with other children? How has he reacted to his stuttering? How has he reacted to your help and concern about it? Questions such as these provide a picture, albeit somewhat cloudy, of the ways in which the parents have reacted to their child as a "stutterer"; and it often provides an overview of the way in which he may be reacting to himself.

Problem Profile from the Child's Teacher

Inasmuch as the child of this age spends a good many hours in school, it is advisable, if at all possible, to obtain a problem profile from the teacher. Many of the same questions asked the parents can also be asked the teacher with regard to the child's performance in school and the teacher's opinion about it. You can thus compare and contrast the attitudes of some of the more important "interactors" in the child's environment.

Problem Profile from the Child

Information should be obtained from the child concerning his views of his verbal interactions both at home and at school. It is not uncommon, however, when a clinician asks a child from approximately 6 to 11 years of age questions about his "stuttering problem" for the child to respond with "I don't know," a shrug of the shoulders, or an apparent lack of interest. You must keep in mind that the child has not had many years of experience in stuttering. He has not spent a great deal of time thinking about the specific problems it creates, in contemplating what it would be like if he didn't do it, or in evaluating in any detail people's reactions and their "attitudes" toward him. He pretty much just accepts people and himself as "the way things are." Ordinarily he is not trying to be defensive; he just doesn't have much to talk about. Meaningful information about people's reactions to him and his feelings about them can be obtained by asking the child about his experiences in talking, using questions such as the following:

"Whom Do You Like to Talk to?" Questions   Whom do you like to talk to at home; at school? Whom don't you like to talk to at home; at school? Who do you think likes to talk with you at home; at school? Who do you think doesn't like to talk with you at home; at school? Questions of this kind can also be asked in terms of a 3-point scale, such as, who likes to talk to you best at home, the next best, the least best? After each answer you can obtain additional information by asking questions such as "Why do you think this is so?"

"Who Talks the Most?" Questions   Who talks the most (the least) at home? Whom do you talk to the most (the least) at home; at school? Whom does your father, mother, brother, teacher talk to the most (the least) at home? Again, these questions can be put on a scale whereby the child ranks the relative amount each member of the family talks. The same scale can be used to find the relative amount the child talks in comparison with other children at home or at school. Where appropriate, follow his answers with "Why?"

"Who Interrupts?" Questions   Who interrupts the most at home, school, play? Who interrupts the least? This question can be pursued by asking who interrupts father, mother, brother the most? Who interrupts you the most (the least)? Whom do you interrupt the most (the least) at home; at school? An answer obtained to any question can be pursued by asking "why" questions.

"Who Are Good Talkers?" Questions   Who's the best talker at home? Who's the next best talker? Who's the poorest talker at home? Why do you consider him or her to be a good talker? Why do you consider (the ones named toward the bottom of the list) not to be very good talkers? If the child has not included himself, you can ask directly about where he puts himself on the scale of "good talker" or "poor talker." The same questions can be asked about his school environment.

"When Do You Want to Talk Well?" Questions   Are there times when you want to talk extra well? Where? Why? Are there times when you don't care particularly how you talk? Where? Why? Do you think this is true about other people who talk?

"When Do You Want to Talk More than You Do?" Questions   In school, on the playground, at parties, when company comes, do you talk more than, less than, or about the same as other children in your class? Are there times when you wish you could talk more but you aren't permitted to? Why do you think this is so? Does this happen with other children? Why?

"Who Listens?" Questions   Who pays the most (the least) attention to you when you talk at home; at school? What do you like listeners to do when you talk to them? How do you want them to listen? For example, do you want them to look down; to look at you; to smile; to frown; to interrupt you; to talk for you? Who does the most and the least of those things that you (like) (don't like) at home; at school? Why do you think they do it?

The above are examples of questions that can be asked the child in order to assist you in understanding his view of the talking world and his place in it. When evaluated in relation to the information received from the parents and the teacher, a composite problem profile begins to form.

HIGH-SCHOOL-AGE OR ADULT STUTTERER

The stutterer of high school age has been grouped with the adult because, for both, the main emphasis at these ages is on the effect stuttering has had on their lives and the ways they have reacted to it. Also more often than not the stutterers in this age group are the main informants for the history.

When you ask questions applicable to an adult from the basic clinical speech case history outline, attitudes and experiences in the following areas should be explored:

Onset and Early Development of Speech Problem

You should make a reasonably thorough, but considerate, effort to find out from the stutterer his account of the onset and early development of the problem. Be sure to note if the report of when stuttering "began" refers to the first instance that *he* remembers (this may be a rather traumatic speaking situation in second or third grade), whether it is a second- or third-hand account told to him by others, or whether it is a family legend without documented reference to dates, places, or other details. Tied to the questions of when it began should be an exploration of his beliefs of why it began. What did his parents believe was the cause of his stuttering? Now that he is older, what does he believe was the cause of it? Careful exploration of these areas will permit you to assess the attitudes and beliefs that he has held about the nature of stuttering and therefore the orientation with which he has operated in growing up and from which he has attempted to cope with the problem.

Speaker's Experience with the Problem Educationally, Socially, and Vocationally

First you will want to obtain information about his level of education, grades received, participation in extracurricular activities, extent of social activities, and vocational preparation, as well as plans and hopes for the future. As you obtain this information, however, you should pursue his expressions of beliefs and attitudes about the ways in which his stuttering either interfered with or facilitated progress in these areas. How does he believe he would have performed differently in classroom activities if he had not stuttered? Would he have been in more or fewer extracurricular activities, would he have dated more or less, would he have gone to more or fewer parties if he hadn't stuttered? To what extent has his stuttering influenced his vocational plans? What does he want to do in life? To what degree have his aspirations been influenced by his stuttering?

Outlook

What is the stutterer's outlook on the future? How hopeful is he about improving the way he talks or "eliminating" the problem? What has been his past experience with clinical treatment or with do-it-yourself therapy? To what degree has it left him with a degree of discouragement and perhaps with certain unfortunate ideas about himself and his problem that must now be counteracted if he is to make a sustained effort to improve?

His attitudes and beliefs about previous therapy experiences will affect directly the ways he is likely to respond in future therapy. What previous therapy has he had? For how long has he received therapy? What does he remember about the specific aspects of therapy? What were, to him, the most helpful things he did in therapy? What were the least helpful? What does he expect from therapy? What does he believe should be the role of the clinician in therapy?

Many adult stutterers have had considerable experience in therapy of some kind. The therapy the individual has had has served to shape and mold beliefs about himself and about what he can do about the problem. Therefore, information in this area constitutes an important part of any case history for the adult stutterer.

Supplementary
Case History
Outline

HEARING
LOSS

Charles V. Anderson and
Julia M. Davis

GENERAL INFORMATION ABOUT THE DISORDER

Unlike many other communication disorders, hearing loss may have its onset at any time during life and may be caused by a wide variety of conditions. In addition, the type of hearing loss may vary from conductive to central and the degree may range from mild to profound. Therefore, a complete case history is an essential part of the appraisal of any individual who exhibits hearing loss.

A loss of hearing may be the result of damage to or a disease of any portion of the auditory system. Occlusion of the external canal, malformation of external canal or middle ear, damage to middle ear structures, or disease of the middle ear may result in a conductive loss of hearing. This type of loss involves poor conduction of sound through the outer or middle ear, but it does not involve damage to the receptors of hearing located in the inner ear. Therefore, conductive hearing loss results primarily in reduced sensitivity to sound. Furthermore, it is usually amenable to medical or surgical treatment and is not necessarily permanent.

When a lesion occurs in the inner ear or the neural pathways from the inner ear to the central nervous system, the loss is sensorineural in type; it does involve the sensory receptors of the inner ear or the nerve fibers of the VIIIth cranial nerve. This type of damage usually results in both a reduction in sensitivity to sound and a disturbance of hearing acuity which in turn results in what we interpret as distortion of the sounds received. At the present time, only a small percentage of sensorineural hearing losses are amenable to medical or surgical treatment and are therefore usually permanent.

The effects of hearing loss on the individual who suffers it depends on the age of onset of loss, the type of loss, and the degree of loss sustained. Hearing loss that occurs in the first few years of life affects the language development and subsequent academic and social development of the patient. Hearing loss that fluctuates (conductive loss) and occurs repeatedly during childhood may affect language development selectively and may also interfere with the learning of academic concepts if exposure to them occurs during periods of reduced hearing.

A hearing loss which has its onset in adulthood affects the ability to communicate even though speech and language skills are already firmly established. The reception of spoken language becomes the major difficulty, although changes may occur in the person's articulation and voice patterns. In view of these differences, it is usually wise to ask different questions when assessing children who exhibit hearing loss than when assessing adults.

SOME POINTS TO BE EMPHASIZED

1. Appropriate medical and surgical care must be accomplished as soon as possible. Not only is this necessary for the restoration of hearing in cases of hearing loss but it also may be important in the prevention of further hearing impairment.
2. The degree of permanent hearing impairment will weigh heavily in recommendations concerning all aspects of habilitation.
3. Amplification is a vital part of the hearing-impaired person's habilitation. Details should be sought concerning any experiences with hearing aids or auditory training units.
4. The effect of any given hearing loss upon a person varies with personality, vocation, and communication needs. In other words, it is not enough to know how much or what kind of hearing loss the person has; we must know how this hearing loss interacts with the important aspects of the person's basic life-style.

SUPPLEMENTARY QUESTIONS—CHILDREN

History of the Hearing Problem

When was hearing loss first suspected? Describe the behavior that caused concern. What action has been taken to determine whether a hearing loss exists? If other professionals have been consulted, what were their conclusions? What advice was given for management of the child? Do other persons in the family have hearing losses?

Describe the speech and language development of the child. At what age did she begin to use words, phrases, sentences? Is her speech intelligible? How does she communicate her needs to others (gestures, speech)? How do others communicate with her? Does she respond to loud sounds, soft sounds, vibrations? Can she understand what is said to her without gestures; with gestures? Does she watch the face of the speaker? Are there words she seems to understand that she cannot say? (If the child is older, these questions are to be modified accordingly.)

Has the child ever worn a hearing aid? Who recommended it? Manufacturer and model of hearing aid worn? When was it purchased? Has it been satisfactory in performance? Describe child's reactions to hearing aid. In which ear is it worn? How consistently?

Developmental History

Did the mother have any of the following diseases during pregnancy: rubella (German measles), toxemia, "flu," other viral diseases? At what point in the pregnancy did the disease occur? Is there a blood incompatibility (Rh factor) between mother and father? During the pregnancy did the mother take any medications known to be ototoxic?

Medical History

Obtain a detailed description of serious illnesses, particularly those involving high fevers, such as measles, mumps, scarlet fever, meningitis, or encephalitis. Has the child experienced ear infections (how often, how treated?), tonsillitis, allergies, chronic or repeated upper respiratory infections?

Social History

Does the child play with other children? How does she communicate with them? How does she participate in group activities? Is she easily managed at home? Does she have temper tantrums? What form of discipline is used? Is it successful? Describe her personality. How does she react to strangers or new situations? Does she separate from the parents easily? How much independence does she have in her neighborhood?

Does anyone other than immediate family live in the home? Is the child expected to behave generally like the other children in the family?

Educational History

Is the child presently enrolled in an educational setting? Describe the setting and the child's achievement there. Is she in a special classroom? If not, does she receive resource help from a teacher of the hearing-impaired? What are her grades? Does her teacher have concerns about her academic achievement? Where is child seated in the classroom? Describe the classroom. Does she use special auditory training equipment at school?

SUPPLEMENTARY QUESTIONS—ADULT

History of the Hearing Problem

When was a hearing loss first suspected? What circumstances brought it to the attention of the patient? Did any event such as illness or accident occur which was related to the onset of the hearing loss, or has it appeared gradually? If this occurred in childhood, what special educational and rehabilitation services were provided? What action has been taken to determine the degree and cause of the hearing impairment? What advice has the person received as to services available to him? What services has he used? Has he had speechreading training or other aural rehabilitation? What has been his evaluation of these services?

Describe the communication behavior of the person. In what situations does he hear best? Worst? Can he hear and understand some people better than others? What seems to him to make the difference? If he wears a hearing aid, in what situation is it helpful or detrimental? How? What does he do to hear and understand better? Does he feel his articulation and voice have changed? Does he use manual communication such as American Sign Language?

Developmental History

Questions in this area are dependent upon the age of onset of the problem. If the onset is assumed to be in early childhood or congenital, it may be important to ask questions given in the section on children; if not, it may be necessary only to determine whether development was considered normal.

Medical History

Has the patient had earaches or drainage from the ear? When? Does the patient experience dizziness? How would he describe this dizziness? Does he note any changes in his hearing in relation to dizziness? Does he have tinnitus? What does it sound like? When does it occur? Where does he hear it? Has he received any medical or surgical treatment for his hearing problems, tinnitus, or dizziness? Was this treatment provided by an otolaryngologist? What was the treatment? How did it affect his hearing?

Has he ever taken ototoxic drugs? Specifically ask about quinine, streptomycin, dihydrostreptomycin, kanamycin, and other medications which may come to be known as ototoxic.

Has he noted changes in his hearing in relation to any medical or health problem?

Social and Vocational History

Get a description of daily communication needs. Is he basically a person who enjoys or depends upon oral communication socially or vocationally? Has he changed his life-style as a result of his hearing impairment? How? Has he changed or does he feel he needs to change his vocation as a result of his hearing loss? Whom does he communicate with primarily? If this group is small or restricted, is it because of his hearing loss? What kinds of leisure-time activities does he engage in? Have these changed as a result of his hearing loss?

Educational History

If the hearing loss occurred prior to the patient's leaving school, refer to the section on educational history for children.

Supplementary Case History Outline

CLEFT PALATE

**Hughlett L. Morris
and D. C. Spriestersbach**

GENERAL INFORMATION ABOUT THE DISORDER

Cleft palate and cleft lip are the result of some factor or factors which interfere with the normal development of the mouth and face during early embryonic life. The exact nature and mode of operation of these factors are not fully known, but they must be in operation by the third month of fetal life because by the end of that time the lips, upper dental arch, and palate have been completely formed.

The speech problems exhibited by persons with clefts vary, of course, from person to person. The most frequent cause of the speech problems is palatopharyngeal incompetence. In such instances the speech is usually characterized by slighted, omitted, distorted, or substituted fricatives, affricates, or plosives; by audible emission of air through the nose; and by hypernasal voice quality. Sometimes a glottal stop is substituted for a fricative or a plosive. The speaker may depress the alae of the nose in an attempt to keep the air from escaping through the nose in order to build up sufficient intraoral breath pressure to produce the consonant phonemes. In addition, the speech problem may be complicated by other abnormalities within the oral cavity such as the misalignment of the dental arches and crooked or missing teeth. Moreover, the speaker may misarticulate for reasons that are related to learning rather than to the structures of the oral cavity.

A child with a cleft palate may have difficulty in nursing and eating, and these feeding problems can sometimes be upsetting to parents. Sucking may be difficult. Liquids and soft and sticky foods may get into the nasal passages and come out through the nose during chewing and swallowing. Sometimes the child will sneeze as a way to clear the clogged passageways. Dental problems rarely cause difficulties in mastication although they may place special demands on brushing the teeth to remove bits of food caught in the dental irregularities.

Frequently these children have middle ear disease and, as a result, hearing is impaired. One of the major reasons for the high incidence of hearing problems in persons with clefts is that the mechanism for opening the pharyngeal orifice of the eustachian tube may be faulty, with a resulting impairment of the aeration or ventilation of the tube and increased danger of infection within the tube and middle ear. Other possible reasons may be that, in the absence of a normally functioning palate, the eustachian tube may be unusually susceptible to infection because of undue exposure to foreign bodies and bacteria. Because of this lack of sterility the tube may even undergo structural changes which prevent it from functioning properly.

Obviously a facial disfigurement or a severe speech problem can result in emotional disturbances and special problems of adjustment for the child and the parents as well. Parental rejection or overprotection may result. Children with clefts may find it hard to accept their problems and live happily if associates do not understand and accept them. They may gradually withdraw from social relationships. Manifestations of such withdrawal may be obvious (refusal to meet people or participate in social activities, or reduction in verbal output) or more subtle (failure to speak loudly enough, or reduction in the activity of the articulators in speaking). Adjustment problems may be intensified during adolescence; in adulthood they may take on importance in relation to vocational development and marriage.

SOME POINTS TO BE EMPHASIZED

1. Usually it is helpful to obtain information about possible etiologic factors related to the presence of the cleft. Is there a history of clefts in the family? During the first trimester of pregnancy was the mother's health seriously affected as the result of illness, injury, or emotional trauma? Usually other professional persons will already have taken histories covering these topics. But because the parents may have been counseled about the importance or lack of importance of these events by professionals whom they have already seen and because they are likely to have attitudes about the relationships of these events to the presence of the cleft, it is important for you to have your own documentation of them for perspective on the counseling which will subsequently be done.
2. Some of the information about the cleft and the associated speech problem is obtained by examination of the speech mechanism or by consulting medical records, if available, rather than by questioning the parents or the child, or by observing the child's speech behavior.

Whatever sources you use, you should obtain (a) a description of the cleft and any associated abnormalities, (b) an account of any physical management procedures (surgical or dental) that have been performed together with an evaluation of their effectiveness, and (c) documentation of any additional physical management procedures that are scheduled or contemplated and why. You may want to get the names and addresses of medical and dental specialists who have provided diagnosis and treatment for the patient. This information is for future reference in case you need to correspond with them directly, with patient or parent consent, about management.

3. The social history should indicate how the patient feels about himself and how he is being treated by his parents, siblings, and associates. You should give special attention to his semantic environment and reactions.

SUPPLEMENTARY QUESTIONS

History of the Speech Problem

Describe the speech problem. If the patient is a child, can the parents usually understand what he is saying? Do other members of the family and close associates understand him? When he wants something, does he use words or point? In the opinion of his parents did he begin to speak at the same time as the other children in the family? Did he at first and does he now speak as much as the other children? As the child grew older did his speech improve, become worse, or remain the same? How have the parents tried to help him with his speech? Has he received any professional help with his speech? Does he feel that he speaks differently from other children? If so, how has he shown this realization? Has his speech given him any problems in school? If so, what is their nature? (If the patient is an older child or adult, these questions are to be modified accordingly.)

Which of the following structures were involved in the cleft: the lip, alveolar ridge, hard palate, soft palate? Was the cleft unilateral or bilateral, partial or complete?

What surgery has been performed? (Be specific.) Did it involve the lip, alveolar ridge, hard palate, soft palate? Did it include a pharyngeal flap operation or other secondary surgical procedure for improving palatopharyngeal competence? Has any plastic surgery been done to improve the cosmetic appearance? At what age was each operation performed? What further surgical procedures, if any, are contemplated?

Has the patient been seen by an orthodontist or prosthodontist? Has he ever been fitted with a prosthetic device ("speech appliance," or obturator)? If he is now wearing it, does it consist of a palatal bulb, a replacement for missing teeth, or both? Do the parents and the child feel that the appliance has been helpful in his eating and speaking? Is the child fitted with an orthodontic appliance or will he be? If he has been fitted with one, is he having any problems with it that seem to affect his eating or speaking? Is any additional dental management contemplated?

Developmental History

What difficulties were there in feeding the child as an infant or as a young child? How were these handled? Does he have any difficulty in eating now?

Medical History

Are there other known birth defects besides the cleft? Is there a history of earaches and ear disease? As a baby was the child unusually fussy? Were there frequent colds and upper respiratory infections? Was there a history of running ears, or of tonsillitis and sore throat? If there is a history of ear disease, what is the past and contemplated medical treatment program?

Is the patient currently under the care of a surgeon because of the cleft? If so, when was he last examined by the surgeon? What did the surgeon say about the status of physical management of the cleft? What further surgical procedures are planned and when? Do the parents or the patient feel that there are unresolved physical management problems related to the cleft or accompanying birth defects?

Social History

What does the child do during the course of the day? Does his mother consider him to be more trouble to her than the other children? More dependent? How is the child punished when he misbehaves? Does he play much with his brothers and sisters or other children? Do the parents take him along when they go out? Does he enjoy going places and meeting people? Do the other children make fun of him because of the way he talks or looks? If so, how have the parents handled such incidents?

What do the parents think caused the child's problem? Is there a history of clefts in the family? Are they concerned about having more children? If so, is the concern the result of the care required by this child, or because of the possibility that subsequent children may also have clefts? Do they think that clefts tend to "run in families"? What reading have they done on the subject of cleft palate? Do they feel that they are in any way responsible for the child's problems? Do they have guilt feelings about them? Are they oversolicitous; rejecting? What do they think will be the probable outcome of the child's problem? (If the speaker is an older child or adult, these questions are to be modified accordingly.)

How do the speakers feel about themselves; the way they look; the way they talk; their ability to cope; their chances of making friends, of being loved?

If the speaker is an older child or adult, are there problems concerning the selection of vocation? Are the vocational goals realistic? Has the choice been influenced by the attitudes of others concerning the place of persons with clefts; by the patient's own attitudes concerning his or her "place"? If married, does he or she feel that the cleft has affected the marriage in any way?

Supplementary
Case History
Outline

CEREBRAL
PALSY

Frederic L. Darley

GENERAL INFORMATION ABOUT THE DISORDER

The brain consists of a number of parts which interact in a complex fashion. Certain parts of the brain control the voluntary movements of parts of the body used in such acts as walking, speaking, and writing. The muscles concerned move as a result of impulses coming from what are called the motor projection areas of the brain. These impulses do not pass directly from the motor areas of the brain to the muscles but are subject to modification en route by the activity of other parts of the central nervous system; then pass through certain relay stations of the brain and brain stem before they arrive at the muscles.

When these motor control centers, modification areas, or relay centers do not function properly because they have been damaged or have not developed normally, control of bodily movements is impaired. This result and its causes, taken together, are designated cerebral palsy. Cerebral palsy is not a result of damage to the spinal cord or the peripheral nerves leading from the spinal cord or brain stem but is due entirely to impairment of the brain's motor control centers, modification areas, or relay stations.

The disturbance of motor control may be widespread and affect all four limbs, the muscles of speech and breathing, and the muscles of the trunk, head, shoulders, or it may be limited to one or more specific sets of muscles. If the cerebral palsy involves the muscles employed in producing speech, speech will not be normal. Articulation may be disturbed because of the slow, weak, or uncoordinated action of the articulators. Various aspects of voice may be affected: pitch may be too high or low, markedly monotonous, or perhaps uncontrolled; rate will probably be slower than average; the voice may be louder than normal; impaired voice quality such as harshness or breathiness may appear; rhythm may be disturbed. Breathing may be shallow and exhalation may be poorly controlled, with consequent gasping, attempts to speak on residual air, and faulty phrasing and rhythm.

Associated with the motor disability implied by the term cerebral palsy there may be other problems, some of them concomitant results of the brain damage, others the result of the patient's reaction to his condition or to his treatment by others. Some of the physical and psychological problems of persons with cerebral palsy are these: convulsions, mental retardation, visual impairments, hearing loss (especially in persons with athetoid cerebral palsy), other impairments of sensation, strong fears and adjustment difficulties, perseveration, uninhibited responsiveness to stimuli, distractibility, and hyperactivity.

The great majority of cases of cerebral palsy fall into four main clinical types. These categories are somewhat arbitrary, since many cases represent mixed types.

1. Spastic cerebral palsy characterized by impairment of voluntary movement, increase in deep reflexes, increased muscle tone, resistance to manipulation, and an exaggerated stretch reflex (elicited when a muscle is suddenly stretched, with a consequent blocking of the movement because of the reflex contraction of the antagonistic muscle).
2. Athetosis, the essential characteristic of which is the presence of unpatterned, unrhythmical, involuntary wriggling and writhing movements overlaid on voluntary bodily movements and interfering with them.
3. Ataxia, characterized by incoordination, the individual being unable to control the magnitude, direction, and timing of voluntary movements.
4. Rigidity, characterized by a more continual and more pronounced degree of increased muscle tone than is found in spastic cerebral palsy.

SOME POINTS TO BE EMPHASIZED

1. Some speech-retarded children have been diagnosed as cerebral palsied before coming to the speech examination, In such cases, you should determine from parents or medical records the clinical type and the probable etiologic factors.
2. In undiagnosed cases of speech retardation with a suspected physical basis for the problem, you should obtain full details concerning past and present speech and physical symptoms, the birth and developmental history, and the medical history. Minimal cues picked up from a detailed history may prompt a referral for a neurologic examination,

which in turn may indicate whether a clear diagnosis of brain damage is warranted.

3. The social history should indicate how the speaker feels about himself and how he is treated by his family and associates. Scrutinize closely the speaker's semantic environment and his semantic reactions. Explore here particularly, as well as in the developmental history, for indications of what the family has done to develop independence in the patient and consider what this manner of treatment suggests concerning the family attitude toward the patient and his problem.

4. Most cerebral palsied persons have multiple handicaps; it is necessary, therefore, to determine the nature of the many obstacles that confront each such patient and his or her potential for overcoming them.

SUPPLEMENTARY QUESTIONS

History of Speech Problem

Describe the speech problem. If the patient is a child, when she wishes something, does she ask for it by using words or does she simply point? Can others understand what she means? Does the family make an effort to require her to speak when she wants something? In the opinion of the parents, did she begin to speak at the same age as the other children in the family? As the child grew older, did her speech improve, become worse, or remain the same? Does the child's speech become worse at certain times? Under what circumstances? Have the parents tried to help the child with her speech? Does she like to be read to? Can the parents hold her attention in reading, conversation, and game playing? Does she usually seem to understand what is being said to her? (If the patient is an older child or adult, these questions are to be modified accordingly.)

Developmental History

Pregnancy During pregnancy did the mother have any of the following: severe nausea and vomiting; toxemia; hypertension; any acute disease (especially virus infections such as German measles); anemia; bleeding, x-ray treatments in pelvic region; nutritional deficiency; metabolic disturbance? Did she take insulin, thyroid, drugs? Specify during what part of the pregnancy the above conditions, if any, occurred. Is there a parental Rh incompatibility?

Birth and Neonatal Period Duration of labor. Labor induced? Breech delivery? Cesarean section? Forceps used? Placenta previa? Was there a drop in maternal blood pressure during delivery? Was the mother given morphine or barbituates?

Concerning the baby, is there a report of jaundice; blueness; pallor;

weak cry; convulsions; twitchings; drowsiness; listlessness? Was the baby considered premature? Was there evidence of head trauma; kinking of umbilical cord; strangulation by cord; blockage of respiratory tract by mucus or fluid? Was blood transfusion necessary; administration of oxygen; incubator? Birth weight. (Birth weights of other children in family and of the parents themselves.)

Physical Growth and Development   At what age was the physical incapacity noticed? Was there a persistence of the tonic neck reflex? Was baby hypertonic? Was there excessive crying; trouble swallowing or sucking; vomiting; refusal to nurse? Was baby a feeding problem; a "colic" baby; a "tongue-pusher"? How were eating and drinking problems handled? Describe present diet. Appetite at first and now? Much drooling; when ended?

Was the baby a "back-archer"? Did she resist a slow pull upward from supine to sitting position? Was she able to hold head up when supine; when prone? Age of sitting; of standing? Age when rolled over? Age, manner, and disturbance of creeping or crawling?

Age when the child stood with support; stood alone; walked with support; walked alone? Did she fall much? Was she able to move easily from lying to sitting or standing? How is her sitting balance; kneeling balance, standing balance? Does she stand wide-based? Position of knees while standing (flexed, hyperextended)? Does she climb stairs? How? Does she walk on toes; have scissors gait? Does she have more trouble with hands or feet? How much time has been spent in teaching her to walk?

What is patient's handedness? At what age did child develop grasp and release? Can she turn pages; write with crayons or pencils; use scissors?

What degree of self-help has patient developed? Is she able to feed self; use spoon, fork, knife; wash; dress; button; tie shoelaces; brush teeth; go to bathroom unaided; comb hair? What articles can't she handle? If certain skills have not been developed, to what extent have opportunities been afforded her to develop them? How much time has been spent in teaching her self-help?

Medical History

Secure full details concerning each early serious illness; duration; high fever; diagnosis; known sequelae. Has speaker suffered any violence to head; possible skull fractures; convulsions? Give age at each, sequelae, and medication.

Has patient had any operations? Have braces ever been recommended or fitted? How successful were they? Are eyes involved? How? Impression of hearing. How has hearing been tested? Does patient startle easily?

Does he or she respond to loud noises; soft noises; loud voices; soft voices; whispering? Does the patient attempt to localize sounds?

Have tremors been noted; involuntary movements in tongue or extremities; rhythmical or unrhythmical involuntary movements; increased tone of muscles; muscle weakness; paralysis? Has speaker ever been described as spastic, athetoid, or ataxic? Has anyone suspected or diagnosed cerebral palsy?

Social History

What does the patient do during the course of the day? How much freedom does he have to choose his activities? If patient is a child does the mother consider him to be more trouble to her than the other children? Is the child more disobedient, dependent, quiet, withdrawn, irritable, impulsive, distractible, hyperactive? Does he have a shorter attention span?

How is the child punished when he misbehaves? Does he play with his siblings or other children very much? Does he get around the neighborhood alone or accompanied to meet other children? Do the parents take the child with them when they go to church or the movies or visiting friends? Does he enjoy going places and meeting people? Do other children ever make fun of him because of the way he speaks, walks, or acts? If so, how have the parents handled such incidents? Does the child seem motivated to improve in walking, self-help, speech? (If the patient is an older child or adult, these questions are to be modified accordingly.)

What do the parents think is wrong with the patient? If they have heard of cerebral palsy, what do they think causes it? What reading have they done on the subject? Do they feel that they are in any way responsible for the patient's problems? Do they seem to have guilt feelings about the condition? Are they ashamed of the child or of themselves? Are they oversolicitous; rejecting? What do they think will be the probable outcome of the problem? Are they optimistic; pessimistic?

Supplementary Case History Outline

APHASIA

Frederic L. Darley

GENERAL INFORMATION ABOUT THE DISORDER

Aphasia is a disorder of language function—a disturbance of the ability to recognize and use the symbols by means of which we relate to our surroundings and to other people. It is not the result of paralysis of the speech musculature nor of deafness or other sensory loss. It is a specific dysfunction in the recognition and expression of language symbols. It results from damage to the brain. The damage (whether the result of a hemorrhage, thrombosis, embolism, infection, tumor, bullet wound, concussion, or other cause) involves part of the so-called association areas of the brain, which constitute complex mechanisms by means of which sensory complexes are correlated, integrated, and resolved into motor complexes. The damage may result in a complete loss of language, but the more usual effect is a less than complete impairment of language function (sometimes designated dysphasia).

Aphasia is not only a disorder of language but may also involve one or more of a large number of nonlanguage effects, including physical and personality changes. No one statement can describe aphasia adequately; not only is each aphasic person different originally from every other, but the changes that result from brain injury are also numerous and assume a variety of patterns. However, in the following paragraphs we offer, for purposes of general orientation to the problem, an oversimplified description of some of the principal changes recognized in the language, personality, and physical behavior of persons who have become aphasic.

Language Disturbances

Sufficiently detailed questioning and testing will probably reveal that the language difficulty is both receptive and expressive in nature.

Aphasic persons cannot express themselves adequately. For example, a patient may wish to say, "I want a glass of water," and be unable to say "water"; she may substitute another word for "water"; or her sentence may be incomplete or incorrectly organized. This inability to express herself may be so severe that her speaking vocabulary is limited to a few automatic expressions or to a few meaningfully used words such as "yes" and "no." In some cases the person may be unable to produce voluntarily even the phonemes of the language (probable evidence of an associated apraxia of speech). Difficulty in expression will include disability in writing.

Aphasic persons have difficulty in understanding what is said to them. For example, if a patient is told to point to a pencil, he may point to some other object or in some way respond incorrectly. He is likely to manifest increasing difficulty in responding as the instructions increase in length and complexity. Difficulty in comprehension will extend to understanding written or printed language.

These are only a few examples of the ways in which language behavior may be affected. It should be remembered that aphasic patients typically have some degree of difficulty in all modalities of language and that these disabilities are present in varying degrees of severity in different persons.

Personality Changes

These changes may be extreme or comparatively mild. A person whose family would have described her formerly as generally complacent may come to exhibit extreme irritation and anger on slight provocation. On the other hand, a tense driving individual may become passive.

Since aphasic persons are less able to do certain things that they formerly could do with ease, they are likely to experience repeated frustration. For example, a patient may be unable to understand clearly what is said to her, to speak her name or the names of her family, to ask or answer questions, to name objects, to read the newspaper, or to write even her own name. It is not difficult to understand, therefore, why emotional outbursts may occur in aphasic individuals.

Some aphasic persons become depressed or anxious as a result of their condition. Tearfulness, discouragement, and worry are not uncommon reactions. Other patients, however, show an abnormal unconcern and even cheerfulness (euphoria). The patient's ability to concentrate attention on a particular task for a given period of time may also be reduced; memory may be poor; judgment, initiative, and organizing ability may be impaired; and the patient may become withdrawn, impulsive, or even infantile.

Physical Disturbances

There may be motor and sensory impairments associated with the aphasic difficulties. The person may be paralyzed, for example; if the paresis involves the speech and breathing musculature, the resulting speech disturbance is called dysarthria. Vision may be impaired. The patient is likely to tire easily. He may experience feelings of dizziness, fainting, severe headaches, and sudden losses of consciousness. He may be subject to convulsive seizures.

SOME POINTS TO BE EMPHASIZED

1. Prognosis in aphasia depends upon a number of physical and psychological factors. Therefore, in order to plan a program of therapy and estimate its probable success, you need a description of the patient's premorbid abilities and personality characteristics, together with an account of the changes noted in language, personality, and physical behavior.
2. An aphasic patient may be expected to progress faster in therapy if the clinician uses familiar materials related to his or her former occupation, interests, and hobbies and in line with his or her educational background. Therefore, it is desirable to obtain information about these matters.
3. The environmental aspects of the aphasic person's life are crucial. Progress may be determined by the reactions of the persons with whom he or she is in daily contact. Try to find out what the patient's associates know about his or her problems and what insights they have into them. Try to determine whether their everyday, moment-by-moment treatment of the patient is such as to facilitate or to hinder recovery. An aphasic person's semantic environment and semantic reactions deserve close scrutiny.
4. The term aphasia does not denote disturbed sensory or motor dysfunction, but associated incidentally with aphasia there may be either sensory or motor impairments or both. It is necessary to determine the nature of all the obstacles that confront each patient and his or her potential for overcoming them.
5. The term aphasia denotes specific language dysfunction which is disproportionate to impairment of other cognitive functions. It does not include those language changes which are seen in more comprehensive impairments of mentation, for example, dementia and confusion states. Try to discern whether the patient's problems are language-specific (therefore properly designated aphasia) or include impairment of calculation, recall of general information, long-term memory, orientation in space and time, and other nonlanguage functions.

SUPPLEMENTARY QUESTIONS

History of Language Disorder

What has been regarded as the cause of the patient's aphasic condition? When did the accident (operation, illness, etc.) occur? Obtain details of the subsequent course of events: initial symptoms or behavior, "spontaneous recovery," nature and rate of changes noted.

Secure information concerning the initial language behavior and the reactions to this behavior by members of the family and associates. Were these people eager to have him start talking? Did they talk to him or at him but without asking or expecting a response? Did they urge him to answer them? Did they show concern or impatience if he failed to answer adequately? How did they handle fragmentary and incorrect answers? Similarly describe current practices and expectations.

Has he had any remedial help? What kind? Results? Is language therapy currently available? Has medical clearance for it been given?

Expressive Aspects

Does the patient try to use words; sentences? When she wants something, does she ask for it in words (or try to ask) or does she just point? Does she use the right words? Does the family understand what she is saying or is she difficult to understand because she mixes up the words or misarticulates them? If she speaks in sentences, does she leave out the little words such as "if," "of," "the," and "and"? Can she recall the names of persons and things? Can she use nouns; verbs; adjectives; prepositions; conjunctions; articles? Is her speech halting or fluent?

Does she say greetings and farewells? How well can she repeat the alphabet; count; say the days of the week; swear? Does she remember parts of prayers or poems or scripture passages? Is she able to sing?

Does the family include her in their conversation or, as a rule, pay little attention to her? Does the family let her talk for herself or do they try to talk for her? (For example, when someone asks her a question, is she allowed to answer it as best she can or is the answer supplied for her?) Does the family try to help her by supplying words when she encounters difficulty in expressing herself? Does the family anticipate her needs and wishes or try to guess what she wants? (For example, at meals are dishes passed to her at her request or in anticipation of her request?) Do her associates correct her when she says the wrong word?

Does she begin conversations herself without first being addressed by someone else? Does she do as much talking now as she did before her accident (operation, illness, etc.)? How well is she able to write? What special disabilities in writing does she show?

Receptive Aspects

Can the patient follow simple requests and instructions (for example, "Turn on the radio") or does he seem not to understand what is said to him? Can he carry out more complicated instructions? Does he understand when someone tells him of some incident or of something in the paper? How does the informant know he understands?

How much does he read? What does he read? How well does he apparently grasp what he reads? How well does he grasp what he hears on radio and TV?

Does he know what the different table utensils are (for example, does he distinguish between a knife and a fork)? Can he recognize parts of the body; colors; forms? Can he make change?

Medical History

Who is the physician in charge of the case? Does the patient have any paralysis or weakness? What treatment is being used for the paralysis? With what results?

Has the patient had any operations? What? When? Has she ever had a plate inserted in her head? Does she ever complain of headaches? Severity? Frequency? Does she ever complain of faintness? Dizziness? Does she ever lose consciousness? Does she ever have convulsive seizures? What kind? What medication has been prescribed for them? Results of medication?

Does she seem unusually fatigable? How much sleep does she get daily? Does she spend most of her day resting or is she usually active? How much walking does she do? How is her appetite? Does she have any difficulty in eating; in dressing herself? Does she have a sense of direction? Does she distinguish between right and left? Does she know where she is? Does she know the day and the date?

Does she ever complain that she cannot see, hear, or feel things properly? Estimate her auditory and visual acuity.

School History

How far did the patient go in school? What kind of grades did she make in school? Has she ever studied any particular subject since she left school? Has she maintained an interest in intellectual pursuits?

Social History

What is or what was the patient's occupation? Did he like his work? Would he like to return to it? Does he expect to? Is he worried that he may not be able to? Are the members of his family worried that he may cease to be their breadwinner? Have they discussed this matter with him? Has he changed jobs often? What hobbies and other interests has he had outside of his job? Does he still show an interest in these? What did he formerly do for recreation? What clubs, fraternal organizations, or other groups did he belong to? How active has he been in them? How active is he now?

What kind of movies did he formerly like to go to? Does he go now? What did he formerly like to read in the newspaper? Does he read papers now? Did he and does he now like to read books and magazines or to be read to? Describe his radio- and TV-listening habits.

Did he formerly take a great deal of interest in his family—spend much time with them? Does he now take an interest in the family? (For example, if he has children or grandchildren, does he play with them quite often?)

Does he like card games? Which ones? How frequently does he play them now? Is he interested in his friends? Does he like to see them? How often does he see them? Has he indicated that he would like them to visit him? When there are visitors in the home, does he seem interested in them and what they are saying? Does he understand and laugh at jokes? Does he try to carry on conversations? How well does he succeed?

Has his personality changed? How? Describe his present personality. Does he ever lose his temper suddenly or become very angry or highly emotional? If so, does the informant know of any reasons why he should become as upset as he does? Does he become angry when members of the family try to help him with something? Is he depressed or anxious about his condition, or perhaps too cheerful and unconcerned about it? Has he ever indicated in any way that he desires to do something about his problem? Does he trust his ability and judgment?

When he has difficulty in doing something such as dressing himself, does the family help him or allow him to do it for himself and assist him only when he asks for help? Do they think it would be a good idea to allow him to do as many things as possible for himself? Are they oversolicitous?

Has anyone ever explained aphasia to the family? Have they read about it? How do the members of the family feel about the patient? Have they ever expressed opinions about his condition and his present characteristics? What opinions? Were they expressed in his presence? Do members of the family become angry or impatient with him or criticize him in any way? How do they act when he becomes angry or upset? Do they try to reason with him or scold him, or do they leave him alone and hope he will soon get over it? Do they or does he for any reason feel guilty about his condition or the causes of it? Do they seem to want to spend time with him and try to help him? Are they optimistic or pessimistic about the outcome?

Supplementary Case History Outline

POSTLARYNGECTOMY SPEECH PROBLEM

Frederic L. Darley
and D. C. Spriestersbach

GENERAL INFORMATION ABOUT THE PROBLEM

Total removal of the larynx is commonly resorted to in cases of cancer of the larynx. The problem occurs most often among persons over 50 years of age and more often in men than in women. In learning to speak without a larynx, a person must, of course, learn to speak in a manner somewhat different from that in which normal speech is produced. He can no longer use the air from the lungs to set the vocal folds into vibration. He may be taught to take air (most appropriately called an "air charge") into the esophagus and then to expel it in such a way that certain structures near the top of the esophagus at approximately the level of the cricoid cartilage are set into vibration. The sound produced is then articulated. Because of changes due to irradiation of the tissues of the neck, or the reactions of the patient to the use of the air charge, or his inability to control the air charge, it may be necessary for him to use an artificial larynx of some type. In such instances tone is produced by an electrically powered vibrator, reed or pneumatic, and the articulators are used in the normal way to produce phonemes.

SOME POINTS TO BE EMPHASIZED

1. Has medical clearance for the starting of speech therapy been given?
2. Determine how much information the patient has about his condition. Does he understand why it was necessary to have his larynx removed? Does he have some idea of how speech is produced? Does he realize that the vibrators that normally produce the sound necessary for speech have been removed? Does he know that it is

possible to produce speech even though the larynx has been removed? Was any information given to him about alternative methods of speech production before the operation? Has he talked to any other laryngectomized person?

3. Success in mastering a wholly new way of speaking depends to a considerable degree upon the patient's motivation and adjustment. Successful acquisition of skill in using esophageal speech requires much experimentation on the part of the patient. How willing is he to devote time and effort to experimenting in an effort to master a new skill? How likely is he to be discouraged by initial failure? Is he likely to be easily embarrassed while attempting to learn eso-phageal speech? Before his operation how talkative was he, how socially inclined, how extrovertive? Is he currently disturbed by insecurity regarding future employment or by fears of the recurrence of cancer? What information has he been given about his physical condition? Is he able to continue doing the same work that he was doing before the operation? Does he have other problems of read-justment?

4. Have his wife and other members of his family been counseled con-cerning the effects of his laryngectomy on his speech? Are they encouraging, impatient, overprotective, solicitous, matter-of-fact, embarrassed, optimistic, pessimistic? How has the patient's laryn-gectomy changed their relationship with him?

5. Does the patient have information about groups and agencies that will be interested in helping him, such as the local division of the American Cancer Society, or the International Association of Laryn-gectomees (219 E. 42nd Street, New York, New York 10017)? Does he know about IAL News, which will be mailed to him by the Asso-ciation upon request? Does he know about the existence of Lost Chord Clubs? Has he tried to find out if one exists in his locality?

3

GENERAL EVALUATION OF ORAL COMMUNICATION

D. C. Spriestersbach
and Hughlett L. Morris

It may seem trite to observe that first there are people and only secondarily people with problems—oral communication problems in the context of this book. And yet the point is frequently overlooked. So often, as professional speech pathologists and audiologists, we make initial contacts with clients whose communication problems have already been identified. Our task becomes that of studying the problem in enough depth to be able to plan a therapy program that will alleviate the problem. In our haste to get from here to there we may forget to observe the client as a speaker with many attributes, some most likely acceptable—possibly even superior—and one or two that are deviant enough to create barriers to effective communication. We need to view these attributes in perspective, whatever the presenting problem is. We include this chapter early in the appraisal section of this book to stress the importance of this total view.

The general examination of oral communication that we describe here (Form 1) has several uses. For instance, you may wish to use it as a screening device to identify those members of a school or class who have speech problems which need to be observed more extensively. Used in this way the examination will give you an indication of the gross clinical needs of groups of speakers and provides a basis for the important initial stages of program planning.

You may also want to use the examination with those persons referred to you with specific problems. As we have already indicated, you will want to place the problem in perspective with the other attributes of oral expression. Further, you will want to make some preliminary observations concerning any possible relationships that may exist between the several attributes, for example, pitch level and harshness. Finally, and perhaps the most important, you will want to evaluate the speaker's oral expression in the relatively unstructured speaking situation used for this examination. The way one typically speaks is, in the final analysis, the "proof of the pudding."

We have devised the General Speech Behavior Rating form (Form 1) for use in summarizing your observations, which, incidentally, you may wish to make again for comparative purposes following a period of remedial work. It should be noted that the set of ratings involved is designed for speakers who have developed some proficiency in the use of language. While no minimal age limits have been established, it is unlikely that it would be used with speakers below the age level of first grade. The rest of this chapter deals with the administration of the test and the completion of the rating form.

OBTAIN A SPEECH SAMPLE

a. If the speaker is old enough to read, observe him while he reads aloud some nonemotional prose. Also observe his extemporaneous and conversational speaking. You are interested in describing his typical speaking behavior rather than his ability to read aloud per se.
b. If the speaker is a nonreader, elicit a speech sample by having him talk about some pictures, tell what he did yesterday, or talk about the TV programs he enjoys watching.
c. If it suits your purpose, you may, of course, use the procedures described in Chapter 4 for obtaining samples of speech.

RECORD YOUR OBSERVATIONS AND EVALUATIONS

a. Remember that you are making a record not only for your own future reference, but also for other interested individuals who will not have heard the speaker. Your observations and impressions must therefore be recorded clearly and fully enough to be meaningful and useful to others.
b. Rate the speaker on each of the eight attributes identified on the form. Circle one of the numbers for each attribute using the following definitions of the four categories:
1. Adequate, within the normal range.
2. A deviation which does not make for a communicative handicap.
3. A deviation which occasions a moderate communicative handicap that should be given clinical attention.
4. A deviation which results in a serious communicative handicap that requires immediate clinical attention.
Keep in mind as you make the ratings that you are basing your judgments on your estimate of the reaction of the average listener to the speaker's oral expression.
Rate each stutterer twice, once on the basis of typical speech

behavior including stuttering, and once on the basis of fluent or nearly fluent speech. In the first instance place the letter S over your ratings and in the second instance place the letters NS over your ratings. The two ratings of the stutterer are required if you are to observe not only the nature of speech behavior while stuttering, but also the nature of the speech behavior when the speaker does not stutter. If the speaker stutters sufficiently to make it difficult to obtain an adequate sample of nonstuttered speech, you may instruct him or her to read in chorus with you or, preferably, with a third person. The speaker will be able to do this with little or no stuttering. The use of chorus reading may distort, of course, certain aspects of speech behavior. However, under this condition you should be able to make a reasonably valid assessment of voice quality, articulation, and those aspects of pitch and loudness not influenced by the speech pattern employed.

You may choose to rate the speaker by tentatively judging each of the attributes separately as you go along or to complete the ratings when you have finished observing the complete speech sample. If you find it difficult to categorize the articulation errors as you go along, you may wish to make marginal notes of observed articulation errors and categorize them at the end of the period of observation.

c. Substantiate your overall ratings of the various attributes by checking the appropriate items listed below the main headings. Refer to the appropriate chapters of this book for discussions of attributes and items listed on the form that you do not understand. In particular see Chapter 9 for definition of the terms listed under *Fluency* and Chapter 4 for background information useful in making the judgments called for under *Language*. Whenever you rate an individual above 1 on any attribute, you should check at least one of the listed items, or after the word *Other* write in one or more things that were observed but not listed on the form. The point is that if you feel that a speaker is deviant in some respect, you must have a reason. To rate a speaker 3 or 4 on an attribute without providing substantiating information is to cast doubt on the validity of your rating.

Listed under the attributes are such wordings as "too high," "too low," "too weak," "too loud." These terms are used in evaluating the usual or modal performance of the speaker. Thus, if you rate a male speaker's pitch as "too high," you are saying that in your judgment his usual pitch level is inappropriate for his sex and age and the speaking occasion and is likely, therefore, to interfere with his general effectiveness as a speaker.

d. In rating the *General Adequacy* of a speaker, represent the overall impression which he or she makes on you. This rating is not an average of the ratings you have given the various attributes. In this instance the meaning of each of the numbers on the scale will depend upon the use you propose to make of the results, and therefore each number must be defined in terms of the practical decisions to be made on the basis of your findings. For example, a rating of 4 might signify that you recommend intensive clinical instruction for the individual, and 3 might mean that the individual is recommended for assignment to a class or section in which attention will be given to the correction of the deviation but in which intensive remedial work will not be provided. The meanings of the various numbers in this rating scale will be determined, therefore, by the nature of the instructional and clinical programs to be provided, and these will vary from one situation to another.

e. Use the *Remarks* section to note any assets of the speaker which may be profitably exploited in trying to bring about improvement; diagram any pattern of speaking, such as rising inflections, that you observe; describe affectations and facial or bodily mannerisms; specify any regional or foreign dialect observed; describe the circumstances under which a voice quality deviation or any other fault is particularly noticeable or diminished; indicate whether the speaker appears to be a stutterer, have a cleft palate, or have some other notable condition of clinical significance; suggest further particular tests that you feel are needed.

f. Indicate possible relationships among the deviations you have observed. For example, if you have noted a jerky rate and you feel it is due to part-word repetitions, draw an arrow between those two items to show the suspected relationship. Or if there is breathiness that seems to be associated with a low loudness level, use an arrow to relate these two variables.

g. Finally, remember that this set of ratings is frequently done to summarize momentary impressions that may be based upon inadequate observations. Obviously, then, the ratings may and often should be changed as you observe the speaker more systematically in additional and varied speaking situations. As a first careful approach to an understanding of an individual's problems, however, this rating procedure will provide you with valuable cues for diagnosis and important leads for the first stages of remedial work.

ASSIGNMENTS

1. Complete the General Speech Behavior Rating, Form 1, for ten female and ten male adult speakers, at least five of whom have speech deviations.

2. Complete the General Speech Behavior Rating, Form 1, for yourself, serving as your own listener and making use of a mirror and a tape recorder. Ask a classmate or a friend to rate you also, and compare your ratings with those of the other observer.

FORM 1
General Speech Behavior Rating

Name _____   Age _____ Sex _____
Examiner _____   Date _____

Pitch: 1 2 3 4

_____ Too high
_____ Too low
_____ Pitch pattern
_____ Monotonous
_____ Pitch breaks
_____ Other

Loudness: 1 2 3 4

_____ Too loud
_____ Too soft
_____ Monotonous
_____ Loudness pattern
_____ Other

Rate: 1 2 3 4

_____ Too rapid
_____ Too slow
_____ Rate pattern
_____ Monotonous
_____ Jerkiness
_____ Other

Voice Quality: 1 2 3 4

Laryngeal Function:
_____ Breathiness
_____ Harshness
_____ Hoarseness
_____ Glottal attack
_____ Other
Resonance:
_____ Hypernasality
_____ Hyponasality

Articulation: 1 2 3 4

_____ General misarticulations
_____ Plosives misarticulated
_____ Fricatives misarticulated
_____ Semivowels misarticulated
_____ Nasals misarticulated
_____ Glides misarticulated
_____ Vowels misarticulated
_____ Diphthongs misarticulated
_____ Substitutions
_____ Distortions
_____ Omissions
_____ Voicing errors
_____ Nasalization errors
_____ Other

Language: 1 2 3 4

_____ No response to examiner
_____ Brief responses
_____ Responses grammatically incomplete
_____ Responses slow
_____ Responses irrelevant
_____ Lack of spontaneity in verbalization
_____ Limited vocabulary
_____ Incorrect use of case of pronouns
_____ Incorrect use of verb tense
_____ Responses vague or ambiguous
_____ Responses seemingly invalid, inconsistent, implausible, bizarre, incoherent
_____ Excessive verbal output
_____ Glib use of platitudes and clichés

Fluency: 1   2   3   4

_____ Interjection of sounds, sylla-
bles, words, or phrases
_____ Part-word repetitions
_____ Word repetitions
_____ Phrase repetitions
_____ Revisions
_____ Incomplete phrases
_____ Broken words
_____ Prolonged sounds
_____ Unvocalized intervals
_____ Other

Reaction to Self and Situation:
1   2   3   4

_____ Apparent tension and strain
_____ Visual evasiveness
_____ Distracting postures
_____ Distracting bodily move-
ments
_____ Apparent uneasiness or em-
barrassment
_____ Distracting laughter or
giggling
_____ Blandness
_____ Other

General Adequacy: 1   2   3   4

Remarks:

4

APPRAISAL OF CHILD LANGUAGE ACQUISITION

Margaret C. Byrne

Everyone has a language. Some people have more than one. Since we all have at least one language, you might think that we would have no difficulty in defining what it is and how we got it. However, the task isn't easy. At present we can describe language and its acquisition, but we can only speculate on how we have acquired it.

There are many theories about how a child acquires a language. McNeill (44) has hypothesized that language develops as a result of an interaction between a child's linguistic experiences and his or her innate linguistic capacities. He says that a child learns to relate the words he or she hears and uses to their meanings. Brown (10) points out that the child hears many language samples and he must induce from what he hears a grammar or a set of rules that he then applies to his own speech. Braine (7) postulates that a child learns and puts into his linguistic structure a relationship between defined entities, such as *big red* and *house,* and their correct slots in a grammar. Schlesinger (57) maintains that meanings come first, followed by acquisition of grammar. He stresses the relationship of cognitive ability to the learning of language. According to Staats (62) language is a form of behavior and is therefore learned within a stimulus-response-reward paradigm.

One of the most provocative studies that can be interpreted to support either the concept of innateness of language acquisition or a learning theory is one that analyzes the movements of newborns (ages 12 hours to 14 days) when an adult talks to them. In a study by Condon and Sander (18) microanalysis of sound films of babies' movements indicated that specific configurations of movements were elicited by the speech of adults, whether live or on tape. There were fewer sequential patterns, however, when disconnected vowels and tapping sounds were presented to them. When the child was already in motion, he made specific movements that seemed to be synchronized with the adult speech. Since the speech was organized and the movements of the babies were also organized, the authors concluded that patterning for the rhythm of language starts at the beginning of life. As a result of these motor patterns and their development in relationship to the organized speech of those in his environment, the infant participates developmentally in millions of repetitions of speech patterns long before he uses them in speaking.

Whichever theory we choose as our tentative frame of reference will determine to some extent how we assess a child's language acquisition and how we evaluate his or her linguistic skills.

In this chapter we shall define language as an organized system of symbols that has meaning and is used for inter- and intrapersonal communication. Oral language, which is our main concern, develops within an environment that encourages a child to experiment with words to express wishes and ideas. When a child learns a language, he learns a set of lexical items—a vocabulary. Each word or word group has a semantic, a phonological, and a grammatical representation. The child's first words may be imperfect representations at any of these levels, but we expect him to modify his utterances as he matures.

A description of a language is called a grammar, a set of principles that tells us about its structure. There are grammatical rules which govern the class structure of the vocabulary, phrase structure, transformations, and inflections. As the child develops his language, we observe his application of these rules. We might conceptualize the grammar as the vehicle which enables us to arrange words in an orderly fashion to convey an idea.

LANGUAGE ACQUISITION

Much of what we have learned about normal language acquisition has come from studies of children in their natural environments. Many linguists say that this is the way to learn how a child develops and processes language. Some linguists and speech-language pathologists have gone a different route. Some gather limited language samples and analyze them for specific grammatical and lexical features. Others have constructed tests or tasks to measure selected linguistic features. Many of us depend on parent recall of how the child's language has developed. In this section we will use information from all of these approaches.

The Environment

Since language is acquired, we will consider first the nature of the linguistic environment in which a child is listening and learning. A mother or a mother-substitute is talking to the baby from the first days of life. Listen to a mother as she leans over the baby's crib and talks to her child. She is asking him questions for which she doesn't expect any verbal response, such as, *Are you hungry, honey? Are you mommy's big boy? Have you lost your bottle? I'll get it for you.* The child responds with smiles, gurgling, different intonations of vowel and consonant sounds and combinations. Mother says: *He understands me.* She continues to talk to the child, to ask him to perform tasks; eventually she gives meaning to the child's early utterances.

The role of the mother or mother-substitute in the child's language acquisition is extremely important. She supplies the child's words for names of things and actions. The name she gives to an object is short and is the one most frequently used in her environment. The animal is called a *dog* or *cat*, not a *four-legged creature.*

Not only is the mother the model for the child's early vocabulary, but she may also be responsible later for the frequency with which the child uses sentence types. When Brown and his students (*10*) classified the sentences spoken by three mothers to their young children, they found a high percentage of simple affirmative active declarative sentences. An example would be: *It's time for your nap, Bobby.* The child also uses this type of sentence most often in preschool years. Of course, it could also be that this is the type we use a great deal, regardless of whether or not we're talking to young children. Brown also noted that mothers ask young babies a great many questions, but the child's early utterances are not in the form of questions.

In the early acquisition stage the meaning of the words must be obvious to the child. Most adults will match what they are identifying to what the child can see, hear, or feel. Parents are redundant, and the words they use are put together in short, meaningful sentences. Usually these utterances are syntactically correct, but not always.

One way of organizing the types of language interactions between the mother and child is to fit them into a set of processes. In Table 4.1 the processes are identified and examples of each have been included.

Observations suggest that adults use antecedent modelling a great deal as a method of initiating discussion and providing information to the child during their mutual talking time. When the child's remark is not grammatically correct, the mother may use expansion alone or with consequential modelling to correct the grammar and at the same time supplement the child's knowledge of a topic. The following exchange between a mother and her 3-year-old son illustrates how these two processes of modelling and expansion intertwine.

1. *Mother:* Why don't you find the new book grandma brought you for your birthday?
   Son: I going to get it now.

TABLE 4.1
Adult Processes in Child Language Acquisition

I. *Modelling:* Adult engages in conversation with the child.

  Antecedent: The adult initiates a conversation with the child.

  Example: I'm going to make some cookies. Do you want to help me?

  Consequential: The adult comments on what the child has said, without correcting or repeating the child's statement.

  Examples

Child	Adult
The dog bite me	He's really playing with you.
Stove hot	Be careful. The cookies are baking in the oven.

II. *Expansion:* The adult corrects the child's grammar.

The dog bite me	The dog bites you.
Stove hot	The stove is hot.

III. *Echoing:* An "echo" begins with an utterance from the child that is partially unintelligible. The adult echoes the child's comments but replaces the unintelligible part with a Wh-word (what, when, where, who).

I ate the _____	You ate the what?
The ball is _____	The ball is where?

---

  2. *Mother:* You're going to get it. It has a picture of the new space ship on the cover.
  Son: Here it is. That my space ship.
  3. *Mother:* When you get big, maybe you'll have one, but at least you can ride in one.
  Son: This mine.
  4. *Mother:* The book is yours, but you don't have a real space ship yet.

In this exchange the mother's first comment is an example of antecedent modelling. Her second is a combination of expansion (correcting his grammar) plus consequential modelling. The third and fourth are consequential modelling, including a clarification of his semantic error about ownership of the spacecraft.

Echoing or prompting is a device we use when we have understood a part of the child's statement but not all of it. When Susan says: *It's my turn to (unintelligible words)*, the adult may inquire: *It's your turn to what?* She is able to attend to the answer to *what* when the child makes her second attempt, and Susan has to concentrate on intelligibility for only one word or a phrase.

Imitation is one of the child's major devices in the early stages of language learning. The term refers to a process whereby a behavior is acquired by copying the behavior of a model. When the model identifies the family's animal as a *dog*, the child may say *da*. The model says: *No, it's a dog*. The child imitates again, and the model accepts his production whether or not it is an exact replication of hers. Additional factors, many of them still unidentified, are now influencing his learning. Eventually the child uses the word *dog* spontaneously when the dog is in view, and the model understands his use of the term. Later the child uses the word *dog* when the object isn't around, but the model associates the word to the correct referent. Finally the child achieves adult pronunciation of the word and uses it appropriately in the presence or absence of the original or similar stimuli. All of these stages may occur within a few minutes or a few days depending upon the child's ability to process and recall the correct representation, and whether he has opportunities to use it.

Several characteristics of the model's speech will influence the exactness of the child's imitation. One of these is the type of word used. When Scholes (58) repeated a series of sentences to preschool children (3 to 4½ years old) without any stress pattern, he found that they retained the content words (nouns, pronouns, verbs, adjectives, and adverbs). They dropped the function words (articles, prepositions, conjunctions). If the words name or describe things or designate actions, the child is more likely to imitate them when he echoes back a sentence. Others (6) have suggested that children 28 to 39 months of age attend to and imitate the most stressed and the final items in an utterance. Length of the sentence or phrase also determines what the child imitates. For the most part the young child does not imitate exactly what the model has said.

Vocabulary

A vocabulary is one essential feature of language. Most children are using a few single-word utterances between 12 and 18 months. Many parents have reported that their children have used combinations of sounds or syllables that represent words as early as 6 months of age. When Darley and Winitz (20) reviewed studies completed up to 1961, they found that the investigators had used a variety of definitions of *first word* and many different procedures in collecting data. Mead (45), for instance, defined the first word as one that associated an idea with an object. Denhoff and Holden's criterion was the time at which a child *said* single words (21). Other investigators did not specify how they defined the first word. Data were gathered primarily in one of four ways:

1. An interview procedure primarily with mothers.
2. Examination of records and files in doctors' offices.
3. Written reports of mothers.
4. Actual examination of children as they interacted with adults.

As a result of the diversity of definitions, procedures for data collection, and the types of children studied, the mean and median for ages of first words varied considerably. The range in this report was 9.8 months (the median for children living near a university [60]) to more than 60 months in a population studied by Abt, Adler, and Bartelme (1). The latter were children with I.Q.'s below 70 and included a sample of children with tumors on the tongue, deafness, and cleft palate. Darley and Winitz consider the age range for first words for most normal children to be between 12 and 18 months.

Any operational definition we select for identifying first words will have some weaknesses. However, when we depend on parental reporting for our information, we might incorporate in our definition two principles that Darley and Winitz discussed. These are: (1) sound, syllable, or "word" is consistently used in reference to an object or situation; and (2) the structure or form of the word resembles the adult form. That description of a word has several pitfalls. For instance, the *word* should be used in reference to the same object or situation 90 to 100 percent of the times the child uses it. Yet we can't be sure that parents have that idea in mind when they record the *words* in the child's baby book. The other problem is the degree of approximation to the adult pronunciation that we should accept as a first word. Can it be a syllable like *wa* for water or *da* for doll? We often accept *mum* for *mommy* or *mother*. In any event, be aware of these problems when you read the report of the parents about their child's age when he spoke his first words.

The child's original pool of vocabulary items consists of basic elements—the contentives. Contentives are words that fit into the grammatical categories of nouns and pronouns, verbs, adjectives, and adverbs. Children use them probably because of their immediate high semantic value. However, a word as used by the child may be conveying a great deal more meaning than we attribute to it when we merely classify it as a noun or a verb. Bobby's word *water* may have multiple meanings, such as *Give me a drink, I want more water*, or *I spilled the water*. We can interpret its meaning only when we know the situation in which he uttered the word. Even then we can't be sure sometimes.

Most of these early utterances are linked to actions and usually express the child's emotional state. The child says the word *car* as she opens its door; her vocal intonation and facial expression as she says it connote her pleasure and excitement. She may repeat *car, car* with the same inflections as she jumps up and down on the front seat or leans out the window.

Within a few weeks or months the child is adding a second kind of word to his or her list—functors. The functors are all the grammatical categories except the contentives and include articles (the, a), prepositions (to, in), and conjunctions (but, and). These are also the categories children leave out when they imitate a model's sentence or when they are trying to tell us something.

TABLE 4.2
Grammatical Category of Words Appearing 100 or More Times in Anthony's Samples

Category	Words and Frequency
Nouns and pronouns	Bobo (132) blanket (125) it (103)
Verbs	is (167) go (90)* jump (31) get (20)
Adjective	that (121)
Article	the (394)
Conjunction	and (105)

Source: Compiled from the lists in the Appendix of Weir, 67.

* These were included because of their designations of actions even though they did not occur 100 times.

There are some published lists of both words and phrases used by individual children. These are gleaned from the transcriptions of language samples and should be evaluated in light of the information we have about such samples. Both the situation and the stimuli available contribute to what the child says and does. When Anthony (67) talked to himself and to his Bobo before he fell asleep, he used some words that appear on the "most frequent" lists of adults as well as some indigenous to his play activity in his crib. They are given in Table 4.2.

Another way of referring to these words of Anthony's is to call them *morphemes*. A *morpheme* is the smallest unit of a language that has meaning and is grammatically pertinent. All of the words in Table 4.2 are morphemes. There are two classes of morphemes: (1) roots or free morphs and (2) inflections. The word *jump* in Table 4.2 is a free morph; we can't reduce it any further and have a meaningful unit. However, we can expand it by adding an inflection—an ending /t/—and transform that free morph to *jumped,* which now has two morphemes. Since we will be referring to morphemes and to the mean morpheme length of utterances, it will be helpful for you to know these terms.

Menyuk's (50) analysis of the vocabulary of children 2½ to 3 years old revealed that they were using a form of the verb *to be* plus a predicate, prepositional phrases of location such as *in the box,* the first and second person pronouns *I* and *you,* the article *the,* and locations *here* and *there.* At age 3 years the following words were appearing: *maybe, will,* and *can.*

Class Structures of the Vocabulary

When a child has acquired a few contentives and functors, he is usually entering the two- or three-word utterance step of language acquisition.

More than a thousand such combinations can appear in a six-month period. Analysis of many of these first phrases has shown that for some children the words can be categorized in two classes: pivot and open (*11*). The pivot class consists of key words that occur frequently in the child's speech in juxtaposition to many different words. The open class includes a wide variety of words that either go with a pivot or may be combined with another from the open class. A child who says *Here the book, Here the car, Here mommy, Here shoe, Here baby* has selected from his repertoire the word *here* as a pivot to be combined with words in the open category. In this instance they are different names of things. At another time he might choose another pivot: *Get car, Go car, Dump car* with the word *car* as his pivot, *get, go,* and *dump* being from the open category.

Brown (*10*) has gone a step beyond classifying the parts of these early combinations as pivot and open classes. He interprets each utterance in terms of its structured meaning. Using the utterance and cues from the environment in which the child said the phrase, Brown identified four types of pivots which cover most of them:

1. Nominations: that + car, dog, bottle
2. Notice: hi + daddy, baby, mommy
3. Recurrence: more + more, water, grandma
4. Nonexistence: no + car, milk, cereal

In later reports Brown has replaced the *Notice* category with two others, each of which is quite specific. They are *Self-references,* like *me* or *I* or a name; and *Mother reference,* like *Mommy.* These classifications are useful in that they tell us what types of semantic relationships the child is expressing in these pivot-open two-word arrangements.

Many two-word utterances can be classed as open-open types or as expressions of semantic functions or relations. Many of these expand in later stages of development into noun phrases, verb phrases, and sentences. The most prevalent semantic relations expressed in the two-word utterances of a group of 12 children were identified by Brown (*11*). He reported that 70 percent of all utterances fell into the following categories:

Agent-action	daddy go
Action-object	drink milk
Agent-object	daddy lunch
Action-locative	go school
Entity-locative	daddy home
Possessor-possession	mommy's coat
Entity-attribute	big book
Demonstrative-entity	that dress

The early utterances are related to what the child is doing now or are observations about herself or her surroundings. When she says *all gone sticky* while washing her hands, or *hot burns* after she touches the warm stove, we know what she means. Even though she hasn't heard these particular combinations, she is putting together meaningful and appropriate words from her own vocabulary to tell us something. A further analysis of early phrases shows that she is following the word order of the sentences she has heard.

Grammar

Phrase Structure Grammar   Once the child is using utterances involving two or more words, it is possible to look at the arrangement of the words in another way. We are now dealing with embryonic sentences, which are series of words arranged in a specific order. The term *phrase structure grammar* has been used by linguists to identify two groupings of words in sentences—noun phrases and verb phrases. Although we see the rudiments of both even in the two-morpheme utterances cited above, children soon are expanding both parts of the elementary sentence. The above example of an attribute, *Big book*, becomes *The big book has pictures*, a simple affirmative declarative sentence. Using that sentence we can identify its parts in the following manner:

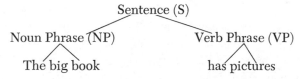

We use the symbols S = NP + VP, with S for sentence, NP for noun phrase, and VP for verb phrase for convenience in plotting the relationship of the two structures to a sentence.

Menyuk (49) found that nursery children 3 to 4½ years of age were all using the phrase structure level of grammar for simple active declarative sentences correctly as well as in many other types of sentences. During this period there are inconsistencies: the child may leave out a part of the noun or verb phrase, misuse the forms of the verb or noun, and show redundancies.

Inflections   Inflections are affixes, that is, units added to a word or a morph to change its number, tense, or degree. Adding /t/ to *cook* changes the verb from present to past tense but does not change the grammatical class of the word *cook*. Inflections begin to appear on nouns, verbs, possessives, and adjectives at the time when children are putting two words together in a phrase, usually about 18 to 24 months of age. By age 6 the majority of children have acquired all of the inflections, but they are not necessarily using them correctly in all utterances. The rules that govern these inflections are applied correctly at first, but as the vocabulary increases and the child figures out more of the rules, he tends to overgeneralize in his application of them. For instance, plurals appear early in the speech of children. They may pluralize the nouns such as *dresses* and *coats* correctly but also pluralize *foot* by adding /s/ to make *foots*.

In general we can expect that children will be using the inflections in the following order within the noun, verb, and adjectival categories:

1. Inflections on nouns
   a. Possessive (boy's, boys')
   b. Plural of regular nouns (cars, dresses)
   c. Plural of irregular nouns (feet, children)
2. Inflections on verbs
   a. Present progressive
      (1) He going
      (2) He's going
   b. Future (will go, will see)
   c. Past
      (1) Regular verbs (jumped, pushed)
      (2) Irregular verbs (ate, gave)
3. Comparative and superlative inflections on the adjective
   a. Comparative (bigger, taller)
   b. Superlative (biggest, tallest)

Mastery of all of them will be occurring simultaneously in the speech of some children. Sarah, one of the children about whom Cazden (*16*) reports, was using all of these except adjectival inflections by the age of 4, and at that time her Mean Length of Utterance of morphemes (MLU) was only 3.50.

Overgeneralization is not uniform in the use of these inflections. Slobin (*61*) found that it occurred one out of five times on the past tense of irregular verbs where there was a vowel change, as in the pair *take–took*. Children said *taked*. It occurred only once in 20 times when there was a vowel change plus /d/ or /t/, as in *bring–brought*. In the latter instance the children tended to use the correct form, *brought*.

Transformations   Just as there is an order in the development of phrase structure and inflections, so there is order in the appearance of transformations. Transformations make it possible to change and add to the word orders so that we can express negation, interrogation, and other grammatical classes. Even though a simple affirmative declarative sentence is the type we use most frequently, it isn't sufficient to express or explain all of our linguistic needs. Children begin to use the simple transformations when they are about 2 years of age, or when they have an MLU of 2.0.

Many children will be 10 or 12 years old before they are using all of the transformations we associate with adult language. Some aren't interpreted correctly when the sentence is ambiguous. However, the following are among the first to appear in the child's grammatical structures:

Transformation	Example
Negation	I am not.
Question	Who is it?
Contraction	That's my hat.
Got	He's got my hat.
Verb auxiliary, *be*	She is kicking my dog.
Do	I do want it.
Possessive	It is Susan's turn.
Pronoun	He has it.
Adjective	It is a blue dress.
Infinitive complement	She wants to read.
Nominal compound	The baby book is here.

The child may start out asking a question *What you buy me* with a rising vocal intonation, instead of *What did you buy me?* He may get negation in his sentence by adding a *no* somewhere or by shaking his head. However, by the time a child is 5 years old he is using all of the above transformations.

When children enter kindergarten, they seem not only to have learned the major types of syntactic structures but to be using them in longer and longer units. Loban (*41*), and O'Donnell, Griffin, and Norris (*55*) were interested in describing the types of subject-verb-object relationships noted in the language samples of school children and also in finding a more accurate method of describing the length of the utterances. O'Donnell et al. devised the T-unit, a minimal terminal syntactic unit, to measure length. It is one main clause plus any subordinate clauses attached to it or embedded in it. He found that T-length increased as the children got older (Figure 4.1). We will be analyzing some utterances using this procedure later in the chapter.

A composite list of the types of syntactic structures that they identified is given in Table 4.3, with a simple example of each. O'Donnell et al. reported that Types 1 and 2 accounted for 80 to 85 percent of all the T-units in their samples. Lohan, who obtained samples from children in kindergarten through twelfth grade, reported that all of these types were present in the speech of some children at each grade level, but not all of them were used by all of the children.

We are all aware of the wordiness which clutters our talking. O'Donnell et al. used the word *garbles* to describe these frequent unnecessary fragments. An example would be: *When I was going home, and have to, I*

FIGURE 4.1
Word length of T-units by grades. (From R. D. O'Donnell et al., *Syntax of Kindergarten and Elementary School Children: A Transformational Analysis.* Research Report No. 8. NCTE Committee on Research, 1967.)

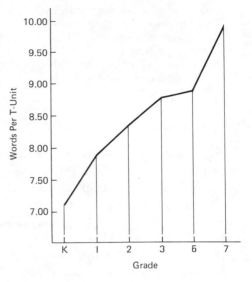

TABLE 4.3
Types of Syntactic Structures Used by Children in Kindergarten Through High School

Types	Examples
1. Subject-verb	John went.
2. Subject-verb-object	John jumps rope.
3. Subject-verb-predicate nominal	John is a big boy.
4. Subject-verb-predicate adjectival	John is big.
5. Subject-verb-indirect object-direct object	John gave Mary his book.
6. Subject-verb-object-object complement	He considers Mary his friend.
7. Subject-verb-object-object adjectival	He considers Mary pretty.
8. Expletive-verb-subject	Here comes John.
9. Any question	What is that?
10. Use of passive voice	John was given a book.
11. Commands or requests	Give it to me.
12. Partials	Any incomplete unit.

Source: From O'Donnell et al. 55.

saw John on his bike. The phrase *and have to* is the garble. Garbles decrease as children move from kindergarten through twelfth grade. Children whom teachers and tests classify as high in language competence display fewer garbles (42).

Loban (42) summarized his analyses of the language of school-age children and adolescents in the following paragraph:

The difference between effective and non-effective users of language does not appear in their control of the grammatical sentence patterns, for all pupils know these before they enter school. Not grammatical sentence pattern but what is done to achieve greater flexibility and modification of ideas within these patterns proves to be the real measure of proficiency with language.

Comprehension

Children hear and comprehend much spoken language before they make their first attempts to talk. You can ask a child to bring you a book and she will do it even though she doesn't use the words herself. Children understand morphologic, syntactic, and semantic forms before they use them orally. They have the basic concepts of these forms by the time they are 5 or 6 years old.

Observations and analyses of the specific decoding skills of children have been limited. There are a few tests of comprehension which we will examine in the section on tests. Other work deals with the influence of ambiguities on the understanding of sentences and the age at which the refinements and intricacies of grammar are apparent. When syntax gets enmeshed with semantics, it takes a lifetime to comprehend all of the possible combinations.

From the information available to date we can say that children do not comprehend one category of form classes before another, but they are understanding many items from several simultaneously. Carrow (12) has hypothesized that comprehension is probably dependent upon several variables. One of these is the frequency with which the linguistic items are used in the environment. Another is the concreteness of the referent for a word. A third is that the earliest items to be learned are those that are not marked. Unmarked words are those without inflections. We referred to these earlier in the chapter as free morphs. For instance, the word *baby* is used frequently in the home; the referent is a child who can be seen and heard; and the noun is not marked. The words and phrases with these characteristics are among the first that children understand.

Chomsky (17) gave a task to school children that probed their understanding of the syntactic structure of the sentence, *The doll is easy to see.* She placed a blindfolded doll in front of the child and asked: *Is the doll easy to see or hard to see?* If the child answered: *The doll is hard to see,* she asked why. A typical reply was *Because you have a blindfold over her eyes.* Only one in four children at age 5 years and three out of four at age 7 gave the correct answer. Evidently they could not use the necessary transformation to come up with a syntactic order that would help them to understand the sentence. By age 9 years all of them "understood."

The work of Kessel (34) shows that children's understanding is influenced by the particular structuring of sentences. He found that children are 7 or 8 years old before they are able to assign the complement subject correctly to sentences such as *John asked Bill what to do* and *John told Bill what to do*. By age 7 they have acquired the syntactic distinction between *John is easy to please* and *John is eager to please*.

Kessel also found that children don't recognize ambiguities in sentences until they are about 12 years of age. He asked them to point to the correct picture for an ambiguous sentence and then to explain why they chose that picture. All the sentences could be interpreted in two ways, depending upon how they were said. It might be presumed that the child who detected the different meanings could explain why. Actually, Kessel found that only the fifth graders succeeded. Sentences like *They fed her dog biscuits* and *He told her baby stories* were more likely to be identified correctly when the readings stressed *dog biscuits* and *baby stories* as noun phrases with a modifier and a noun, rather than identifying *dog* and *baby* as indirect objects. Kessel suggests that the degree of abstraction of a sentence's meaning is an important variable contributing to the child's understanding of it. He found that children comprehended ambiguities when they could perceive relationships that are not tied to the here and now, the concrete externals, and this ability is emerging at about 12 years of age.

Summary

There are some basic principles that summarize what we know at present about language development. First, children are attaching words they have heard in their environment to objects or situations. Someone has given meaning to those words, many of which have been embedded in sentences. Second, children presumably hear the adult sentences but express themselves in a form that is at first brief but not simple. Third, in those first utterances they have shown semantic relationships of possession, negation, location, attributes, agent-action, agent-action-object, and many others without the formal inflections they will use later on. Fourth, these complex grammatical relationships are learned and interpreted in an environment, usually with the parents and siblings providing the original and continuing models. Fifth, the speed of acquisition is phenomenal. Most children move from a meaningful utterance of one word at 12 to 18 months to oral competence in the basic syntactic and inflection forms by 6 years of age. Their understanding of language units surpasses their use, and their vocabulary has been estimated at several thousand words at the receptive level and a minimum of two or three thousand at the expressive level at the time they enter kindergarten. Sixth, further refinements in comprehension and use of linguistic structures and their semantic interpretations will continue throughout their lives.

LANGUAGE DEFICITS

Our ability to predict how fast a child will master our language is almost nil because we have so few longitudinal studies for guidelines. Sharf (59) followed a group of 13 children at two- to four-month intervals and analyzed their language samples according to verbal output and structural complexity. The children at the beginning of the study ranged in age from 17 to 24 months. Some showed a slow but steady progression in both mean length of response and number of different words used. There was an increment in the language complexity and developmental sentence types. Other children started out with higher scores in each of these measures but then progressed more slowly over the period of the study. In most instances children whose phrase structure became more complex demonstrated longer mean length of response and a larger number of different words. As a group they moved through the simpler phrase structures of noun phrase followed at some point by the verb phrases and then by the combination of the two. However, no single measure predicted where they would be in language usage a year or so after the first evaluation.

There are many ways of describing the language problem of a child. We can use general or specific criteria. The first definition given below is concerned with the relationship of a child's language to his purpose and to the group with whom he lives. The second is an empirical one.

A child has a language deficit when he experiences consistent difficulty in understanding others or his listeners do not comprehend what he says. His deficit is determined by the criteria that his environment has set with regard to the age of the child. The extent of the deficit will be decided by the dictates of the social group. We compare the child's spoken language with that of Standard English, the dialect spoken by the educated middle-class American and the one taught in our schools.

Weiner (65) identifies a child as deficient in language when he has a prorated verbal I.Q. 15 or more points below his nonverbal I.Q. as measured by selected subtests of the Wechsler Intelligence Scale for Children (WISC) (64). In other words, the child's verbal skills are approximately one standard deviation below his nonverbal performance on a specific test.

Most authors of tests provide information about the mean score for different age groups; some indicate percentile ranks; others tell us the age at which 60, 75, or 90 percent of a sample of the population passed individual test items. In a language sample we can identify what structures are omitted or for which ones substitutions were made. We can obtain a language score.

The reference point for all of these is the performance of the average individual of a particular age. We can then determine how far below the average scores a child must be before he or she is considered to be deficient in any or all facets of language comprehension and use.

When we want to know whether a child has a language deficit, we have several optional courses of action. We can obtain and analyze spontaneous language samples, ask him to imitate whatever language unit we present to him, or give him standardized tests. Usually we use a combination of these three procedures. We shall discuss each of these three.

LANGUAGE SAMPLES

We obtain language samples for different purposes. One is to be able to describe the language use of an individual. Another is to compare a child's linguistic performance with that of his peers of similar age in his community. A third and fourth follow from the first two: the information should enable us to plan specific programs of remediation and to evaluate a child's progress in therapy.

The first of these purposes requires that we make some preliminary judgment about the level of language the child is currently using. Then we must have a system for obtaining the sample. The language must then be analyzed according to some set of specific principles or attributes of language.

If we have assumed for the moment that a child is using primarily one- and two-morpheme utterances, we can show her pictures or toys and say: *Tell me what you see.* If we want to know whether the child can name parts of her body or ours, such as nose, ears, eyes, hands, arms and legs, we can point to our own and to hers and say *What is this?* The large colorful cards in the Peabody Language Development Kits (23) organized in categories such as People, Activities, Foods, Clothes, Numbers, and Colors are appropriate for eliciting both labels and other short responses.

If we decide to obtain a free-flowing speech sample, we have several possible approaches. Brown and his students (10) obtained tape recordings of children in their natural environments—the home. For some they recorded all of the oral interchanges of a child for several hours on different days. Weir (67) recorded the presleep verbalizations of her 2½-year-old son in his crib every night for several weeks, with no adult present. Clinicians have used many different procedures and materials to elicit "spontaneous" language samples. In the early studies (43, 63) children were asked to tell about toys and pictures that were presented to them. In addition to this procedure clinicians ask questions about an individual's favorite TV programs, books he is reading, his work at school, sports that interest him, recent movies, space travel, wishes, and others. O'Donnell et al. (55) showed children some animated cartoons of Aesop's fables with the sound track off and asked each one to tell an interviewer the stories and answer some questions following the presentations. Hubbell et al. (30) using the puzzles for the WISC asked the parents of 3- and 6-year-old children "to help" them put the puzzles together. Although Myklebust developed his Picture Story for analyzing written language, Wilson (68) used it as the stimulus for her study of the oral language of children. On the Verbal Expression subtest of the Illinois Test of Psycholinguistic Abilities (35), four objects are presented one at a time to the child. The examiner can prompt the child on a demonstration item by asking questions to elicit information about the name, use, size, color, category, parts, and other characteristics.

When we obtain this sample, we are assuming that it is representative of an individual's usual speech performance. Therefore, the kind of stimuli and the size of the sample are important considerations. Loban (42) found it essential to use different stimulus materials in his longitudinal language studies of children as they progressed from kindergarten through twelfth grade. Topics that interested a child at age 5 held little meaning for him six or twelve years later. Weir (67) found that the nature and frequency of the words which her son used were a function of the items in his environment. From Table 4.2 you can see that he used *Bobo* and *blanket* more frequently than any other words except the article *the*. These were the two favorite things that he always wanted in his crib when he went to bed, and he talked about and to them a great deal.

When we are getting this sample, we must follow a standard set of instructions in order to be able to compare the child's performance with that of his peers or with his own later language usage. These directions, however, can be limiting, as Brannon and Murry (9) found in their analyses of samples of deaf, hard of hearing, and normal 12-year-olds. They required that the child stop at the end of each sentence. This instruction no doubt contributed to the type and length of the utterance. The children responded to their pictures using simple declarative sentences averaging only six or seven words in length.

Wilson (68) provides additional evidence of the wide range of responses we get from children in spite of the fact that instructions are standardized and the same stimulus pictures are used for all of them. She reported that Total Words Correct, a measure similar to Number of Different Words, ranged from 13 to 895, and her total number of sentences ranged from 2 to 61. She reported on a group of children aged 3 to 17. It seems unlikely that the wide range is due only to the age factor. This study reflects the difficulty in using picture stimuli which are appropriate for a group of young people ranging in age from 3 to 17. The particular picture used in this situation is one of a young boy at a table working with doll figures and furniture. The fact that the picture stimulus is the same and the directions are the same does not mean we are getting a typical language sample particularly from those at the low end and the high end of the age range studied.

We should also be aware of what kinds of responses we may obtain when we use certain types of questions. If we use a tag question, all the child can do is respond with a *yes* or *no* verbally or motorically. For instance, if you say to a child *You like apples, don't you?* you give her little choice. She must respond either affirmatively or negatively. On the other hand, if you ask the child any question beginning with a Wh-word, she must respond with either a phrase or a sentence. When you say to her *What did you do at school today?* the child's language response may be lengthy or brief but it cannot be *yes* or *no*.

You can predict whether or not the child's response will be *yes* or *no* or optional by the type of verb with which you introduce your question. The questions *Is your bicycle broken?* and *Do you have my pencil?* require a *yes* or *no* response. It may be that an individual child will tell you a great deal more about his bicycle or about the pencil, but his first response will be *yes* or *no*. If the child is unable to make the differentiation between an affirmation and a negation, his responses will be inappropriate either because he doesn't understand the question—a semantic problem—or doesn't know the syntactic rule.

Leach (*36*) notes that we place several constraints upon an individual when we question him. Some questions require that the referent be present. For instance, if we say *What is he doing?* either an individual is present or a picture or an object is being referred to. In other questions the presence of a referent may be optional. The question *How do you play baseball?* does not require that a baseball or a softball be in view. It does require, however, that the child understand the term *baseball*. Some questions in addition require that the clinician accompany the question with a gesture. A question such as *What is this?* requires the clinician to point to the referent for *this* as well as to ask the question. On the other hand the question *How do you play baseball?* requires only the linguistic cues.

Both the nature of our questions and the words we use in the questions should be related to the child's level of language acquisition. For instance, Brown and Bellugi (*10*) have reported that adults use cues that are in the immediate environment when they are talking to a young child. We have a tendency to ask questions such as *What's your*

name? and *How old are you?* which are related to the individual to whom
we are talking. We use more abstract comments and questions in dealing
with older children. We expect the older child to be able to recall events,
sequence information he gives us, and use a vocabulary which does not
necessarily reflect anything in the immediate environment of the adult-
child interaction. We use questions that require more mature children
to understand the present, past, and future tenses and to be able to
apply them appropriately in answering our questions; we expect them
to differentiate the singular from the plural forms and to understand
our use of personal pronouns. A child may pick up the cues as a
result of his or her syntactic knowledge or by a combination of syntax
and semantics.

Leach (36) categorized the questions raised by mothers of children
who ranged in age from 26 to 60 months. The most popular questions
were those which used the interrogatives *what, who,* and *which.* This
type of question required the child either to name an action, give a
yes or *no* response, or imitate the adult. With the older children the
mothers used a larger variety of questions than they did with the younger
children. Table 4.4 provides a list of the types of questions used frequently
and rarely by mothers.

We don't know how large a sample we need to be sure that it is representative. Brown (*10*) wanted six hours of tape on each child. Lee and

TABLE 4.4
Types of Questions Used by Mothers

Questions	Examples
Types Used Most Frequently	
1. Tag	You like apples, don't you?
2. Auxiliary + infinitive	Do you want to eat it?
3. Auxiliary + no infinitive	Do you like apples?
8. Wh-location, space	Where is the apple?
9. Wh-nominal (what, who, which)	What is this?
10. Wh-adjectival (what, how)	What kind of apple is this?
11. Wh-verbal (*do* is the main verb)	What are you doing?
13. Wh- (*why* and *how*)	Why do you play ball?
Types Used Rarely	
Auxiliary + embedded wh-modifier	Do you read when you're in school?
Wh-locate, time (when)	When do you go home?
Wh-adverb (how)	How soon will you go?
Auxiliary +	Can you tell me about this picture?

Source: Compiled from data in Leach, *36.*

Canter (39) obtain a one-hour tape recording of a preschool language-deficient child in the clinic room. Most clinicians get a three- to ten-minute sample. Some clinicians are not concerned with a time measure but use 50 to 100 utterances in their analyses. In any event the additional time required to transcribe the sample and to establish the reliability of the transcriber is an important consideration that cannot be minimized.

Since we have to make transcriptions of our tapes and since we want representative samples, we should create a recording setting that will be conducive to ease and accuracy of transcribing as well as to spontaneous speaking. We should experiment with the use of rugs to eliminate scraping of chairs on the floor, use of fabrics such as felt on the table when we suspect that a child will bang toys on it, and even different kinds of toys. With many children we want to conceal the microphone as a protection against its being handled and possibly damaged, or put it in an unobstrusive place so that it won't deter a child from talking naturally.

The type of recording equipment needed will depend to some extent on the types of analyses we want to make and where we are recording. If we want a careful analysis of morphemes or inflections, then we want the highest possible fidelity for only in this way can we make an accurate transcription. With young children and those with minimal language, it's difficult to say whether a professional tape recorder is any better than a cassette. Usually the former is easier to listen to on playback. However, the latter is easier to conceal and is less expensive. If the recordings are being made in a clinic setting where the equipment is part of the permanent or semipermanent installations, we won't have any choice. When it is possible, use a high fidelity tape recorder and microphone.

Let's assume for the moment that you have obtained a language sample. We're ready to make a typescript of it. We should put into the typescript everything the individual says—all audible pauses (ah, uh, er), false starts, contractions used, redundancies, repetitions, single-word responses, and phrases. It is helpful to indicate what the clinician said, so that you have an intelligible reference upon which to focus if necessary. This will be particularly important when the individual is partly unintelligible. Also the questions and comments of the clinician may cue you as to why the child spoke so little or so much. You should also know what toys, pictures, or games were presented so that you can make a judgment about whether or not these were appropriate to elicit at least an average sample of language.

Now that you have the first copy of your typescript, compare it carefully with the tape recording. The best typescript is one that provides 100 percent of all the utterances of the individual. In any case you want to double-check your own reliability as both transcriber and typist.

With your completed, checked typescript, you are now ready to analyze it. The analyses will provide information about the questions we asked in the first place. Does this individual have a language deficit? If he does, in what aspects of our linguistic system is he deficient? Is it in the area of understanding or in the area of expressing language? If the latter, we should be able to obtain an organized pattern of where he is from our language sample.

If our language sample shows that this child is using primarily one-word responses, we should analyze the sample in two ways. First, make a list of the words you have elicited and indicate whether these were used spontaneously as a result of the general situation or whether you had to elicit them with repeated questions and toys. Second, classify the words as contentives or functors.

How does he use these words? Does it appear that he conveys an idea with just a single word? Or is he perhaps just naming objects and pictures? How much time did you spend in getting your language sample? Did you elicit all the words—and more—that the parents had indicated he used at home?

Many children who are still primarily at the one-word level use some two-word phrases. A guideline that you might use to determine whether his communication fits into the single-word or the short phrase category is to determine what percentages of his utterances fall into the two classes. If single-word utterances constitute 60–70 percent of his over-all speaking, then he's at this stage. It is rare for children whose language is developing normally to be at the single-word stage as defined much beyond the age of 24 months. The child's world is becoming so complex by 2 years of age that he has to put some words together to express himself.

If a child is functioning at the two-word phrase level, we determine what words he puts together. Then we can categorize them as to pivot or open categories. Remember that the *pivot* is the frequently occurring word he uses to which he attaches one labeled *open*. Usually he will have a few pivots and many in the open category.

After you have listed them and classified them as pivot-open, open-open, or open-pivot, you are ready to determine the purposes for which he used them. Refer back to the categories and examples in the previous section on language acquisition. You may have difficulty making judgments about where to put these two-word phrases, because the clues you've recorded about what you were doing or saying at the time aren't sufficient. Also the child may have been talking spontaneously about something that happened in his home that morning or in the car on his way to see you, and you haven't a clue as to what he means. If you have many of these, make an additional note about "unclassifiable" two-word utterances. Use the same percentage figures suggested for the single-word class (60–70 percent) to decide if he's in this stage.

Most children will have left behind them this phase of language learning by the time they are 30 to 36 months of age. By the latter time many normally developing children will already be using full-blown sentences. Many of the sentences may not be grammatically correct, but the words are in the adult order of words.

From your transcript identify the syntactic units, that is, the noun phrase and the verb phrase. We expect children 3 years old to be proficient in the use of both types of phrases. Therefore, you should determine which of his utterances are "mini sentences," how he is expressing the verb phrase and the noun phrase. The key questions at this stage of development are whether he is putting these phrases in the correct order, how complete the phrases are, whether or not there is subject-verb agreement, and whether there is evidence of some inflections on nouns and verbs. Is the vocabulary of use primarily concrete? Does it seem to be of sufficient size to enable him to express himself as other 3-year-olds do? If 60–70 percent of his utterances can be classified within this phrase structure type of analysis, you can say he's at this level. There is such a wide range among children that it's difficult to say how sophisticated the structures themselves must be to be considered average or below average. As yet we have only some clinical hunches about their makeup.

We have indicated earlier, and you will recognize from your talking to them, that normal 4-year-olds are using sentences quite adequately. They are demonstrating the concept of a sentence, but they may be making errors in their use of transformations, inflections, and subject-verb agreement. The sentence as a unit of expression will become more and more complex as a result of increase in vocabulary and intricacy of the thoughts to be expressed.

You may want to determine first what percentage of the utterances are sentences. If your percentage isn't at least 50 percent, you may want to return to an analysis of NP-VP as directed above. If you have a large number of sentences—75, for instance—you may want to analyze all of them, or only 50. If you don't analyze all 75, it's a good idea to drop the first 15 and the last 10. Many times it takes a child a few minutes to "warm up"; by eliminating the early responses you may get a more accurate measure of his or her performance. The last few responses may be influenced by fatigue, lack of interest in the task, or something else.

Earlier in the chapter we referred to the work of O'Donnell et al. (55) and their measure of sentence length, the T-unit. If your language sample is composed primarily of sentences, you can analyze it according to their rules. The following definitions will be helpful, since you will want to obtain information about each of them.

A. A T-unit (terminal unit) is a "single independent predication together with any subordinate clauses that may be grammatically related to it. It may be a simple or a complex sentence, but *not* a compound sentence." (55)

Example: 1. The girl has a book.
2. The girl who lives next door has my book.
3. When you want a book, go to the library.

B. A garble is any element that can be classed as a false start, abnormal redundancy, or a word tangle.

Example: 1. *Next time,* tomorrow I'll get it.
2. *He in the out* he went home.
3. The bird saw the cat—*I have a cat named Sparky*—so he flew away.

C. Audible pauses are the sounds we produce that are extraneous to the communication unit.

Example: 1. Uh
2. m-m-m
3. a-a-a

D. Single-word, noun-phrase, and verb-phrase utterances are to be separated from the T-unit.

It is useful to place all garbles in parentheses and to draw a line through the audible pauses. Draw two lines through single-word and short phrase responses. All the rest constitute T-units.

With the T-units identified, count the number of words in each one, and score it according to the following directions:

A. Garbles and audible pauses receive *no* points.
B. Each word has a count of 1.
C. Each contracted word has a count of 2.

Example: 1. wasn't
2. he's
3. they're

D. If the T-unit begins with *and,* the word *and* has a count of 1.

You are now ready to determine the mean number of words in the T-units. When you have found the mean, compare the mean of your child with those of others at his grade level (Table 4.5). Also determine the range of his utterances. Does he usually have T-units of four words, or does he have a range of three to ten words?

Next you are ready to count the number of garbles. Compare the number with those of other children (Table 4.5).

In making your comparisons keep in mind that O'Donnell et al. used the same stimulus movies for all subjects. In addition, each child was asked exactly the same questions and no additional ones. Even though you use a different number of utterances and a different set of stimulus materials, you will find it useful to make the comparisons, particularly with children whose language is deficient.

You can also classify these same T-units according to Table 4.3. In that table are listed the types of sentences in the repertoire of children

TABLE 4.5
Normative Data on T-Units

	K	1	2	3	5	7
				Grades [*]		
Mean number of words in a T-unit	7.1	8.0	8.3	8.7	8.9	9.8
Range in mean number of words per T-unit	4.0–9.5	5.2–10.1	6.3–9.8	7.4–10.8	7.6–11.5	8.1–12.7
Percent of T-units less than nine words long	75.1	67.4	64.2	60.3	60.8	54.2
Mean number of garbles	11.3	8.8	16.1	13.5	10.8	11.1
Range of numbers of garbles	3–40	0–26	1–52	2–43	1–25	0–40

Source: O'Donnell et al., 55.
[*] Thirty children in each grade level, all from white middle-class environments.

from kindergarten through adulthood. The only one for which you won't have information is the *Partial*, because you've eliminated those phrases and words from your above analyses. However, you can now go back and count those in your transcripts. They will be the ones through which you drew two lines.

Lee (39, 40) has provided a different approach to the analysis of language samples. She obtains a 50-sentence sample of spontaneous speech. She has defined a sentence as an utterance that has a subject and a predicate. Noun phrases or verb phrases alone do not fit her definition. In analyzing the language sample she identifies the following eight grammatical features:

1. Indefinite pronouns or noun modifiers such as *it, this, that*
2. Personal pronouns
3. Main verbs
4. Secondary verbs
5. Negatives
6. Conjunctions
7. Interrogative reversals
8. Wh-questions

Lee postulates that these are the most important structures for determining a child's ability in formulating sentences. Each is given a certain number of points. Table 4.6 lists the structures and their corresponding

TABLE 4.6
Structures and Weights Assigned to Them in Developmental Sentence Scoring

	Indefinite Pronouns or Noun Modifiers	Personal Pronouns	Main Verbs	Secondary Verbs
1	it, this, that	1st and 2nd person: I, me, my, mine, you, your(s)	A. Uninflected verb: I *see* you. B. copula, is or 's: *It's* red. C. is + verb + ing: He *is coming.*	
2		3rd person: he, him, his she, her, hers	A. -s and -ed: *plays, played* B. Irregular past: *ate, saw* C. Copula: *am, are, was, were* D. Auxiliary: *am, are, was, were*	Five early-developing infinitival complements: I wan*na see* (want *to see*) I'm gon*na see* (going *to see*) I got*ta see* (got *to see*) Lemme [*to*] see (let me [*to*] *see*) Let's [*to*] play (let [us *to*] *play*)
3	A. no, some, more all, lot(s), one(s), two (etc.) other(s), another B. something, somebody, someone	A. Plurals: we, us, our(s) they, them, their B. these, those		Non-complementing infinitives: I stopped *to play.* I'm afraid *to look.* It's hard *to do* that.
4	nothing, nobody, none, no one		A. can, will, may + verb: *may go* B. Obligatory do + verb: *don't go* C. Emphatic do + verb: I *do see.*	Participle, present or past: I see a boy *running.* I found the toy *broken.*
5		Reflexives: myself, yourself, himself, herself, itself, themselves		A. Early infinitival complements with differing subjects in kernels: I want you *to come.* Let him [*to*] *see.* B. Later infinitival complements: I had *to go.* I told him *to go.* I tried *to go.* He ought *to go.* C. Obligatory deletions: Make it [*to*] *go.* I'd better [*to*] *go.* D. Infinitive with wh-word: I know what *to get.* I know how *to do* it.

Negatives	Conjunctions	Interrogative Reversals	Wh-Questions
it, this, that + copula or auxiliary is, 's, + not: 　It's *not* mine. 　This is *not* a dog. 　That is *not* moving.		Reversal of copula: *Isn't it* red? *Were they* there?	
			A. who, what, what + noun: 　*Who* am I? *What* is he eating? 　*What book* are you reading? B. where, how many, how much, what . . . do, what . . . for 　*Where* did it go? 　*How much* do you want? 　*What* is he *doing*? 　*What* is a hammer *for*?
	and		
can't, don't		Reversal of auxiliary be: *Is he* coming? *Isn't he* coming? *Was he* going? *Wasn't he* going?	
isn't, won't	A. but B. so, and so, so that C. or, if		when, how, how + adjective 　*When* shall I come? 　*How* do you do it? 　*How big* is it?

TABLE 4.6 (continued)

	Indefinite Pronouns or Noun Modifiers	Personal Pronouns	Main Verbs	Secondary Verbs

6		A. Wh-pronouns: who, which, whose, whom, what, that, how many, how much
		    I know *who* came.
		    That's *what* I said.
		B. Wh-word + infinitive:
		    I know *what* to do.
		    I know *who(m)* to take.
			A. could, would, should, might + verb: *might come, could be*
			B. Obligatory does, did + verb
			C. Emphatic does, did + verb	

7	A. any, anything, anybody, anyone
	B. every, everything, everybody, everyone
	C. both, few, many, each, several, most, least, much, next, first, last, second (etc.)
		(his) own, one, oneself, whichever, whoever, whatever
		    Take *whatever* you like.
			A. Passive with *get*, any tense
			Passive with *be*, any tense
			B. must, shall + verb: *must come*
			C. have + verb + en: *I've eaten*
			D. have got: *I've got* it.
				Passive infinitival complement:
				With *get*:
				    I have *to get dressed.*
				    I don't want *to get hurt.*
				With *be*:
				    I want *to be pulled.*
				    It's going *to be locked.*

8			A. have been + verb + ing had been + verb + ing B. modal + have + verb + en *may have eaten* C. modal + be + verb + ing *could be playing* D. Other auxiliary combinations: *should have been sleeping*	Gerund: *Swinging* is fun. I like *fishing.* He started *laughing.*

Source: Reproduced with permission from Lee, *40.*

Negatives	Conjunctions	Interrogative Reversals	Wh-Questions
	because	A. Obligatory do, does, did: *Do they* run? *Does it* bite? *Did*n't *it* hurt? B. Reversal of modal: *Can you* play? Won't *it* hurt? *Shall I* sit down? C. Tag question: It's fun, *isn't it?* It isn't fun, *is it?*	
All other negatives: A. Uncontracted negatives: I can *not* go. He has *not* gone. B. Pronoun-auxiliary or pronoun-copula contraction: I'm *not* coming. He's *not* here. C. Auxiliary-negative or copula-negative contraction: He was*n't* going. He has*n't* been seen. It could*n't* be mine. They are*n't* big.			why, what if, how come how about + gerund *Why* are you crying? *What if* I won't do it? *How come* he is crying? *How about* coming with me?
	A. where, when, how, while, whether (or not), till, until, unless, since, before, after, for, as, as + adjective + as, as if, like, that, than I know *where* you are. Don't come *till* I call. B. Obligatory deletions: I run faster *than* you [run]. I'm *as big as* a man [is big]. It looks *like* a dog [looks]. C. Elliptical deletions (score 0) That's *why* [I took it]. I know *how* [I can do it]. D. Wh-words + infinitive: I know *how* to do it. I know *where* to go.	A. Reversal of auxiliary have: *Has he* seen you? B. Reversal with two or three auxiliaries: *Has he been* eating? *Could*n't *he have* waited? *Could he have been* crying? *Would*n't *he have been* going?	whose, which, which + noun *Whose* car is that? *Which book* do you want?

weights (*40*). These weights range from one to eight; the weight given to a grammatical feature is based on the general development order of syntactic structures. For instance, in the sentence *I'm playing,* the verb (auxiliary + playing) appears early in children's speech. In the Lee scoring system that verb receives a count of *one.* In the sentence *I should have been playing,* the auxiliary is more complex and appears later so the verb is given *eight* points. In addition, each utterance that is a correct complete sentence receives a score of *one.* Each of the above examples would be credited with a sentence point. The utterances *Where you going, he eat the candy,* and *her don't have any* have errors of order, inflection, or incorrect form. None of them would receive a sentence point, but each would be analyzed and points given to the grammatical features in it that are correct. Appendix A to this chapter provides a hypothetical corpus of 30 sentences and shows how each sentence would be scored and the scores totaled and averaged.

The Developmental Sentence Score (DSS) is the mean sentence score of the 50-sentence sample. See Figure 4.2 for norms for DSS for children 1½ through 6½ years old. One difficulty with using a total score is that it can be a reflection of the complexity of the child's language, or it may be high just because of the number of words he or she uses. The score itself is difficult to defend statistically. We add together weighted points for categories of nouns and verbs, for instance, without knowing that a given score in each of the eight categories is comparable.

The major strength of this procedure is that it enables us to prepare a profile of the child's linguistic structures. Since it is a clinical tool, the information we get from the profile can be used immediately in program planning for the individual child. It is especially useful in helping to identify what structures are not present and the type of substitution a child is using for the correct form.

Another system for analyzing linguistic output involves categorizing all words in one of 14 classes (*32*). Although the system was originally used to analyze the language of adult aphasic patients, others (*8*) have used it with language samples of children. The system uses the word as a single unit. As a result you can take any spoken language sample, transcribe it, and count the total number of words in the sample and the number in each of the categories. The categories are the following:

Nouns	Relative pronouns	Prepositions
Verbs	Articles	Conjunctions
Adjectives	Indefinites	Interjections
Adverbs	Auxiliaries	Unclassified
Pronouns	Quantifiers	

Such a system points up the word classes that are missing and those that are most frequently used. However, it does not provide information

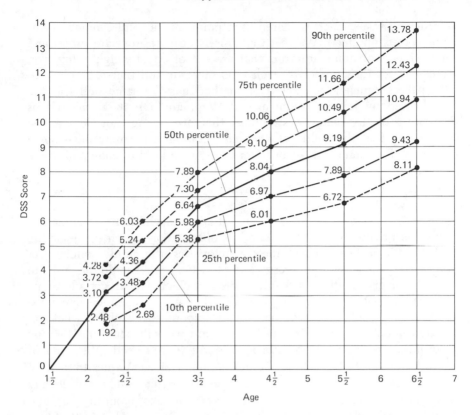

FIGURE 4.2
Norms for developmental sentence scoring (reweighted, 1972). (From L. L. Lee, *Developmental Sentence Analysis,* Evanston, Ill.: Northwestern University Press, 1974.)

about the nature of the syntactic structures themselves because of its emphasis on the single word. In fact, many of the words could be used inappropriately, a matter we have no way of checking.

McCarthy (*43*) and Templin (*63*) were among the first child psychologists to develop procedures to describe a language sample. They were concerned with the mean length of a sentence, size of vocabulary, and percentages of different grammatical features in the sample. The problems involved in determining when a sentence ends has been a serious drawback when others have tried to use their criteria. Detailed instructions for this type of analysis are included in the first edition of this text (*31*).

Myklebust (*53*) has devised a different system of analysis. He has classified all syntactic errors as word additions, omissions, substitutions, or order mistakes. Each is scored as a point and a total syntactic error score is thus obtained. We feel that this is an inappropriate procedure, since we cannot summate errors that are not of equal weight. However, we can count the number of each type of error and plot a graph indicating the frequency of each. This method has the same faults as the one devised by Jones, Goodman, and Wepman (32): it doesn't tell us the nature of the syntactic structures that are wrong, nor does a low score mean that the child has adequate grammar. He may have none; he may be functioning at the one-word utterance level of communication.

Summary

As clinicians become more adept at listening to children's language, it should be possible to use the period of observation which precedes the evaluation as a time to check the characteristics of a child's communication. Once we know the gross characteristics, we should be able to select a few grammatic or semantic units for which we can get additional information in the testing situation. Whether we do complete language analyses or partial ones, we will still be hypothesizing about what linguistic competence the child needs most and we will begin our therapy program to test out our preliminary hypothesis. A considerable amount of work remains to be done in the development of techniques to analyze language samples. In our opinion the most valuable system for dealing with phrase structures is the analysis of verb phrases, noun phrases, and emerging noun phrase–verb phrase utterances. Sentence level utterances can be analyzed by the O'Donnell et al. T-unit for length, or one can classify the sentences as to types and analyze the sample using the Lee procedure but not her total mean score. A further analysis of the sample of sentences would involve classification of types of errors—omissions and substitutions—with regard to personal pronouns, the inflections of verbs and nouns, and subject-verb agreement.

IMITATION OF SENTENCES

Another way to measure the child's language involves having him or her imitate a set of sentences each of which demonstrates one of the primary characteristics of English grammar. The sentences developed and used by Menyuk (51) are short, ranging in length from three to ten words. (See Appendix B to this chapter for a list of her sentences.) When she asked a group of 3- to 6-year-old children with normal and another group with deviant language to repeat these sentences after her, she found some major differences. She classified the repetitions of the sentences as being either correct, having omissions, or displaying other kinds of modifications. Figure 4.3 indicates that children with normal

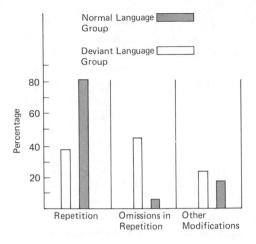

FIGURE 4.3
The percentage of sentences repeated correctly, repeated with
omissions, and repeated with
other modifications by normal-
speaking children and deviant-
speaking children. (From P. Menyuk, *Sentences Children Use*,
Research Monograph No. 52,
Cambridge, Mass.: The M.I.T.
Press, 1969.)

language development repeated 80 percent of the sentences correctly.
About 5 percent of the sentences had some omissions and another 15
percent showed other modifications. The accurate reproduction of so
many of the sentences is an indication, according to Menyuk, that
children have acquired the rules of grammar demonstrated in the list
of sentences. The role of auditory memory in the reproduction of the
sentences is extremely important. We can observe the effect of short
memory span in the poor reproduction of these same sentences by the
deviant-language children. The younger ones tended to repeat only the
last words that they heard.

Although the children were able to reproduce the sentences containing selected grammatical structures, they did not necessarily use those
structures in their language samples. It may be that the children understood and reproduced the forms in this particular task but did not have
sufficient control of the grammar to be able to use it in their own
communication of ideas. It may also be that the language sample was
too short and as a result the children could not demonstrate all of these
rules. Perhaps imitation of sentences is a much easier task for the child
and therefore his success rate is high. We know from studies of articulation that children's imitation of the clinician's production of a phoneme
in a word is more often correct than their spontaneous production of
the same phoneme. In any event, we can say that the child has a
degree of control over the rules but is still not using those forms fully.

When we ask a child to repeat an utterance, we need to structure
that utterance to take into account both syntactic and semantic features
and at the same time be aware of the child's limited capacity to remember long sentences. Based on Miller's (52) work concerning the
length of an utterance that can be repeated, many investigators use the

formula of seven words plus or minus two words to construct utterances. In other words, the range would be five to nine words per sentence. Young children have difficulty processing and reproducing a long sequence of words or one that has too many chunks in it. (A "chunk" is an organized unit of what we hear and is related to short-term memory span.) Even when the order of words approximates an English utterance, children of 4 and 5 years have many errors of omission when they repeat a string of words.

To test the accuracy of reproduction of utterances among 4- through 7-year-olds, Carrow and Mauldin (*15*) structured five-word utterances that reflected four levels of approximation to English. Their first-order strings were unrelated words: *does part color paper height*. The second-order sets had some words that could be chunked: *room size of time is*. Third-order utterances included words that were more clearly related to one another: *it may happen to corner*. Fourth-order sets made the most sense: *if I were captain of*. They hypothesized that the children would make fewer errors as they progressed from the first-order set through the fourth-order set, and that for all four orders there would be a diminishing number of errors from the youngest to the oldest group.

The results indicated that the overall accuracy of reproduction was indeed a function of age. In the fourth-order sets 4-year-olds made more omission errors than the 6- and 7-year-olds. Carrow and Mauldin interpret this result by suggesting that semantic growth does not begin until age 5. However, this explanation cannot be applied to the performance of these same 4-year-olds in their repetition of third-order sets: the children recalled these with greater accuracy than they did the fourth-order strings of words. Presumably the correct grammar of the fourth-order utterances and the natural groupings of words didn't help the 4-year-olds to reproduce the utterances accurately. On the other hand, it could be that these words were not familiar to the children but that the third-order words were. In any event, repetition per se does not tell us about the linguistic cues used by young children, particularly if they make mistakes.

When young children are asked to repeat strings of words, they tend to hold in memory and repeat back the contentives. Evidently they are familiar with the contentives and hold them in short-term memory for a longer period. If the child can assign meaning to the utterance, he will delete the functors. If he cannot assign meaning to it, he will treat all the words alike and the deletions will be governed more by his capacity than by a linguistic strategy.

Scholes (*58*) feels that the young child has classified words into two major groups: contentives and functors. He does this at an early age and then uses this rule when he repeats units of utterances. He treats the two classes differently even when stress patterns are eliminated. Scholes hypothesizes that the child is using the strategy "identify and retain contentives."

There is still another variable that we must be aware of in interpreting the child's imitation of sentences: children will change verb forms so that they match those with which they are familiar. Jordan and Robinson (33) studied this problem using preschool children of middle-class and working-class origin. They found that the children imitated accurately the sentences with verb forms used by children of their own social class. However, when they were presented with sentences whose verb forms were those of the other class, the children altered the verb forms and produced those with which they were familiar. The authors conclude that a child filters imitations through his or her own grammatical productive system.

Summary

In both the construction and presentation of utterances we must be aware of what we want to measure. When is an utterance to be imitated too long or too complex for the child to handle? If we could be sure that accurate imitation was a reliable indicator that the child had a linguistic rule, it would certainly simplify our task of measurement.

LANGUAGE TESTS

The number of language tests available to the clinician is limited. Published tests that have been standardized to some degree will be reviewed in this section. To administer these tests, you must be knowledgeable about testing procedures in general as well as those specific to the test. In addition, we recommend that you practice giving them several times to children and young adults to become familiar with the materials, the recording of responses, and procedures for interpreting the results.

One advantage in giving a standardized test is .that it is an objective measure. Also you can compare the child's performance with that represented in the norms provided. A disadvantage of many language measures is that their standardization has been inadequate and therefore the norms are in question. According to Weiner and Hoock (66), adequate standardization of a test requires several procedures:

1. Selection of the variables that affect scores on the behavior being tested. Examples would be age, hearing, socioeconomic level of the family, and ethnic background.
2. Adequate sample size. For instance, if the norms are to apply to children who live in cities, small towns, and rural communities, samples must be obtained from these areas.

3. Random samples. Ideally each person should have as much chance to be included in the tested population as every other person.
4. Testing must be completed in a limited time span. Data gathered over a four-year period are subject to question unless they are longitudinal. All of our test norms are cross-sectional in nature.
5. Statistical treatment of the data should be complete. Providing mean scores without either the standard deviations or the ranges is an example of inadequate statistical information.

When you read the manuals that accompany most of these tests or the articles in which the tests have been described, you should check for each of these criteria in order to evaluate how much you can rely on the data the author has provided. Whatever interpretation you place on a given child's scores must be tempered by the procedures used in standardization.

Most tests are given with the general understanding that a "normal" rate of speaking will be used. As clinicians, however, we need to recognize that when we request a child to point to items, as we do on the Peabody Picture Vocabulary Test (22), slower rates of giving directions produce more correct answers. When we talk too fast, children become confused and may make more errors because of our rate rather than because of lack of correct information.

When Berry and Erickson (5) presented the items of the receptive section of the Northwestern Syntax Screening Test (38) at five different rates to kindergarten and second-grade children, they found that the slower rates of 2.6 and 3.4 syllables per second produced more correct answers. The normal or above normal rates of speaking seemed less comprehensible to the children, and they made more errors in comprehension.

The following review of each test includes the rationale, the language aspect it measures, for whom it is appropriate, how it is administered, and some comments about its limitations where appropriate.

The Illinois Test of Psycholinguistic Abilities

The Illinois Test of Psycholinguistic Abilities (ITPA) (35) was conceived as a diagnostic instrument that would identify the strengths and weaknesses of children with communication problems. The developers postulated that once the weaknesses were determined, a remediation program could be structured to eliminate the child's specific inadequacies. They hypothesized that the subtests they used tapped most of the major skills needed for communication. Additional ones were added in the revised edition to measure abilities not assessed in the first edition, and several of the original ones were modified.

The theoretical model for the ITPA is an adaptation of Osgood's communication model (56). Osgood hypothesized that communication has three dimensions: (1) three processes—receptive, organizing, and expressive; (2) two levels of organization—representational and automatic; and (3) several channels—auditory, visual, motor, and vocal. Within this framework he attempted to identify the steps involved when a person receives a message, interprets it, and in turn sends his or her own comments to a listener.

The test provides information about each of the processes mentioned above: reception, or the ability to recognize or understand what is being seen or heard; expression, or the ability to disclose ideas either vocally or motorically; and organization, which assigns meaning to what is spoken, seen, or heard. Performance in each of the three is evaluated at the two levels: representational or automatic. The representational level requires the use of symbols that carry the meaning of an object. The automatic level is concerned with less voluntary but well-organized methods of functioning. Four channels are tapped: two of sensory input (visual and auditory) and two of response output (verbal and motor).

The test was designed for children 2 years 4 months through 10 years 3 months of age. From the results the examiner can obtain a language age based on the total test, as well as a language age for each of the subtests. Both of these psycholinguistic ages (PLA) provide an indication of the level of performance of a child with reference to other children of the same age. The subtest PLA scores can be used to a greater degree for program planning for the child than the composite or total PLA because the program can be made specific to the inadequacies of a child.

The revised edition also permits the examiner to obtain scaled scores which take into account not only the mean of the group scores but also their variances. As a result the examiner can compare an individual's performance across subtests. The scaled score should be used in plotting the profile of a child's performance and in planning a remedial program.

To determine whether or not a child needs special help, we obtain a mean or median scaled score (SS) of all the subtests and then compare that SS to the SS for each subtest. A discrepancy of plus or minus 6 is not an indicator of difficulty or excellence because about 66 percent of all children fall within that range. A difference of plus or minus 7, 8, or 9 constitutes borderline performance, and plus or minus 10 is indicative of a substantial strength or deficit.

We should note the pattern as well as the individual scores. Keeping in mind the theoretical model upon which the test was based, the examiner should be able to determine whether the successes and failures are at one or both levels, in which channels, and in which processes. This information can be noted graphically on the profile of abilities completed for each child.

This test can point up areas where additional testing is needed. For instance, if a child's SS for the Grammatic Closure subtest is –10, we will want to obtain additional information about his grammatical structures. We must determine more specifically which grammatic units are missing or deviant and plan accordingly.

Some clinicians want information about only the auditory input and verbal output channels. If our observations and other reports support our clinical hunches, then we can give the following subtests only: Verbal Expression, Grammatic Closure, Auditory Association, and Auditory Reception. In this way we can compare a child with his or her peers on these sections. We will have sampled all three processes at two levels and in two channels and can plan a program accordingly.

Peabody Picture Vocabulary Test

One of the few measures of the comprehension of vocabulary that a speech-language pathologist can administer is the Peabody Picture Vocabulary Test (22). It consists of 150 plates on each of which four pictures appear. The child is asked to look at all of the pictures on the sample plate, the examiner then says a word, and asks the child to put a finger on the appropriate picture. Older children who can read are asked to give the number of the picture that identifies the word. Practice items insure that the child has understood the instructions. The test has no time limit and can be given in sections if the child is not able to attend long enough to complete the task. It has two forms that can be given in alternate sessions to check the reliability of the score obtained. It is suitable for those in the age range of 2 years 3 months to 18 years. Tables in the manual provide information about the MA, I.Q., and percentile rank of an individual.

Clinicians need no special training to administer this test. You must read the manual of instructions carefully and follow the directions for administering and scoring the test. Usually it takes 10 to 15 minutes to give it and another 5 to score and record the necessary information on the test form.

Although this test is considered by its authors to be a measure of the intelligence of a child, there is sufficient evidence that clinicians should use it only as a measure of receptive vocabulary. We can refer to a child's mental age based on the test results as a receptive language age.

When it is used with environmentally different children, the results should be viewed with caution. The vocabulary is culture-bound and may not be in the repertoire of such children. When we use it with young black children and with others from low-middle and low socioeconomic backgrounds, we should be aware that the scores we get may not be valid. One explanation for test errors is that these children don't hear and use these words in their environments. We need to ask ourselves, therefore, whether these scores are a valid measure of the receptive language of kindergarten and first-grade black children. Since more than one-half of our clinicians and the majority of teachers of classes of children with learning disabilities use this test, we should interpret the data cautiously.

Full-Range Picture Vocabulary Test

The Full-Range Picture Vocabulary Test (2) is a short test of verbal comprehension. Although it too was designed as a measure of intelligence, we can consider it a measure of auditory comprehension of language. Norms are available from age 2 years through adulthood. It has two forms. It requires only a pointing response. The test consists of 16 cards each with four line drawings on it. The testee points to the picture which represents the particular word given by the examiner. All items are scored as either right or wrong.

Reliability has been determined by comparing the scores on Form A with Form B. The range of the correlations is from 0.86 to 0.99. The populations upon whom the reliability studies were based were quite diverse, from preschool children to children from ethnic groups or with special kinds of problems. Validity has been determined by comparing scores on this test with scores obtained on the Stanford-Binet, the WISC, and the Ravens Progressive Matrices. The range of the correlations is from 0.47 to 0.91, depending upon the size of the population and the nature of the population being studied.

Because the test provides only a limited number of items to which an individual can respond, it has limited application. In addition, most studies dealing with the reliability and validity of this measure were completed approximately 20 years ago. The references which accompany this test suggest that little research has been completed with it since 1955.

Test for Auditory Comprehension of Language

One of the first major attempts by a speech-language pathologist to develop an auditory test of language comprehension was made by Carrow (12). The experimental version became available in 1969 and the most recent revision appeared in 1973. The author's purpose in developing the experimental version was threefold: to assess the auditory comprehension of English language structures in children; to determine the sequence in which children comprehend the grammatical and lexical aspects of English; and to obtain the same information on Spanish-speaking children. The test consists of a set of plates, each with three black-and-white drawings. One drawing represents the referent for the linguistic form being tested, and the other two are referents for contrasting linguistic forms or decoys. For example, for the stimulus sentence *The doll is in the box*, a plate shows a doll beside a box, one in a box, and one on top of a box. The child's task is to point to the referent for *The doll is in the box*. It requires no oral expression from the child. He gets one point for each correct response.

The original version was given to children aged 2 years 10 months through 7 years 9 months. Carrow used the age at which 60 percent of an age sample comprehended the item as the norm for that structure. Three-year-olds understood about 25 nouns; three verbs; some qualitative adjectival contrasts; the colors *red, brown,* and *blue;* the adverbs *up* and *down;* the prepositions *on, under,* and *in;* and the interrogatives *who* and *what*. Negatives were understood by age 3½ years; gender and number of pronouns, except for the contrast she/he/they, by age 4. The children had a wider comprehension of nouns than the other form classes, probably because of the extent of their exposure to them and their dependence upon them.

The 1973 edition, Test for Auditory Comprehension of Language (TACL), has 101 plates which test comprehension of selected nouns, morphological structures, and principles of grammar and syntax (*14*). In addition four plates provide practice in following directions; for instance, the child must *find the rabbit, point to the cookie, select the basket with flowers, point to fish*. Only the referent may be given to him later in the test. The entire test must be administered since the items are arranged by grammatical category and not by level of difficulty. It takes 20 to 30 minutes to administer.

Norms are provided for children aged 3 through 6 years who come from middle-class backgrounds. It is possible to compare a child's raw score with the average score for his age or to find his age-equivalent score. A child's score can also be compared with the norms for his age group to determine his percentile rank. You can analyze the classes of errors a child has made and use the information in planning language therapy. You can also determine which items should be in his repertoire according to his age.

On the response sheet the lowest age level at which 75 and 90 percent of the children passed each item is provided. No age group had mastered 13 of the 101 items at the 75 percent level. These include some items in each of the four categories, for example, the referents *pair, easily,* and *gently* in the vocabulary section; *bicyclist* and *pianist* in the morphology section; verb tenses in the grammar section; and direct-indirect object in the syntax section.

A screening version (STACL) of this test is also available (*13*). It uses 25 items from the longer version. The author says in the manual that these items were chosen "on the basis of the author's and experts' opinions as to which were best suited to evaluate knowledge of specific grammatical structures." Norms are available for children aged 3 through 6 years. The procedure for administering the 101-item version is used for this one also. The screening version can be given to small groups if there are sufficient monitors to check and help the children follow the directions. If it is given to groups, each child has a set of plates and draws a line through the line drawing he or she considers to be correct.

You can determine whether or not a child needs to be given the longer version by determining his percentile rank. If his score falls in the lowest 10 percent for his age, he probably needs further study of his language deficits. You can use either more or less stringent cutoff scores if you wish, depending on the composition of your sample and your purpose in administering this form.

At present no norms are available for the Spanish version for either the screening or the full test. In the Spanish version about one-third of the directions to the children are either different from the English directions, or they may be ambiguous because of the Spanish words used. Therefore, use caution in your interpretation of the results if you give both versions to children who comprehend both English and Spanish. The scores may not be an indication of just auditory comprehension.

The 1973 edition (TACL) is quite different from the 1969 and 1970 editions. More than a third of the items of the earlier versions have changed. New forms have been added, others replaced, and many items, particularly nouns, omitted. Also the order in which items are presented has changed. As a result, the reliability data in the manual should be interpreted with caution because some of them are not based on the 1973 edition but rather on the earlier editions. Also works are cited to support the high reliability of test-restest scores but the authors used the 1968 and 1969 editions for evaluation of reliability. Test-retest data for the screening version (STACL) were obtained on 100 children; the reliability was 0.60.

Like most tests of this kind, this one has limitations. However, it provides a great deal of information about a child's comprehension of the structures of English. Further work on reliability, use of the test with larger and different samples of the population, and prediction of change in comprehension following therapy programs based on initial test results are necessary.

Assessment of Children's Language Comprehension

Assessment of Children's Language Comprehension (ACLC), developed by Foster, Giddan, and Stark (26), also is concerned with a child's understanding of grammatical units. It is suitable for children aged 3 through 7. The authors made three assumptions when they constructed their test: (1) the learning of language proceeds from simple to complex units; (2) children with language impairments have short auditory memory spans; (3) because of limited auditory memory these children don't process adequately what they hear.

To administer the ACLC, you need the 50 plates and a recording sheet (25). The clinician tells the child to point to pictures for items she will say. It provides information about the child's understanding of a core vocabulary and his ability to process an increasing number of critical elements. A critical element is a grammatical unit, a word. For instance, when the clinician asks the child to point to *shoe*, the word *shoe* is one critical element. Asked to find the *big shoe*, he has a two critical-element item to which he must respond. If the child is cooperative, the entire test can be completed in from 10 to 15 minutes.

The test has four sections. Part A consists of 50 words which require the identification of selected nouns, verb forms, prepositions, and modifiers. Each is presented to the child as one critical element. The child may be required to pick out *balloon* on a plate with five pictures; or he may point to *eating* on a card that shows a boy doing five different tasks. If he misses many of these, the testing is terminated.

Parts B, C, and D use only these same words, but the words are put together as two, three, and four critical-element items respectively. Each part requires ten responses. In Part B the child responds to one of the four items on each plate. The two critical elements may represent agent-action (dog eating); attribute-agent (broken cup); or compound agents (chair and horn). Part C requires the child to point to pictures that represent three critical elements. Again he selects the appropriate picture from the four on each plate. Constructions such as the following are used: attribute-agent-action (happy lady sleeping); agent-action-object (baby pulling the wagon). In Part D the child selects from among five pictures on a plate. The four critical elements represent longer declarative type utterances, using the agent-action relations and expanded noun phrases. An example of the former would be *cat standing under the bed* and for the latter *broken boat on the table*.

The norms for this edition were based on the responses of 365 children aged 3-0 and 6-5. The means for each of the four sections show an increase in correct responses with age. Each part is progressively more difficult, however; as a result, the percentages of correct responses decrease across parts. For the age group 3-0 to 3-5 the mean percentages for the four parts are 84, 82, 66, and 50 respectively. For the age group 6-0 to 6-5 the percentages are 96, 98, 92 and 70. Included in these means are the scores of some children diagnosed as neurologically or educationally handicapped.

Several problems arise in using the normative and nonnormative data. The samples on whom the norms were based were small and not random. The nursery children who represented almost one-third of the total were drawn from nurseries in Florida and California representing all levels of socioeconomic and educational family backgrounds; 20 percent were black. The rest of the sample were kindergarten children from low- to middle-income families in one school district in California. The ethnic backgrounds of children in this school district were diverse, with almost half of the schools' population having Spanish, Asian, Indian, or black backgrounds.

The scores of only a small sample of children with language impairments (N = 51) have been reported. They show greater difficulty than the normal sample on all four parts, but the differences except for Part D were not great. Since they performed almost as well on Part A, the core vocabulary, as the normal sample, they represent one group on a continuum of children with language deficits. Many children won't know the core vocabulary; as a result the test must be terminated. The authors don't report how many of the children in either of their samples could not proceed through the four parts.

A second edition of the ACLC was published in 1973. Four of the original pictures were changed and others improved. No new data were gathered on the 1973 edition when it was published. Therefore, when you use it, be cautious in your comparison and interpretation of a child's scores based on the earlier edition.

A screening test, using items from the longer version, is also available for group testing. However, no normative data have been provided on this test.

Detroit Tests of Learning Aptitude

Two subtests of the Detroit Tests of Learning Aptitude (3) may be useful to the clinician. The Oral Commissions subtest consists of a set of commands that the child must execute in the order in which they are given. The rationale is that ability to remember sequences is one of the skills needed for learning. The subtest begins with one command, *Show me the window,* and ends with a sequence of four: *Open the door, then put a mark on this paper, then bring me that book, then stand by the window.* This subtest is appropriate for children aged 3 through 8-3. The examiner says to the child: "I am going to tell you something to do. You listen and do just what I tell you to do after I get all through. Listen." Unless you feel that the child didn't hear you, you cannot repeat the commands. Scoring is a bit tricky; therefore, it's a good idea to have sufficient space on your recording sheet to write the order in which the child carries out the commands. For instance, if the commands are all carried out in order, the child gets a point for each command. If she reverses the order of a two-command unit, she gets no credit. If she gives the correct response for command 1 and reverses 2 and 3 in a three-command unit, she gets only one point. In a four-command item, she might reverse the order of items 1 and 2 and give 3 and 4 in correct order, thus obtaining a score of two. The items and the norms are provided in Appendix C at the end of this chapter.

The Auditory Attention Span for Related Syllables subtest is an imitative task which uses sentences. The child listens to each of its 43 sentences and is supposed to repeat each one exactly. This, too, is a test of memory. The authors make the assumption that with increasing mental age one's ability to remember and repeat sentences of longer length and complexity improves. Thus the first few sentences are simple affirmative declarative sentences, averaging six words each. The last sentence is a complex affirmative declarative sentence of 22 words. Those who do well on this task are using the concept of chunking, that is, they listen for word groupings rather than for successive single words. This subtest has norms for those with MA's of 3 to 19 years.

To administer this subtest the clinician says: "I am going to say something to you. When I get all through, you say just what I said." You start with sentence 1 if the child is in the first grade or below, with sentence 5 if he is in the second grade, and with sentence 10 if he is in third grade or higher. If the child fails, you can move back to a simpler level unless you have started with sentence 1. Continue the administration until there are three successive sentence failures. A sentence is failed if the indiviudal makes three or more errors. Errors may be a word omitted, a word added, or an unsuitable word substituted.

In scoring this subtest you give three points for a sentence with no errors, two points if the sentence is repeated with one error, one point if it has two errors, and no credit if it has three or more errors. Scoring will be easier for you if you again leave sufficient space on your test form to draw a line through any words omitted and to write in any words added or substituted. If you are a beginner, you may find it easier to tape-record the individual's sentences and do your scoring from the tape later. The items and the norms are included in Appendix D at the end of this chapter.

Test of English Morphology

A few tests measure a child's knowledge of morphologic rules. One of the first was developed by Berko (4). After studying the language of first-grade children to determine which features of morphology they used most frequently, she selected the following for study:

Plurals
Two possessive forms of the noun
Third person singular of the verb
Present progressive and past tenses of the verb
Comparative and superlative forms of the adjective

She tested each feature with colored pictures which she identified with nonsense words, like *wug, niz,* and *spow.* The words followed the rules for possible sound combinations and thus were "believable." In fact, some of the children thought the words were ones they hadn't learned yet!

Figure 4.4 provides an example, indicating what the clinician says and what the child is to do. It is a simple but unique sentence completion test. The task requires that the child inflect some forms and derive, compound, or analyze compound words. It was administered to children aged 4 through 7 years.

Berko's primary concern was to determine what rules the children knew, whether they mastered these rules in any order, and whether they generalized the rules from the *real* to the *nonsense* words. She reported that they verbalized what she wanted them to do and even told her that some of the problems were hard. They would emphasize the inflection as they said it and might even correct the inflection after the initial try. She says, "The answers were not always right so far as English is concerned, but they were consistent and orderly answers." She concluded that children in this age range have some simplified morphologic rules. The younger group seemed to have control of fewer rules, and the older ones were still in the process of perfecting their application of the rules.

To form a plural the children followed the rule that a voiceless sibilant after a voiceless consonant except for sibilants, and a voiced sibilant after a voiced consonant constituted *plural*. However, they didn't always use the rule. For instance, 75 percent of the younger and 99 percent of the older children gave the correct plural for the word *glass*. They didn't generalize the rule to the nonsense word *tass* as we might have expected. Only 28 percent of the younger and 39 percent of the older children used the rule correctly in this instance. They had similar problems with *gutch*.

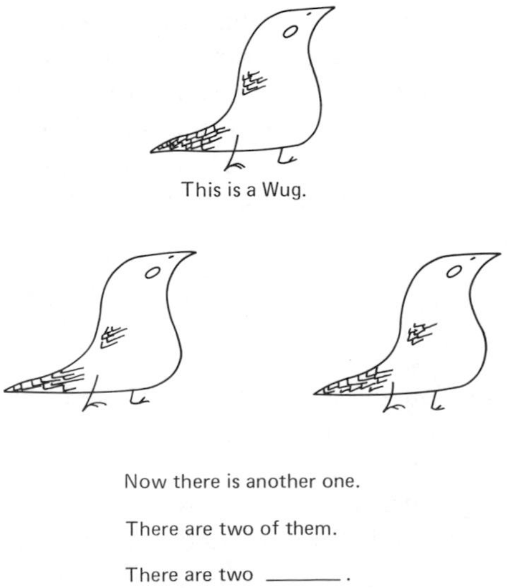

This is a Wug.

Now there is another one.

There are two of them.

There are two _____ .

FIGURE 4.4
The plural allomorph in /-z/. (From J. Berko Gleason, The child's learning of English morphology, in A. Bar-Adon and W. F. Leopold, eds., *Child Language: A Book of Readings,* Englewood Cliffs, N.J.: Prentice-Hall, 1971.)

Three transformations require the addition of the allomorph /-s/: third person singular of the verb, the possessive, and the plural form of the regular nouns. Since this inflection represents different meanings when added to the morphs, we would expect that a child's proficiency would vary as a function of time of learning the meaning. Berko found just that—that the verb form and possessive were correct more frequently than the plural.

The present progressive form of the verb seems to be among the most frequently correct of the verb inflections. Children's speech reflects present time for the most part; and since all present progressives are formed by adding the single inflection -ing, children demonstrate use of the rule most of the time.

The rule they seemed to have for forming past tense was not sufficient to handle irregular verbs. Evidently the children use the rule that past tense is formed by adding /-d/ to the present.

The comparative and superlative forms of the adjective were the most difficult for these children. Unless they were given both the adjective and its comparative, they tended not to give the correct superlative inflection.

On the basis of the information from this test Berko found the following order of development of the selections, although there was a great deal of variation both as they were used by individual children and as applied to individual items on the test:

1. Present progressive
2. Possessive form of the noun
3. Plurals
4. Past tense
5. Comparative-superlative forms of the adjective

Pictures to illustrate these morphologic rules are not available commercially, but a set can be constructed from the information provided in the author's report. The list of the tested structures and related information are given in Appendix E at the end of this chapter. Others (54) have used the same items to study the responses of other groups of children. This test can be a model for constructing detailed evaluations of the various morphologic structures.

Imitation-Comprehension-Production Tasks

The Imitation-Comprehension-Production Tasks were developed by Fraser, Bellugi, and Brown (28). The authors wanted to know the order in which these three processes developed in relation to a set of grammatical problems. The grammatical problems they selected were those that were not mastered completely until children were about 4 years of age. In addition, they used problems capable of being represented pictorially.

The ten grammar problems were set up as contrasts. For instance, if they wanted to study the child's mastery of the singular/plural inflection, they drew pictures that showed one and more than one of an object doing something. They tested his mastery by giving him the problem to solve in each of the three procedures: Imitation (*I*), Comprehension (*C*), and Production (*P*). The ten problems are given together with additional information in Table 4.7; further information about the tasks is presented in Appendix F at the end of this chapter.

Fraser et al. constructed six pairs of utterances for each of the ten problems—two pairs to be used for the *I*, two for the *C*, and two for the *P* procedure. The utterances for each grammatical contrast were equivalent to one another. For the *I* task no pictures were used. For the *C* and *P* tasks colored line drawings illustrate the grammatical contrasts. The utterances and their pictures for the *C* and *P* tasks were divided into two sets—A and B.

The authors used these sets of tasks with a group of 12 children (6 girls and 6 boys) who ranged in age from 37 to 43 months (mean 40 months). The children attended preschool in Cambridge, Massachusetts. Sample selection favored children who would cooperate.

In the *I* task the examiner recited two utterances while the child listened. Then the examiner repeated one of the utterances and the child copied him. The second utterance was then given by the examiner

TABLE 4.7
Task Scores on Grammatical Problems in Order of Increasing Total Difficulty

| | *Tasks* | | | |
Problem	*Imita-tion*	*Compre-hension*	*Produc-tion*	*Total Score*
Affirmative/Negative	18	17	12	47
Singular/Plural of third-person possessive pronoun	23	15	8	46
Subject/Object, in active voice	19	16	11	46
Present progressive tense/Future tense	20	16	6	42
Singular/Plural marked by *is* and *are*	20	12	7	39
Present progressive tense/Past tense	17	13	6	36
Mass noun/Count noun	12	13	1	26
Singular/Plural marked by inflections	14	7	1	22
Subject/Object in passive voice	12	7	2	21
Indirect object/Direct object	11	5	3	19

Source: From Fraser, Bellugi, and Brown, 28.

and the child imitated him. In the C task the examiner showed two pictures, recited the two utterances that matched the two pictures, but didn't indicate which sentence belonged to each picture. Then the examiner repeated one of the utterances and asked the child to point to the correct picture. The second utterance was given and the child was again requested to point to the correct picture. In the P task, the examiner said the two sentences, said them again in reverse order, then pointed to one picture at a time and asked the child to describe it as he had done.

There were 60 problems, 20 for I, 20 for C, and 20 for P. In the I and P tasks a child received a point for each correct imitation and each correct production of a grammatical contrast; in the C task he obtained a point for each correct pointing to represent the grammatical contrast. Thus each child could get a score of 60. Since there were 12 children and two items for each grammatical contrast, the highest possible score for each problem was 24.

The study shows first that in nine out of ten problems, imitation precedes comprehension, and in all ten production appears last. These 3-year-olds tended to have the least difficulty in imitating the spoken grammatical contrasts. Yet they apparently comprehended only some of the contrasts, and they could produce even fewer of them.

No child had a perfect score for any of the three tasks. The range was 7 to 18 on the I task, 3 to 17 on C, and 9 to 12 on P. Two children had identical I and C scores, but all the others had scores that showed a decrement as they moved from the I to the C to the P tasks.

There was a range of difficulty among the ten grammatical contrasts, as shown in Table 4.7. The easiest problem was the affirmative/negative contrast, if we look at the total scores. The most difficult was the indirect object/direct object.

Even though Fraser et al. were not concerned with clinical problems, the rationale they deleveped and the procedures they used have had considerable influence on speech pathologists. They provided a model for testing aspects of morphology and syntax, and their work has raised important questions about the role of imitation as a testing procedure for measuring a child's rules of grammatical structures.

Northwestern Syntax Screening Test

The Northwestern Syntax Screening Test (NSST) (38) was developed as a screening device to evaluate the comprehension and use of syntax of young children. The ideas for the test were generated by the earlier work of Brown and his students on the order in which imitation, comprehension, and production figured in the development of a child's grammar. Lee's students (37) worked out this test as part of independent projects she directed. The section on imitation was dropped in order to shorten the test.

The test consists of 20 sentence pairs that a child identifies with corresponding pictures as a measure of comprehension; and a similar set of 20 sentence pairs that the child produces as responses to pictures. The following grammatical structures are included in both sections of the test, although the contentives are different in the two sections:

Subject-verb agreement	Negative
Prepositions	Possessive
Pronouns	Passive
Question/statement contrasts	Indefinite pronoun
Verb tenses	Grammatical confusions
Wh-questions	Singular/plural contrasts

These items are arranged on the two sections of the test in order of increasing difficulty. The order is different for the two sections.

To administer the comprehension portion the examiner shows a page with four black and white line drawings and says: *"I'm going to tell you about these pictures. When I'm done, you show me the right picture."* The examiner shows page one and reads the sentences in the order they are given on the form. Then he repeats the asterisked sentence and the child points to the correct picture. The examiner does the same with the other sentence. Then he continues with page two, following the same format.

For the expressive section the examiner says: *"I will tell you about these. When I am done, you copy me. Say just what I say."* The examiner shows page one, which has two pictures, and says the sentences in the order of their appearance on the form. Then he points to the asterisked one and asks: *Now what's this picture?* After the child has replied, the examiner asks the same question for the nonasterisked sentence.

This test has been devised for children between 3 and 8 years of age. Scores obtained on 344 children have been arranged to show the scores for the 90th, 75th, 50th, 25th, and 10th percentiles for each six-month age group. A clinician can compare a child's performance with that of others of his age and determine whether he needs a more comprehensive test of his grammatical structures. Lee suggests that children who fall two standard deviations below the mean for their age group should be studied further.

When large numbers of children are to be screened, Lee suggests that when a child reaches a receptive or an expressive score that places him in the 10th percentile for his age, the test can be terminated. You may wish to select a different cutoff point depending upon the purpose of the screening.

This is a useful test for clinicians. Follow the directions carefully for both administration and scoring. Otherwise, the latter can be subjective. Although some children can complete the test in 15 minutes, we have found that many young children in day care centers require a longer time, usually in two sittings, and some fail to understand the tasks.

Concept-Comprehension-Use Tasks

No test has been standardized to determine whether knowledge of the concept related to an inflection precedes comprehension and use of the inflection. However, Eyre (24) has developed a series of tasks to see in what order and at what age the basic concepts, the understanding, and the use of five inflections were appearing. She hypothesized that the concept of numbers would be basic to the plural inflections, the concept of time placement would be necessary for verb tenses, and discrimination of differences would be basic to the adjective forms of comparative and superlative.

Three concepts were tested both receptively and expressively. For instance, for number identification the child has six blocks placed in front of him and the examiner asks him to give her one, two, or three of them. The expressive aspect of that same concept involves the examiner's picking up one, two, or three blocks in random order and asking the child: *How many blocks do I have?* For same-different concepts the examiner places three objects in front of the child; she hands him one of the three and asks him to give her *one like the one I gave you.* The expressive section requires the child to tell the examiner whether a pair of items he was given are the same or different. The time tasks involve placing actions dealing with dressing and eating activities in time. In the dressing sequence the examiner places three pictures in front of the child and says: *This boy just got up and he's getting dressed. Show me which of these things he does first. What does he do next? Which does he do last?* For the expressive half the child is asked: *Tell me when each of these happens.* Situations such as learning to walk, getting a job, going to college, were presented to him. If he failed to respond or made an irrelevant response, a prompt such as the following was used: *When you were a baby, now or when you get big?*

For each of the five inflections—plurals, present progressive and past tenses, and comparative and superlative forms of the adjectives—eight tasks were designed to measure understanding and eight for using each. For example, the examiner would give the child a statement such as *All of these candles are tall. Point to the one that's tallest.* Appropriate items from the Grammatic Closure subtest of the Illinois Test of Psycholinguistic Abilities (35) plus others following the same principles were used for measuring the use of the inflections. All the items and the answers are given in Appendix G at the end of this chapter.

On the basis of the limited testing of children 2 through 5 years of age we can say that the concept underlying an inflection is appearing concurrently or prior to the comprehension of the inflection, and that the use of the inflection comes either at the same time or following the comprehension of the inflection. Clinical hunches based on observations of children would also support this relationship. We need more comprehensive work, however, that will examine not only these relationships but others in order that the clinician will know whether lack of use of an inflection is due to lack of the necessary concept or to inadequate learning of an inflection.

SCREENING TESTS AND SCALES

We have few standardized tests that tap the early vocal and verbal skills of children from birth to about 2½ years of age. However, with current interest in "high-risk" babies several groups have used rating scales, interview techniques with the parents, or selected evaluation items in the clinic, home, or physician's office (47). The items cover a wide range of expressive and receptive skills. Some require a vocal or a verbal response, while others involve pointing or some other motor act.

Most authors of these measures have taken items from other tests and incorporated them within their scale. Reliability and validity data are either limited or nonexistent.

The Early Language Assessment Scale (29) uses the early signs of communication familiar to all of us. The clinician obtains descriptive information about crying, laughing, smiling, babbling, responses to noises and the human voice, word imitation, and vocabulary items that are learned and used during the child's early years. Directions for providing credit for each item are explained in the manual. However, the question of what constitutes normal, usual smiling or crying is not easy to answer. We expect newborns to cry a great deal, but we don't expect the same behavior in the 1-year-old. For a firstborn child the mother may not know what is "normal" crying or babbling, and until we can provide adequate guidelines, it is difficult to use these types of items.

The *Preschool Language Scale* (69), developed in 1969 for children 2 through 7 years old, has three sections; one deals with auditory comprehension, a second with verbal ability, and the third with articulation. Neither reliability nor validity data are provided.

The auditory comprehension section has a total of 40 items, each requiring only a pointing response. For instance, an item at the 18-month level is the following: *Show me the dolly's hair, mouth, eyes, feet.* Items for children 7 years of age include ones like the following: You show him Picture No. 17 which has the numbers 5, 10, 15, 20, 25, and 50 printed on it plus the numbers in sequence from 1 through 9; in addition, you show him a dime, nickel, quarter, and half-dollar. You say to the child, *Look at this money. Can you tell me how many pennies are in a dime, nickel, quarter, half-dollar?* The child may point to a written representation of the correct number or he may verbalize the correct answer.

The verbal ability checklist starts with items for children at the 18-month level and continues in six-month increments to age 7 years. You can obtain information about one-half of the items for the 18-month and 24-month levels from parental reports or by observing the child. Item 1 in the 18-month level requires that the child use ten words. We don't know whether those are words that everyone in his environment can understand nor how close they are to adult production, nor whether these words have specific meaning to the child. Item 3 in the same age range can likewise be answered through interviewing the parents: does the child ask for simple needs? Items at the two-year level provide information about the child's use of pronouns and his own name. From the 30-month level on up to 7 years, much of the verbal ability is measured as a result either of repetition of what the clinician says or questions that can be answered with single-word responses. Some items like the following require that you write down everything the child says: you ask him to tell you about pets or about his brothers or sisters or baby. Presumably the child is conversing in sentences at this point but he may not be.

Included in the articulation section are items that deal with production of phonemes. The major phonemes are presented by the clinician and the model is imitated by the child. At age 7 he is expected to repeat sentences like the following: *Space ships race around the earth* or *Alligators never brush their teeth.* The first sentence is such a tongue twister that the child may miss several phonemes. Many of the phonemes are presented within the developmental order determined by Templin (*63*). However, others do not follow developmental learning sequence.

Although this Preschool Language Scale is used widely by paraprofessionals with little or no training in speech and language, it does not provide adequate information about either language comprehension or use. For the most part, the items on a scale such as the Gesell and those from the Stanford-Binet do not have item validity. They have been set up to be presented at certain age levels within a pattern of other items.

The revised edition of the *Utah Test of Language Development* (*47*) consists of 51 items selected from various standard sources like the Gesell Scale, the Vineland Social Maturity Scale, the Peabody Picture Vocabulary Test, and the Stanford-Binet. For each test item there is information about the presentation of the item and also about scoring the item plus or minus. Administration of the test requires the manual of instructions, a set of plates, and some miniature items. Both the plates and the toys are fragile. The plates themselves have many pictures on each of them, many more than are suitable for young children. Several pictures are confusing.

The language age equivalents range from 9 months to 16 years. However, most of the items are at the preschool level. Therefore, it may be of most value for preschool-age children, particularly if we use it as a screening instrument and recognize that it has the same limitations as other tests which are compilations of items from other sources.

The *Houston Test for Language Development* (19) was developed in two parts: Part I for children 6 to 36 months of age, Part II for those between 3 and 6 years. Part I stresses general developmental items, such as social-motor, vocal, and receptive. Since a child can get a point for a single response, such as a random production of a back vowel, the total score can be spuriously high and inappropriate.

Part II has sections on vocabulary, identification of body parts and gestures, counting, geometric designs, and drawings. It also provides for a language sample of ten responses. The nature of the items is such that a child can give primarily one-word responses to the majority of the items. Scoring of the language sample is also gross.

These two forms were standardized on small samples of white children in Houston, Texas, 113 for Part I and 100 for Part II. There are no validity studies and only one limited report on the test-retest reliability of Part I. Many subjective judgments must be made by the clinician who administers this test; as a result its value either as a measure of current or predictive performance is questionable.

There are situations in which it is not possible to obtain an adequate language evaluation for a child. For the difficult-to-test child there is the *Verbal Language Development Scale* (46), which will provide some information. It uses items dealing with communication from the Vineland Social Maturity Scale plus additional ones. From the scale you can obtain a language age equivalent based on information provided usually by the parents.

The items have been identified as those which can be classified as (1) listening, (2) speaking, (3) reading, and (4) writing. Like the Vineland Social Maturity Scale it provides information about the current skills of an individual. When we administer this scale, we ask the adult what the child is doing now, not what he has done in the past. The author has defined each item in the manual. For instance, Item 10 at the 1–2 year level asks the adult if the child recognizes names of familiar objects. A follow-up question would have to deal with what common objects he recognizes. In order to get credit for that item, the child should be recognizing a dozen or more common objects when he hears their names.

The test has 50 items which provide information about children from 1 month to 16 years of age. Each item can receive a score of one if the informant indicates that the child is routinely performing that item. Where it seems that the child's skill is emerging on a particular item, the child gets one-half point. When the clinician judges that the performance on an item is primarily absent, the child gets zero credit.

In administering this test, you should start one year below the child's chronological age. For instance, if he is 3 years of age, start with the level designated as 2–3 year level. Mecham has not provided information about when we should stop the administration. Presumably we know on the basis of the informant's answers when to stop. This is one of the weaknesses of the scale. Once you have obtained a score on a child, a table in the manual provides the child's equivalent language age.

As with all scales administered through informants, there are problems in interpreting the information we get. The information may be either overevaluating or underevaluating the child's performance. In addition, we do not know whether the items on the scale are the best ones for obtaining a language age. It may be that there are many others that should have been selected. There has been little research relating to the validity of this scale. The author reported a rank order correlation of 0.91 between clinical ratings of language development of normal children and their scores on this scale and a 0.94 correlation between clinician ratings and scores on this measure for a sample of retarded children. Such correlations, based on gross performance, should be interpreted with caution.

For clinicians who wish to obtain information about overall development of a child, the *Denver Developmental Screening Test* (27) is useful. It provides information about the four general categories of social, fine-motor-adaptive, gross motor, and language skills of children. It can be administered to children aged 1 month through 6 years. All items have been taken from other tests.

The recording form has been organized in such a way that the examiner can see at what age each item was passed by 25, 50, 75, and 90 percent of the children upon whom the test was initially standardized. To make it easier for you to see at a glance in which of these four areas the child is average, above, or below, you draw a line through these four areas at his or her chronological age level. Mark each item as either passed or failed. Wherever possible, the authors recommend that you observe the behavior that you are measuring. However, it is possible for a parent to provide this information.

There are 21 items in the language area. Some items deal with basic hearing (responding to a bell, turning to a voice). Others deal with comprehension, such as comprehending three prepositions or adjectives like *cold* and *hungry*. Others require expressive language like defining words and indicating the composition of items like *spoons*.

This scale has been widely used particularly to identify children who are considered high-risk babies. Often it is given by a nurse, medical student, or aide. If the clinician is not the one to administer the language portion, she should at least be aware of the nature of the test and be able to demonstrate procedures for giving, scoring, and interpreting it.

Summary

This section has provided some basic information about the tests and scales available to us. You should evaluate each one to determine its strengths and weaknesses.

There is no expressive vocabulary test in this review. The only ones we would recommend are those that are subtests of the Stanford-Binet or the WISC. Since most speech clinicians are not qualified to administer either of these intelligence tests, we should refer children to clinical psychologists when we want this type of information.

ASSIGNMENTS

1. What evidence do McNeill, Staats, and others provide to support their hypotheses about language acquisition? Check the references on this topic for your answer.
2. Define single-word responses according to various writers. Tape-record the utterances of one or two children between the ages of 12 and 24 months, identify their "words," and determine whether they are contentives or functors.
3. In the above sample indicate which words referred to objects and people in the child's immediate environment. With which ones did the child use gestures? Did any of them refer to items or people who were not present?
4. If you wish to classify words as pivots, what rule do you follow? Put one line under the pivots and two lines under the opens in each of the following.

1.	A coat	2.	A celery
3.	A Becky	4.	A hand
5.	The top	6.	My mommy
7.	That Adam	8.	My stool
9.	Two sock	10.	Two knee
11.	Dirty knee	12.	Little man
13.	Big man	14.	Go car
15.	Daddy car	16.	My car
17.	Adam car	18.	Pretty girl
19.	Nice baby	20.	Sue big

5. Obtain a language sample from a child whose sentence structures are just emerging. Identify on the transcript the noun phrases and the verb phrases.
6. Place one line under each noun phrase and two lines under each verb phrase in the following sentences:

   1. The mommy cat wasn't here.
   2. He wouldn't come down for his milk.

3. No, he runned up a tree—oh—my toe.
4. Look at the man.
5. You remember, that's just like the ocean, isn't it?
6. Now look at the sailboats and the steamboat and the birds and all the animals, the crabs, the seagulls, the lizard.
7. You must remember it, the kind of animal that you don't like to eat it.
8. A lighthouse has a light shining all night to protect the ships so that they won't get off their course and run into a rock.
9. Why did you let her do it?
10. A young girl with pretty blue eyes wants to buy the pink dress she is trying on.

7. For the following language samples find the mean T-units and classify all sentences using Table 4.3 as your guide. Do this for both the clinician and child.

Clinician (age 22)

1.

2. Bill, what have you been doing in class?

4. Where are you going for Mother's Day?

6. Who will you have for company?

8. How many brothers and sisters do you have?

10. What else have you been doing in school?

Child (first grader)

1. My sister has one of these, 'cept hers is little.

3. Work.

5. We're gonna stay at home and have company over—and then go skating.

7. Uh, my aunts and cousins but my aunt's boyfriend won't come.

9. One brother.

11. I play and sometimes I draw pictures.

8. Plan how you want to obtain a child language sample, being sure to utilize the principles for superior language sampling.
9. Obtain a language sample on a 7-year-old child, and analyze your transcript using the Lee procedures.
10. How will you define a language deficit?
11. After reading the test manual for the Peabody Picture Vocabulary Test (22), define the following: basal, ceiling, raw score, percentile rank, forms.
12. Administer all of the tests at least twice to peers who simulate responses of a child. What problems did you face in administering and scoring these?
13. Interview at least two sets of parents of children under 2 years of age to obtain information about children's early vocal and verbal behavior. Discuss the problems you encounter.

14. Select, administer, and score a set of tests and tasks appropriate to a child reported to be nonverbal; to a child whose parents report she rarely talks; to a child with grammatical errors. What information may each of these test batteries give you?
15. According to Siegel, what essentials must one keep in mind when using tests of language? See Siegel, G. M., The use of language tests. *Language, Speech, and Hearing Services in Schools,* 1975, 6:211–217.
16. Discuss the rationale upon which each of the tests and scales is based.

REFERENCES

1. Abt, I. A., Adler, H. A., and Bartelme, P., The relationship between the onset of speech and intelligence. *Journal of the American Medical Association,* 1929, 93:1351–1355.
2. Ammons, R., and Ammons, H., *Full-Range Picture Vocabulary Test.* Missoula, Mont.: Psychological Test Specialists, 1958.
3. Baker, H., and Leland B., *Detroit Tests of Learning Aptitude.* Indianapolis: Bobbs-Merrill, 1935.
4. Berko, J., The child's learning of English morphology. *Word,* 1958, *14:*150–177. Reprinted in Bar-Adon, A., and Leopold, W. F., eds., *Child Language: A Book of Readings.* Englewood Cliffs, N.J.: Prentice-Hall, 1971.
5. Berry, M. D., and Erickson, R. L., Speaking rate: Effects on children's comprehension of normal speech. *Journal of Speech and Hearing Research,* 1973, *16:*367–374.
6. Blasdell, R., and Jensen, P., Stress and word position as determinants of imitation in first-language learners. *Journal of Speech and Hearing Research,* 1970, *13:*193–202.
7. Braine, M. D. S., The ontogeny of English phrase structure. The first phase. *Language,* 1963, *39:*1–13. Reprinted in Bar-Adon, A., and Leopold, W. F., eds., *Child Language: A Book of Readings.* Englewood Cliffs, N.J.: Prentice-Hall, 1971.
8. Brannon, J. B., Jr., Linguistic word classes in the spoken language of normal, hard-of-hearing, and deaf children. *Journal of Speech and Hearing Research,* 1968, *11:*279–287.
9. Brannon, J. B., Jr., and Murry, T., The spoken syntax of normal, hard-of-hearing, and deaf children. *Journal of Speech and Hearing Research,* 1966, *9:*604–610.
10. Brown, R., ed., *Psycholinguistics: Selected Papers.* New York: Free Press, 1970.
11. Brown, R., *A First Language: The Early Stages.* Cambridge, Mass.: Harvard University Press, 1973.
12. Carrow, Sister M. A., The development of auditory comprehension of language structure in children. *Journal of Speech and Hearing Disorders.* 1968, *33:*99–111.

13. Carrow, E., *Screening Test for Auditory Comprehension of Language; Test Manual.* Austin, Tex.: Urban Research Group, 1973.
14. Carrow, E., *Test for Auditory Comprehension of Language: English/Spanish.* Austin, Tex.: Urban Research Group, 1973.
15. Carrow, E., and Mauldin, M., Children's recall of approximations to English. *Journal of Speech and Hearing Research,* 1973, *16*:201–212.
16. Cazden, C., The acquisition of noun and verb inflections. *Child Development,* 1968, *39*:433–448.
17. Chomsky, C., *The Acquisition of Language from Five to Ten.* Cambridge, Mass.: The M.I.T. Press, 1969.
18. Condon, W. S., and Sander, L. W., Neonate movement is synchronized with adult speech: interactional participation and language acquisition. *Science,* 1974, *184*:99–101.
19. Crabtree, M., *Houston Test for Language Development.* Houston, Texas: Box 35152, 1963.
20. Darley, F. L., and Winitz, H., Age of first words: review of research. *Journal of Speech and Hearing Disorders,* 1961, *26*:272–290.
21. Denhoff, E., and Holden, R. H., The significance of delayed development in the diagnosis of cerebral palsy. *Journal of Pediatrics,* 1951, *38*:452–456.
22. Dunn, L. M., *Peabody Picture Vocabulary Test.* Circle Pines, Minn.: American Guidance Service, 1965.
23. Dunn, L. M., Smith, J. O., and Horton, K. B., *Peabody Language Development Kits.* Circle Pines, Minn.: American Guidance Service, 1965.
24. Eyre, N., Concept learning in the acquisition of inflectional endings. Ph.D. dissertation, University of Kansas, 1971.
25. Foster, R., Giddan, J. J., and Stark, J., *Assessment of Children's Language Comprehension* (Plates). Palo Alto, Calif.: Consulting Psychologists Press, 1973.
26. Foster, R., Giddan, J. J., and Stark, J., *Manual for the Assessment of Children's Language Comprehension.* Palo Alto, Calif.: Consulting Psychologists Press, 1972.
27. Frankenburg, W. K., Dodds, J. B., and Fandal, A. W., *Denver Developmental Screening Test Materials.* Denver: University of Colorado Medical Center, 1970.
28. Fraser, C., Bellugi, U., and Brown, R., Control of grammar in imitation, comprehension, and production. *Journal of Verbal Learning and Verbal Behavior,* 1963, *2*:121–135. Reprinted in Brown, R., ed., *Psycholinguistics: Selected Papers.* New York: Free Press, 1970.
29. Honig, A. S., and Caldwell, B. M., *Early Language Assessment Scale.* Syracuse, N.Y.: Syracuse University Children's Center, 1966.
30. Hubbell, R. D., Byrne, M. C., and Stachowiak, J., Aspects of communication in families with young children. *Family Process,* 1974, *13*:215–224.
31. Johnson, W., Darley, F. L., and Spriestersbach, D. C., *Diagnostic Methods in Speech Pathology.* New York: Harper & Row, 1963.
32. Jones, L. V., Goodman, M. F., and Wepman, J. M., The classification of parts of speech for the characterization of aphasia. *Language and Speech,* 1963, *6*:94–107.
33. Jordan, C. M., and Robinson, W. P., The grammar of working and middle

class children using elicited imitations. *Language and Speech,* 1972, 15:122–140.

34. Kessel, F. S., The role of syntax in children's comprehension from ages six to twelve. *Monograph of the Society for Research in Child Development,* 1970, 35, #6, Serial #139.

35. Kirk, S. A., McCarthy, J. J., and Kirk, W. D., *Illinois Test of Psycholinguistic Abilities.* Rev. ed. Urbana: University of Illinois Press, 1969.

36. Leach, E., Interrogation: A model and some implications. *Journal of Speech and Hearing Disorders,* 1972, 37:33–46.

37. Lee, L. L., A screening test for syntax development. *Journal of Speech and Hearing Disorders,* 1970, 35:103–112.

38. Lee, L. L., *Northwestern Syntax Screening Test.* Evanston, Ill.: Northwestern University Press, 1971.

39. Lee, L. L., and Canter, S. M., Developmental sentence scoring: A clinical procedure for estimating syntactic development in children's spontaneous speech. *Journal of Speech and Hearing Disorders,* 1971, 36:315–340.

40. Lee, L. L., *Developmental Sentence Analysis.* Evanston, Ill.: Northwestern University Press, 1974.

41. Loban, W. D., *The Language of Elementary School Children.* Res. Report #1. NCTE Committee on Research. 508 S. 6th Street, Champaign, Ill., 1963.

42. Loban, W. D., *Language Development During the School Years.* Kansas Studies in Education. Lawrence: University of Kansas Publications, 1968.

43. McCarthy, D., The language development of the preschool child. Institute of Child Welfare Monograph Series, No. 4. Minneapolis: University of Minnesota Press, 1930.

44. McNeill, D., *The Acquisition of Language: The Study of Developmental Linguistics.* New York: Harper & Row, 1970.

45. Mead, C. D., The age of walking and talking in relation to general intelligence. *Pedagogical Seminary,* 1913, 20:460–484.

46. Mecham, M. J., *Verbal Language Development Scale.* Circle Pines, Minn.: American Guidance Service, 1958.

47. Mecham, M. J., Jex, J. L., and Jones, J. D., *Utah Test of Language Development.* Rev. ed. Salt Lake City, Utah: Communication Research Association, 1967.

48. Meier, J., *Screening and Assessment of Young Children at Developmental Risk.* Washington, D.C.: DHEW Publications No. (OS) 73–90, March, 1973.

49. Menyuk, P., Syntactic structures in the language of children. *Child Development,* 1963, 34:407–422. Reprinted in Bar-Adon, A., and Leopold, W. F., eds., *Child Language: A Book of Readings.* Englewood Cliffs, N.J.: Prentice-Hall, 1971.

50. Menyuk, P., Comparison of grammar of children with functionally deviant and normal speech. *Journal of Speech and Hearing Research,* 1964, 7:109–121.

51. Menyuk, P., *Sentences Children Use.* Research Monograph No. 52. Cambridge, Mass.: The M.I.T. Press, 1969.

52. Miller, G. A., Magical number seven, plus or minus two. *Psychological Review,* 1956, 63:81–97.

53. Myklebust, H., *The Psychology of Deafness.* New York: Grune & Stratton, 1964.

54. Newfield, M. U., and Schlanger, B. B., The acquisition of English morphology by normal and educable mentally retarded children. *Journal of Speech and Hearing Research,* 1968, *11:*693–706.

55. O'Donnell, R. D., Griffin, W. J., and Norris, R. C., *Syntax of Kindergarten and Elementary School Children: A Transformational Analysis.* Res. Report #8. NCTE Committee on Research, 508 S. 6th Street, Champaign, Ill., 1967.

56. Osgood, C. E., A behavioristic analysis of perception and language as cognitive phenomena. In *Contemporary Approaches to Cognition,* pp. 75–118. Cambridge, Mass.: Harvard University Press, 1957.

57. Schlesinger, I. M., Production of utterances and language acquisition. In Slobin, D. I., ed., *The Ontogenesis of Grammar: A Theoretical Symposium.* New York: Academic Press, 1971.

58. Scholes, R. J., On functors and contentives in children's imitations of word strings. *Journal of Verbal Learning and Verbal Behavior,* 1970, 9:167–170.

59. Sharf, D. J., Some relationships between measures of early language development. *Journal of Speech and Hearing Disorders,* 1972, 37:64–74.

60. Shirley, M. M., *The First Two Years: A Study of 25 Babies.* Vol. II. *Intellectual Development.* Institute of Child Welfare Monograph Series, No. 7. Minneapolis: University of Minnesota Press, 1933.

61. Slobin, D. I., ed., *The Ontogenesis of Grammar.* New York: Academic Press, 1971.

62. Staats, A. W., Linguistic-mentalistic theory vs. an explanatory S-R learning theory of language development. In Slobin, D. I., ed., *The Ontogenesis of Grammar.* New York: Academic Press, 1971.

63. Templin, M., *Certain Language Skills in Children.* Institute of Child Welfare Monograph Series, No. 26. Minneapolis: University of Minnesota Press, 1957.

64. Wechsler, D., *Wechsler Intelligence Scale for Children.* New York: Psychological Corp., 1949.

65. Weiner, P., The cognitive functioning of language deficient children. *Journal of Speech and Hearing Research,* 1969, *12:*53–64.

66. Weiner, P., and Hoock, W. C., The standardization of tests: Criteria and criticisms. *Journal of Speech and Hearing Research,* 1973, *16:*616–626.

67. Weir, R., *Language in the Crib.* The Hague: Mouton, 1962.

68. Wilson, M. E., A standardized method for obtaining a spoken language sample. *Journal of Speech and Hearing Research,* 1969, *12:*95–102.

69. Zimmerman, I. L., Steiner, V. G., and Evatt, R. L., *Preschool Language Manual and Scale.* Columbus, Ohio: Merrill, 1969.

APPENDIX A

Hypothetical Corpus of 30 Sentences Illustrating Developmental Sentence Scoring

	Categories									
	Indefinite Pronoun	Personal Pronoun	Main Verb	Secondary Verb	Negative	Conjunction	Interrogative Reversals	Wh-Question	Sentence Point	Total
1. Boy eat.			—						0	0
2. Boy eat cookie.			—						0	0
3. The boy is eating a cookie.			1						1	2
4. The boys are eating cookies.			2						1	3
5. They ate them.		3,3	2						1	9
6. They didn't eat them.		3,3	6		7				1	20
7. Didn't they eat them?		3,3	6		7		6		1	26
8. Why didn't they eat them?		3,3	6		7		6	7	1	33
9. Why didn't they?		3	inc.		7		6	7	1	24
10. All the cookies were eaten.	3		7						1	11
11. I want to eat some cookies.	3	1	1	2					1	8
12. I want him to eat some cookies.	3	1,2	1	5					1	13
13. I tried to find some cookies.	3	1	2	5					1	12
14. Could you find them?		1,3	6				6		1	17
15. You couldn't find them, could you?		1,3	6		7		6		1	24
16. Nobody knows where to find them.	4	3	2	5		8			1	23
17. Who knows where she keeps them?		3,2	2,2			8		2	1	20
18. I looked but I couldn't find them.		1,1,3	2,6		7	5			1	26
19. I like eating cookies.		1	1	8					1	11
20. Nobody told me that I shouldn't eat them.	4	1,1,3	2,6		7	8			1	33
21. I only ate a few.	7	1	2						1	11

APPENDIX A (continued)

22. Somebody else must have eaten all the rest.	3,3	8		1	15
23. Let's eat some more.	3,3	1	2	1	10
24. Mommy said, "Don't eat those cookies."	3	2,4	4	1	14
25. That isn't what she said.	1	6,2	1,2	5	1	18
26. Him can't have some.	—	4	4	0	8
27. What you eating?	1	—	—	2	0	3
28. Her don't gots any.	7	—	—	—	0	7
29. Mommy find out.	—	—	0	0
30. You want to get spanked?	1	—	7	—	0	8

Total: 409

409/30 = 13.63 DDS

Source: From Lee, *40.*

APPENDIX B
Sentences Used by Menyuk (51)

Transformation	Sentences
1. Passive	1. He got tied up.
2. Negative	2. He isn't a good boy.
3. Question	3. Are you nice?
4. Contraction	4. He'll be good.
5. Inversion	5. Now I have kittens.
6. Relative Question	6. Where are you going?
7. Imperative	7. Don't use my dough.
8. Pronominalization	8. There isn't any more.
9. Separation	9. He took it off.
10. Got	10. I've got a lollipop.
11. Auxiliary Be Placement	11. He is not going to the party.
12. Auxiliary Have Placement	12. I've already been there.
13. Do	13. I did read the book.
14. Possessive	14. I'm writing daddy's name.
15. Reflexive	15. I cut myself.
16. Conjunction	16. Peter is over here and you are over there.
17. Conjunction Deletion	17. I see a red book and a blue book.
18. Conjunction If	18. I'll give it to you if you want it.
19. Conjunction So	19. He saw him so he hit him.
20. Conjunction Because	20. He'll eat the ice cream because he wants to.
21. Pronoun in Conjunction	21. David saw the bicycle and he was happy.
22. Adjective	22. I have a pink dog.
23. Relative Clause	23. I don't know what he's doing.
24. Complement	24. I want to play.
25. Iteration	25. You have to drink milk to grow strong.
26. Nominalization	26. She does the shopping and cooking and baking.
27. Nominal Compound	27. The baby carriage is here.

APPENDIX C
Detroit Tests of Learning Aptitude (3)

Oral Commissions Subtest

Items

1. a. *Show* me the window.
    b. *Stand* up straight.

2. a. *Walk* to the door; *then bring* me that book.
    b. *Walk* to the window; *then put* this book on a chair.

3. a. *Put* this pencil on the table; *then open* the door; *then fold* your hands
        behind you.
    b. *Bring* me that piece of paper; *then close* the door; *then stand* on this
        line.

4. a. *Walk* to the window; *then tap* the floor once with your foot; *then put*
        this penny in my hand; *then tell* me your name.
    b. *Open* the door; *then put* a mark on this paper; *then bring* me that
        book; *then stand* by the window.

Norms

Age Level	Raw Score	Age Level	Raw Score
3-0	2	5-9	10
3-3	2	6-0	11
3-6	3	6-3	12
3-9	4	6-6	13
4-0	4	6-9	14
4-3	5	7-0	15
4-6	6	7-3	16
4-9	6	7-6	17
5-0	7	7-9	18
5-3	8	8-0	19
5-6	9	8-3	20

APPENDIX D
Detroit Tests of Learning Aptitude (3)

Auditory Attention Span for Related Syllables Subtest

1. My doll has pretty hair.
2. We will go for a walk.
3. My dog chases the white cat.
4. Our new car has four red wheels.
5. Henry likes to read his new book.
6. Bring the broom and sweep the front room.
7. The bell on the engine rings loudly.
8. On Sundays all of us go to church.
9. In summer we go North where it is cool.
10. Green leaves come on the trees in early spring.
11. The airplane makes a loud noise when it flies fast.
12. We saw a little fire on the way to school.
13. The sun shone brightly today and it hurt my eyes.
14. The men painted our new house white with dark green blinds.
15. They gave me some pretty shoes for by birthday last month.
16. The art teacher comes to our own school three days a week.
17. Ten persons went to a party where there was lots to eat.
18. Three boys spent a happy day last week on a fishing trip.
19. On Tuesday for lunch we had some fresh bread which our mother baked.
20. Father must buy some new license plates for his car once each year.
21. When the train passes the whistle blows for us to keep off the track.
22. In the summer time the nights are very short and the days are very long.
23. We had a party for Jean last Monday with cake and ice cream to eat.
24. At eight we go to bed and mother reads to us from our story books.
25. Each year when the big circus comes to town Father takes the whole family.
26. Many boys and girls go to the movies on nights at the end of each week.
27. My sister Mary has a pretty new doll which shuts its eyes and goes to sleep.
28. The man who lives next door is a good neighbor and invites us for many rides.
29. Last winter we made a big round snow man and put a little black hat on his head.
30. In my uncle's home there was a soft red carpet on the floor of the living room.
31. The day of the football game the weather was clear but chilly and the wind blew briskly.
32. Because there were a few vacant lots the police roped off our street so that we might be safe.
33. On the Fourth of July my father puts on his army suit and joins his friends on parade.
34. In fair weather and at high tide ships from many nations set sail for their own distant ports.

35. The baseball team from our high school played fifteen games; they lost six but ended in second place.
36. Last night there was a large banquet at the hotel where many people dined and had a pleasant time.
37. Our reading books at school have many fine stories which are short but very full of life and action.
38. In the north country the days are very short in winter and the sun hangs low in the southern sky.
39. China closets filled with all kinds of dainty dishes and cut glass lined the large walls of the dining room.
40. On cold, clear nights hundreds of thousands of twinkling stars shine brightly from their cradles far up in the sky.
41. In the heart of the Congo there are many kinds of beasts which are a nightly terror to the black natives.
42. Down near the bank of the river is an estate from which sound the shouts of happy children hour after hour.
43. Each four years voting takes place which results in many men being placed in office for terms of two years or more.

Detroit Tests of Learning Aptitude

Auditory Attention Span for Related Syllables Subtest

		Norms		
Test Score	*Mental Age*		*Test Score*	*Mental Age*
12–15	3-0		74–75	11-0
16–18	3-3		76	11-3
19–21	3-6		77–78	11-6
22–24	3-9		79	11-9
25–27	4-0		80–81	12-0
28–30	4-3		82	12-3
31–33	4-6		83–84	12-6
34–36	4-9		85	12-9
37–38	5-0		86–87	13-0
39–40	5-3		88	13-3
41–42	5-6		89–90	13-6
43	5-9		91	13-9
44–45	6-0		92–93	14-0
46	6-3		94	14-3
47–48	6-6		95–96	14-6
49	6-9		97	14-9
50–51	7-0		98–99	15-0
52	7-3		100	15-3
53–54	7-6		101–102	15-6
55	7-9		103	15-9
56–57	8-0		104–105	16-0
58	8-3		106	16-3
59–60	8-6		107–108	16-6
61	8-9		109	16-9
62–63	9-0		110–111	17-0
64	9-3		112	17-3
65–66	9-6		113–114	17-6
67	9-9		115	17-9
68–69	10-0		116–117	18-0
70	10-3		118	18-3
71–72	10-6		119–120	18-6
73	10-9		121–122	18-9
			123 up	19-0

APPENDIX E
Berko Test of English Morphological Rules (4)

The following is the order in which the cards are presented. Included is a statement of what was being tested, a description of the card, and the text that was read. Pronunciation is indicated by regular English orthography; a phonemic transcription is included for first occurrences of nonsense words.

1. Plural. One birdlike animal, then two. "This is a wug /wʌg/. Now there is another one. There are two of them. There are two _____."

2. Plural. One bird, then two. "This is a gutch /gʌtʃ/. Now there is another one. There are two of them. There are two _____."

3. Past tense. Man with a steaming pitcher on his head. "This is a man who knows how to spow /spou/. He is spowing. He did the same thing yesterday. What did he do yesterday? Yesterday he _____."

4. Plural. One animal, then two. "This is a kazh /kæz/. Now there is another one. There are two of them. There are two _____."

5. Past tense. Man swinging an object. "This is a man who knows how to rick /rɪk/. He is ricking. He did the same thing yesterday. What did he do yesterday? Yesterday he _____."

6. Diminutive and compounded or derived word. One animal, then a miniscule animal. "This is a wug. This is a very tiny wug. What would you call a very tiny wug? _____. This wug lives in a house. What would you call a house that a wug lives in?" _____.

7. Plural. One animal, then two. "This is a tor /tɔr/. Now there is another one. There are two of them. There are two _____."

8. Derived adjective. Dog covered with irregular green spots. "This is a dog with quirks /kwɚks/ on him. He is all covered with quirks. What kind of dog is he? He is a _____ dog."

9. Plural. One flower, then two. "This is a lun /lʌn/. Now there is another one. There are two of them. There are two _____."

10. Plural. One animal, then two. "This is a niz /nɪz/. Now there is another one. There are two of them. There are two _____."

11. Past tense. Man doing calisthenics. "This is a man who knows how to mot /mɑt/. He is motting. He did the same thing yesterday. What did he do yesterday? Yesterday he _____."

12. Plural. One bird, then two. "This is a cra /krɑ/. Now there is another one. There are two of them. There are two _____."

13. Plural. One animal, then two. "This is a tass /tæs/. Now there is another one. There are two of them. There are two _____."

14. Past tense. Man dangling an object on a string. "This is a man who knows how to bod /bɑd/. He is bodding. He did the same thing yesterday. What did he do yesterday? Yesterday he _____."

15. Third person singular. Man shaking an object. "This is a man who know how to naz /næz/. He is nazzing. He does it every day. Every day he _____."

16. Plural. One insect, then two. "This is a heaf /hif/. Now there is another one. There are two of them. There are two _____."

17. Plural. One glass, then two. "This is a glass. Now there is another one. There are two of them. There are two _____."

18. Past tense. Man exercising. "This is a man who knows how to gling /glɪŋ/. He is glinging. He did the same thing yesterday. What did he do yesterday? Yesterday he _____."

19. Third person singular. Man holding an object. "This is a man who knows how to loodge /ludʒ/. He is loodging. He does it every day. Every day he _____."

20. Past tense. Man standing on the ceiling. "This is a man who knows how to bing /bɪŋ/. He is binging. He did the same thing yesterday. What did he do yesterday? Yesterday he _____."

21. Singular and plural possessive. One animal wearing a hat, then two wearing hats. "This is a niz who owns a hat. Whose hat is it? It is the _____ hat. Now there are two nizzes. They both own hats. Whose hats are they? They are the _____ hats."

22. Past tense. A bell. "This is a bell that can ring. It is ringing. It did the same thing yesterday. What did it do yesterday? Yesterday it _____."

23. Singular and plural possessive. One animal wearing a hat, then two. "This is a wug who owns a hat. Whose hat is it? It is the _____ hat. Now there are two wugs. They both own hats. Whose hats are they? They are the _____ hats."

24. Comparative and superlative of the adjective. A dog with a few spots, one with several, and one with a great number. "This dog has quirks on him. This dog has more quirks on him. And this dog has even more quirks on him. This dog is quirky. This dog is _____. And this dog is the _____."

25. Progressive and derived agentive or compound. Man balancing a ball on his nose. "This is a man who knows how to zib /zɪb/. What is he doing? He is _____. What would you call a man whose job is to zib?" _____.

26. Past tense. An ice cube, then a puddle of water. "This is an ice cube. Ice melts. It is melting. Now it is all gone. What happened to it? It _____."

27. Singular and plural possessive. One animal wearing a hat, then two. "This is a bik /bɪk/ who owns a hat. Whose hat is it? It is the _____ hat. Now there are two biks. They both own hats. Whose hats are they? They are the _____ hats."

28. Compound words. The child was asked why he thought the following were so named. No pictures were used for these items. The purpose is to see if the child is aware of the separate morphemes in each word.

1. afternoon
2. airplane
3. birthday
4. breakfast
5. blackboard
6. fireplace
7. football
8. handkerchief
9. holiday
10. merry-go-round
11. newspaper
12. sunshine
13. Thanksgiving
14. Friday

Answer sheet for the Berko Test:

1. wugz
2. gutchez
3. spowd
4. kazzez
5. rickt
6. wuggy, wug house
7. torz
8. quirky
9. lunz
10. nizzez
11. motted
12. craz
13. tassez
14. bodded
15. nazzd
16. heavz or heafs
17. glassez
18. glingd
19. loodzez
20. bingd
21. niz'z, nizzez'
22. rang
23. wug'z, wugz'
24. quirkier, quirkiest
25. zibbing, zibber
26. melted
27. bik's, biks'

APPENDIX F
Imitation-Comprehension-Production Tasks (28)

Following are the ten grammatical contrasts and the accompanying utterances for each in Set A. The ten contrasts and the scoring will be the same for all three tasks (I, C, and P), but the examples of the contrasts differ from Set A to B and in the set used for the Imitation Task.

For a child's response to be considered correct, it must include the criteria given for each grammatical contrast.

1. Contrast: Mass noun/Count noun.
   Utterances: Some *mog*/A *dap*.
              Some *pim*/A *ked*.
   Correct: Some/A + any nonsense syllables or appropriate English words.

2. Contrast: Singular/Plural, marked by inflections.
   Utterances: The boy draws/The boys draw.
              The kitten plays/The kittens play.
   Correct: Noun without inflection and verb with -*s*/Noun with -*s* and verb without inflection.

3. Contrast: Singular/Plural, marked by *is* and *are*.
   Utterances: The deer is running/The deer are running.
              The sheep is eating/The sheep are eating.
   Correct: *Is/Are*.

4. Contrast: Present progressive tense/Past tense.
   Utterances: The paint is spilling/The paint spilled.
              The boy is jumping/The boy jumped.
   Correct: *Is* and verb with -*ing*/No auxiliary and verb with -*d*.

5. Contrast: Present progressive tense/Future tense.
   Utterances: The girl is drinking/The girl will drink.
              The baby is climbing/The baby will climb.
   Correct: *Is* and verb with -*ing*/*Will* and verb without inflection.

6. Contrast: Affirmative/Negative
   Utterances: The girl is cooking/The girl is not cooking.
              The boy is sitting/The boy is not sitting.
   Correct: Absence of *not*/Presence of *not* + some assertion.

7. Contrast: Singular/Plural, of third-person possessive pronouns.
   Utterances: His wagon/Their wagon.
              Her dog/Their dog.
   Correct: *His* or *her/Their*.

8. Contrast: Subject/Object, in the active voice.
   Utterances: The train bumps the car/The car bumps the train.
              The mommy kisses the daddy/The daddy kisses the mommy.

Correct: Noun₁ + active form of verb + noun₂/Noun₂ + active form of verb + noun₁.

9. Contrast: Subject/Object, in the passive voice.
   Utterances: The car is bumped by the train/The train is bumped by the car.
                The daddy is kissed by the mommy/The mommy is kissed by the daddy.
   Correct: Noun₁ + verb + -*d* + by + noun₂/Noun₂ + verb + -*d* + by + Noun₁.

10. Contrast: Indirect object/Direct object.
    Utterances: The girl shows the cat the dog/The girl shows the dog the cat.
                 The boy brings the fish the bird/The boy brings the bird the fish.
    Correct: Any verb + noun₁ + noun₂/Any verb + noun₂ + noun₁.

APPENDIX G
Test Items for Inflection Tests (24)

I. *Receptive Inflection Test*

Instructions: I am going to show you some pages with pictures on them. Each time I show you a page, I'll ask you to point to *one* of the pictures on the page. Listen carefully and point only to the one picture that I say.

Demonstration 1: Point to the boy who's sitting.
Demonstration 2: Point to the mouth that's closed.

1. All of these people are old. Point to the one that's oldest.
2. Point to the coffee that's been poured.
3. Point to the picture of clocks.
4. Both of these ladies are happy. Point to the one that's happier.
5. Point to the picture of glasses.
6. Point to the one who's swinging.
7. Both of these snowmen are fat. Point to the one that's fatter.
8. Point to the person who's throwing.
9. All of these candles are tall. Point to the one that's tallest.
10. All of these seats are big. Point to the one that's biggest.
11. Point to the boy who's sleeping.
12. Both of these ladies have long hair. Point to the hair that's longer.
13. Point to the picture of irons.
14. Point to the boys who finished their sodas.
15. Point to the boy who raised his hands.
16. All of these people are mad. Point to the one who's maddest.
17. All of these men have full arms. Point to the arms that are fullest.
18. Point to the picture of pictures.
19. Both of these people are ugly. Point to the one who's uglier.
20. Point to the house that burned.
21. Point to the dog that's resting.
22. Point to the boy who's carrying bottles.
23. Both of these ladies have curly hair. Point to the hair that's curlier.
24. All of these pans are small. Point to the one that's smallest.
25. Point to the picture of lamps.
26. Point to the man that fished.
27. Point to the room that has been cleaned.
28. Point to the picture of chair.
29. All of these fish are thin. Point to the one that's thinnest.
30. Both of these boys have dark hair. Point to the hair that's darker.
31. Point to the one who's sliding.
32. Point to the dog that knocked over the house.
33. Point to the man who's painting.
34. All of these rockets are short. Point to the one that's shortest.
35. Both of these people are busy. Point to the one who's busier.
36. Point to the one that pounded.
37. Both of these bowls are dirty. Point to the one that's dirtier.
38. Point to the picture of TV set.

39. Point to the duck that's swimming.
40. Point to the picture of cups.

II. *Expressive Inflection Test*

Instructions, demonstration items, and items 1 to 22 on this test can be found in the Examiner's Manual for the Illinois Test of Psycholinguistic Abilities (35).

23. Here is a hat. Here are two _____.
24. These Indians like to dance. Here they are _____.
25. Mother is cooking dinner. Here the dinner has been _____.
26. This shelf is not high. This shelf is high. This shelf is even _____.
27. And this shelf is the very _____.
28. This bear likes to sleep. Here he is _____.
29. This boy is not sad. This boy is sad. This boy is even _____.
30. And this boy is the very _____.
31. This fox likes to sit. Here he is _____.
32. Here is a ball. Here are two _____.
33. This girl likes to paint pictures. Here are some pictures that she _____.
34. This boy likes to kick the ball. Here is the ball that he _____.
35. This boy likes to fly his kite. Here he is _____.
36. Here is a pan. Here are two _____.
37. This girl likes to row the boat. Here she is _____.
38. This mouse likes to scare the cat. Here is the cat that he _____.
39. This boy likes to run. Here he is _____.
40. Here is a spoon. Here are two _____.
41. This string is not short. This string is short. This string is even _____.
42. And this string is the very _____.
43. This girl is not close. This girl is close. This girl is even _____.
44. And this girl is the very _____.
45. This lady is boiling meat. Here is the meat that she _____.
46. This girl likes to ride the horse. Here she is _____.
47. This animal is not heavy. This animal is heavy. This animal is even _____.
48. And this animal is the very _____.
49. Here is a ring. Here are two _____.
50. This swimming suit is not warm. This coat is warm. This coat is even _____.
51. And this coat is the very _____.
52. Grandmother likes to receive letters. Here are some letters she _____.

53. Here is a shoe. Here are two _____.
54. This house is not fancy. This house is fancy. This house is even

_____.

55. And this house is the very _____.

Test Items for Related Concepts (24)

1. Number Identification I (Expressive): How many blocks do I have?

1. (2) _____	4. (3) _____	7. (3) _____
2. (3) _____	5. (1) _____	8. (1) _____
3. (1) _____	6. (2) _____	9. (2) _____

2. Number Identification II (Receptive): Give me _____ blocks.

1. (3) _____	4. (1) _____	7. (3) _____
2. (2) _____	5. (3) _____	8. (2) _____
3. (1) _____	6. (2) _____	9. (1) _____

3. Same and Different Test I (Expressive): Are these the same or different? How are they different (the same)?

1. (toothpaste-thread D) _____	6. (rings S) _____
2. (spoons S)	7. (plates D) _____
3. (earrings D)	8. (pins D) _____
4. (soap S)	9. (bandaids D) _____
5. (blocks D) _____	10. (balloons D) _____

4. Same and Different Test II (Receptive): I gave you one. Now, you give me one like the one I gave you.

1. Pencil: pencil   pen   ruler
2. Straight pin: nail   thumbtack   straight pin
3. Circle: circle   square   triangle
4. Rectangle: square   rectangle   triangle
5. Big circle: little circle   big circle   square
6. Little square: little square   big square   medium square
7. Red sucker: red sucker   green sucker   orange sucker
8. Blue balloon: pink balloon   blue balloon   green balloon
9. Thin paper: thin paper   thick paper   medium paper
10. String: twine   thread   string

5. Time Placement Test I (Receptive): Which of these things does (he, she) do first? Which does (he, she) do next? Which does (he, she) do last?

	1st choice	2nd choice	3rd choice
1. This boy just woke up, and he's getting dressed. (123)	_____	_____	_____
2. This girl is eating. (231)	_____	_____	_____
3. This man is washing the car. (321)	_____	_____	_____
4. This woman is shopping. (312)	_____	_____	_____
5. This boy is swimming. (213)	_____	_____	_____

6. This boy is climbing the stairs. (132)

_____ _____ _____

7. This girl is unwrapping a present. (231)

_____ _____ _____

8. This boy is building a tower. (312)

_____ _____ _____

9. This mother is doing the dishes. (213)

_____ _____ _____

10. This girl is drawing a picture. (321)

_____ _____ _____

6. Time Placement Test II (Expressive): Tell me when each of these happens. Prompt: When you were a baby, now, or when you get big?

1. Going to college _____
2. Being born _____
3. Talking to me _____
4. Wearing _____ (name something child is wearing) _____
5. Getting a job _____
6. Being a mommy (daddy) _____
7. Learning to walk _____
8. Being a girl (boy) _____
9. Wearing diapers _____
10. Driving a car _____

Answer Sheet (24)

Inflection Tests:

1. Receptive Inflection Test

Demo 1-1 _____
Demo 2-3 _____

1. (super-1) _____	15. (past-1) _____	28. (pl-2) _____
2. (past-2) _____	16. (super-1) _____	29. (super-1) _____
3. (pl-3) _____	17. (super-2) _____	30. (comp-2) _____
4. (comp-1) _____	18. (pl-1) _____	31. (prog-3) _____
5. (pl-1) _____	19. (comp-1) _____	32. (past-2) _____
6. (prog-3) _____	20. (past-2) _____	33. (prog-2) _____
7. (comp-2) _____	21. (prog-1) _____	34. (super-3) _____
8. (prog-1) _____	22. (prog-1) _____	35. (comp-1) _____
9. (super-1) _____	23. (comp-1) _____	36. (past-2) _____
10. (super-3) _____	24. (super-3) _____	37. (comp-2) _____
11. (prog-3) _____	25. (pl-3) _____	38. (pl-2) _____
12. (comp-2) _____	26. (past-1) _____	39. (prog-3) _____
13. (pl-2) _____	27. (past-3) _____	40. (pl-3) _____
14. (past-3) _____		

2. Modified Grammatic Closure Subtest (ITPA)

1. (1-dogs)	_____	29. (sadder)	_____
2. (4-barking)	_____	30. (saddest)	_____
3. (5-dresses)	_____	31. (sitting)	_____
4. (6-opened)	_____	32. (balls)	_____
5. (9-wrote)	_____	33. (painted)	_____
6. (15-bigger)	_____	34. (kicked)	_____
7. (16-biggest)	_____	35. (flying)	_____
8. (17-men)	_____	36. (pans)	_____
9. (18-planted)	_____	37. (rowing)	_____
10. (20-more)	_____	38. (scared)	_____
11. (21-most)	_____	39. (running)	_____
12. (22-feet)	_____	40. (spoons)	_____
13. (23-sheep)	_____	41. (shorter)	_____
14. (24-better)	_____	42. (shortest)	_____
15. (25-best)	_____	43. (closer)	_____
16. (26-hung)	_____	44. (closest)	_____
17. (27-stole)	_____	45. (boiled)	_____
18. (28-women)	_____	46. (riding)	_____
19. (30-leaves)	_____	47. (heavier)	_____
20. (31-children)	_____	48. (heaviest)	_____
21. (32-mice)	_____	49. (rings)	_____
22. (33-themselves)	_____	50. (warmer)	_____
23. (hats)	_____	51. (warmest)	_____
24. (dancing)	_____	52. (received)	_____
25. (cooked)	_____	53. (shoes)	_____
26. (higher)	_____	54. (fancier)	_____
27. (highest)	_____	55. (fanciest)	_____
28. (sleeping)	_____		

5

APPRAISAL OF ACQUIRED LANGUAGE DISORDERS

Frederic L. Darley

Just as the clinician must be equipped to assess the status of a child's language acquisition and to appraise specific language skills, so the clinician must be equipped to appraise the dissolution of the language function. With the passage of years insidious or sudden deterioration of function may occur. Sometimes the impairment of function that we observe is language-specific—that is, the dysfunction is restricted to language processing or at least it is disproportionate to impairment discernible in other intellective functions. At other times the language dysfunction is embedded in a more comprehensive disorder, and the patterns of disorder may suggest any of several ongoing pathologic processes.

The clinician who is asked to appraise the communication status of a patient with a suspected language impairment is interested, to put it in general terms, in the patient's ability to process the arbitrary language code which we use for communication. How well can the patient decode (interpret) the language that he hears and reads? How well can he encode (formulate and express) his ideas into the symbol system in order to share those ideas with others? The clinician needs to know whether there has been a breakdown in what has been called the central language process (4), also known as symbolic formulation.

According to Brown's model of the central language process (4), the learning and the efficient use of language involve four components: (1) a body of words, the vocabulary or lexicon, which we acquire as children and which continues to grow in size as well as in richness and depth of meaning throughout our lives; (2) syntax, a set of rules whose mastery allows us to put words together properly and produce efficient sentences; (3) auditory retention span of sufficient duration to allow us to process what we hear; and (4) channel selection, the ability to arrange competing inputs or alternative outputs in some hierarchical order, and the selection of the appropriate signal to attend to or the verbal response to emit. In *aphasia* all of these components of the central language process are impaired. We define aphasia as a multimodality reduction in the capacity of a patient to process the language code and associate old learning with new stimuli. We do not include within aphasia single-modality impairments, for in aphasia the problem is not modality-bound; it implicates the central integrative process. Furthermore, the language dysfunction is disproportionate to other observed impairments in cognitive processes.

In some patients communication is specifically impaired because of single-modality input or output problems of nonsymbolic nature. Their behavior indicates interruption of input along one modality (for example, auditory) whereas input along another modality (for example, visual) is uninterrupted. Likewise, some patients demonstrate inability to perform in one modality (for example, speaking) but show intact performance in another modality (for example, writing). If the person is stimulated or allowed to respond through an alternative modality, he or she may perform well. This type of modality-bound input or output difficulty has been called by Wepman et al. (25, 26) a transmissive type of problem to differentiate it from the central problem of symbolic formulation demonstrated by aphasic patients, who have difficulty understanding and formulating language no matter which input and output modalities are used. The patient with a transmissive problem will demonstrate an agnosia or an apraxia, whereas the patient with the central problem will demonstrate an aphasia. *Agnosia* is defined as failure to recognize the import of sensory input. *Apraxia* refers to an inability to perform a skilled voluntary act in spite of the fact that there is no impairment of muscular control.

Still other patients do not display a language-specific disorder either of the central language process (aphasia) or of a specific input or output language modality (agnosia or apraxia) but demonstrate a more comprehensive "thinking" disorder one aspect of which may be aberrant language function. In these patients we observe faulty application of language in problem solving and social interaction. These more comprehensive disorders which implicate language together with other cognitive processes include senile and presenile dementia, confusion, and various psychiatric disorders.

In order to get a handle on a patient's ability to cope with language and to determine whether the central language process or specific input and output modalities are impaired, we ordinarily evaluate a spectrum of language behavior. We want to know how efficiently the patient recognizes, retains, and comprehends various kinds of input—auditory, visual, and tactile; how well he integrates and interprets this input and formulates some sort of response to it; and how well he produces various types of output—oral, graphic, and gestural—both imitatively and spontaneously. The spectrum of possible stimuli and responses is vast, encompassing several levels of complexity. The responses to be evaluated are multifaceted and must be interpreted with regard to such characteristics as completeness, promptness, accuracy, and efficiency. To evaluate comprehensively every conceivable type of language content and structure with every possible mode of input coupled with every possible mode of output would tax one's ingenuity and result in a test battery so lengthy that no patient could bear it. A sampling procedure is necessary. The sample must be restricted enough to permit evaluation within the practical time limits of a clinicial situation but comprehensive enough to reveal significant deficits in communicative behavior and allow differential diagnosis of aphasia from nonaphasic language disorders.

CONSIDERATIONS IN SELECTION AND ADMINISTRATION OF LANGUAGE TESTS

You are free to develop for your individual use a battery of language-sampling procedures which answer your questions about a patient's degree of language intactness or impairment, or you may draw upon a pool of published tests. A good many tests are commercially available today, many of them identified as tests of aphasia, others designated more generally as tests of language or communication, which permit fairly precise description of a patient's skills in handling the symbol system. As you study this array of tests, you can see that the materials used and the procedures recommended tend to be rather similar although the theories behind the tests vary considerably and the classification systems of patterns of impairment derived from the results of the administration vary considerably. In this textbook we do not propose to counsel you to develop any certain type of language battery, nor do we advocate the use of specific commercially available tests. You will want to learn the usefulness and the limitations of many of the tests listed at the end of this chapter, and you may well be motivated to make certain modifications or additions to such a ready-made battery with some creations of your own. Our intent is to alert you to the problems inherent in language testing and to suggest certain considerations that you should keep in mind when you choose a test, administer it, interpret the results, and use those results in diagnostic decisions and therapy planning.

1. The Purposes of Language Testing

Language evaluation may be accomplished with more than one purpose in mind, and scrutiny of the tests available will reveal that test makers had different purposes in mind when they designed their instruments. Exploration of language impairment was originally motivated by interest in brain mechanisms in the search for anatomic correlates of behavior. Some tests today still have information of this sort as their primary goal. For example, the designers of the Boston Diagnostic Aphasia Examination have indicated that the design of their test is "based on the observation that various components of language may be selectively damaged by aphasia and that this selectivity is a clue to: (1) the anatomical organization of language in the brain, (2) the localization of the causative lesion, and (3) the functional interactions of various parts of the language system" (9, p. 2). Other tests have less to do with differentiating patients from one another and deriving localization information but are geared more to provide clinical information (7, 14, 18, 21, 24). Some attempt to provide a realistic view of how the patient uses language in confronting the problems of everyday life; the Functional Communication Profile (15) is such a measuring instrument.

Test makers have generally not gone through a validation step, that is, demonstrating that results on their tests significantly relate to outside measurements of the patient's adequacy in social communication. Their goals have primarily been to describe patterns of ability and disability on the basis of which predictions of recovery can be made and plans for meaningful therapy can be based. For example, the Minnesota Test for Differential Diagnosis of Aphasia has been used to assign patients to any of several classifications, with each of which a prognosis of outcome has been developed (19). The Porch Index of Communicative Ability (PICA) (14) allows a contrast between the patient's language behavior on his highest nine subtests and his language behavior on his lowest nine subtests and the prediction of what level he will ultimately reach. Both of these tests provide the kind of information that suggests to the clinician where he might start in therapy in terms of relative levels of difficulty within the various language tasks.

Some tests are particularly useful in providing a discrete, quantified representation of the patient's performance in designated language areas. One thus obtains a numerical baseline, and one can trace change with the passage of time, the application of therapy, the use of adjuncts to therapy such as drugs, et cetera. Such tests include the Peabody Picture Vocabulary Test (6), the Token Test (5), the Word Fluency Test (3), and the PICA (14).

No language test can accomplish all possible purposes of language testing. Selection of components for the battery you will use with given patients will be determined by the information you most need to know and the determination of the instruments that best help you accomplish this purpose.

2. Comprehensiveness of Language Evaluation

One can arrive at serious misconceptions about a patient's language performance by sampling it too sketchily. All too often medical practitioners base their impressions of a patient's language facility upon automatic responses to everyday questions such as "How are you?" and "How do you feel?" and to such inevitably repetitious situation stimuli as "Close your eyes," "Stick out your tongue," "Wiggle your toes." Incomplete examinations frequently lead the unwary examiner to the conclusion that the patient "understands everything." Schuell has said that "somehow or other this is something people always say about aphasic patients, particularly when they have no speech and even when they cannot comprehend instructions as simple as 'Put the spoon in the cup.' . . . Sometimes when the patient makes an obvious error the speaking person ascribes it to his own difficulty in communicating with the aphasic patient. This is a very curious phenomenon" (19, p. 21).

Another kind of artifact may emerge from language testing unless you guard against it. Your theoretical bias may lead you to expect certain kinds of problems and indeed self-fulfillingly confirm your prophecy that such problems exist. If an examiner is looking for evidence of the classical category of anomia, he can test the patient's recognition and use of nouns, discover a difficulty, and designate it "anomia" or "nominal aphasia," overlooking the fact that the patient has equal trouble with other parts of speech. If a clinician is looking for errors in syntax, she can find them and designate the problem "syntactical aphasia" or "agrammatism," glossing over the fact that the patient also has trouble with lexical items. A person may focus on expressive difficulties to a degree that he overlooks receptive difficulties.

You should test not only for what you are especially interested in but for everything that is important. You should set out not to confirm a theoretical point of view about language deterioration but to derive an accurate description of a particular patient's language deterioration. Obviously a brief screening test will seldom suffice to answer the questions that you are usually out to answer.

3. The Relative Usefulness of Various Language Tasks

With such a spectrum of language tasks available, you should consider what each type of testing activity can contribute to your understanding of a patient. Some tasks will give direct insight into his or her ability to function in activities of everyday life, and these tasks may somehow seem more "relevant" and "valid" than others that require language activity rarely engaged in in everyday life. Thus you may be attracted to such test items as having the patient make change, read road signs, follow recipes, and tell about an event or an activity. Such tasks seem more "real" than asking a patient to spell words aloud, think of all the words she can that begin with a given letter within one minute, indicate by gestures how certain implements are used, or even name pictures and objects. We might expect the patient to cooperate more readily on realistic tasks than on apparently artificial or schoollike tasks.

However, some apparently artificial and nonrealistic tasks provide important shortcuts in language appraisal that save time and allow objective evaluation of performance. A task such as confrontation naming of pictures and objects is a kind of shortcut to evaluation of word-finding difficulty, which is less conveniently and objectively tested by having the patient describe a picture or converse spontaneously about something. Two seemingly nonrealistic tests, the Token Test (5) in which a person points to colored shapes and the Word Fluency Test (3) in which the patient produces in one minute words beginning with each of four letters, have proven to be highly revealing, discriminating effectively between language-impaired and nonlanguage-impaired patients; they pick up minimal deficits that other kinds of tests overlook.

You can seldom confine yourself to tests which have apparent face validity. You must through investigation and experience determine the relative usefulness of various tests, however irrelevant or nonrealistic they may seem to be in achieving your goal in language evaluation.

4. Evaluating Not Only Failure but Success

The purpose of language evaluation is not simply to determine what trouble the patient has in language processing, the nature of his failures, and the severity of his deficit. It should also reveal how the patient manages to respond, what successes he has in using compensatory mechanisms to communicate. It may be important to know that when a patient is given ten commands, she fails to execute eight of them when they are scored simply right or wrong. Even more important may be information as to whether she overcomes some of those eight failures when the command is repeated, or when the command is spoken at a slower rate with insertion of pauses between phrases. It is important to know whether when she is given more time, she self-corrects her error, or whether she manages to write a response that she cannot utter.

By way of illustration, in his test *Examining for Aphasia* (7), Eisenson has a test item whose purpose is to assess the ability of the patient to recognize common objects (spoon, penknife, fork, key, quarter, comb). The examiner is invited to use multiple methods: "Patient is asked to do one of the following: name object to which examiner points; point to object named by examiner; demonstrate the object's use; or select the name from choices given orally by examiner." Obviously these different modes of response indicate different levels of efficiency in language performance, but for the purpose of the test item any of them can be used and all of them should be used before the examiner concludes that the patient cannot recognize the objects. Every test should provide maximum information about the ability of the patient to perform, and you should do enough things in your testing to derive this information. If you find that standardized tests do not accomplish this, after you use the standardized test in the prescribed way do other things with it to derive more information about the patient's behavior. The test is not sacrosanct. Your discrimination and decisions are more important than the test; the thinking you do about the patient's behavior is more important than simply going through the motions of administering any certain test in any certain way.

This goal may be reached in part by including parallel sets of items in various parts of the test which allow you to see how the patient performs on identical items in different modes of stimulus and response. One can use a limited number of items, such as the ten objects used in the PICA (14), to learn a great deal about how a patient performs when he or she is given different amounts and kinds of information.

5. Reliability of Language Evaluation

A commonly heard myth about aphasic behavior is that aphasic patients are highly variable in their responses to testing and that test results are consequently highly unreliable. Porch (14), Schuell (18), and others who devised specific standardized procedures for testing have demonstrated that more usually the variability lies in the examiner. When he is tested in the same way from time to time, the aphasic patient demonstrates quite consistent behavior. It is true that from day to day a patient may pass or fail different items within a test battery, but his overall performance in terms of percentage correct is reasonably stable.

One lesson for the clinician administering a language evaluation battery, then, is to see to it that in any given subtest a generous number of items be included to allow for diurnal variability within a representative sample of behavior. A second lesson is to adopt and maintain standardized procedures, administering given items in the same way from test situation to test situation, using uniform scoring procedures, and restraining oneself from inserting irrelevant though well-meant comments. Thus we help to guarantee that any variability recorded in the level of performance from test to test is attributable to the patient's variability and not to the examiner's inconsistency.

6. Range of Difficulty

The tasks within the test battery we select will inevitably cover a range of difficulty for most aphasic patients. In some tests the subtests are arranged in order of difficulty, from most to least difficult. In an early test in the series, the patient is provided little information around which to structure his or her response; later tests build upon the earlier ones which have provided certain bits of information about the test items used. Other tests have not been structured in this way but still provide for a range of difficulty within each of the modalities examined.

You will want to consider the difficulty level of given items. It is desirable on some tests to make sure that the requirements for performance are extremely simple, such as simply touching an object, pointing to a picture, or matching a picture to an object, in order to be sure that failures in performance can be attributed to language dysfunction and not to the patient's level of intelligence. One of the primary advantages of the Token Test (5) of auditory comprehension is that performance does not depend upon level of intelligence but only upon the patient's ability to grasp the nonredundant message which increases in length or complexity from Part I through Part V.

On other subtests of a test battery, however, you will probably want to include items representing a range of difficulty. In a picture- or object-naming test, for example, you will want to include items which are highly familiar and commonly used, and also include less familiar items the names for which occur less frequently in the language. You may include well-known objects which everyone might be expected to name but also include less familiar names of parts of those objects: for example, hand plus fingers, thumb, nail, knuckle, wrist, and palm; watch plus stem, second hand, numerals; coat plus sleeve, buttons, and lapel. In oral and written tests of spelling a range of difficulty will similarly provide additional information that one would not gain if all items were of similar difficulty. Thus within given subtests one may build in enough "top" to pick up lesser degrees of aphasic impairment.

7. Testing for Other Cognitive Processes

The purpose of language testing is not only to detect aphasic impairment but to differentiate what is properly considered to be a language-specific impairment from other impairments which involve as well as functions other than language. Therefore, you will probably want to include in your testing some subtests directed less specifically at language processing and more at the appraisal of cognitive processes. You will find it useful to include a battery of questions about general information, items about which even poorly educated subjects might have some information, such as when we celebrate Christmas, how many states there are in the Union, where the capital of the United States is, who discovered America, who the president is, who the president was before him, and the like. You will probably also want to include tests of mental and written calculation graduated from easy through harder items involving all arithmetic processes. You may want to include a test of the patient's recognition of absurdities. You may want to include a subtest in which the patient is asked to explain the general meaning of proverbs, the purpose being to see whether he is able to generalize or whether his analysis remains on a concrete level.

One cannot usually include a large sample of such tests of general intellectual function, but at least a sample of these should be included so you will have some inkling as to whether you are dealing with a problem of generalized intellectual impairment or a language-specific disability. In the end the differentiation will probably depend upon psychometric testing for which the patient will be referred to the proper examiner.

8. Analyzing the Fluency Dimension

In building a battery of tests for language evaluation you should not confine yourself to highly structured tests which require limited and easily scored responses. Be sure to include tasks which permit a subject to produce contextual speech within the limits of his or her ability. This can be done by having the patient describe pictures, talk about home and family, explain the meanings of words and proverbs, or describe what he has done today. You should then appraise these samples of contextual speech in terms of what can be called a fluency dimension. (The assessment of this dimension is highlighted in the Boston Diagnostic Aphasia Examination [9].)

Goodglass, Quadfasel, and Timberlake (10) concluded that an analysis of the pattern of speech output deficits provides the most significant differentiating clue among several types of aphasia. Benson (2) used the set of scales shown in Table 5.1 for evaluating the speech output of aphasic patients. He concluded that patients could be divided into two main groups: a group with nonfluent speech presented sparse, effortful perseverative speech with many pauses, disturbances of rhythm, abnormal pronunciations, short phrases, and word substitutions. These patients would make a low score on the scale, with a total close to 10. A second group of speakers, identified as having a fluent aphasia, produced a great deal of speech easily with little pausing, normal rhythm, and a lack of perseveration, abnormal pronunciation, and word and speech sound substitutions; their scores were closer to 30. Benson related the fluency of a group of patients to the site of their cerebral lesions and found that the fluent speakers presented primarily posterior lesions (temporo-parietal) whereas the nonfluent speakers presented more anterior lesions (frontal, fronto-temporal).

Such an analysis of the contextual speech of the patient helps to determine to what extent his language processing is contaminated by a

TABLE 5.1
Variables and Rating Scales for the Evaluation of Spontaneous Speech

1. *Word Choice*		6. *Pauses*	
Nominal or fragments of words	− 1	Many	1
Normal	0	Medium	2
Many relational words, cliché, etc.	+1	Normal	3
2. *Rate of Speaking*		7. *Prosody*	
Very slow (0–50 wpm)	1	Marked disturbance	1
Slow (51–90 wpm)	2	Slight disturbance	2
Normal (>90 wpm)	3	Normal	3
3. *Articulation*		8. *Verbal Paraphasias*	
Marked dysarthria	1	Many	1
Moderate dysarthria	2	Some	2
Normal	3	None	3
4. *Phrase Length*		9. *Phonemic Paraphasias*	
Predominantly 1–2 word phrases	1	Many	1
Predominantly 3–4 word phrases	2	Some	2
Predominantly >4-word phrases	3	None	3
5. *Effort*		10. *Perseveration*	
Marked	1	Severe	1
Moderate	2	Moderate	2
None	3	None	3

Source: From Benson, 2.

problem in the motor programming of speech. Further testing (see Chapter 11) can confirm the presence and determine the severity of apraxia of speech in association with or even independent of aphasic impairment.

9. Consider the Importance of Attitude

The performance of the patient on a language test can be importantly influenced by the attitude of the examiner toward the patient and his performance. Stoicheff (22) has shown that the attitudinal "set" established by different kinds of instructions given to patients causes significant variation in their performance. Patients subjected to an encouraging condition in which they received much favorable feedback, expressions of approval, and predictions of success from the examiner did significantly better than an equated group of patients subjected to a discouraging condition in which they received negative feedback and were reminded of how poorly they had done and would probably continue to do. It would be desirable in the language-testing situation to try to insure that we are eliciting an optimum performance from the subject. That probably means that we should let subjects know that we are interested in them, expect them to do well, and appreciate their best efforts. We can provide positive feedback and let them know when they are succeeding or at least when they are making efforts that we appreciate and commend. (Keenan and Brazzell [13] emphasize this requirement of adequate testing.)

Creation of this kind of attitudinal set must be balanced against the need for standardized procedures in testing, particularly when testing is to be repeated in order to trace the patient's change from time to time. We do not want our findings to be contaminated by wide variations in test administration. At least one test, the PICA (14), specifies every word that the examiner is to say and specifically forbids his injecting evaluational comments, either encouraging or discouraging. Some users find this test feature inordinately restricting and complain that the standardized procedures prevent their providing the patient with even that minimum feedback which gives him or her a feeling of security for performing appropriately.

Our suggestion is that you as examiner be highly alert to the mood of the patient and aware of the fact that a feeling of panic is usually at the threshold with the language disordered patient. You should through your demeanor indicate acceptance and sympathetic understanding of difficulties and convey a feeling of encouragement for best efforts. Putting these attitudes into action should not be carried to the extent that the rules of test administration prescribed by certain test makers are violated.

10. Reducing Observations to Quantified Terms

Some language tests provide a system of quantification that can be used in statistical investigations and for convenient reference in serial studies. The PICA (14) provides an overall numerical score as well as separate numerical scores on the verbal, gestural, and graphic groups of subtests. The Boston Diagnostic Aphasia Examination (9) allows for converting individual scores to profiles and to z-scores, which indicate how a patient's performance on a certain subtest in comparison to a large group relates to how well he does on another subtest in comparison to a large group. It also provides for a translation of a patient's total test performance to a 6-point "aphasia severity rating scale." The Minnesota Test of Differential Diagnosis of Aphasia (18), using a 7-point rating scale of adequacy of performance, for each of four areas tested—understanding what is said, speech, reading, and writing, provides for conversion into clinical ratings of information derived from testing.

Whatever the test or tests used, you may want to convert your impressions about the patient's performance to a scale of adequacy using numbers and descriptive terms which may communicate to others his level of performance. The "descriptive continuum of language responses in aphasia" illustrated in Table 5.2 was devised by Lucille Kaplan (*12*) as an effort to present an "orderly description of the behavior of aphasic patients."

TABLE 5.2
Descriptive Continuum of Language Responses in Aphasia

I. Effectiveness of Auditory Stimulation
  A. No observable response to verbal or nonverbal auditory stimulation
  B. Response to audio-visual stimulation
    1. Primary incorrect responses
    2. Inconsistent accuracy of responses
    3. More consistent accuracy of responses to simple sentences, questions, and commands
    4. Responses to complex auditory stimulation
      a. some errors
      b. little or no observable error

II. Nature of Speech Response
  A. No oral response
  B. Oral expression without communication
    1. Repetitive, stereotyped sounds, nonsense syllables, words, or phrases
    2. Jargon
    3. Jargon with occasional recognizable words or phrases emerging
    4. Correct production of words only after repetition
    5. Incoherent statements because of misuse of recognizable words or unrelated to subject
  C. Oral expression with communication
    1. Conditioned, situational responses
    2. One-word responses:
      a. poorly articulated
      b. correctly articulated
    3. Telegraphic style
    4. Sentence formation but difficulty encountered because of:
      a. inability to call forth specific words or supply information
      b. articulation disorder (inconsistent or consistent)
      c. word substitutions or associations
    5. Breakdown of complicated language occurs when:
      a. a too complex language pattern is required and/or
      b. presence of audience is too threatening

TABLE 5.2 (continued)

III. Effectiveness of Visual Stimulation
   A. No observable response to any visual stimulation
   B. Responses to visual-verbal stimulation
      1. Can match letters or words only
      2. Responds to words when the printed symbol is combined with oral spelling
      3. Matches printed word with spoken word or with objects
      4. Reads primarily nouns and verbs:
         a. errors usually occur on prepositions, conjunctions, etc.
         b. errors made on words which look alike
      5. Responds appropriately to single sentences only
      6. Responds appropriately to paragraphs
      7. Frequency of error increases with complexity of printed material
      8. Responds appropriately to complex materials with no observable difficulty

IV. Nature of Written Response
   A. No observable response to stimulation
   B. Writing responses to stimulation
      1. Illegible copying of letters
      2. Copying of letters and figures
      3. Writes or prints name only
      4. Writes only when word is spelled by or for him
      5. Writes name and a few words
      6. Writes phrases and/or simple sentences but errors may occur in spelling, word use or sentence structure
      7. Writes sentences but errors increase with increased complexity
      8. Writes better to dictation than spontaneously
      9. Little or no observable impairment in writing ability

Source: From Kaplan, *12.*

Another dimension of patient behavior which one may want to scale is a patient's ability to self-correct his or her errors. Wepman (23) has devised a scale of the patient's capacity for self-criticism and his ability to withdraw or improve a response when he recognizes its inadequacy (Table 5.3). He suggests that the prognosis for the patient's language recovery depends more upon his rate of progress to successive better levels within the scale than it does upon his initial status on the scale.

11. Obstacles to Valid Language Evaluation

The subjects whom the clinician will test are typically older patients with various kinds of cerebral dysfunction, a variety of impairments of health, and a wide range of emotional reactions to their situation. Ob-

TABLE 5.3
Wepman Self-Correction Scale

Level 1.   Fails to recognize errors made in any modality. Cannot recognize errors when they are pointed out and therefore cannot correct them.

Level 2.   Fails to recognize errors in any modality. Can recognize them when they are pointed out, but cannot correct them.

Level 3.   Fails to recognize errors in *either* speech or writing. Can recognize errors when pointed out, but cannot correct them.

Level 4.   Fails to recognize errors in *either* speech or writing. Can recognize the errors when pointed out and can correct them with assistance.

Level 5.   Recognizes errors made in *both* speech and writing. Cannot correct them without assistance.

Level 6.   Recognizes errors in *both* speech and writing. Can correct errors in one without assistance, but not in both.

Level 7.   Recognizes errors made in *both* speech and writing. Can correct them without assistance most of the time but only with considerable effort and even then with some mistakes.

Level 8.   Recognizes errors made in both speech and writing. Corrects them easily without assistance. May subvocalize as a means of self-correction before exposing his speech efforts.

Source: From Wepman, 23.

viously many hazards arise in trying to test such patients and interpret the results. The examiner needs to be highly conscious of the following factors and their influence upon test performance:

a. The responsiveness of the patient may be impaired by his being generally *obtunded*. A patient with organic brain syndrome or one emerging from coma following stroke or trauma may be unaware of his environment and unable to relate to the examiner and focus upon stimulus materials presented to him. One should not interpret his behavior as aphasic since his impaired responsiveness is to his total environment and not simply to language stimuli within it. Valid language testing must wait until he is in touch with his environment and able to relate to the examiner and to the materials presented to him.

b. A patient who is severely *depressed* may be almost as unresponsive as a patient who is obtunded. He may look at the examiner blankly, respond inordinately slowly, or respond not at all and be unable to verbalize why he cannot respond. When his mood is elevated, his cooperation will improve and a more accurate analysis of his language status can be made.

c. Depending upon his level of *panic* and *frustration* and his perception of many threats to his self-esteem and intellectual intactness, the patient may reject the testing situation as a threat not to be endured. Sometimes an explanation of why language testing is in order will serve to assuage the anxiety of the patient and permit him to cooperate.

d. The effect of *fatigue* may have been overemphasized in descriptions of the problems of aphasic patients, but it should be recognized that patients in the early stages of recovery from a stroke and elderly patients may find the task of participating in language evaluation tiring. Testing may need to be divided into several sessions in order to avoid the deleterious effect of fatigue during prolonged testing.

e. Patients with various kinds of cerebral dysfunction may display more than usual *emotional liability*. Pseudobulbar crying and laughing may intervene during test performance. The realization of his difficulty in performing what appear to be simple tasks may at times overwhelm the patient and cause him to break down. Words of reassurance may help, or the examiner may choose to move to a less threatening task until the patient's emotional equilibrium is restored.

f. *Sensory deficits* may interfere with valid evaluations of language function. The examiner should be alert to the possibility of a hearing loss, visual field defect, and reduction of visual acuity in the patients he is testing. He should, if possible, do this testing in quiet surroundings free of distractions to which the patient might not be able to refrain from reacting.

TESTS OF LANGUAGE FUNCTION

The following tests are available commercially or are of such nature that you can make them yourself, following the descriptions provided by the test makers in the references indicated.

The Minnesota Test for Differential Diagnosis of Aphasia (18) contains 47 subtests for exhaustive testing in five major areas of possible disturbance: 9 subtests of auditory recognition, retention, and comprehension; 9 of visual and reading performance; 15 of oral function and oral expression; 10 of visual motor and writing skills; and 4 of numerical concepts and arithmetic processes. Subtests range in length from 5 to 32 items. A clinical rating scale from zero to 6 can be used to quantify the patient's performance in the areas of comprehension, eliciting comprehension, speaking, reading, and writing. On the basis of the Minnesota Test, the classification of patients into one of five major groups and several minor groups can be made, the major groups being simple aphasia, aphasia with visual involvement, aphasia with sensorimotor involvement, aphasia with scattered findings compatible with generalized brain damage, and irreversible aphasic syndrome. A short form of the Minnesota Test (16), consists of selected subtests from the longer battery found to have high diagnostic and prognostic value; Schuell (17) later deplored publication and general use of the short test as she felt it was not reliable or comprehensive enough. Administrative manual, test booklet, two packs of stimulus cards. (Publisher: University of Minnesota Press, Minneapolis, Minnesota 55455.)

The Porch Index of Communicative Ability (PICA) (14) quantifies a limited sample of language behavior. The trained examiner rates performance on ten items in each of 18 subtests on a 16-point multidimensional scale that captures details of the completeness, accuracy, promptness, responsiveness, and efficiency of the patient's communicative efforts. An overall test score is obtained, as well as separate scores on the verbal, gestural, and graphic subtests. Percentile scores show how a given patient compares with a large sample of aphasic patients on whom the test was standardized. Comparison of the mean score of the patient's best nine subtests with his mean score on his poorest nine subtests reveals the range of language disability which it is hoped can be narrowed by therapy. Other long-term predictions of recovery outcome can be derived from the test data. (Publisher: Consulting Psychologists Press, 577 College Avenue, Palo Alto, California 94306.)

The Language Modalities Test for Aphasia (24) uses filmstrips for presenting visual stimuli and the voice of the examiner for auditory stimuli. Aural and graphic responses are scored on a 6-point scale. Matching responses are scored as passed or failed; the patient's difficulties in handling free-response items are summarized by the examiner. Test results can be used for placement of the patient into one of five classifications of aphasia: syntactic, semantic, pragmatic, jargon, and global. Manual, film strips, record booklet for Forms I and II. (Publisher: Education-Industry Service, 1225 East 60th Street, Chicago, Illinois 60637.)

The Functional Communication Profile (15) measures the ability of the patient to use language functionally in activities of everyday life. In informal interaction with the patient in a conversational situation the clinician rates the patient's ability to use his or her residual communication skills in 45 activities. Ratings are made on a 9-point scale and a percentage score can be derived to indicate the general language ability of the patient. Manual, form sheets. (Publisher: Institute of Rehabilitation Medicine, New York University Medical Center, 400 East 34th Street, New York, New York 10016.)

The Boston Diagnostic Aphasia Examination (9) explores comprehensively a wide range of communication skills by means of a battery of 31 subtests and evaluation of conversational speech which yields seven additional scores, plus supplementary groups of 13 language and 14 nonlanguage tests. Scores can be derived which allow comparison of various subtest scores with the performance of a standardized group. Patient profiles are presented which the authors consider to be characteristic of each syndrome of the "classical" classification system (Broca's, Wernicke's, anomic, conduction). Manual, stimulus cards, record booklet. (Publisher: Lea & Febiger, 600 Washington Square, Philadelphia, Pa. 19106.)

Aphasia Language Performance Scales (ALPS) (*13*) consists of four 10-part subtests, one for each modality (listening, talking, reading, writing). Each subtest permits scaling of performance within the modality from 1 to 10, different levels of performance being defined in terms of message length and complexity—single words, phrases, sentences, and multi-sentence groups. Test instructions emphasize exploiting the clinician-patient relationship so as to elicit the patient's best responses on all tasks. Patient profiles indicate optimum levels at which to initiate therapy. Manual, score sheet, packet of reading materials. (Publisher: Pinnacle Press, P.O. Box 1122, Murfreesboro, Tennessee 37130.)

The Sklar Aphasia Scale (*20*) provides for evaluation of auditory and visual decoding and oral and graphic encoding. A percentage of impairment profile is drawn for classification of the patient into categories of no impairment, mild, moderate, severe, and global impairment. Manual, protocol booklet, test materials. (Publisher: Western Psychological Services, 12031 Wilshire Blvd., Los Angeles, California 90025.)

The Neurosensory Center Comprehensive Examination for Aphasia (*21*) contains 20 language tests and 4 control tests of visual and tactile function which are designed to detect deficits that might affect performance on the language tests. One can construct a profile of percentile scores for performance on all parts of the test for any patient, corrected for age and educational level. Manual, record forms. (Publisher: Neurosensory Laboratory, University of Victoria, Victoria, British Columbia.)

Examining for Aphasia (*7*) is a shorter test which provides for screening evaluative and receptive disturbances (Part I) and productive and expressive disturbances (Part II). Most items are scored as pass or fail; some open-ended items require individual evaluation. Manual (including some stimulus materials), record entry form. (Publisher: Psychological Corp., 304 East 45th Street, New York, New York 10017.)

The Token Test (*5*) is a highly discriminating test designed to detect minimal auditory comprehension deficits. It uses 20 tokens—two shapes (circles, rectangles) of two sizes (large, small) and five colors—arranged before the patient, who is given progressively longer and more complex instructions to manipulate given tokens. Part I requires the processing of two bits of information; Part II, three bits; Part III, four bits; Part IV, six bits; Part V, linguistically more complex tasks. Test materials are simple, test performance is independent of the patient's level of intelligence, and the test requires the patient to grasp the significance of each word in each completely nonredundant message. (Not commercially available but readily made by any clinician.)

The Word Fluency Test (3) requires the patient to list within a minute all words he can think of which begin with a given letter of the alphabet; four letters are tested. The test is quite discriminating between those with normal and disturbed language function. (Not commercially available; no special materials are required.)

Language tests ordinarily used for purposes other than evaluating acquired language disorders in adults may be useful. These tests include the *Peabody Picture Vocabulary Test* (6), the *Ammons Full-Range Picture Vocabulary Test* (1), *Gray's Standardized Oral Reading Paragraphs* (11), and the *Gates Primary Reading Test* (8).

REPORTING THE RESULTS OF LANGUAGE EVALUATION

The domain of acquired language disorders is particularly beset by terminological problems. It behooves us to choose carefully the language we use to report the language problems we discover in the patients we test.

As we pointed out in Chapter 1, the language we use may do our thinking for us and foster habits in our thinking that are elementalistic, either-orish, absolute, vague, or inaccurate. The language of science is calculated to help avoid these pitfalls. It seeks a close correspondence between the language and the territory to which the language relates. It tries to get the speaker and the listener on the same wavelength. It uses techniques that remind us that the world is in flux, that our view of it is at best only partial, and that the classifications applied to data under investigation may importantly determine one's view of the data and their implications.

The area of acquired language disorders provides an excellent example of the need for terminological hygiene. When Henry Head entitled his 1926 volumes *Aphasia and Kindred Disorders* (rather than simply *Aphasia*), he reminded us that several kinds of impairments of communication can result from lesions of the brain, that these may exist separately or in combination, and that they are differentiable and require differential management. (Chapter 17 particularly, and Chapters 18, 19, and 20 as well, discuss the various disorder entities which must be differentiated.) The hazard we particularly run into is a premature identification of a language problem as aphasia and the application of one of a myriad of labels which proliferate in the literature of aphasiology.

Depending upon what test(s) they have been using, what books they have been reading, and what theoretical framework their studies have slanted them toward, examiners may be driven to call almost any language aberration *aphasia* and then to append an adjective to "clarify" the term. They may want to call it Broca's or Wernicke's or conduction or amnesic; sensory or motor; receptive or expressive; fluent or non-fluent; syntactic, pragmatic, or semantic. They may call it anomic, nominal, verbal, auditory, acoustic, subcortical, transcortical, central, or jargon. They may specify alexia, agraphia, or acalculia. One can find all of these words used by experts and can quote lengthy definitions provided by their authors to justify the nomenclature.

Regrettably these labels for what in some opinions are different "types" of aphasia turn out to mean different things to different people. Special definitions and "clarifications" of these words are continually being offered; their use without an intervening step of explanation may fail to communicate the user's intent.

Also regrettably, the use of certain terms may seem to imply that certain language functions are intact when in actuality they are not. When one goes to the trouble to identify a problem as "expressive," a possible implication is that receptive functions are unimpaired. When one highlights a lexical problem by calling the patient's aphasia "amnesic" or "nominal" or "anomic," one inevitably throws into shadow the patient's troubles with syntactic aspects of language. If one does not specifically allude to "agraphia," is the reader to assume that writing functions are intact?

Finally and also regrettably, the use of these labels all too often totally fails to convey any *useful* information. Chances are that the reader to whom our report of language dysfunction is directed needs clinically practical information about the patient's level of functioning in various modalities, how he manages to respond as well as he does, and if and on what tasks one should plan to initiate therapy—information never implicit in any label.

As a clinical speech-language pathologist, you will be much better off if, on completion of language evaluation, you *describe the behavior* you have observed. You should not try to encapsulate your wealth of observations in a word or two and hope that the nurses, physicians, and family members you are addressing will have enough background in aphasia to interpret your labels meaningfully. Rather you should share some of that detail, using adequately descriptive words, in order to provide a map of the territory that any reader can decipher. The most useful information will ordinarily reveal the length and the complexity of the message the patient can handle in the input modalities of listening and reading and in the output modalities of talking and writing. Specific details about the patient's need for repetition or cueing, the nature of his self-corrected and unrecognized errors, and his degree of insight and level of emotionality will also likely be helpful.

Only after this kind of description is provided should you indulge in the application of a label if one is necessary, in full awareness of the booby traps that abound in linguistic nomenclature.

ASSIGNMENTS

1. Why is it important to determine whether a patient has a multi-modality (central) communication problem or a modality-bound (transmissive) communication problem? Reading the following articles will help you develop your answer: Wepman, J. M., and Van Pelt, D., A theory of cerebral language disorders based on therapy. *Folia Phoniatrica*, 1955, 7:223–235. Wepman, J. M., Jones, L. V., Bock, R. D., Van Pelt, D., Studies in aphasia: background and theoretical formulations. *Journal of Speech and Hearing Disorders*, 1960, 25:323–332.

2. Obtain a copy of the Minnesota Test for Differential Diagnosis of Aphasia (*18*). How comprehensive does this test appear to be? What separate clinical groupings of patients did Schuell delineate through administration of the test and patient follow-up? See also reference *19*.

3. For what specific reasons did Schuell regret that she ever published her short examination for aphasia? See reference *17*.

4. Obtain a copy of the Porch Index of Communicative Ability (*14*). Of what subtests does the Index consist? Why are these subtests arranged in the order in which they are? How is the 16-point multi-dimensional scoring scale designed? How might this scale be adapted to other kinds of speech or language appraisal?

5. Why is use of the terms "receptive" and "expressive" redundant in describing a patient as follows: "He has both a receptive and an expressive aphasia"?

6. How long should a test for aphasia be?

7. Compile a bibliography of recent publications dealing with the administration and interpretation of the Token Test (*5*). How has the test been revised over the years? What questions and problems have arisen in connection with its use?

8. Is the Word Fluency Test (*3*) a test of aphasia?

9. Obtain a copy of the Boston Diagnostic Aphasia Examination (*9*). How comprehensive does this test appear to be? What is meant by nonverbal agility and verbal agility? How are the patient's conversational and expository speech evaluated?

10. Consider the findings of the Stoicheff study (*22*). What implications do they hold for you as a clinician? How can you apply the outcome of the study to your own practice in language evaluation?

11. Contrast the "permissiveness" of test procedure suggested by Keenan and Brazzell (*13*) and the "rigidity" of procedure demanded by Porch (*14*). Can you reconcile the points of view?

12. Read one or more of the following books which deals with the feelings and experiences of patients who have suffered severe impairment of language function. What insights do these books provide which can improve your efficiency in language evaluation and

treatment? McBride, C., *Silent Victory.* Chicago: Nelson-Hall, 1969. Moss, C. S., *Recovery with Aphasia: The Aftermath of My Stroke.* Urbana: University of Illinois Press, 1972. Ritchie, D., *Stroke.* Garden City, N.Y.: Doubleday, 1961. Wulf, H. H., *Aphasia, My World Alone.* Detroit: Wayne State University Press, 1973.

13. Consider the classification systems which "emerge" from use of the following tests: the Boston Diagnostic Aphasia Examination (9), the Language Modalities Test for Aphasia (24), the Minnesota Test for Differential Diagnosis of Aphasia (18). How are the classification systems different? Can they be consolidated? Why does the Porch Index of Communicative Ability (14) not yield a classification system?

14. Compare and contrast the "quantification" feature of the following instruments for language evaluation, that is, how patient performance is translated into numerical scores: the Functional Communication Profile (15), the Porch Index of Communicative Ability (14), the Minnesota Test for Differential Diagnosis of Aphasia (18), the Boston Diagnostic Aphasia Examination (9), and Aphasia Language Performance Scales (13).

REFERENCES

1. Ammons, R. B., and Ammons, H. S., *Full-Range Picture Vocabulary Test.* Missoula, Mont.: Psychological Test Specialists, 1948.
2. Benson, D. F., Fluency in aphasia: correlation with radioactive scan localization. *Cortex,* 1967, 3:373–394.
3. Borkowski, J. G., Benton, A. L., and Spreen, O., Word fluency and brain damage. *Neuropsychologia,* 1967, 5:135–140.
4. Brown, J. R., A model for central and peripheral behavior in aphasia. Paper presented at Academy of Aphasia, October 1968. Reviewed on p. 249 in Perkins, W. H., *Speech Pathology: An Applied Behavioral Science.* St. Louis: Mosby, 1971.
5. DeRenzi, E., and Vignolo, L. A., The Token Test: a sensitive test to detect receptive disturbances in aphasia. *Brain,* 1962, 85:665–678.
6. Dunn, L. M., *Peabody Picture Vocabulary Test.* Circle Pines, Minn.: American Guidance Service, 1965.
7. Eisenson, J., *Examining for Aphasia.* Rev. ed. New York: Psychological Corp., 1954.
8. Gates, A. I., *Manual of Directions for Gates Primary Reading Test.* New York: Teachers College, Columbia University, 1942.
9. Goodglass, H., and Kaplan, E., *The Assessment of Aphasia and Related Disorders.* Philadelphia: Lea & Febiger, 1972.
10. Goodglass, H., Quadfasel, F. A., and Timberlake, W. H., Phrase length and the type and severity of aphasia. *Cortex,* 1964, 1:133–153.
11. Gray, W. S., *Standardized Oral Reading Paragraphs.* Bloomington, Ill.: Public School Publishing Co.

12. Kaplan, L. T., A descriptive continuum of language responses in aphasia. *Journal of Speech and Hearing Disorders*, 1959, 24:410–412.
13. Keenan, J. S., and Brazzell, E. G., *Aphasia Language Performance Scales*. Murfreesboro, Tenn.: Pinnacle Press, 1975.
14. Porch, B. E., *Porch Index of Communicative Ability*. Palo Alto, Calif.: Consulting Psychologists Press, 1967.
15. Sarno, M. T., *The Functional Communication Profile: Manual of Directions*. New York: Institute of Rehabilitation Medicine, New York University Medical Center, 1969.
16. Schuell, H., A short examination for aphasia. *Neurology*, 1957, 7:625–634.
17. Schuell, H., A re-evaluation of the short examination for aphasia. *Journal of Speech and Hearing Disorders*. 1966, 31:137–147.
18. Schuell, H., *Differential Diagnosis of Aphasia with the Minnesota Test*. Minneapolis: University of Minnesota Press, 1965.
19. Schuell, H., Jenkins, J. J., and Jiménez-Pabón, E., *Aphasia in Adults: Diagnosis, Prognosis, and Treatment*. New York: Harper & Row, 1964.
20. Sklar, M., *Sklar Aphasia Scale: Protocol Booklet*. Beverly Hills, Calif.: Western Psychological Service, 1966.
21. Spreen, O., and Benton, A. L., *Neurosensory Center Comprehensive Examination for Aphasia*. Victoria, B. C.: Neurosensory Laboratory, University of Victoria, 1969.
22. Stoicheff, M. L., Motivating instructions and language performance of dysphasic subjects. *Journal of Speech and Hearing Research*, 1960, 3: 75–85.
23. Wepman, J. M., The relationship between self-correction and recovery from aphasia. *Journal of Speech and Hearing Disorders*. 1958, 23:302–305.
24. Wepman, J. M., and Jones, L. V., *Studies in Aphasia: An Approach to Testing; Manual of Administration and Scoring for the Language Modalities Test for Aphasia*. Chicago: Education-Industry Service, 1961.
25. Wepman, J. M., Jones, L. V., Bock, R. D., and Van Pelt, D., Studies in aphasia: background and theoretical formulations. *Journal of Speech and Hearing Disorders*, 1960, 25:323–332.
26. Wepman, J. M., and Van Pelt, D., A theory of cerebral language disorders based on therapy. *Folia Phoniatrica*, 1955, 7:223–235.

6

APPRAISAL
OF RESPIRATION
AND PHONATION

Hughlett L. Morris
and D. C. Spriestersbach

THE NATURE OF VOICE DISORDERS

Many students and beginning practitioners in speech pathology consider voice problems, particularly voice quality problems, to be among the more nebulous aspects of the field of communication disorders. Some attributes of voice, such as pitch, loudness, and pitch variability, are readily recognized after brief instruction and seem to cause little difficulty for even the more naive student. The major difficulty is with disorders which have to do with voice quality. The reason is probably that voice quality is more difficult to define and, consequently, so are labels of normal or deviant. In addition, while listeners are relatively quick to detect differences in voice quality, a disorder of this aspect of communication must be rather extreme before it significantly interferes with the communication process. This apparent lack of specificity in the consideration of voice disorders causes some special problems in diagnosis that are encountered less often in other aspects of clinical speech pathology.

There is indeed some confusion in the labels used to describe voice quality. However, it is our general impression that most of that confusion arises in discussions which are more technical than the one to be presented here. Consequently, while we recognize the controversy, we will use four categories of voice quality disorders here: *breathiness, harshness, hoarseness,* and *disorders of nasality* (the latter category is discussed in Chapter 7).

Now for some definitions of voice disorders, somewhat simplified for purposes of this discussion:

1. *Disorder of pitch:* A pitch level that appears either to the listener or to the clinical speech pathologist as being inappropriate for the

speaker's age and sex (in the case of the listener) or inappropriate for the laryngeal mechanism (in the case of the clinical speech-language pathologist). The pitch level may be inappropriate because it is too low or too high.

2. *Disorder of loudness:* May be a habitual loudness level that appears to the listener to be inappropriate (either too low or too high) for the specific communication setting. There may also be sporadic bursts of loudness or cyclic alteration in loudness (observed in some neurologic disorders).

3. *Disorder of pitch variability:* A pattern of pitch usage so monotonous that it distracts the listener from the message. (Conceivably, the same interference might result from a pattern of excessive variability, but that does not seem very likely).

4. *Disorders of voice quality:* [1]
   a. *Breathiness:* Characterized by a perceptible escape of "unused" air during phonation. Sounds "whispery," "soft." Often associated with low loudness levels.
   b. *Harshness:* Characterized by aperiodic noise, with listener perception of tension and tightness during phonation. Generally associated with an unusually low pitch level.
   c. *Hoarseness:* As conventionally used, seems to include a variety of voice quality deviations. Includes elements of both breathiness and harshness. Typically characterized as a symptom of a common cold or respiratory infection. May also be the result of vocal abuse. Some specialists, objecting to the label of hoarseness on the grounds that it is somewhat vague, prefer a label such as roughness.
   d. *Disorders of nasality:* May be either hypernasality or hyponasality. Hypernasal speakers seem to be talking through their nose, and indeed they are. Hyponasal speakers demonstrate less nasal component in the speaking voice than we are accustomed to; they sound as if they have a severe head cold or nasal congestion.

An integral part of diagnosis is a consideration of etiology, so we need to describe briefly some aspects of the causes of voice disorders. For purposes of this discussion, we will identify some causes that may be described as structural and some that may be considered functional. Structural bases for voice disorders are physical conditions, sometimes related to disease, which have such an adverse effect on voice production that a voice disorder results. Functional bases for voice disorders are factors which apparently relate to behavioral patterns of voice production; the emphasis is on *how* voice is produced, rather than on the physical mechanism that is used to produce it.

Note that we said factors which *apparently* relate to behavioral pat-

[1] We have adopted here essentially the definitions offered by Fairbanks (4).

terns. In general our methods are more reliable for detecting physical bases for voice disorders than they are for detecting functional bases. Sometimes, for a specific patient, we conclude that the basis of the voice disorder is functional only by the process of elimination. Central to the discussion of functional causes for voice disorders is the problem of vocal abuse, which we will discuss later in this section.

While the structural-functional dichotomy is a useful scheme for thinking about causes of voice disorders, frequently the scheme is not very satisfactory in the real world. That is because for some patients a structural condition, which at the time of examination appears to be causing a voice disorder, in turn may have been the result of long term vocal dysfunction.

In this discussion a distinction is made between respiration-phonation and resonance. We recognize the dangers of oversimplifying our consideration of the various components of voice production, but for purposes of clarity it seems helpful to describe separately aspects of voice and voice quality which arc associated primarily with the *production* of the voice (respiration and phonation) and those which are associated with one kind of modification of the signal (resonance). For that reason, resonance, while referred to occasionally here, is considered primarily in the following chapter.

Finally, we need to make some special comments about the important relationship in diagnosis of voice disorders between the speech-language pathologist and members of other professions, notably the otolaryngologist. The relationship comes about as the result of the fact that both structural and functional factors may contribute to the development and maintenance of voice disorders. In our society only the physician is trained to diagnose and treat physical problems. On the other hand, the speech-language pathologist is trained in matters of function or behavior. As indicated earlier, in many instances of a voice disorder, comprehensive diagnosis must include both kinds of procedures and so services from both professions are needed. Thus the relationship between the otolaryngologist and the speech-language pathologist must be a cooperative, interdependent one, with each of the two professionals making appropriate contributions.

THE PROCESS OF DIAGNOSIS FOR VOICE DISORDERS

The Complaint

An important first step is determining what the complaint is. As indicated in Chapter 2, usually the best way to obtain this information is simply to ask the patient. If the patient has been referred by another professional worker, you will already know some things about the problem. However, it is important that you obtain this information firsthand also.

Several kinds of information may be available from the patient's discussion of the complaint. First, you will get some notion of what the patient thinks is wrong, and his estimate of its severity. In the majority of cases, though certainly not always, in his response to the question about the complaint he will focus on the matter which is uppermost in his mind and for which he expects some assistance. Again, in most instances, whatever else the diagnostic procedures reveal, the clinician needs to address the matter reported in the complaint before the diagnostic interview is terminated.

Second, as a general rule, the patient demonstrates by his language and general affect his feelings about the problem. Some impressions will be obtained about the degree to which he is anxious or upset about the problem. Observations of this sort are particularly useful in instances in which psychological stress seems to have etiological significance.

Third, some early impressions are gained in this first portion of the examination about the nature of the voice disorder and its severity. These impressions are frequently valuable in making decisions about which diagnostic tests seem to be indicated for the patient.

In the case of voice disorders associated with respiration and phonation, the complaint is likely to be simply a difficulty in talking, either in general or at specific times. If the patient has been referred by another specialist, the patient may not even recognize that he has a voice disorder, but that is not usually the case.

The History of the Problem

Many experienced clinicians proceed immediately with the history-taking phase of the examination since that process allows the patient additional opportunity to talk about the problem and allows the clinician additional opportunity to evaluate the voice during conversation. Since the history-taking process has already been described in considerable detail (Chapter 2), we will not repeat that material here. However, we need to emphasize here the special importance of material about the history of the problem, medical history, and, in those instances where psychological stress may be relevant to the phonatory disorder, social and family history.

The Examination of the Voice

With special reference to the patient's comments about what he or she considers to be the voice disorder, we now proceed to the task of describing the patient's voice production patterns. In general, the task is threefold: to identify and label the disorder, to estimate the relative severity of the disorder, and to estimate the variability of the disorder.

Identification of the Disorder Some voice disorders are more easily identified and labeled than others. For example, disorders of pitch, loudness, and nasality, when they occur singly, are not difficult either to recognize or identify. In contrast, other disorders, notably hoarseness, are relatively easily recognized as deviant from normal but may be difficult to label. That is particularly the case when a patient presents a voice that appears to demonstrate several possible disorders at once. A beginning practitioner should not feel defeated by this problem. On the contrary, one should simply do one's best to identify what one hears, with less concern about attempting to apply a single label which describes the combined effect.

Estimating Severity of the Disorder The task of estimating relative severity of voice disorders is troublesome. In that regard, we share with many other clinical professions the difficulties in measuring a clinical event. (As pointed out in Chapter 1, clinical judgments enter into the assessment of the nature and severity of all speech and language pathologies.) The problem is that our principal measuring stick in the clinic is the process of clinical judgment and, for several reasons, clinical judgments are not optimally reliable. That is to say, agreement about severity of disorder between judges and for one judge at different times is not as high as we would like. (Notice that the problem is mainly with estimating relative severity, not whether or not there is a disorder. Reliability of clinical judgment of the latter appears to be sufficiently high for most purposes.)

There is a procedure by which reliable values for relative severity of a voice disorder can be obtained: psychological scaling. That procedure has been used by many to assess the relative severity of a variety of voice disorders as well as of other kinds of speech problems.[2] The difficulty is that several aspects of the psychological scaling procedure are incompatible with the mechanics of most clinical speech pathology practice. For example, for psychological scaling procedure, extraneous material (such as the examiner's voice or room noise) must be eliminated from the sample to be judged. The speech samples must be relatively equal in length. The samples must be presented in consecutive order. Some training-orientation procedures are generally needed for the judges. And, finally, a number of judges are needed for the judging procedure so that measures of central tendency and variability may be obtained.

It is apparent, then, that for most clinical needs we must use clinical judgments for estimating severity of a voice disorder. Our major objective is to make the judgments in as reliable a fashion as circumstances permit and to consider the matter of reliability in using them.

---

[2] See reference 7 for the original application of the method to voice disorders and reference 3 for a description of recent methodology.

As a clinician you can take several steps to make your clinical judgments somewhat more reliable:

1. Identify the aspect of voice to be judged for severity, and make every attempt to disregard other attributes. In judging voice quality it may be necessary to play the tape recordings backwards in order to avoid being influenced by articulation skill or some other aspect of the speech sample under consideration (7).
2. If feasible, tape-record samples of speech to be judged along with other samples at a later time. (This practice is particularly useful when the judgments are to be used for evaluating the results of treatment.)
3. Ask a colleague to make judgments independently for an "outside" opinion.
4. For the sake of consistency, use a single severity-rating scale in all your clinical practice. Indications are that the smaller the number of points on the scale, the more reliable the scale is for clinical judgments. Typically, a 5-point scale proves to be adequately discriminating yet fairly reliable. Probably the labels used for the points on the scale are not crucial. Some clinicians use labels such as none, somewhat, moderate, marked, and severe. Others use numbers to identify the midpoints and label only the extremes of the scale.
5. Devise a method for periodic auditory retraining of yourself with the clinical judgment scale that you use. Construct a training tape which contains extremes for each voice disorder that you deal with. Listen to the tape periodically so that you may attempt to "calibrate" your clinical judgments.

Variability of the Disorder   Estimating the variability of the disorder is of considerable value in diagnosis since from such information inferences can be made about the relative severity of the problem, its etiology, prognosis for voice therapy, and specific procedures for voice therapy that may prove effective.

Observations about variability come from several sources. First, some information about variability is available from the sample of contextual speech produced by the patient during the discussion of the complaint and during the history-taking process. There will be information also from the history about variability: When is the disorder most evident; at what time of the day; after or during what activities?

Finally, the clinician must make some direct observations about variability as the patient performs certain vocal tasks on instruction. The purpose of the instruction is to find out whether attempts to change a certain parameter of voice production results in a change in the perception of the voice disorder. Variations in pitch level, loudness level, and "laryngeal function" patterns are commonly assessed. The first two, pitch and loudness, are relatively easy to assess. The third, "laryngeal function," is more difficult and merits some special consideration in this discussion.

In general, the hypothesis is that there is a range of laryngeal function relating mostly to patterns of adduction and abduction of the vocal folds. The extremes of function are hypofunction (relative abduction, resulting in breathy voice quality) and hyperfunction (relative adduction, resulting in harsh voice quality.) [3] Clearly, this view of laryngeal function is an oversimplification, yet the notion is helpful in clinical practice. For example, a patient with harsh voice quality related to laryngeal tension may show relatively normal quality on a vocalized sigh because during the vocalized sigh the phonation pattern moves away from hyperfunction and toward hypofunction. Likewise, a patient with a breathy voice related to a vocal cord paralysis may demonstrate a more normal voice quality during certain physical effort, particularly of the torso, because during such effort the phonation pattern moves away from hypofunction and toward hyperfunction.

Following are some tasks which many clinicians use for the purpose of assessing variability:

1. Count to 20, beginning with a very soft voice, increasing loudness with each number, and ending with a very loud voice. Then reverse the process, going from very loud to very soft.
2. Count to 20, beginning with the lowest-pitched voice possible, using a higher pitch level with each number, and ending with the highest-pitched voice possible (including falsetto). Then reverse the process, going from highest to lowest.
3. Perform a series of vocalized sighs.
4. Initiate phonation with simultaneous exertion of physical effort, which especially involves the torso (the so-called pushing exercise).
5. Count to 10, using as much effort as possible.
6. Count to 10, using as little effort as possible but maintaining consistent phonation.
7. A stressful task, such as counting to 200 (or even 500), or repeating a vowel such as /ɑ/ at the rate of 1 or 2 per second, to provide information about the effects of fatigue on phonation.
8. Cough with as sharp a glottal coup as possible.

The clinician will probably ask the patient to perform each of these (and possibly other) tasks several times until a reliable observation has been made. Inexperienced clinicians frequently find it difficult to judge whether there are indeed variations in voice quality during these tasks. With practice, however, the judgments become easier to perform.

At the conclusion of this part of the examination the clinician has

---

[3] For further information about this notion see the original paper by Froeschels (5) and the later publications of Brodnitz (2) and Boone (1).

some relatively clear notions of the nature and severity of the voice disorder as well as its variability and conditions causing variability.

Respiration Patterns

There clearly is a relationship between patterns of respiration and voice production. One requirement for adequate voice production is sufficient pulmonary air pressure and respiratory flow rate to set the vocal folds in motion. In addition, the respiratory support system must be capable of sustaining levels of pressure and flow for as long as the individual needs them for voice production.

Individuals who make unusual demands on the voice, such as professional singers, actors, or speakers, usually need to pay careful attention to the use of the respiratory system which drives the vocal mechanism. Consequently there is considerable information in the literature (some of it speculative) about criteria for voice production related to respiratory function, methods for assessing respiratory function, and treatment procedures for improving respiratory function associated with voice production.

Within certain limits, and they can be defined relatively well by even a beginning clinician, respiratory function of many voice patients can be regarded as normal and there is no need to devote extensive time, effort, and resources in assessing that aspect of the behavior. (Do not confuse respiratory function with laryngeal function. Although the two are probably interrelated, we need to distinguish carefully between what happens to the air supply at the level of the glottis—laryngeal function —and factors which contribute to the buildup and maintenance of the air supply—respiratory function.)

As indicated in the preceding paragraph, there are indeed some instances in which we need to consider carefully the possible contribution of respiratory function to voice problem. In general, these are patients for which the "power supply" does indeed seem to be part of the problem. The voice may be described as weak or thin, and the patient may appear to show or even report chronic shortness of breath. The general practice clinician should refer such patients to a specialty clinic for further study. In addition to the need for special diagnostic procedures, such as those described by Boone (1, p. 84), there may also be a need for a specialized medical examination, especially in the case of patients who have a complaint involving general pulmonary function.

Pitch Level

We have referred several times in this discussion to pitch level. For the majority of purposes, the practicing speech pathologist can make the necessary observations about pitch level as clinical judgments, especially after the clinician has had some experience doing so. However, there are assessment techniques which are considerably more precise than the judgments; an excellent review of some of them is presented by Boone (*1*, p. 89). Some of them do not require much specialized equipment or technical experience while others do. As in the case of respiratory function, the clinician seeking extensive information about pitch level may choose to refer the patient to a specialty clinic.

The Physical Examination

Aside from an examination of the speech mechanism which is described in Chapter 11, the speech pathologist has license to make relatively few specific observations about physical status that are relevant to voice disorders. That is because, as indicated several times in earlier discussion, we are dealing with the physical examination of the larynx which is the province of the physician, specifically the otolaryngologist. There are, however, a few simple observations the speech pathologist can make which may have immediate diagnostic value:

1. In a patient who demonstrates harshness, where vocal production seems characterized by laryngeal tightness or strain, the clinician should attempt to determine whether there is indeed evidence of muscular tension in the throat during phonation. The tension may be evident by visual observation in which case the external surface of the throat, particularly in the area of the thyroid notch, almost seems to contract abruptly with efforts to phonate. The larynx may be in an unusually elevated position. The tension may not be visible but may be detectable by the fingertips.
2. Patients who have voice problems associated with anxiety may exhibit physical symptoms of that anxiety during the examination. Sometimes the symptoms are in body movements: patients may be unusually agitated or restless, they may perspire heavily during the examination, or they may show other signs of stress. At the other extreme, patients with this kind of disorder may be unusually controlled in their body movements. Either extreme is worthy of note.
3. The clinician needs to be alert for other signs of unusual physical activity of the oral mechanism which may not be related to anxiety but which may be relevant to the voice problem. Examples are generally oral inactivity, restricted mouth opening, and transient involuntary movements of the mouth and face. While such patterns are usually associated with articulation proficiency, they are also contributory to voice production as they affect the vocal tract in general.

Referrals to Other Professionals

We have already discussed the role of the otolaryngologist in the diagnosis and treatment of voice disorders. In general, that role is the specification of physical findings which appear to contribute to the development and maintenance of the voice disorder and, where indicated, the treatment of physical disorders and disease. Although there sometimes are exceptions to the rule, referral to the otolaryngologist is typically made as part of the diagnostic process, and management decisions made by the speech pathologist are delayed until the medical consultation is completed and a report received.

The main purpose of the medical referral is to find out whether there is a problem for which medical treatment seems indicated and, if so, to determine what the nature of the treatment program will be. This information is needed before plans can be made about voice training. Sometimes the notion of medical clearance for voice training seems to be included in the language used in making medical referrals for voice patients. We agree with the temporal sequence: we need information about the physical aspects of the problem *before* we can make decisions about behavioral management. However, it is clearly the responsibility of the speech pathologist to decide whether therapeutic voice training is to be initiated. Consequently, the intent of the language used in the referral should be to request information, not to ask whether voice therapy may be begun.

Generally, we think of a referral as being time-limited, with the referral, the examination, and the report all taking place in the period of only several weeks. In many cases initial referral leads to a series of discussions between the speech pathologist and the otolaryngologist which continues until sufficient information is obtained for management decisions or until the patient's condition has stabilized. In such cases the referral process may be continued over an extended period of time.

There are other professionals to whom voice patients may be referred. Some of these are in the medical profession, such as the neurologist and the endocrinologist. Generally, such referrals are for specific medical purposes and are made by the family physician [4] or the otolaryngologist. Another general category of professional expertise that may be needed pertains to mental hygiene and personality adjustment. Depending on the resources available in the community, the age of the patient, and the nature of the problem, referral may be made to either the clinical psychologist or the psychiatrist, or in some situations, the psychiatric social worker. Typically, consultation with the family physician or pediatrician, local school authorities, the local mental health service program, or even speech pathology colleagues will assist a speech pathologist in deciding what the appropriate referral may be.

---

[4] It is important in all clinical speech pathology and audiology to work closely with the family physician in all matters which pertain to the health status of the patient. Certainly it is the family physician who will be of greatest assistance in helping the patient and his or her family obtain consultation with medical specialists of all types.

The criteria for making such a referral are somewhat less well defined than are those for making a referral for medical reasons. In general, there should be some rather obvious evidence that anxiety and psychological stress are serving to create and maintain a voice disorder and may be interfering with the patient's ability to function generally. In addition, there should be indications that the anxiety and stress are sufficiently severe that professional treatment, of a kind that the speech pathologist is not trained to provide, is needed before changes in behavior—vocal or otherwise—can be effected.

The discussion of this kind of referral with patients must be held in such a way that it is clear to them that seeking such consultation is a voluntary action on their part. The speech pathologist should not attempt to persuade a patient to seek that kind of consultation; for maximal effectiveness, a patient should seek assistance because he or she feels it necessary and certainly not just at the direction or even as a favor to the speech pathologist!

It should be clear from this discussion that the need for this kind of consultation may not be apparent during the initial examination, and indeed, may be apparent only after some voice training is provided. The discussion is included here, however, because of the relevance of the referral to the total diagnostic process.

FORMULATING THE CLINICAL IMPRESSION AND RECOMMENDATIONS

This step in the process of diagnosis represents the summarization of each set of observations and an attempt to relate and interpret the various observations. The clinical impression is a brief concise statement which in general contains information about the nature and severity of the problem and the nature of the etiology of the problem. The clinical impression is generally accompanied by management decisions, typically referred to as the recommendations.

The recommendations are of course the end result of the entire diagnostic process. This is the point at which the clinician considers carefully the clinical impression and decides what to do about the problem.

There are three general outcomes of diagnosis for voice disorders. All are focused on the question of voice training to be performed by either the examining speech pathologist or a colleague in that profession. (In this way we avoid any language that suggests we are prescribing to another profession.) The outcomes, simply stated, are voice training, no voice training, or recommendation deferred.

In the first instance, voice training recommended, decisions have been made which indicate that (1) there is a "significant" disorder, (2) the physical conditions underlying the disorder are stable and do not contraindicate voice therapy, (3) there is reason to expect favorable response to therapy, (4) the patient is motivated to change his or her voice production behavior, and (5) no further information about the problem is needed before voice therapy can be started.

The second instance, voice training not recommended, might be based on a variety of decisions. Perhaps the disorder is not viewed as important enough to indicate therapy. It may be that there are clear indications of poor motivation and cooperation on the part of the patient. Or perhaps the results of previous therapy programs indicate that there is little chance of improvement. The important point here is that the clinical speech pathologist has obtained all the information he or she deems necessary for making a management decision and the decision of no speech pathology management has been made. The decision may be reconsidered at a later date if there are reasons to suspect that circumstances have changed, but for the present the case is closed.

In contrast, when recommendation is deferred, the decision has been made that in spite of all the observations made during the diagnostic process, the information about the problem and the patient is not sufficient for making the final decision about whether voice therapy is to be provided. Perhaps more referrals to other professional workers are needed or perhaps the referrals already made have not been completed. An example might be a case in which the otolaryngologist wishes to explore further the physical findings or the results of medication. It is also possible that the patient is not ready to make a commitment for voice therapy and the speech pathologist wants to know more about motivation level before making a decision about therapy. In any case, further consideration of the problem and the patient is required before the recommendations are formulated.

An outline (Form 2) for the examination of voice quality is presented at the end of Chapter 7.

ASSIGNMENTS

1. Listen carefully to the voice characteristics of three public speakers (teachers, ministers, newscasters, actors, politicians). What variations in voice quality do you observe? What voice qualities stand out? Do you find those voice qualities pleasing or objectionable?

    Repeat the assignment, using friends or members of your family. What differences are there between the two groups?
2. Ask three friends to describe their notion of a "pleasing" voice. Encourage them to be as specific as possible. What differences are there among the three descriptions?

    Repeat the assignment, asking this time for descriptions of a voice that's not "pleasing." What differences are there between the two sets of descriptions?

REFERENCES

1. Boone, D., *The Voice and Voice Therapy*. 2nd ed. Englewood Cliffs, N.J.: Prentice-Hall, 1977.
2. Brodnitz, F. S., *Vocal Rehabilitation*. Rochester, Minn.: Whiting Press, 1967.
3. Carney, P. J., and Sherman, D., Severity of nasality in three selected speech tasks. *Journal of Speech and Hearing Research*, 1971, *14*:396–407.
4. Fairbanks, G., *Voice and Articulation Drillbook*. Rev. ed. New York: Harper & Row, 1960.
5. Froeschels, E., Hygiene of the voice. *Archives of Otolaryngology*, 1943, 37:122–130.
6. Johnson, W., *People in Quandaries: The Semantics of Personal Adjustment*. New York: Harper & Row, 1946.
7. Sherman, D., The merits of backward playing of connected speech in the scaling of voice quality disorders. *Journal of Speech and Hearing Disorders*, 1954, *19*:312–321.

7

APPRAISAL
OF RESONANCE

Hughlett L. Morris
and D. C. Spriestersbach

The phenomenon of vocal resonance is exceedingly complex and perhaps not fully understood even by specialists with unusual expertise. For purposes of this text, it seems sufficient to acknowledge that voice quality is influenced to an important extent by resonance and that, indeed, it may be the effects of resonance that determine importantly the individuality of each voice.

The phenomenon of resonance has to do with selective amplification of frequency bands in the acoustic spectrum produced by the vibration of the vocal folds. Although we are not entirely certain about the matter, it is reasonable to assume that dimensions and configuration of the vocal tract, conditions of the walls of the tract, and characteristics of passages which are connected to the vocal tract are all relevant to consideration of the resonating system of human voice production.[1]

Certain of these variables, notably the dimensions and configuration of the vocal tract and the conditions of the walls of the tract, are difficult to assess. For practical purposes, they are not included in the typical examination of the speech mechanism except indirectly. Our primary concern is with the resonance contributed by the nasal cavity and the relative effect of that resonance in making the voice more or less nasal in quality.[2]

For purposes of this discussion, we want to make a distinction between hypernasality and nasal emission. Hypernasality is a phenomenon of excessive nasal resonance, occurring primarily during vowel production; nasal emission refers to the direction of the airstream through the nasal cavity rather than the oral cavity, occurring primarily during consonant

[1] For a technical discussion of resonance of the human voice, see Brackett (1).
[2] Curtis (3) provides a general discussion of the acoustics of nasalized speech.

213

production. Making such a distinction in contextual speech is sometimes difficult even for the trained examiner (for example, voiced consonants in reality are inseparable from the vowels which follow them); nevertheless the concept of a difference between the two is useful in many aspects of appraisal.

THE PROCESS OF DIAGNOSIS

In the preceding chapter we considered the process of diagnosis for voice disorders in general, so that discussion will not be repeated here. There are certain special additional considerations to be made, however, for disorders of resonance.

The Complaint

Typically the complaint includes statements which refer directly to nasalization of speech. There also may be comments about a physical condition, such as cleft palate.

The History of the Problem

For patients who demonstrate hypernasality, there may be special relevant developmental and medical history. For obvious reasons, specific questions should be asked about a congenital orofacial cleft. In that regard, the beginning clinician must be alert to the disorder commonly labeled congenital palatal incompetence.[3]

While sometimes there are no visible signs of a palatal deficit, careful examination clearly reveals palatopharyngeal[4] dysfunction. Some patients show minimal signs of clefting, such as bifid uvula (an indication of a submucuous cleft palate) or congenitally missing incisors. For many patients the palatal disorder does not become obvious in early childhood, presumably because hypertrophied adenoids serve to compensate for the palatal deficit. After adenoidectomy the deficit is demonstrated in palatopharyngeal incompetence for speech.

The Examination of the Voice

Much the same procedure is used for examination of disorders of resonance as that outlined previously for disorders of phonation and respiration. The task is essentially the same: to identify and label the disorder, to estimate severity, and to estimate variability. Form 2, at the end of this chapter, provides an outline to follow in this examination.

[3] This is discussed in Chapter 15. See also the discussion by Bradley (2) regarding congenital and acquired palatopharyngeal incompetence.
[4] The terms palatopharyngeal and velopharyngeal are synonymous. The former is used throughout this text.

Identification   There is usually not much difficulty, even for the beginning clinician, in identifying and labeling disorders of resonance. Voices that demonstrate excessive nasal resonance are hypernasal; voices that demonstrate insufficient nasal resonance are hyponasal. In the majority of instances, a voice disordered by resonance imbalance is either one or the other. Sometimes, but not often, we see patients with specific deficits of the palatopharyngeal mechanism who seem to demonstrate both hypernasality and hyponasality in their speech production. Mainly, they are patients with a pharyngeal flap structure or a dental prosthetic device (obturator) which provides insufficient occlusion of the palatopharyngeal mechanism for normal orality of speech, yet the mechanism is occluded too much for normal speech resonance. These are special cases, however.

Some medical references use terms such as rhinolalia aperta and rhinolalia clausa to attempt to distinguish between two kinds of hypernasality. While there is some basis for such a distinction for certain types of disorders, in general the distinction is not very useful in typical speech pathology clinical practice.

Estimation of Severity   The same procedures are used as outlined for disorders of phonation and respiration. A word of caution is needed, however, about the matter of selecting speech tasks to be used for this purpose, particularly for the patient with a relatively mild disorder of hypernasality. There is considerable documentation that speakers with mild or marginal disorders are perceived as more hypernasal during speech tasks which include many nasal consonants than they are if the speech task includes no nasal consonants. That is probably true because the presence of the nasal consonants makes it physiologically more difficult for the speaker to use the palatopharyngeal mechanism appropriately. For such patients, the clinician needs to include both kinds of speech tasks in the examination.

Variability   The same considerations must be made for disorders of resonance as for disorders of phonation and respiration. In addition, the clinician will need to assess variability related to phonetic context, as indicated above. Other tasks might include an overexaggerated articulation pattern and an overexaggerated mouth opening, since both tasks appear to result in greater amounts of oral activity, which in turn sometimes lessen the degree of hypernasality.

In general, variability may be expected to be greater in patients who are hypernasal than in those who are hyponasal.

The Physical Examination

The major concern about physical findings for a hypernasal speaker is the degree to which the palatopharyngeal sphincter serves to separate the oral and nasal cavities. That aspect of diagnosis is discussed in some detail in Chapter 11.

In cases of hyponasality the clinician must be observant of physical findings that appear to contribute to occlusion of the nasopharynx or the nasal airway. One such finding is hypertrophied adenoids often evident in children. Usually the speech pathologist cannot provide as definitive a description of adenoidal size as can the physician. However, sometimes—particularly in a patient with postoperative cleft palate—if the adenoids are very large they can be visualized below the curtain of the soft palate. If the adenoids are not observable, enlarged tonsils in combination with history of chronic upper respiratory illness or chronic middle ear disease may lead to the conclusion that the adenoids are enlarged. Observed or reported chronic mouth breathing may also be indicative of enlarged adenoids.

Another finding of interest in connection with hyponasality is the presence of a pharyngeal flap structure or an obturator. If a hyponasal speaker has either, it may be that there is insufficient palatopharyngeal opening for the normal production of nasal consonants and those vowels which normally include some nasal resonance. In these cases, there also may be mouth breathing.

Finally, in the case of hyponasality some consideration must be given to the presence of obstruction in the nasal cavity. One example is extreme nasal congestion, usually readily detectable by the examiner. The examiner also needs to be aware of the possible effects of a deviated nasal septum, nasal polyps, and retropharyngeal tumors. Sometimes there is obvious evidence of such a structural problem (a patient who has suffered a broken nose, for example), but more often a medical examination is required for definitive description.

As we have pointed out before, frequently it is difficult to relate any one of these findings causally to a resonance disorder yet the combined effect of a number of physical findings may be relevant.

REFERRALS TO OTHER PROFESSIONALS

Clearly there may be need for referral to an otolaryngologist for examination of treatment of diseases or physical disorders related to problems of resonance. In addition, in some centers other surgical specialists, notably plastic surgeons, may be involved in matters which require surgical intervention. Frequently problems of this sort are managed by a team of specialists (of which the speech pathologist is a member) in a medical center. In that case, the local speech pathologist may simply refer the patient to a professional colleague on the team for ultimate diagnosis and management by the team at the center.

The criteria for referrals are described in some detail in Chapter 6.

FORMULATING THE CLINICAL IMPRESSION
AND RECOMMENDATION

The criteria for arriving at the clinical impression are described in Chapter 6.

Since many problems of resonance imbalance are causally related to physical diseases and disorders, the recommendations made by the speech pathologist must take into account management decisions by the physician. In general, in either hypernasality or hyponasality, speech pathology treatment procedures alone cannot be expected to yield normal speech. Rather, such procedures will be effective only as they assist the patient to compensate as well as possible for the physical deficit. (An exception, of course, is the patient for whom hypernasality is a dialectal trait.) If normal speech is the objective, it is highly probable that the treatment regimen must include physical management, usually surgery.

ASSIGNMENTS

1. Complete Form 2 for two speakers whose voice quality is deviant.
2. Experiment with your voice, attempting to read a passage with hypernasality, and again with hyponasality. Some practice may be necessary. What differences do you hear?
3. Ask a friend to do the same. What differences do you hear?
4. Ask your instructor to comment about the differences between simulated and pathological hypernasality and hyponasality.
5. If pathological speakers or recorded speech samples from such speakers are available, describe their resonance characteristics. What differences are there between the simulated and pathological resonance patterns?

FORM 2

Examination of Voice Production: Respiration, Phonation, and Resonance

1. Complaint
2. Primary voice problem
   breathiness _____ harshness _____ hoarseness _____ hypernasality _____ hyponasality _____ pitch _____
   loudness _____ other _____
3. Pertinent history
   a. History of the problem:
      Nature of onset:
      Duration of the problem:
      History of vocal misuse (talking in a noisy environment, excessive
      speaking, shouting, screaming): yes _____ no _____. If *yes*,
      describe the circumstances:
      Description of how voice is used in daily work:
      Variations in the severity of the problem noted by the speaker and
      circumstances when variations occur:
      Has speaker had voice therapy? yes _____ no _____. If *yes*,
      what was the nature of the therapy?
   b. Family history of voice and speech problems:
      Other members of the family with voice or speech problems?
      yes _____ no _____. If *yes*, describe the nature of the prob-
      lem and relation of person to the speaker in each case.
   c. General physical development and health:

	Yes	No		Yes	No
allergies	___	___	hormone therapy	___	___
anemia	___	___	diphtheria	___	___
glandular			influenza	___	___
imbalance	___	___	typhoid fever	___	___
hyperthyroidism	___	___	rheumatic fever	___	___
hypothyroidism	___	___	scarlet fever	___	___
chronic colds	___	___	orofacial cleft	___	___
chronic rhinitis	___	___	head and neck surgery	___	___
sinus infection	___	___	head and neck trauma	___	___
chronic			excessive smoking	___	___
laryngitis	___	___	broken nose	___	___
ear disease	___	___	mouth breathing	___	___
incoordination			retarded sexual		
of face or			development	___	___
tongue			other	___	___
muscles	___	___			
gait peculiarities	___	___			
random					
purposeless					
movements	___	___			

If the answer to any of the items above is *yes*, give relevant details:

4. Examination of pertinent physicial mechanisms
   a. Respiratory mechanism:
      Breath supply and control appears to be adequate? yes _____
      no _____
      Any apparent muscular tensions of the chest and neck? yes _____
      no _____
      Any history or complaint of respiratory disorders? yes _____
      no _____
   b. Larynx:
      History of laryngeal pathology (growths, inflammations, chronic pain,
      or tickling) _____ Complaint of "tired throat" _____ Mus-
      cular contractions exhibited during phonation which are similar to
      those exhibited during swallowing _____
      If the answer to any of the items above is *yes,* give relevant details:
      Does the speaker exhibit any of the following during phonation?
      hard glottal attack _____ diplophonia _____ infrequent
      pitch breaks _____ frequent pitch breaks _____ phonation
      interspersed with whispering _____ tremulous voice _____
      sporadic bursts of loudness _____ cyclic alterations in loudness
      _____ deterioration of loudness with prolonged effort _____
      increase of hypernasality with prolonged talking _____ unusually
      short phrases _____ audible inhalations _____
      If the answer to any of the items above is *yes,* give relevant details:
      Has speaker done any formal singing? yes _____ no _____. If
      yes, describe his activities.
      Can speaker sing up and down the musical scale? yes _____
      no _____
      Can speaker imitate inflectional patterns? yes _____ no _____
      Does pitch usage appear appropriate? yes _____ no _____
   c. Articulatory mechanism:
      Activity of lips and jaws (extent of mouth opening) while speaking:
      immobile and clenched _____ slight movement _____
      average movement _____ above average movement _____
      Quality when nostrils are occluded during sustained phonation of
      vowels: changed _____ unchanged _____
      Any indications of palatopharyngeal incompetence? yes _____
      no _____
      Tonsils: none _____ small _____ moderately large _____
      very large _____
      Nasal obstruction:
      right nostril: none _____ some _____ complete _____
      left nostril: none _____ some _____ complete _____
      Discuss the significance of any deviations noted above:
   d. Posture:
      Is overall posture of the body generally adequate? yes _____
      no _____
      Is head held in reasonably upright position during speaking?
      yes _____ no _____
      Is the position of the larynx in the neck symmetrical? yes _____
      no _____

If the answer to any of the items above is *no,* describe the deviation and discuss any possible relationship it may have to the voice problem:

5. Associated variables

  a. Pitch, loudness, and effort:

    Is quality changed under any of the following conditions?

    lower than habitual pitch level: yes _____   no _____

    higher than habitual pitch level: yes _____   no _____

    softer than habitual loudness level: yes _____   no _____

    louder than habitual loudness level: yes _____   no _____

    less than habitual effort level (a simulated breathy voice): yes_____ no _____

    greater than habitual effort level (a simulated sudden vocal onset): yes _____   no _____

    prolongation of speaking effort: yes _____   no _____

  b. Personal and social adjustment:

    What is the degree of apparent concern that the speaker has about his voice problem? none _____   some _____   marked _____

    Does the language which the speaker uses tend to be well qualified, normally cautious, specific, or does it tend to be rigidly either-orish, absolute, inappropriate to the situation?

    Does the speaker's interpretation of objective events tend to be competent, impersonal, factual, or does it tend to be exaggerated, self-defensive, vague?

    Does the speaker tend to have a relaxed appearance, a smooth, rhythmical gait, firm handshake, direct gaze, or tend to appear physically tense, move jerkily, remain quietly at ease only with difficulty, refuse to look directly at the examiner?

    Does the speaker tend to appear hostile (curt, cryptic, indifferent), extremely dependent, generally insecure, or cooperative, pleasant, helpful, interested?

    In talking about the voice problem itself is the speaker reticent, apologetic, embarrassed, depressed, and defensive, or able to discuss it freely in a forthright manner, with an interested, objective problem-solving attitude?

    Specify and discuss any other aspects of the speaker's behavior which appear to be indices of his or her adjustment:

    Do the speaker's maladjustments, if any, appear to be related largely to specific problems and situations or do they appear to be characteristic of his or her behavior generally? List any situations to which the speaker appears to adjust poorly.

    How would you rate the speaker's overall adjustment? above average _____   average_____   below average _____

6. Relationship of the voice quality problem to other variables, if any, not discussed above:

7. Summary of the relationship of findings recorded under "Associated Variables" to the voice quality problems revealed by the General Speech Behavior Rating:

REFERENCES

1. Brackett, I. P., Parameters of voice quality. In Travis, L. E., ed., *Hand-book of Speech Pathology and Audiology*, pp. 441–463. Englewood Cliffs, N.J., Prentice-Hall, 1971.
2. Bradley, D. P., Congenital and acquired palatopharyngeal insufficiency. In Grabb, W. C., Rosenstein, S. W., and Bzoch, K. R., eds., *Cleft Lip and Palate*, pp. 658–669. Boston: Little, Brown, 1971.
3. Curtis, J. F., The acoustics of nasalized speech. *Cleft Palate Journal*, 1970, 7:380–396.

8
APPRAISAL
OF ARTICULATION
Frederic L. Darley

Of all the aspects of speech, voice, and language that will engage your attention as a clinician, the one that you are likely to examine and evaluate in the greatest proportion of cases is articulation, how speakers produce the phonemes of their language. A comprehensive nationwide sampling of public school speech clinicians has reported that children with so-called functional articulation problems constituted 81 percent of their average current case load (26, pp. 37–38). It is likely that a considerable proportion of the remaining children in the average case load also present articulation problems; children with delayed speech development (4.5 percent), hearing loss, (2.5 percent), clefts of the palate (1.5 percent), and cerebral palsy (1.0 percent) swell the total percentage of children with articulation problems in the average current case load to 90.5 percent. It is clear that testing procedures which can help you define the problems of these children and point the way to economical and effective remedial services for them are highly important. In this chapter we present essential information about the development of phoneme articulation and procedures for examining and describing a person's articulation patterns.

HOW PHONEME ARTICULATION DEVELOPS

There are between 45 and 50 phonemes used in the three main dialects of English spoken in the United States. The way in which children acquire these phonemes has been the subject of considerable research, some of the most enlightening of which has been reported by Irwin and his associates (10, 11, 12, 13, 14, 15, 16, 45). They studied 30-breath samples of vocalization obtained at monthly intervals from a sizable group of infants from birth to age 2½ years, using the International Phonetic Alphabet to record the sounds heard during these observations. Analyzing the 30-breath samples in terms of two main measures, the number of different phonemes produced on the average in the samples (phoneme type) and the total number of phonemes produced (phoneme frequency), Irwin derived curves indicating an impressive orderliness in phoneme development in the babbling and speech of infants. Figure 8.1 indicates that at the first age level (months 1 and 2 combined) the average child produces seven different phonemes in a sample of 30 breaths. By the fifteenth age level (months 29 and 30) the average child is producing 27 different phonemes. This is a decelerating curve, with the faster acquisition of new phonemes being demonstrated at the earlier ages. Children begin with a meager repertory, gradually adding phonemes which they hear about them. Figure 8.2 shows that the growth in total number of different phonemes produced in the 30-breath sample accelerates with increase in age.

For each of the measures mentioned above there is considerable variability among children (*11*). Data based upon groups of children are highly stable, but Winitz and Irwin (*45*) reported that the individuals studied did not consistently maintain their positional standings in the group with respect to the two measures of phoneme development.

Most parents and speech clinicians, wanting to determine whether a child's articulation is satisfactory for his or her age, are less interested in the number of phonemes the child can produce in babbling and contextual speech than they are in the correctness of articulation of phonemes in context. The Irwin data demonstrate that by 30 months children use all the English phonemes *noninstrumentally*—producing all the articulatory gestures—but it takes much longer for them to integrate these phonemes into their language system and use them *instrumentally*—to convey meaning.

Four research studies portray the sequence in which children master the instrumental use of phonemes. Wellman et al. (*43*) studied the ability of 204 children ranging in age from 2 to 6 years (only 15 were 2 years old) to produce 133 items on an articulation test. They report the earliest ages at which various phonemes (in three positions—initial, medial, and final) and consonant clusters were produced correctly by 75 percent of the children tested. Davis (*5*) administered an articulation test to more than 20,000 preschool and school-age children and reported the earliest ages at which 23 consonant phonemes in three positions were produced correctly by 100 percent of the children tested. Templin (*34*) administered a 176-item articulation test to a total of 480 children, 60 (30 boys, 30 girls) at each of eight age levels from 3 through 8 years old; she reported the earliest ages at which 75 percent of the children correctly produced each of 24 consonant phonemes in three positions. Prather, Hedrick, and Kern (*25*) tested 147 children distributed at seven

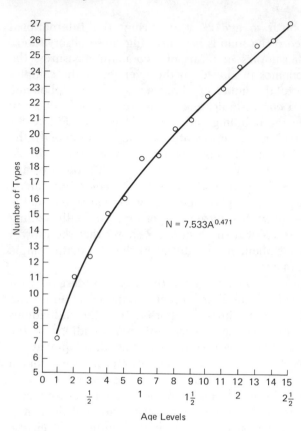

FIGURE 8.1

Curve of development derived from mean numbers of different phonemes (types) produced during 1622 observation periods of 30 breaths each by a total of 95 infants at the designated age levels. Circles represent the obtained values and the solid curve is described by the indicated equation. (From Orvis C. Irwin and Han Piao Chen, Development of speech during infancy: curve of phonemic types, *Journal of Experimental Psychology*, 1946, *36*:431–436. Copyright 1946 by the American Psychological Association; reprinted by permission.)

age levels between 2 and 4 years of age and reported the earliest ages at which 75 percent of the children produced each of 25 consonant phonemes in two positions (initial and final only). Table 8.1 summarizes the data from these four studies. The sequences of phoneme development revealed by the four studies are quite similar. A primary difference between the studies is the finding of consistently earlier age levels for

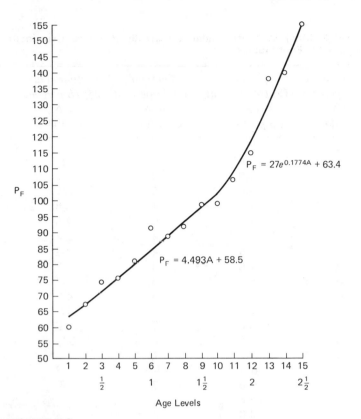

FIGURE 8.2
Curve of development derived from mean phoneme frequencies (numbers of speech sounds of all types produced)
during 1622 observation periods of 30 breaths each by a
total of 95 infants at the designated age levels. Circles
represent the obtained values and the solid curve is described in its lower and upper portions, respectively, by
the indicated equations. (From Orvis C. Irwin and Han
Piao Chen, Development of speech during infancy: curve
of phonemic types, *Journal of Experimental Psychology,*
1947, 37:187–193. Copyright 1947 by the American Psychological Association; reprinted by permission.)

correct phoneme productions in the most recent of the four studies, that
of Prather et al.

Having just presented the ages at which children can be said to
produce given consonant phonemes, we must assert that this description
of phoneme acquisition is somewhat artificial and arbitrary. These "facts"
are in actuality artifacts of the presentation of a particular statistical
treatment of the data and of particular definitions of acquisition. They

TABLE 8.1
Ages (in Years and Months) at Which Children Correctly Produced Consonant
Phonemes, as Reported in Four Studies

Phoneme	Wellman et al. (43) 75 percent of N 3 positions	Davis (5) 100 percent of N 3 positions	Templin (34) 75 percent of N 3 positions	Prather et al. (25) 75 percent of N 2 positions
m	3	3-6	3	2
n	3	4-6	3	2
ŋ	*	4-6	3	2
p	4	3-6	3	2
b	3	3-6	4	2-8
t	5	4-6	6	2-8
d	5	4-6	4	2-4
k	4	4-6	4	2-4
g	4	4-6	4	3
f	3	5-6	3	2-4
v	5	5-6	6	4+*
θ	*	6-6	6	4+*
ð	—	6-6	7	4
s	5	5-6	4-6	3**
z	5	5-6	7	4+*
ʃ	—	6-6	4-6	3-8
ʒ	6	6-6	7	4
h	3	3-6	3	2
w	3	3-6	3	2-8
r	5	8	4	3-4**
l	4	6-6	6	3-4**
tʃ	5	—	4-6	3-8
dʒ	6	—	7	4+*

 * = Phoneme tested but not produced correctly by 75 percent of children of oldest
     age tested.
— = Phoneme not tested or reported.
 ** = Reversal reported at earliest age level if only one reversal occurred and per-
     centage at all older age levels exceeded 75 percent. Reversal indicated when
     criterion for appearance of a phoneme was achieved at an age level but not
     achieved at a later age level.

reveal something about phoneme *mastery* and reflect upper age limits
rather than average performance. Sander (29) has suggested that a less
stringent and more meaningful way to describe phoneme acquisition is in
terms of ranges of customary production. For example, the range for
acquisition of a given phoneme can begin at the earliest age at which a
phoneme is correctly produced in two positions by 51 percent of the
children and can extend to that age at which 90 percent of the children
produce it correctly. This manner of representation is certainly true to

the facts of the process of phoneme development, characterized as it is by considerable variability. We are less likely to misunderstand the process if we think of it as encompassed within definable ranges rather than encapsulated in absolute numbers.

Figure 8.3 displays in such form the developmental data presented in

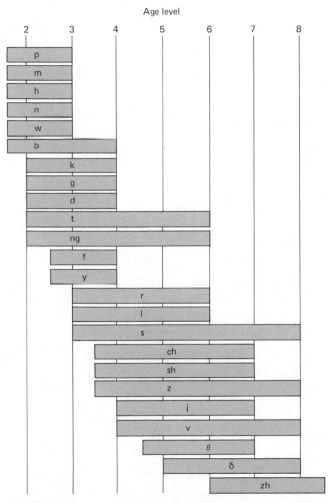

FIGURE 8.3

Average age estimates and upper age limits of customary consonant production. The solid bar corresponding to each sound starts at the median age of customary articulation; it stops at an age level at which 90 percent of all children are customarily producing the sound. (From E. K. Sander, When are speech sounds learned? *Journal of Speech and Hearing Disorders*, 1972, 37:55–61.)

the Wellman et al. and Templin studies. As a supplement to it, Figure 8.4 presents data from the more recent study of children from 2 to 4 years of age by Prather et al.

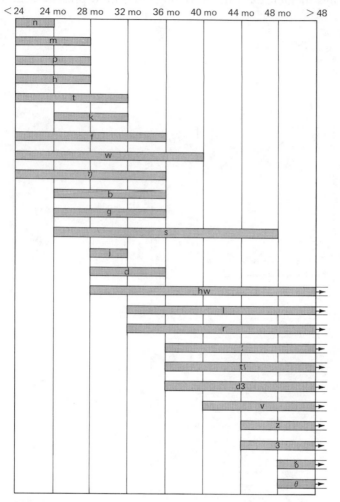

FIGURE 8.4

Average age estimates (50 percent) and upper age limits (90 percent) of customary consonant production by 147 children aged 24 to 48 months studied by Prather et al. (25). When the percentage correct at 24 months exceeded 70 percent, the bar extends to the left 24; when the 90 percent level was not reached by 48 months, the bar extends to the right 48. (From E. M. Prather et al., Articulation development in children aged two to four years, *Journal of Speech and Hearing Disorders*, 1975, 40:179–191.)

By scanning from the top to the bottom of these figures one can abstract a general sequence of phoneme development—which phonemes are mastered early, which later. No single list which establishes a hard and fast order of acquisition can be derived. It is evident that we need more data on phoneme development of young children—from 18 months on—and that these data be secured from children representing small discrete age groupings. The data then deserve analysis not only at phonemic but at subphonemic level; analysis by distinctive feature usage such as has been reported by Menyuk (22), Crocker (4), and Prather et al. (25) should ultimately better specify the sequence of phoneme acquisition and the reasons underlying it.

As a final word regarding how articulation develops, we can look at the other side of the coin and consider which phonemes are reportedly most frequently misarticulated by children and adults. Studies (8, 28, 30) are in good agreement that the fricatives /s/, /z/, /ʃ/, /ʒ/, /θ/, and /ð/; the affricates /tʃ/ and /dʒ/; and the semivowels /r/ and /l/ are the most frequently misarticulated phonemes revealed in screenings of both children and adults. The phonemes /k/, /g/, /t/, and /d/ are also frequently misarticulated by children.

THE SPEECH SAMPLE

As in any other type of speech test, a sample of speech is necessary in a test of articulation. The nature of the sample depends upon the purpose one has in testing. We may have any of several purposes in testing a child's articulation:

(1) Sometimes we wish to assess the general accuracy of his articulation, in which case we use a screening test. Such a test is used frequently in school speech surveys or in other initial contacts with children to detect those who probably will need speech correction because their articulation is inadequate for their age. It need test only those sounds and sound clusters which are associated with significant progress in the development of articulation.

(2) At times we need to know whether and with what consistency the child can produce speech elements of a given type; for example, consonants requiring substantial intraoral breath pressure for their efficient production, or clusters of consonants involving a given phoneme adjacent to a series of varying phonemes which may facilitate its correct production. For this purpose we use special groupings of selected items, concentrating our attention on only those elements immediately relevant to our questions.

(3) We may wish to obtain a detailed description and analysis of a child's articulation, for which purpose we use a diagnostic test. Such a test may be used in deciding whether a child needs speech therapy, but more frequently it is used with children already identified as having articulatory problems to aid in prescribing the nature of speech therapy. It provides detailed information

about a child's ability to produce a wide range of speech sounds in a variety of positions and phonetic contexts. (37, p. 1)

When we test articulation in an adult we may have similar purposes in mind, or in the case of an acquired articulation problem we may be more interested in obtaining a general impression of the subject's articulatory precision and the nature and frequency of his articulatory breakdowns in order to determine what type of dysarthria he manifests. For this we will probably not need an articulation inventory but will structure our observations differently (see pp. 246–247).

Whenever you want specific information about a speaker's ability to produce the phonemes of his language, whether that information is to be limited or detailed, you must have a method of eliciting the desired phonemes and a systematic method of recording what you hear when the speaker attempts to produce them. You may elicit the phonemes in any one of several ways. You may hold a conversation with the individual you are testing and note the correctness of his production of the various phonemes as they occur in his speech. Obviously, however, this procedure is inefficient and time consuming. You may have to wait a long time for some of the less common phonemes to appear. At best the observations would not be systematic and probably the conclusions drawn from them would lack precision.

You may ask the subject to read sentences prepared to contain given phonemes in specific positions and phonetic contexts. The procedure will prove effective in the case of sufficiently good readers, but many individuals given articulation tests read poorly if at all.

With most preschool children or those in early elementary grades you probably will resort to one of two other methods. In one, pictures are used to elicit as spontaneous speech responses words containing the desired phonemes in given positions and contexts. Such a procedure is fairly interesting to most children and is reasonably economical of time. With the other method you have the child repeat after you words containing the desired phonemes. This procedure is even more economical of time, but it is likely to become rather boring to young children. Winitz (44) and Templin and Darley (37, pp. 4–7) have reviewed the contradictory findings from research done on the relative merits of these two methods, which may be called the "spontaneous" and the "imitative," respectively. The latter concluded that when what is desired is the most typical response of the subject—that is, a response influenced as little as possible by prior stimulation—the spontaneous method is probably to be preferred.

In the following paragraphs we present procedures designed to elicit a sample of speech for screening purposes, to record the results of the articulation test making use of International Phonetic Alphabet symbols, and to analyze the results for precise appraisal of the problem and deriving cues for therapy. Frequent reference is made to the work of

Templin (*34*), whose normative research findings give meaning to the results obtained in clinical use of the procedures, and to the articulation test manual developed by Templin and Darley (*37*), in which a more detailed presentation of the rationale for each step of the procedure is presented.

A word of warning: It is well to remind yourself periodically that the results obtained from your articulation testing are based upon a small sample of speech behavior. You cannot generalize safely from one such brief sample to a person's total performance at all times and in all situations. You will want to be alert to the possibility of two important kinds of variation:

1. The subject may vary in articulatory performance from time to time and from day to day in relation to his or her mood, degree of fatigue, interest in communicating, security in the speaking situation, and other factors pertaining to physical, motivational, and emotional conditions. Furthermore, the subject's production of phonemes in one-word utterances must not be assumed to be identical with his or her performance in the rapid flow of contextual speech.
2. Observers or examiners fluctuate, too, in how critical they are and how discerningly they listen. The information we have about the temporal (day to day or time to time) reliability of the examiner in articulation testing indicates that at different times one listens differently depending on what one is tuned to listen for, how hurried or tired one is, how well the person being tested cooperates, or what listening activities one had engaged in prior to the task at hand. It is essential that you appreciate the fact that these statements apply to you as they do to other clinical observers. Depending upon your perceptual set, everyone may seem to have a hissing /s/ or everyone may sound normal.

As a careful examiner, then, you will beware of overinterpreting your data and drawing conclusions that are too sweeping or final about what a speaker can or cannot do.

PREPARATION OF A PICTURE TEST

A number of satisfactory picture articulation tests are commercially available. Eight of these are described in the final section of this chapter. However, you will find it an illuminating and useful enterprise to prepare your own picture materials for eliciting the speech responses of the children whose articulation you are to test. The following instructions pertain to a three-part test battery: the 50-item screening test of articulation developed by Templin (Test 1), a 42-item test of single consonant phonemes in the initial and final positions of words (Test 2), and the 43-item Iowa Pressure Articulation Test (*23*) (Test 3). Tests 1 and 2 together give us a picture of the general adequacy of a child's articulation, allowing scrutiny of every consonant phoneme we are interested in. Test 3 answers our questions about a child's ability to produce specific phonemes requiring substantial intraoral breath pressure and thus gives us a clue to his or her palatopharyngeal competence. You would have to prepare additional materials in order to have a complete diagnostic articulation test, including an inventory of vowel and diphthong production and a more exhaustive analysis of consonant production in various phonetic contexts.

1. Materials

The test will consist of 39 cards of convenient size (3″ x 5″ or 5″ x 7″), each of which will carry two, three, or four pictures. Each picture should be selected to elicit one single phoneme or one consonant cluster, in one position. The items to be included on each card are listed in Chart A. The first 50 items constitute Test 1, the Screening Test; items

CHART A
Arrangement of Items in Picture Articulation Test

Card	No. of Pictures	Test Items (Numbered as on Test Record)	Card	No. of Pictures	Test Items (Numbered as on Test Record)
1	2	1, 2	21	2	51, 52
2	2	3, 4	22	3	53, 54, 55
3	2	5, 6	23	2	56, 57
4	3	7, 8, 9	24	2	58, 59
5	3	10, 11, 12	25	2	60, 61
6	4	13, 14, 15, 16	26	2	62, 63
7	3	17, 18, 19	27	2	64, 65
8	3	20, 21, 22	28	2	66, 67
9	2	23, 24	29	3	68, 69, 70
10	3	25, 26, 27	30	3	71, 72, 73
11	3	28, 29, 30	31	3	74, 75, 76
12	3	31, 32, 33	32	2	77, 78
13	2	34, 35	33	2	79, 80
14	2	36, 37	34	3	81, 82, 83
15	3	38, 39, 40	35	2	84, 85
16	2	41, 42	36	2	86, 87
17	2	43, 44	37	2	88, 89
18	2	45, 46	38	2	90, 91
19	2	47, 48	39	3	92, 93, 94
20	2	49, 50			

marked with an asterisk constitute Test 2, single initial and final consonants; items whose numbers are underlined constitute Test 3, the Iowa Pressure Articulation Test. Some items are used in all three tests.

2. Key for Each Picture

On the back of each card make the following entries:

a. Place the number of the card in the upper right-hand corner.
b. List the numbers of the items on Form 3, the Articulation Test Record, at the end of the chapter, which the pictures on the card are designed to test.
c. Place an asterisk to the right of each number designating an item in Test 2 (single initial and final consonants).
d. Underline each number designating an item in Test 3 (Iowa Pressure Articulation Test).
e. After each number enter the phonetic symbol representing the item.
f. Where appropriate show whether the phoneme being tested occurs in the initial (i), medial (m), or final (f) position.
g. Write the word which each picture is designed to elicit.
h. Write a simple starter question or statement for each item which (if possible) does not contain the phoneme the picture is designed to elicit.

For example, entries such as the following would be written on the back of card number 6:

*13. /z/(i)   zebra   This striped animal is a ＿＿＿＿＿＿＿.
*14. /ʃ/(i)   shoes   We wear ＿＿＿＿＿＿＿.
 15. /ʃ/(m)   washing   What's she doing?
*16. /ʃ/(f)   fish   Let's catch a ＿＿＿＿＿＿＿.

The asterisks show that in addition to being part of the Screening Test, items 13, 14, and 16 are part of Test 2 (consonant singles). The underlinings show that in addition to being part of the Screening Test, items 14, 15, and 16 are part of Test 3 (Iowa Pressure Articulation Test).

Entries such as the following would be written on the back of card number 18:

 45. /tw-/   twins   These girls look alike. They are ＿＿＿＿＿＿＿.
 46. /kw-/   queen   The king's wife is the ＿＿＿＿＿＿＿.

The underline shows that in addition to being part of the Screening Test, item 45 is part of Test 3.

3. Subject Matter of the Pictures

The words you select for use in the test should be appropriate to the vocabulary level of preschool children; they should be words one would reasonably expect young children to know, for this is to be a speech examination rather than an intelligence test. To find out what words occur in the vocabularies of children you may refer to relevant studies (*1, 6, 9, 27, 38, 39, 40*).

Although you will use the norms developed by Templin (*34*) with this test battery, it is not necessary that your test employ the same words Templin used in her normative study. In an earlier investigation Templin (*36*) found that "there is little difference in measured articulation when the same sound is tested in different words. . . . The measure of a specific sound is a measure of the general ability to produce that sound and not to articulate it in a specific word." Hence you are justified in choosing words that you find easily pictured and highly suitable for the age level of the children you expect to test.

Select pictures that are simple in subject matter, clear in detail, and colorful. A common error is that of selecting a picture containing several items of interest or representing a complex and possibly confusing collection of things, thus providing distractions from the one item to which a response is desired. A picture of one simple object is to be preferred. Colored pictures should be used in preference to black and white. You may find them in magazines, catalogues, children's dictionaries, and other common sources.

4. Suggestions

a. You can handle a group of test cards more easily if you orient all the pictures toward either an end or a side than you can if you mix them up with some lengthwise and others sideways on the card.
b. A neat paste job adds greatly to the appearance.
c. Uniformity of design of the pictures (for example, all colored photographs, all colored drawings, all watercolor cutouts from paint books) is preferable.
d. If you like, you may "animate" the test with actual objects (for example, a feather, a button, a miniature knife) which can be affixed flat on the card. You should not use bulkier objects (toy cars, miniature furniture) which make the repeated and hasty handling of a single pack of cards unwieldy.

RECORDING AND ANALYZING RESULTS OF ARTICULATION TESTING

1. Recording

Form 3, the Articulation Test Record, can be used for recording the results of administration of any or all of the three tests in the battery you have made. On the Articulation Test Record space is provided after each test item for you to note the subject's response. Three common types of error are the following:

Substitution: The use of one phoneme in place of another, as of /w/

for /r/ in the pronunciation of "wabbit" for "rabbit," or of /n/ for
/ŋ/ in "singin" for "singing."

Distortion: The faulty production of a phoneme, although the production is recognized as being an example of the desired phoneme. For
example, a whistled or lateral /s/ may be considered a distortion of
the /s/ phoneme.

Omission: The failure to produce a phoneme in the position where it
should occur and the failure to insert any other phoneme in its place.
For example, an omission of final /t/ is noted in the pronunciation of
"ca" for "cat." (We must beware of recording a phoneme as omitted
when in fact it is not. Children may attempt a phoneme but produce
it with inadequate acoustic power so that we do not easily detect it.
If any attempt at a phoneme is perceived, the phoneme should not be
regarded as omitted.)

You will note that the Articulation Test Record provides for entries
derived from the testing of the single consonant phonemes usually in
two but sometimes three positions—initial, medial, and final. We recognize that the traditional concept of three positions of consonants in
words is artificial—an artifact growing out of orthography in disregard
of the dynamics of speech production. We recognize that a more meaningful phonetic analysis would be one related to the findings of Stetson
(33), who showed that the syllable is "the smallest indivisible phonetic
unit." He demonstrated that "the syllable is a puff of air forced upward
through the vocal canal by a compression stroke of the intercostal
muscles. It is usually modulated by the actions of the vocal folds. It is
accompanied by accessory movements (syllable factors) which characterize it. These are the *release* (by the action of either the chest muscles
or the releasing consonant), the *vowel shaping* movements of the vocal
canal, and the *arrest* (by the action of either chest muscles or the arresting consonant)" (33, p. 200). Consonants are properly understood, then,
as serving either a releasing function, initiating the syllable pulse, or an
arresting function, bringing the syllable pulse to a close.

In spite of our conviction that this classification of consonants is
meaningful and descriptive of the dynamics of speech *as spoken,* we
have to some degree retained the traditional classification of consonants
with regard to their position in the written word—initial, medial, final
—in the articulation testing here described. We have done this in order
to permit you to relate your test findings to available yardsticks, especially the normative data reported by Templin, since medial consonants
appear in both the Screening Test and the Iowa Pressure Articulation
Test as originally designed.

Make entries on the Articulation Test Record as follows for each single
consonant in the test battery:

a. If the subject articulates the phoneme correctly, enter a check mark
(√).

b. If the subject substitutes another phoneme, enter the phonetic symbol representing the phoneme produced.

c. If the subject omits the test phoneme in pronouncing the test word, indicate the omission with a dash (—).

d. If the subject distorts a phoneme enter an (x).

e. If the subject produces the phoneme with nasal emission of air, enter *ne*.

f. If you fail to elicit a response to an item, enter *nr*, signifying "no response."

In the case of consonant clusters adapt these entries so that errors and correct productions can be identified readily. For example, if one phoneme of a two-phoneme cluster is produced correctly while the other is omitted or distorted, transcribe phonetically the correctly produced phoneme and indicate the error by a dash or x.

To illustrate, part of the Articulation Test Record might be completed as follows:

    5. /l/ (i)   /w/
   14. /ʃ/ (i)   x
   29. /kr-/   /kw/
   50. /skr-/   /—kw/
   91. /-lf/   /—f/

These entries would be interpreted as follows: the consonant /w/ was substituted for the single consonant /l/ in the initial position. The production of the initial single consonant /ʃ/ was distorted. In the two-consonant cluster /kr-/ the consonant /k/ was produced correctly while /w/ was substituted for the consonant /r/. In the three-consonant cluster /skr-/ the consonant /s/ was omitted, the consonant /k/ was produced correctly, and /w/ was substituted for the consonant /r/. In the two-phoneme cluster /-lf/ the consonant /l/ was omitted while the consonant /f/ was produced correctly.

2. Analyzing

The three picture tests you have made provide information that answers different questions. Test 1 (items 1–50) is the Screening Test developed by Templin to determine the general adequacy of a child's articulation. It consists of those 50 items found to discriminate best between good and poor articulation of preschool and kindergarten children. If a child fails to attain a certain cutoff score, we conclude that his articulation should be studied further and a more thorough inventory made (using perhaps the Templin-Darley 141-item Diagnostic Test [37] or the McDonald Deep Test of Articulation [18]) in order to discern the pattern of the child's errors and thus develop an appropriate remedial plan.

Test 2 shows us how well the child produces each single phoneme in both initial and final positions and thus affords a look at the entire repertory of English consonant phonemes, not covered in Test 1. While a number of articulation measures are probably valid indices of a child's developmental speech status, the measure "number of defective single sounds" on the Templin-Darley Diagnostic Test was found by Jordan (17) to be the measure most highly related to judgments of severity of defectiveness of contextual speech samples of 150 children made by a group of 36 judges. This test, then, provides a measure directly related to how listeners perceive one's speech adequacy. Administration of both Tests 1 and 2 should yield the information you will usually want to know about a given child's articulation status, and use of these tests together is recommended.

Test 3 assesses the production of phonemes requiring significant buildup of intraoral breath pressure and thus allows us to make an inference about the adequacy of a speaker's palatopharyngeal closure. The 43 items comprising it were those items out of the Templin-Darley Diagnostic Test which best differentiated two groups of children, one with demonstrated palatopharyngeal competence and one with demonstrated palatopharyngeal incompetence.

After you administer each of these tests, you must scrutinize the results in such ways as will answer the questions which motivated you to administer the test. Analysis of the outcomes will show how a child compares with his or her peers, what the patterns of error that emerge suggest about the nature of the articulatory problem, if any, and what next step should be taken.

Comparison with Norms

Test 1   Count the number of correctly produced test items and enter the total in the space labeled "Score" on line 1a on the Articulation Test Record Analysis Sheet. Refer to Table 8.2 to determine the mean performance of children of the subject's age and sex, and enter the appropriate value under "Norm" on line 1a. Consult Table 8.3 to determine the cutoff score which separates adequate from inadequate performance at the age of your subject; enter this value in the space labeled "Norm" on line 1b. If the child is over 8 years old, use the 8-year-old values.

Does the child's score fall below, above, or close to the mean of his peers? If below, how far below in terms of standard deviations from the mean? Is it below the cutoff score? If so, he almost surely has a significant articulation problem; he deserves more complete testing to determine in detail the scope of his problem and to plan a remedial program tailored to the needs revealed by the evaluation.

Test 2   Count the number of consonant singles (both initial and final) produced correctly and enter the total under "Score" on line 1c. Refer to

TABLE 8.2
Mean Scores on Test 1, 50-Item Screening Test,
by Age for Boys and Girls

C.A.	Boys (N = 30)		Girls (N = 30)	
	Mean	SD	Mean	SD
3	22.5	13.5	20.1	12.9
3½	25.1	15.2	30.5	13.1
4	34.7	11.2	34.2	10.6
4½	34.3	13.4	37.3	10.3
5	34.7	14.5	40.6	12.0
6	38.5	13.8	44.3	8.7
7	44.0	8.4	47.8	3.9
8	47.8	4.2	47.9	4.6

Source: From Templin (34) and Templin and Darley (37).

Table 8.4 to determine the mean performance for the child's age and sex, and enter this value under "Norm" on line 1c. Also enter the number of incorrectly produced consonant singles (42 minus the number correct) under "Score" on line 1d.

Test 3 Count the items designated by underlined numbers produced correctly and enter the total under "Score" on line 1e. From Table 8.5 determine the mean performance for the child's age and sex, and enter this value under "Norm" on line 1e. These norms are based on normal children with presumably adequate palatopharyngeal closure and so reflect only the developmental status of the phonemes tested in the children of the sample. No norms are available which are based on samples of children with cleft palates or palatopharyngeal incompetence, nor can a cutoff score be suggested which can be interpreted as separating adequate from inadequate intraoral breath pressure or palatopharyngeal closure.

Types of Errors Note all the single initial or final consonant phonemes on which errors were noted on Test 1 and Test 2. List these phonemes in section 2 in the appropriate column as omissions, substitutions, distortions, or nasal emissions, indicating the position of the error

TABLE 8.3
Cutoff Scores for Test 1, Screening Test, at Eight Age Levels

C.A.	3	3½	4	4½	5	6	7	8
Cutoff Score	12	18	23	26	31	34	39	44

Source: From Templin (35) and Templin and Darley (37).

TABLE 8.4
Mean Scores on Test 2, Consonant Singles,
by Age for Boys and Girls

C.A.	Boys (N = 30)		Girls (N = 30)	
	Mean	*SD*	*Mean*	*SD*
3	26.5	8.0	24.9	7.6
3½	27.2	7.6	29.9	5.8
4	32.4	6.0	31.7	5.5
4½	31.3	8.1	34.2	5.7
5	31.9	9.5	35.6	6.8
6	35.6	7.1	38.7	3.4
7	38.9	4.6	40.6	2.6
8	40.7	2.2	40.9	4.6

Source: From Templin and Darley (37).

(initial or final). A number of research studies (*17, 28, 31, 34, 43*) have shown that omission is the articulation error consistently associated with the most immaturity and a good predictor of judged severity of articulation impairment. The data suggest that children who have difficulty in articulation may progress from errors of the omission type to substitution errors and then to distortion errors on their way toward mastery of the phonemes. It is important, then, to determine the phonemes on which a child makes errors and the type of error he or she is making. Analysis of

TABLE 8.5
Mean Scores on Test 3, Iowa Pressure Articulation Test,
by Age for Boys and Girls

C.A.	Boys (N = 30)		Girls (N = 30)	
	Mean	*SD*	*Mean*	*SD*
3	26.4	12.5	23.6	11.6
3½	28.8	12.5	32.9	9.6
4	35.1	9.7	33.5	8.8
4½	34.1	9.4	35.0	8.8
5	33.8	11.2	37.5	8.6
6	35.5	10.3	39.5	6.5
7	39.6	5.7	41.6	3.0
8	42.0	3.3	41.7	2.9

Source: From Templin and Darley (37).

errors according to this system indicates something of the severity of a child's problem and helps in deciding where to begin in therapy.

On Test 3 an important type of error is nasal emission, since that is an indication of palatopharyngeal incompetence for speech. See Chapters 11 and 16 for additional discussion of the interpretation of this test.

Consistency of Errors   Note which of the consonant singles produced incorrectly in at least one position (initial or final) were produced correctly in the other position or elsewhere in the tests in a consonant cluster. Perhaps a phoneme omitted in the final position was produced correctly in the initial position; or perhaps a phoneme misarticulated in both positions as a single was produced correctly when it appeared as one element of a consonant cluster. Note which phonemes were never produced correctly in any position or phonetic context. List all the misarticulated phonemes under the appropriate heading in section 3 as inconsistently or consistently misarticulated phonemes.

Investigations summarized by Spriestersbach and Curtis (32) have shown that when children misarticulate certain consonant phonemes, they tend to misarticulate them inconsistently. That is, sometimes a child produces a correct /r/ or /s/ phoneme while at other times he does not. Given a large enough sample of speech, an examiner would presumably find that almost any child sometimes articulates correctly the phonemes which he or she usually misarticulates. The inconsistency appears to depend in part upon the phonetic context of the phonemes in question; for example, a child may produce /r/ correctly when it follows the consonant /t/ in the cluster /tr-/, as in the word "tree," but not when it occurs as a single, as in the word "Mary." Possibly the inconsistency also depends partly on the child's ability to discriminate between incorrect and correct forms of a given phoneme.

Response to Stimulation   In testing a speaker's articulation performance, you will be interested in determining the ease with which he can correct his incorrect phonemes following intensive auditory stimulation. After noting those phonemes which the speaker has produced incorrectly throughout the tests, go back over each of these with him. Present each of them three times in isolation (for example, t—t—t) slowly and distinctly, and ask him to imitate your production as closely as possible. Then present the phoneme in a syllable, in a word, and in a consonant cluster in a word. List the results of stimulation in the appropriate space in section 4, showing which phonemes were produced correctly in which modes and which were never produced correctly.

It will pay you in several ways to make such an examination of a subject's ability to produce his faulty phonemes. For one thing, if the subject is producing a phoneme correctly a considerable part of the time or if he can produce it rather easily following stimulation, you can be reasonably certain that his speech mechanism is structurally adequate for production of the phoneme, at least in those contexts. (You should not assume, however, that his speech mechanism is physiologically capable of producing it at all possible rates at which he might speak.) Then, too, other things being equal (and excepting particularly the influence of mental subnormality), the prognosis should be more favorable for speakers whose misarticulations are not consistent or who can produce the phonemes correctly following a limited amount of stimulation than for those who are consistent in their misarticulations. Speakers who are inconsistent must at least be aware of the phoneme which they have misarticulated in some contexts, but not in others, and so they should not require as much ear training as persons who never produce the faulty phonemes correctly. With a view to economy in subsequent retraining, it is worthwhile to determine the phonetic contexts in which a speaker correctly produces the phonemes that he or she sometimes misarticulates. You may find, for example, that you need not teach /r/ "from scratch." After showing a child that she does produce the phoneme correctly in saying certain words, you can more readily and quickly motivate her to go from the correct productions to attempts at producing the phoneme in other phonetic contexts.

Comparison with Contextual Speech We have mentioned that it is unsafe to assume that a speaker's articulation of phonemes in the one-word responses elicited by a picture articulation test is representative of his or her articulation generally. It is quite possible for a person to fail to maintain this degree of articulatory competence in various kinds of contextual speech. A cerebral palsied child, a dysarthric adult, or a speaker with palatopharyngeal incompetence may be able momentarily to attain correct placement of the articulators and impound adequate intraoral breath pressure for satisfactory consonant production in single words, but contextual speech with its usual requirements of quick adjustments of the articulators may place excessive demands upon muscles limited in precision, speed, and extent of movement. Children without organic limitations may also display a considerable discrepancy between their careful, attentive production of phonemes in single words and their production of the same phonemes when they are "just talking."

You should scrutinize, if possible, different speech samples to see how the child's articulation varies with the task and the situation. Engage him in conversation about some toys or his favorite TV shows; have him tell you about some pictures containing lots of action; look at a book with him and get him to comment on what's happening in the story. Note any articulation errors which were not evident on the articulation test and list these in section 5 of the Articulation Test Record Analysis Sheet.

Search for Patterns When you have completed all the entries, review the record to see if you can discern any patterns among the errors which might help you understand why they occur or how therapy might be planned. You may note that the misarticulated phonemes have some common requirement which the speaker seems to be incapable of achieving, such as the buildup of a critical amount of intraoral breath pressure or adequate impedance of the breath stream by the anterior maxillary teeth. Voiceless phonemes may be more consistently misarticulated than their voiced cognates. The incorrectly produced phonemes may have high frequency components, and their misarticulation may be related to a possible hearing loss.

Patterns of articulation error will perhaps be most analytically and meaningfully described in terms of distinctive features. Psycholinguistic analysis of phonology posits that each phoneme is not a unitary entity but rather represents a bundle of features that together give that phoneme its identity and its distinctiveness. These subphonemic features are the result of how the phoneme is produced (motor aspects) and how it sounds (acoustic aspects). Chart B lists the 13 features proposed by Chomsky and Halle (2) as adequate to describe English phonemes, with explana-

CHART B
List of Distinctive Features

Vocalic. Two conditions are necessary for a sound to be labeled vocalic: the constriction in the oral cavity can not be greater than that required for the /i/ and /u/, and the vocal cords must be positioned to allow spontaneous voicing. Vocalic sounds include the liquids and the vowels. They are /i/, /u/, /e/, /o/, /r/, /l/, /æ/, /ʌ/, and /ɔ/ (negative-nonvocalic).

Consonantal. Consonantal sounds are made with a narrow constriction as in the fricative consonants. All liquids, nasal consonants, and nonnasal consonants have this feature. Consonants include /r/, /l/, /p/, /b/, /f/, /v/, /ð/, /θ/, /tʃ/, /k/, /g/, /m/, /t/, /d/, /ʃ/, /dʒ/, /n/, /s/, /z/, /ʒ/, and /ŋ/.

Rounded. A narrowing of the lip orifice is a characterization of rounded sounds. They include /u/, /o/, /w/, /ɔ/, /ũ/, /œ̃/, and /ɔ̃/ negative-nonround).

Tense. Tense sounds are produced by supraglottal musculature, with considerable effort in that the articulatory organs maintain their configurations for a relatively long period. The tense feature is present in /u/, /ẽ/, /õ/, /ã/, /œ̃/, /ɨ/, and /ɔ̃/ (negative-nontense).

Nasal. When the velum is lowered to allow the air to be directed through the nose, the nasal feature is present. The sounds with this feature include /m/, /n/, and /ŋ/ (negative-nonnasal).

Continuant. In a continuant sound a partial obstruction to the air flow is present in the vocal tract. Continuants include /l/, /r/, /f/, /v/, /θ/, /ð/, /s/, /z/, /ʃ/, /ʒ/, and /h/ (negative-noncontinuant).

Voiced. In voiced sounds the vocal folds are vibrating. The phonemes /r/, /l/, /b/, /d/, /v/, /g/, /z/, /m/, /n/, /ð/, /ʒ/, /dʒ/, and /ŋ/ have the feature of voicing (negative-nonvoiced).

Strident. A strident sound is characterized by noisiness which is produced

tory comments provided by McReynolds and Huston (*21*). Other investigators have used a lesser number of features in speech analysis. Some have proposed alternative systems of analysis; Walsh (*41*), for example, criticizes the Chomsky-Halle system as dealing with "an abstract idealized level of language, often far removed from the physical surface realities of human speech"; he suggests a feature system based strictly upon how the various parts of the speech mechanism play a role in producing the phonemes.

The distinctive feature system is binary; a given feature is either present (positive, designated +) or absent (negative, designated −) in a given phoneme. By listing the features present and absent in a given phoneme you can see what differentiates it from all others. If a child substitutes another phoneme for that target phoneme, you can list the features of the substituted phoneme and see how the two lists differ. This comparison is more revealing than is the mere identification of the two phonemes.

Psycholinguistic research has shown that we should not consider a

CHART B (continued)

---

when air is passed over a rough surface at the necessary rate of flow and angle of incidence. The phonemes /f/, /v/, /s/, /z/ /ʃ/, /tʃ/, /ʒ/, and /dʒ/ have a strident feature (negative-nonstrident).

Place of articulation is included in the next five features. Four of the features are concerned with position of the tongue and one is concerned with the region of the mouth. The features covered in the tongue positions use as a base of reference the neutral tongue position, which is usually defined as the position of the tongue in producing the /ɛ/ as in *bed*.

Coronal.   In coronal sounds the blade of the tongue is raised from the neutral position. The coronal feature is included in /r/, /l/, /t/, /d/, /θ/, /ð/, /n/, /s/, /z/, /ʃ/, /tʃ/, /ʒ/, and /dʒ/ (negative-noncoronal).

High.   In the high feature the body of the tongue is raised above the neutral position. The phonemes in which the high position is positive include /i/, /u/, /w/, /ɪ/, /ɨ/, /u/, /tʃ/ /dʒ/, /k/, /g/, /ʃ/, /ʒ/, and /ŋ/ (negative-nonhigh).

Low.   In the low feature the body of the tongue is lowered below the neutral position. The sounds with this feature include /æ/, /ɔ/, /h/, /æ/, /ã/, /œ̃/, and /ɔ̃/ (negative-nonlow).

Back.   When the body of the tongue is retracted from the neutral position the sound includes a back feature. The sounds are /u/, /ʌ/, /o/, /ɔ/, /w/, /k/, /g/, /ʃ/, /ɨ/, /ũ/, /õ/, /ã/, and /ɔ̃/ (negative-nonback).

Anterior.   The anterior feature is present when a sound is produced in the region of the mouth in front of where the /ʃ/ is produced. These sounds are /l/, /p/, /b/, /f/, /v/, /m/, /t/, /d/, /θ/, /ð/, /n/, /s/, and /z/ (negative-nonanterior).

Source: From Chomsky and Halle (*2*); explanations and illustrations provided by McReynolds and Huston (*21*).

child's articulation errors simply as idiosyncracies but rather as revelations of his or her grasp of phonologic rules. Crocker (4) and Menyuk (22) have shown that the sequence of normal phoneme acquisition can be accounted for in terms of children's learning of certain distinctive-feature rules of increasing complexity and specificity. Children who deviate from normal phoneme acquisition are shown not to be making random errors but to be operating with somewhat different sets of rules; the rules a given child is using account for his particular set of errors. A child's errors are seen not to be disorderly and lawless, but orderly, lawful, and consistent with the rules on which he is operating; the more bizarre a child's rules, or the larger the number of deviant rules on which he is operating, the more deviant and unintelligible his speech.

This being so, an economy immediately becomes evident: we probably need not deal in therapy with all of the surface manifestations of the child's phonologic problem (that is, each error phoneme individually) but we can reduce the problem to more general terms and deal with the rules (lesser in number than the error phonemes) which account for the errors. Thus Weber (42) reduced the list of errors made by each of 18 children to a smaller number of patterns (each pattern reflecting some deviant rule), the number of patterns in given children ranging from one to six, no two children exhibiting the same set of patterns; and he designed therapy to correct the patterns rather than to improve production of phonemes one at a time. Similarly Compton (3) reduced one child's 20 articulation errors to a set of 12 generalizations, and he reduced the 12 generalizations to seven phonologic rules which accounted for them; therapy directed at altering the child's rules was economical and effective. Other studies by McReynolds and Huston (21), McReynolds and Bennett (19), and Pollack and Rees (24) have confirmed the usefulness of this type of analysis of children's deviant articulation and the development of therapy programs tailored to correct deviant phonologic rules rather than individual phonemes.

We suggest, then, that in your search for patterns of error you scrutinize the child's errors in terms of distinctive features and the phonologic rules which the child appears to be using. You will find helpful suggestions for procedure contained in the book by McReynolds and Engmann (20). See if you can explain the specific errors by some general principles that underlie them. For example, does the child omit the plosive component of affricative phonemes? Does he displace his tongue too far forward in production of lingua-alveolar or lingua-palatal sounds? Does he omit the voiced feature and fail to contrast voiceless and voiced cognate pairs? Does he substitute plosive for fricative phonemes? Does he add a plosive to each nasal consonant? What features does he appear to lack and which features that he has does he appear to use inappropriately?

Enter your observations in section 6 of the analysis portion of the Articulation Test Record.

Rating of Intelligibility   Finally you should arrive at a judgment about the influence a child's articulation status has upon the overall intelligibility of his or her speech. Consider the samples of contextual speech you have observed and scale the speech in terms of how understandable it is to the listener. Use the 4-point scale given in section 7 to conclude whether the speech is readily intelligible, intelligible if one knows the topic, fragmentarily intelligible now and then, or completely unintelligible.

SUGGESTIONS FOR ADMINISTERING AN ARTICULATION TEST

You will inevitably encounter difficulties in testing some young children. The following remarks may alert you to some of these problems and help you cope with them.

1. Some children do not easily become absorbed in an externally imposed task. They may be easily distracted and quickly fatigued. If you are to keep a child attentive, cooperative, and talkative, you must remember Goodenough's statement that the child "can be allured but not coerced" (7, p. 297).
2. Conduct the test with no observers present, if possible. If the child requires the presence of a parent, ask the parent to be unobtrusive and not to prompt a response; the parent may be called upon to interpret if necessary.
3. Don't work too fast. Let the child become accustomed to the testing situation. Direct his attention away from himself; ignore him perhaps for a time; if necessary, interest him initially in things other than the picture cards—for example toys or blocks. Goodenough warns, "Do not urge the child to respond before he is ready. Let the child make the advances when he is ready" (7, p. 300). Of course when you are ready to present the test stimuli, you will remove the play materials, which otherwise might continue to distract him.
4. Throughout the test use the starter questions or statements you have entered on the backs of the cards in order to avoid monotonous repetition of the question, "What's this?" If you find a child to be quite responsive, you may find it possible to omit the starter and simply let the child name the pictures spontaneously. If the starter fails to elicit the desired response, even after two or three presentations, say the word and ask the child to repeat it. A useful technique which reduces the influence of your stimulation of the target word is to ask, "Is it a frog or a fish?" (where *frog* is the desired response).
5. Respond to remarks made by the child. You need not acknowledge

his every response, but react frequently and praise him liberally. Keep him motivated, using his desire for approval and his curiosity.

6. Remember that you are in charge: don't let the child take over, dominate the testing session, or destroy the test materials. It is possible for you to be friendly and participate in the game without surrendering the leadership.

7. Some examiners appear to believe that to make the child feel at home and interested they must descend to the child's level. The resulting foolishness, effusiveness, and childishness sometimes become excruciating and ridiculous, even to the youngster. Other examiners remembering that they must maintain control, mistakenly assume an air that is too austere and aloof, to which the child reacts with cold withdrawal. Others are so conscientious about their task that they hover eagerly over the youngster, like overhanging trees smothering a young sapling, tensely awaiting each response and overwhelming the child.

   You will usually find that the best approach is a straightforward, person-to-person naturalness, quietly communicating to the child a feeling that you like him, consider him your friend, and have some fascinating pictures to show him.

8. You may not always hear the child's response clearly the first time. Ask him to repeat, but avoid asking for too much repetition or you may meet rebellion. It is better to go back later and recheck doubtful responses.

9. The picture articulation test cards constitute a tool, and the tool may prove inappropriate for use with a given child. With younger children and those with short attention spans, small objects which the child may manipulate often prove more successful in stimulating speech responses. Most speech clinicians who work with children collect a set of inexpensive objects for use in testing or for rapport building.

10. The child, not the test, must be central. Don't be afraid to abandon a routine and adjust to circumstances. It is better not to use the test materials at all and just play and talk if that is the only way you can obtain a speech sample.

OBSERVATION OF ARTICULATORY GESTALTS

As mentioned earlier, in cases of other than developmental articulatory disorder, you may not need to administer a complete inventory and thus determine the adequacy of production of each phoneme. A more important observation will be the general pattern of articulatory dysfunction displayed. In all of the dysarthrias and in apraxia of speech (discussed in Chapter 19) articulation is a primary disordered dimension. Your observations may suggest what the nature of the speaker's disorder is, for the various motor speech disorders sound different in many respects.

Ordinarily you will base your observations on a sample of contextual speech. Ask the subject to describe a picture (use a photograph or painting of a situation full of action and many details) or read a paragraph aloud, or both. Let these questions guide you in observing the articulation:

Is the rate of articulation slowed or accelerated and to what degree?

Are the consonant phonemes precisely articulated or are they slighted and indistinct?

Are elements of consonant clusters slighted or even omitted?

Are transitions between the elements of consonant clusters accomplished smoothly and efficiently or effortfully and inefficiently?

Does the precision of articulation deteriorate progressively as the speaking task continues?

Are any certain types of phonemes especially poorly produced—lingua-alveolar phonemes requiring maximum tongue-tip elevation, affricates, "pressure" consonants, lingua-velar phonemes, et cetera?

Does nasal emission of air characterize any consonant productions?

Are vowels ever distorted, suggesting aberrations of tongue placement?

Do the errors on given phonemes occur consistently or are the errors highly irregular in their occurrence?

Do you hear irregularities in the duration of some phonemes—at times a prolongation, at other times a telescoping of the phoneme?

Does the slighting of some phonemes appear to be the result of reduced excursion of the articulators?

Are there repetitions of phonemes?

Are some articulation errors "complications" such as substitutions and additions as opposed to "simplifications" such as distortions or omissions?

Are repeated trials of a word characterized by similar errors from trial to trial or by variable errors?

Do errors occur primarily on longer words or are they likely to occur on any word?

Information you collect about these articulatory dysfunctions needs to be considered together with information derived from evaluations of respiration and phonation (Chapter 6), resonance (Chapter 7), prosodic features of rate and fluency (Chapter 9), and the speech mechanism (Chapter 11). The patterns that emerge are interpreted in Chapter 19.

A SELECTED LIST OF PUBLISHED ARTICULATION TESTS

The emphasis in this chapter has been on development of your personal testing materials and becoming intimately familiar with them and their power and limitations. In your professional work you will no doubt want to make use of other test materials. The following are some of the commercially available articulation tests with which you will want to become acquainted.

A Deep Test of Articulation, 1964. (By Eugene T. McDonald.) Spiral-bound booklets of pictures and sentences (third-grade level) allow for detailed testing of 30 phonemes in multiple phonetic contexts. *Screening Deep Test of Articulation*, 1974, elicits ten productions of each of nine commonly misarticulated consonants. Norms for each phoneme are based on sample of 521 children. (Publisher: Stanwix House, 3020 Chartiers Ave., Pittsburgh, Pennsylvania 15204.)

Arizona Articulation Proficiency Scale, revised ed., 1970. (By Janet B. Fudala.) Consists of 48 picture cards or test sentences. Protocol booklet or Survey Form can be used for recording responses of one or up to ten subjects. Serial testing yields "percentage of improvement" score. Manual provides norms for children 3 to 11 years old based on sample of 45 children. (Publisher: Western Psychological Services, 12031 Wilshire Blvd., Los Angeles, California 90025.)

Fisher-Logemann Test of Articulation Competence, 1971. (By Hilda B. Fisher and Jerilyn A. Logemann.) Contains 109 colored pictures on 35 easel-mounted cards to test all consonant singles and groupings of /s/, /r/, and /l/ clusters; Screening Test covers 11 most frequently misarticulated consonants. Fifteen test sentences are also provided. Manual of instructions explains administration and analysis. Record Forms facilitate analysis of errors according to distinctive features. (Publisher: Houghton Mifflin Co., 110 Tremont St., Boston, Massachusetts 02107.)

Goldman-Fristoe Test of Articulation, 1969. (By Ronald Goldman and Macalyne Fristoe.) The 36 spiral-bound pictures and two stories which child retells provide for evaluation of 23 single consonants and 12 consonant clusters. Stimulability Subtest is provided. Percentile rank norms for ages 6 to 16+ are based on National Speech and Hearing Survey of 38,884 children. (Publisher: American Guidance Service, Inc., Publishers Building, Circle Pines, Minnesota 55014.)

Photo Articulation Test, 1969. (By Kathleen Pendergast, Stanley E. Dickey, John W. Selmar, and Anton L. Soder.) Eight spiral-bound plates contain 72 color photographs, the same pictures also provided in a deck of cards. Manual provides supplementary test words and norms for boys and girls, aged 3 through 12, based on standardization sample of 684 children. (Publisher: Interstate Printers and Publishers, 19–27 North Jackson St., Danville, Illinois 61832.)

Predictive Screening Test of Articulation, 3rd ed., 1973. (By Charles Van Riper and Robert L. Erickson.) Manual (no picture stimuli) describes administration of 47-item test, child repeating words and sentences after examiner. Cutoff scores identify first-grade children unlikely to develop mature articulation by third grade without speech therapy. (Publisher: Continuing Education Office, Western Michigan University, Kalamazoo, Michigan 49001.)

Sequential Inventory of Communication Development, 1975. (By Dona Lea Hedrick, Elizabeth M. Prather, and Annette R. Tobin.) One part of this comprehensive test of language development evaluates articulation. Test was devised for young children between 4 and 48 months of age. Manual reports standardization study of 252 children and provides instructions for test administration and analysis. (Publisher: University of Washington Press, Seattle, Washington 98105.)

Templin-Darley Tests of Articulation, 2d ed., 1969. (By Mildred C. Templin and Frederic L. Darley.) The 57 spiral-bound cards contain 141 colored pictures comprising diagnostic test and including 50-item Screening Test, 43-item Iowa Pressure Articulation Test, and miscellaneous groupings of consonant clusters, vowels, and diphthongs. Test sentences are also provided. Manual explains test procedures and rationale and presents norms for boys and girls at eight age levels, ages 3 through 8, based on sample of 480 children. (Publisher: Bureau of Educational Research and Service, University of Iowa, Iowa City, Iowa 52242.)

ASSIGNMENTS

1. Administer your three articulation tests to five children of preschool or early elementary school age, recording the results of each test on Form 3.
2. On the basis of your administrations of the tests, write a brief evaluation of your test cards, indicating which pictures prove ambiguous or consistently elicit some response other than the desired one, and suggesting desirable changes. Make alterations in your test in accordance with your evaluation.
3. Summarize the impressions you gained from administering the test to five children. What mistakes did you make? What did you do that appeared to foster rapport and make for maximum interest and cooperation on the part of the children? What other approaches will you use next time?
4. Consider the data presented in Table 8.1 and Figures 8.3 and 8.4 which show the sequence in which the articulation of consonant phonemes is mastered by children. What factors can you think of that might account for this sequence? Consider sensory and motor aspects of speech production and the relative frequency of occurrence of the various phonemes in English. Does any single factor adequately account for the sequence or does a summation of several possible factors provide a more reasonable explanation?
5. Study the results you have obtained in administering the articulation tests. On the basis of your findings, which phonemes might you

logically select to start work on in a remedial program with each of the children you tested? Why?

6. Prepare additional picture cards for testing consonant clusters other than those included in your set. Plan an array of items to test often misarticulated consonants in a variety of phonetic contexts. These additional cards, together with your basic set, can constitute a diagnostic test to answer specific questions about the consistency of a child's misarticulations.

7. Compose sentences for testing all the single consonants. Make each sentence brief (less than ten words long), containing one instance of the phoneme in the initial position and one instance in the final position. Do not use words containing the phoneme in a cluster. Your goal is a set of sentences that read smoothly and naturally and are not "loaded" with the target phoneme. Try them out on five adults, recording the results on the Articulation Test Record.

FORM 3
Articulation Test Record

Test 1

Additional Consonant Singles*

Screening Test

1. ɝ	_____	26. br-	_____			
2. ju	_____	27. tr-	_____			
*3. r(i)	_____	28. dr-	_____			
4. r(m)	_____	29. kr-	_____			

Initial / *Final*

51. m _____ 52. m _____
53. n _____ 54. n _____
55. ŋ _____
56. p _____ 57. p _____
58. b _____ 59. b _____
60. t _____ 61. t _____
62. d _____ 63. d _____
64. k _____ 65. k _____
66. g _____ 67. g _____
68. l _____
69. f _____ 70. f _____
71. v _____
72. s _____ 73. s _____
74. z _____
75. ʒ _____
76. h _____
77. w _____
78. dʒ _____

1. ɝ _____ 26. br- _____
2. ju _____ 27. tr- _____
*3. r(i) _____ 28. dr- _____
4. r(m) _____ 29. kr- _____
*5. l(i) _____ 30. gr- _____
*6. v(i) _____ 31. fr- _____
*7. θ(i) _____ 32. θr- _____
8. θ(m) _____ 33. ʃr- _____
*9. θ(f) _____ 34. pl- _____
*10. ð(i) _____ 35. kl- _____
11. ð(m) _____ 36. gl- _____
*12. ð(f) _____ 37. fl- _____
*13. z(i) _____ 38. sm- _____
*14. ʃ(i) _____ 39. sn- _____
15. ʃ(m) _____ 40. sp- _____
*16. ʃ(f) _____ 41. st- _____
17. ʒ(m) _____ 42. sk- _____
*18. j(i) _____ 43. sl- _____
19. j(m) _____ 44. sw- _____
*20. tʃ(i) _____ 45. tw- _____
21. tʃ(m) _____ 46. kw- _____
*22. tʃ(f) _____ 47. spl- _____
*23. dʒ(i) _____ 48. spr- _____
24. dʒ(m) _____ 49. str- _____
25. pr- _____ 50. skr- _____

Additional Pressure Test Items

79. k(m) _____ 87. -gɚ _____
80. g(m) _____ 88. -ʃɚ _____
81. f(m) _____ 89. -ɚk _____
82. s(m) _____ 90. bl- _____
83. z(m) _____ 91. -lf _____
84. -pɚ _____ 92. -sm _____
85. -pt _____ 93. -ks _____
86. -kɚ _____ 94. -mps _____

* Asterisk designates a consonant single used in Test 2.
— Underline beneath item number designates an item used in Test 3.

Analysis Sheet

Score   Norm

1. Comparison with norms:
    a. Test 1: Screening Test (Table 8.2)   _____ _____
    b. Test 1: Cutoff score (Table 8.3)   _____
    c. Test 2: Consonant singles (Table 8.4) _____ _____
    d. Test 2: Number of defective singles   _____
    e. Test 3: Iowa Pressure Articulation Test (Table 8.5)   _____ _____

2. Types of errors: consonant singles incorrectly produced in Tests 1 and 2, with position of error indicated as initial (i) or final (f):

    Omission   *Substitution*   *Distortion*   *Nasal Emission*

3. Consistency of misarticulation:

    Inconsistently Misarticulated   *Consistently Misarticulated*

4. Response to stimulation:

    Produced Correctly Following Stimulation

As a Single	*In a Cluster*	*Never Produced*
In Isolation	*In a Syllable*	*In a Word*	*In a Word*	*Correctly*

5. Other errors noted in contextual speech: _____
    _____
    _____

6. Patterns of error: _____
    _____
    _____
    _____

7. Rating of intelligibility of contextual speech:
    _____ Readily intelligible
    _____ Intelligible if listener knows topic
    _____ Words intelligible now and then
    _____ Completely unintelligible

REFERENCES

1. Buckingham, D. R., and Dolch, E. W., *A Combined Word List*. Chicago: Ginn, 1936.
2. Chomsky, N., and Halle, M., *The Sound Pattern of English*. New York: Harper & Row, 1968.
3. Compton, A. J., Generative study of children's phonological disorders. *Journal of Speech and Hearing Disorders*, 1970, 35:315–339.
4. Crocker, J. R., A phonological model of children's articulatory competence. *Journal of Speech and Hearing Disorders*, 1969, 34:203–213.
5. Davis, I. P., The speech aspects of reading readiness. *17th Yearbook of the Department of Elementary School Principals*, NEA, 1938, 17:282–289.
6. Gates, A. I., *A Reading Vocabulary for the Primary Grades*. New York: Teachers College, Columbia University, 1935.
7. Goodenough, F., *Mental Testing*. New York: Holt, Rinehart and Winston, 1949.
8. Hall, M. E., Auditory factors in functional articulatory speech defects. *Journal of Experimental Education*, 1938, 7:110–132.
9. Horn, M. D., *A Study of the Vocabulary of Children Before Entering the First Grade*. International Kindergarten Union, Child Study Committee, 1928.
10. Irwin, O. C., Development of speech during infancy: curve of phonemic frequencies. *Journal of Experimental Psychology*, 1947, 37:187–193.
11. Irwin, O. C., Infant speech: variability and the problem of diagnosis. *Journal of Speech Disorders*, 1947, 12:287–289.
12. Irwin, O. C., Infant speech: consonantal sounds according to place of articulation. *Journal of Speech Disorders*, 1947, 12:397–401.
13. Irwin, O. C., Infant speech: development of vowel sounds. *Journal of Speech and Hearing Disorders*, 1948, 13:31–34.
14. Irwin, O. C., Infant speech: the effect of family occupational status and of age on use of sound types; on sound frequency. *Journal of Speech and Hearing Disorders*, 1948, 13:224–226, 320–323.
15. Irwin, O. C., Infant speech: speech sound development of sibling and only infants. *Journal of Experimental Psychology*, 1948, 38:600–602.
16. Irwin, O. C., and Chen, H. P., Development of speech during infancy: curve of phonemic types. *Journal of Experimental Psychology*, 1946, 36:431–436.
17. Jordan, E. P., Articulation test measures and listener rating of articulation defectiveness. *Journal of Speech and Hearing Research*, 1969, 3:303–319.
18. McDonald, E., *Articulation Testing and Treatment: A Sensory-Motor Approach*. Pittsburgh: Stanwix House, 1964.
19. McReynolds, L. V., and Bennett, S., Distinctive feature generalization in articulation training. *Journal of Speech and Hearing Disorders*, 1972, 37:462–470.
20. McReynolds, L. V., and Engmann, D. L., *Distinctive Feature Analysis of Misarticulations*. Baltimore: University Park Press, 1975.
21. McReynolds, L. V., and Huston, K., A distinctive feature analysis of

children's misarticulations. *Journal of Speech and Hearing Disorders*, 1971, *36*:155–166.

22. Menyuk, P., The role of distinctive features in children's acquisition of phonology. *Journal of Speech and Hearing Research*, 1968, *11*:138–146.

23. Morris, H. L., Spriestersbach, D. C., and Darley F. L., An articulation test for assessing competency of velopharyngeal closure. *Journal of Speech and Hearing Research*, 1961, *4*:48–55.

24. Pollack, E., and Rees, N. S., Disorders of articulation: some clinical applications of distinctive feature theory. *Journal of Speech and Hearing Disorders*, 1972, 37:451–461.

25. Prather, E. M., Hedrick, D. L., and Kern, C. A., Articulation development in children aged two to four years. *Journal of Speech and Hearing Disorders*, 1975, *40*:179–191.

26. *Public School Speech and Hearing Services. Journal of Speech and Hearing Disorders,* Monograph Supplement No. 8, 1961.

27. Rinsland, H. D., *A Basic Vocabulary of Elementary School Children.* New York: Macmillan, 1945.

28. Roe, V., and Milisen, R., The effect of maturation upon defective articulation in elementary grades. *Journal of Speech and Hearing Disorders,* 1942, 7:37–45.

29. Sander, E. K., When are speech sounds learned? *Journal of Speech and Hearing Disorders*, 1972, 37:55–61.

30. Sayler, H. K., The effect of maturation upon defective articulation in grades seven through twelve. *Journal of Speech and Hearing Disorders,* 1949, *14*:202–207.

31. Snow, K., and Milisen, R., The influence of oral versus pictorial presentation upon articulation testing results. *Journal of Speech and Hearing Disorders,* Monograph Supplement No. 4, 1954, 30–36.

32. Spriestersbach, D. C., and Curtis, J. F., Misarticulation and discrimination of speech sounds. *Quarterly Journal of Speech,* 1951, 37:483–491.

33. Stetson, R. H., *Motor Phonetics.* Amsterdam: North-Holland Publishing Co., 1951.

34. Templin, M. C., *Certain Language Skills in Children.* Institute of Child Welfare Monograph Series, No. 26. Minneapolis: University of Minnesota Press, 1957.

35. Templin, M. C., Norms on a screening test of articulation for ages three through eight. *Journal of Speech and Hearing Disorders,* 1953, *18:* 323–331.

36. Templin, M. C., Spontaneous versus imitated verbalization in testing articulation in preschool children. *Journal of Speech and Hearing Disorders*, 1947, *12*:293–300.

37. Templin, M. C., and Darley, F. L., *The Templin-Darley Tests of Articulation.* 2nd ed. Iowa City: University of Iowa Bureau of Educational Research and Service, 1969.

38. Thorndike, E. L., *The Teacher's Word Book.* New York: Teachers College, Columbia University, 1921.

39. Thorndike, E. L., *A Teacher's Word Book of 20,000 Words.* New York: Teachers College, Columbia University, 1932.

40. Thorndike, E. L., and Lorge, I., *The Teacher's Word Book of 30,000 Words*. New York: Teachers College, Columbia University, 1944.
41. Walsh, H., On certain practical inadequacies of distinctive feature systems. *Journal of Speech and Hearing Disorders*, 1974, 39:32–43.
42. Weber, J. L., Patterning of deviant articulation behavior. *Journal of Speech and Hearing Disorders*, 1970, 35:135–141.
43. Wellman, B. L., Case, I. M., Mengert, I. G., and Bradbury, D. E., Speech sounds of young children. University of Iowa Studies in Child Welfare, No. 5. Iowa City: University of Iowa Press, 1931.
44. Winitz, H., *Articulatory Acquisition and Behavior*. Englewood Cliffs, N.J.: Prentice-Hall, 1969.
45. Winitz, H., and Irwin, O. C., Infant speech: consistency with age. *Journal of Speech and Hearing Research*, 1958, 1:245–249.

9

APPRAISAL
OF RATE
AND FLUENCY

**Dean E. Williams,
Frederic L. Darley,
and D. C. Spriestersbach**

Among the basic dimensions of communicative behavior are those of amount of speaking and of rate and fluency, or disfluency, of speaking and oral reading. Available knowledge and general observations strongly indicate that amount or frequency of disfluency in its various forms, the amount of social speaking or verbal output, and the rate of speaking and of oral reading tend to change in relation to common variations in health and disease, shifts in emotional and psychological states, aging, certain neuropathologies, and various forms of psychopathology.

Speech clinicians are well advised to secure routinely a tape-recorded (audio or video) sample of the speaking and oral reading of each patient served. These speech samples not only provide a baseline from which to quantify changes in behavior as a result of clinical intervention but also assist you in differential diagnosis of various speech and language disorders. It can be of special importance in describing similarities and differences between the various fluency disorders discussed in Chapter 14.

In this chapter we present procedures for measuring or observing the rate, fluency or disfluency, and amount of speaking and oral reading, together with relevant normative data.

MEASURES OF RATE OF SPEAKING AND ORAL READING

Rate of utterance is a basic dimension of speech and of oral reading. As has been suggested above, measures of rate are of general interest in the examination of persons with speech and language problems. They have a particular relevance to the study of stuttering and aphasia. In evaluating the problem sometimes referred to as "cluttering" the measurement of rate is of fundamental importance.

Measurements of rate of utterance may be expressed as words, or as syllables, per minute, or in other ways. In a study of rate of oral reading Darley (2) had each of 200 college students, 80 male and 120 female, read aloud three passages, each of which was 300 words in length. The passages differed in mean number of syllables per word. One passage contained only one-syllable words. One was made up of words which averaged 1.5 syllables in length, a word length reported (1, 9, 11) to be average for representative language samples. The mean word length of the third passage was 2.2 syllables. Darley reported that he perceived a slower rate of reading as the passages increased in word length and as less commonly used words, according to the word count of Thorndike (13) were added to the passages. Darley stated, "This progressively slower perceived rate corresponds directly to the measures of reading rate in words per minute, but bears an inverse relationship to the measures of reading rate in syllables per minute" (2). He concluded that, in this specific sense, a value representing words per minute provide a more valid measure of reading rate than one expressed as syllables per minute.

Franke (3) obtained judgments of "slow," "normal," or "fast" made by seven observers listening to recorded samples of the oral reading of 42 subjects. These ratings correlated highly (r = 0.93) with measurements of rate in words per minute. Rate as measured in words per minute appears, thus, to correspond rather closely with rate as perceived by listeners, at least so far as oral reading is concerned under the conditions of Franke's study. However, Kelly and Steer (8) found that for extempore speaking, listeners' judgments of rate correlated 0.47 with overall measurements of words per minute and 0.62 with measurements of words per minute within sentences.

The measure of words per minute is to be used with due regard to the findings of Kelly and Steer (8). Observing two-minute samples of the extempore speech of 24 college speakers, they measured rate in words per minute for each sentence and computed a mean sentence rate as well as an overall rate for each speaker. The average overall rate of their subjects was 159 words per minute and the average sentence rate was 209 words per minute. Since the sentences contained all the words uttered, it may fairly be said that the mean sentence rate represented more closely than did the overall rate the actual execution of the movements involved in the utterance of words, exclusive of pauses or nonspeaking intervals. Kelly and Steer reported a mean duration of syllables of 0.154 seconds and a correlation of − 0.47 between mean syllable duration and mean sentence rate in words per minute; the faster the mean sentence rate the shorter the mean syllable duration, although the correlation coefficient of − 0.47, while significantly greater than a chance value, indicates that mean sentence rate is by no means to be accounted for wholly on the basis of mean syllable duration. Important also is the proportion of time during which voice is produced. Kelly and Steer found that in producing the average sentence their speakers phonated 71 percent of the total time.

The measure of mean sentence rate is probably more useful in general in evaluating spontaneous or extempore speech than in measuring the rate of oral reading, and in any instance the purposes of your examination should govern your decision as to which rate measure to use. A practical consideration, of course, has to do with the greater time and labor required to make the mean sentence rate measurement. In deciding which of these measures to use at any given time, due consideration is to be given to the correlation of 0.77 between overall rate in words per minute and the mean sentence rate in words per minute.

For many ordinary clinical purposes rate can be meaningfully measured as words per minute. On Form 4 provision is made for computing either or both of the measures of overall rate or mean sentence rate in words per minute. You can make measurements of the rate of oral reading and speaking most adequately by using tape-recorded samples of speech, although the overall rate of oral reading may be readily measured directly by timing the reading of a test passage such as Oral Reading Test Passage No. 1 at the end of the chapter. A procedure for obtaining tape-recorded samples of speaking and oral reading from adults is described below. The basic procedure may be adapted for use with children and adults for whom modified instructions and techniques are needed.

PROCEDURES FOR OBTAINING TAPE-RECORDED SAMPLES OF SPEAKING AND ORAL READING FROM ADULTS

The Job Task

Seat the speaker in full view of the recording equipment and ask his cooperation in speaking into the microphone and following instructions so that a good tape recording may be secured. Turn on the tape recorder and ask the speaker for identifying information such as name, age, and date. Have him tell briefly about any previous experience in having his speech recorded. If necessary, ask additional questions concerning school, family, and home town in order to accustom the speaker to the recording situation. After two or three minutes of conversation turn off the recorder, and instruct the speaker to talk for three minutes or so about his preferred, or possible, future job or vocation. Suggest to the speaker that he briefly describe the vocation, tell why he has chosen it, and say anything else about it that he wishes. If he does not seem able or inclined to talk about a possible future vocation ask him to tell about jobs he has held in the past. Do not encourage a formal speaking performance; a performance resembling a public speech is not what is wanted. The objective is to obtain a sample of the person's representative speaking. Tell him to take a minute or so to think about what to say. When he is ready, turn on the recorder and ask him to begin speaking. If he stops before the end of about three minutes, encourage him by means of leading questions to continue speaking. Make a reasonable effort to obtain a three-minute sample of speech.

When the speaking performance has been completed, turn off the recorder and hand the speaker a copy of the 300-word Oral Reading Test Passage No. 1 reproduced on p. 276. Instruct him to read it aloud as he ordinarily would. It is important that you not give him any more detailed instruction than this, and if he asks questions about the rate or loudness level at which he should read, or what he should do about stuttering or related matters, tell him simply to read as he ordinarily would. When he is ready to begin, turn on the recorder again and ask him to begin reading aloud. Record a reading of the complete passage.

The TAT Task

If you desire, a second speaking task, the TAT Task (5) may be employed. Presumably this task induces somewhat more emotional involvement in some speakers, but the difference between the Job Task and the TAT Task seems not to be very great for most persons. In administering the TAT Task, show the person Card No. 10 from the Thematic Apperception Test (10) and ask him to tell a story based on the picture. Ask him to talk for three minutes about what is happening at the moment in the pictured situation, what events have preceded those represented in the picture, and what the outcome of the story is to be. Allow him up to one minute, while he studies the picture, to prepare his story. At the end of this minute, turn on the recorder again and ask him to begin talking. If he stops talking before the end of three minutes, stimulate him to continue by asking questions. Every reasonable effort should be made to get at least a three-minute sample of speaking.

No observers other than the examiner should be present when these tape recordings are made.

Modifications of Procedure for Children and Atypical Adults

The procedures described above may be adapted for obtaining samples of speaking and oral reading from children—or adults—who are unable to follow exactly the indicated instructions.

A phonetically edited reading passage that is widely used in speech clinics and that is suitable for a large proportion of readers at younger age levels, as well as adults, is "Arthur, the Young Rat" (reproduced as Oral Reading Test Passage No. 2 on p. 276). It contains 180 words, and this number is to be used, therefore, instead of 300, in computations based on data obtained by means of this reading passage.

In securing samples of speaking from children, two types of procedure have been most commonly used. In one the examiner engages the child in conversation of a sort designed to encourage him or her to talk as freely as possible until the child has produced 200 to 300 words or more of representative speech. In the other the child is asked to respond to pictures by talking about what the people shown in the pictures are doing, what they have been doing, what they probably will do next, how it will turn out, whether the child would like to be doing what they are doing, where and when and with whom he or she has done such things, and so on until a sample of some 200 to 300 words or more has been obtained.

It is particularly important in timing children's speech samples for purposes of measuring speaking rate to time only the actual speaking, omitting intervals of unresponsiveness and the speaking done by the examiner in order to encourage the child to begin or to continue speaking.

Procedures for Measuring Rate of Speaking and Oral Reading

The Oral Reading Test Passage No. 1 contains 300 words. When this passage is used, overall oral reading rate in words per minute is computed by dividing the number of words, 300, by the number of seconds required to read the passage, and multiplying the result by 60. For example, if the subject reads the 300-word passage in 200 seconds, you would make the following computations: $300/200 = 1.5 \times 60 = 90$ words per minute. Always take 300 as the number of words read when this passage is used, provided it is completed, even though one or more words may be added or left out in the reading. If the 180-word Oral Reading Test Passage No. 2 is used, 180 is substituted for 300 in making these computations. Use Form 4, Measures of Rate of Speaking and Oral Reading, to record your measurements.

In order to compute either the overall or the mean sentence rate of speaking, it is desirable to make a transcript of the tape-recorded speech sample. It is essential, whether or not a transcript is made, to count the words spoken and to time the speaking of them, preferably with a stop watch, or by means of a watch with a second hand. One reason why it is advantageous to use tape recordings in making rate measurements is that with some speakers it is necessary to do a certain amount of prompting in order to obtain sufficiently long samples. In timing such samples, the use of tape recordings makes it possible to stop the watch with the completion of the last word uttered prior to each prompting and to start it again with the beginning of the first word uttered following the prompting. In each case indicate on the form whether the speaker was prompted while producing the speech sample.

In counting words in speech samples, count only those words that would have been spoken had the speaker performed no disfluencies.

That is, for example, "Uh, when I wuh—wuh—wuh—was 10 years old, I went—I went—I went to New York" is regarded for word-counting purposes as consisting of "When I was 10 years old, I went to New York," a total of 11 words. Count only once each word repeated singly or in a phrase. For example, count "We—we—we went home" as three words rather than five. Do not count sounds or words such as "well," "uh—uh—uh," and the like, which are not integral parts of the meaningful context. In any instance of revision, count only the words in the final form. For example, count "I started to—I went to town and bought some bread" as 8 rather than 11 words, disregarding the false start "I started to."

The computations to be carried out in determining either overall or mean sentence rate in words per minute are indicated on Form 4. Rate data, with which you may compare your rate measurements, are summarized in Table 9.1. (With regard to these norms, you will find it of some interest to read reference 4 for a discussion of apparent increases in average oral reading rate which have been reported in recent years.)

ASSIGNMENTS

Use Form 4 and the procedures described above.

1. For an adult stutterer, one adult with some other speech problem, and one adult with normal speech measure the following:
   a. Overall oral reading rate in words per minute (use Oral Reading Test Passage No. 1)
   b. Overall speaking rate in words per minute (Job Task)
   c. Mean sentence rate in words per minute (Job Task)
   d. Overall speaking rate in words per minute (TAT Task)

Write a report of the information and impressions you obtain by interviewing each subject about the differences and similarities among these performances, and of your observations of the differences and similarities among the speakers. Evaluate your rate measurements by reference to Table 9.1. Discuss the difference between the overall and the mean sentence rate in words per minute, indicating what you consider its implications to be. Comment on the variation in rate from sentence to sentence.

2. For one young stutterer, one youngster with some other speech problem, and one young normal speaker measure the following:
   a. Overall oral reading rate in words per minute (use Oral Reading Test Passage No. 2)
   b. Overall speaking rate in words per minute (use CAT pictures, or other pictures, or conversation)

Write a report of the information and impressions you obtain by interviewing each subject about the differences and similarities among

TABLE 9.1
Ranges and Deciles of Distributions of Values for Speaking and Reading Rates in Words Per Minute for Each of Three Specified Tasks for Adult Subjects

Task	N	Range	Decile [a]								
			1	2	3	4	5	6	7	8	9
Job [b]											
Male stutterers	50	24.7–184.4	39.3	67.1	81.4	92.5	102.0	105.5	121.0	133.0	139.4
Female stutterers	50	12.9–183.3	44.1	64.8	70.6	81.0	98.9	103.1	120.0	148.3	170.2
Male nonstutterers	50	42.3–201.2	105.4	112.6	120.3	129.7	136.2	141.5	146.6	158.1	160.0
Female nonstutterers	50	94.7–198.4	121.8	131.1	135.7	140.9	147.0	150.0	154.8	164.7	185.1
TAT [c]											
Male stutterers	50	18.3–148.6	29.4	48.9	68.2	78.6	86.1	91.8	102.0	119.9	135.7
Female stutterers	50	9.9–177.2	31.7	44.7	56.6	70.4	78.6	84.0	104.7	113.2	141.4
Male nonstutterers	50	72.5–197.8	99.6	101.6	112.3	114.7	119.2	127.2	130.9	138.0	148.6
Female nonstutterers	50	58.6–202.7	108.8	117.1	119.9	122.9	130.5	138.2	144.3	151.4	162.4
Reading [d]											
Male stutterers	50	31.9–200.0	55.4	76.5	102.4	116.7	123.5	131.6	142.9	162.2	181.8
Female stutterers	50	20.3–200.0	53.6	67.7	84.1	92.3	109.8	128.6	146.5	155.2	181.8
Male nonstutterers	50	104.9–217.4	151.5	160.4	164.8	171.4	176.5	179.6	181.8	187.5	202.7
Female nonstutterers	50	135.1–219.0	155.4	163.9	171.4	173.4	176.5	181.6	184.1	187.5	197.4
Normal speakers [e]	200	129–222	148	155	159	162	166	170	175	181	190

Source: Johnson (5); Darley (2).
[a] Computed from ungrouped data.
[b] Speaking for about three minutes about future job or vocation.
[c] Speaking for about three minutes about Card No. 10 of the Thematic Apperception Test (10).
[d] Reading aloud the 300-word Oral Reading Test Passage No. 1.
[e] Darley's (2) 200 college-age normal speakers, 120 men and 80 women.

these performances, and of your observations of the differences and similarities among the speakers.

3. With the cooperation of a classmate or friend, obtain measurements of your own:
   a. Overall oral reading rate in words per minute (use Oral Reading Test Passage No. 1)
   b. Overall speaking rate in words per minute (Job Task)
   c. Mean sentence rate in words per minute (Job Task)
   d. Overall speaking rate in words per minute (TAT Task)

Write a report of your observations and impressions of the differences and similarities among these performances. Evaluate your rate measurements by reference to Table 9.1. Discuss the difference between the overall and the mean sentence rate in words per minute, indicating what you consider its implications to be. Comment on the variation in rate from sentence to sentence.

MEASURES OF DISFLUENCY IN SPEAKING AND ORAL READING

Samples of speaking and oral reading are fluent or disfluent in some degree. There are important differences among speakers—and in any given speaker from time to time, or from one condition or situation to another—in fluency or disfluency. As a practical matter, it is easier to think in terms of measuring disfluency than fluency. A forthright approach consists in identifying instances of disfluency and counting them. We can tabulate all disfluencies without regard to type, or we can classify them into various kinds of disfluency and tabulate each kind separately. We can make various combinations of kinds, or we can count some kinds but not others. Also we can simply tabulate the number of words that are associated with any kind, or with some specified kinds, of disfluency. Several methods of measuring disfluency have been developed in the course of laboratory and clinical work with the stuttering problem. We shall describe these methods here and discuss them in Chapter 10 where their role in the clinical study of the problem of stuttering will be considered.

A system of classification of disfluencies and procedures for computing two measures of disfluency are presented in the following pages.

A System of Classification of Disfluencies

A relatively comprehensive classification of disfluencies is essential to the systematic investigation of the disfluent aspects of speech. Our suggested classification includes the following categories:

Interjections of Sounds, Syllables, Words, or Phrases This category includes extraneous sounds such as "uh," "er," and "hmmm" and extraneous words such as "well" which are distinct from sounds and words associated with the fluent text or with phenomena included in other categories. An instance of interjection may include one or more units of repetition of the interjected material; for example, "uh" and "uh—uh—uh" are each counted as one instance of interjection. (The number of times the interjection is repeated—that is, the number of units of repetition—within each instance may also be noted; "uh—uh" is an example of an interjection repeated once and "uh—uh—uh" is an example of an interjection repeated twice.)

Part-Word Repetitions   Repetitions of parts of words—that is, syllables and phonemes—are placed in this category. (Within each instance of repetition the number of times the phoneme or syllable is repeated may be counted; "buh—boy" involves one unit of repetition and "guh—guh—girl" involves two units.) No attempt is made to draw a distinction between phoneme and syllable repetitions. "Ruh—ruh—run," "cuh—come," "ba—ba—baby," and "abou—bout" are examples of part-word repetitions.

Word Repetitions   Repetitions of whole words, including words of one syllable, are counted in this category. (The number of repetition units within each instance may be counted. "I—I—I," "was—was," and "going—going" are samples of instances of word repetition; the first involves two units of repetition and each of the other two involves one unit.) Under certain circumstances, you may wish to tabulate separately word repetitions that occur on monosyllabic words and those that occur on polysyllabic words. A word repeated for emphasis as in "very, very clean," is not counted as a disfluency. A part-word repetition, or an interjection, does not nullify a word repetition; for example, "going—uh—going" or "guh—going going" is classified as a word repetition. In any such case, the interjected or associated disfluency is also tabulated in the appropriate category.

Phrase Repetitions   Repetitions of two or more words are included in this category. "I was—I was going" is an example of this type of disfluency. (Again, if desired, the number of units of repetition within each instance of repetition may be separately noted.)

Revisions   Instances in which the content of a phrase is modified, or in which there is grammatical modification, are classified as revisions. Change in the pronunciation of a word is also counted as a revision. "I was—I am going" is an example of this category.

Incomplete Phrases   An incomplete phrase is one in which the thought or content is not completed and which is not an instance of phrase repetition or of revision. "She was—and after she got there he came" contains an example of an incomplete phrase.

Broken Words This category is typified by words which are not completely pronounced and which are not classifiable in any other category, or in which the normal rhythm of the word is broken in a way that definitely interferes with the smooth flow of speech. "I was g— (pause) —oing home" is an example of a broken word.

Prolonged Sounds Phonemes or parts of words that are judged to be unduly prolonged are included in this category. It is usually the initial phoneme of a word that is prolonged.

Instances of any of these types of disfluency may be performed with ordinary or unusual degrees of tension, effort, or strain.

The above disfluency classification system has been used in many research investigations. However, in an unpublished manuscript Johnson and Moeller have suggested that the categories of Broken Words and Prolonged Sounds be replaced by the categories of Dysrhythmic Phonation in Words and Tension Pause. These latter two categories encompass certain kinds of speaking behavior that are difficult to categorize in the classification system described above. These two categories are defined as follows:

Dysrhythmic Phonation in Words Dysrhythmic phonation, identified only with words, is that kind of phonation which disturbs or distorts the so-called normal rhythm or flow of speech. The disturbance or distortion may or may not involve tensing and may be attributable to prolongation of a phoneme, an accent or timing which is notably unusual, an improper stress, a break, or any other speaking-behavior infelicity not compatible with fluent speech and not included in another category. Dysrhythmic phonation is a within-word category.

Tension Pause Tension is a disfluency phenomenon judged to exist between words, part-words, and nonwords (i.e., an interjection) when at the between-point in question there are barely audible manifestations of heavy breathing or muscular tightening. The same phenomena within a word would place that word in the category of dysrhythmic phonation.

You are encouraged to use the classification system that best serves your needs.

Procedures for Measuring Disfluency

Follow the procedure described on pp. 258–260 in obtaining the necessary tape-recorded samples of speaking and oral reading. In each case make a verbatim transcription of the tape and then proceed by listening to the tape as you follow along on the transcription, identifying disfluencies for later tabulation on Form 5, Measures of Disfluency of Speaking and Oral Reading. Listen to each tape as often as you like or until you are satisfied that you have identified and properly classified all, or as many as possible, of the disfluencies in the sample.

Total Disfluency Index

The Total Disfluency Index is the total number of disfluencies, of all types, per 100 words read or spoken. This represents the most thorough type of disfluency analysis, in which you identify, classify, and tabulate all the disfluencies in a sample of speech or oral reading. For this purpose, use the entire classification system described on pp. 263–265. Use Form 5 to record your findings and make your computation.

Disfluency Type Index

Form 5 provides for the computation of the number of each of eight types of disfluency per 100 words. Each such number is the Index of Disfluency for the type of disfluency which it represents.

ASSIGNMENTS

Using Form 5 and the procedures for obtaining tape-recorded samples of oral reading and speaking described in the preceding pages:

1. Obtain from one adult stutterer and one adult nonstutterer a tape-recorded sample of oral reading (use Oral Reading Test Passage No. 1) and a 200-word sample of speaking (Job Task). Transcribe the samples; identify and tabulate the disfluencies while listening to the tape; and, using Form 5, determine:
   a. Oral Reading: Total Disfluency Index and Disfluency Type Indexes
   b. Speaking: Total Disfluency Index and Disfluency Type Indexes
      Write a report of the information and impressions you obtain by interviewing each subject about the differences and similarities among these performances, and of your observations of the differences and similarities between the two speakers.
2. Perform the same operations, with oral reading and speaking samples obtained from one young stutterer and one young nonstutterer. Use Oral Reading Test Passage No. 2. Obtain a 200-word speech sample, using the TAT (10) pictures or other suitable pictures as stimulus materials. Write a report of the information and impressions you obtain by interviewing each subject about the differences and similarities among these performances, and of your observations of the differences and similarities between the two speakers.
3. With the cooperation of a classmate or friend tape-record your own reading of "Your Rate of Oral Reading" (Oral Reading Test Passage No. 1) and 200 words of speaking about your future job; and then perform the same operations as for Assignment 1 above, computing your own disfluency indexes. Write a report of your observations and

impressions of the differences and similarities among these performances.

THE ADAPTATION EFFECT

The adaptation effect was first reported and named in 1937 by Johnson and Knott (7). It has been utilized mainly in the study of stuttering. When a stutterer makes several successive oral readings of a passage, there is a tendency for the number of words that are judged as stuttered to decrease from reading to reading. A similar effect is observed in the frequency of disfluencies when a normal speaker reads a passage aloud several times.

The relevance of obtaining adaptation data for each stutterer is discussed in Chapter 10. Their possible use in the differential diagnosis of fluency problems is discussed in Chapter 14.

Procedure for Measuring the Adaptation Effect

Using the procedure described on p. 259, obtain a sample of the oral reading of a stutterer. When he has finished, ask him to read the passage a second time, then a third time, and a fourth time, and a fifth. Time each reading carefully by means of a stop watch or a watch with a second hand.

During the first reading of the passage, follow along on your own copy and write the numeral 1 above each word you judge to be stuttered. During the second reading write a 2, during the third reading a 3, during the fourth a 4, and during the fifth reading a 5, above each word classified by you as stuttered. You may do this while the stutterer is reading, or if you use a tape recorder you may mark the stuttered words—and also time each reading—later while listening to the tape recording.

Count the words you judged as stuttered and enter your totals for the different readings in the appropriate spaces on Form 6, Measures of Adaptation of Stuttering and Oral Reading Rate. Enter the time in seconds for each reading in the spaces provided. Then complete Form 6.

ASSIGNMENTS

Using Form 6 and the procedure described above, do the following assignments:

1. Tape-record five successive readings by a stutterer of either Oral Reading Test Passage No. 1 or No. 2. Mark and tally the words you judge as stuttered in each reading of the passage and enter your tallies on Form 6. Also time each reading and enter the time of each

reading in seconds in the space provided. Complete the computations called for on Form 6.

2. Using the same tape recording and the same procedures, measure the adaptation of disfluency, as disfluency is defined in this chapter. Compute adaptation scores for:

   a. Total disfluencies
   b. Interjections
   c. Repetitions of words and phrases combined
   d. Part-word repetitions, broken words, and prolonged sounds combined.

   Compare these adaptation scores with that for words you judged as stuttered.

3. After a minimal interval of 24 hours, repeat Assignment 1 and Assignment 2.a., with this difference: instruct the stutterer to do his best to read without stuttering. Compare results and discuss their possible implications with your supervisor and with the stutterer.

THE CONSISTENCY EFFECT

Several investigators (6) have observed that when a stutterer reads the same passage several times in succession, he or she tends to stutter on the same words from reading to reading. This finding was first reported by Johnson and Knott (7), who named it the consistency effect. In recent years it has been demonstrated that normal speakers also tend to show the consistency effect. They are more likely than one would predict by chance alone to be disfluent on the same words during successive readings of a passage.

The importance of obtaining consistency data for each stutterer is discussed in Chapter 10. In Chapter 14 we refer to it in the assessment of fluency disorders.

Tate and Cullinan (12) have evaluated the several different methods proposed for computing the degree or strength of the consistency effect. See their article and the publications to which they refer for further information about the various technical problems involved in research on the consistency effect.

A relatively simple procedure for measuring consistency is presented here. It is designed to serve essential purposes in most clinical situations. As computed by means of this procedure, degree of consistency is expressed as a Consistency Index. Form 7, Measures of Stuttering Consistency, is designed for recording your measures. In using this method, you compute in each case the percentage of the words which you have judged as stuttered [1] in a given reading of a passage that are words

---

[1] In the instructions for computing consistency the term "stuttering" is used. For assessing the consistency effect for other populations the word "disfluencies" would be used.

which you also judged as stuttered in one or more specified previous readings of the passage. For example, suppose that you have a subject read a 100-word passage twice, and that you judge her to stutter on 20 words, or 20 percent of all the words, in the first reading and on 15 words in the second reading. (In Form 7, the 20 percent would be entered as *A*.) Suppose, further, that of the 15 words stuttered in the second reading 12, or 80 percent were among the 20 words stuttered in the first reading. Her Consistency Index, therefore, is 80 percent. (In Form 7, the 80 percent would be entered as *B*.)

Relevant studies (6, 7) have shown that in a series of successive readings of a passage the average adult stutterer is about 65 to 70 percent consistent—that is, of the words he or she stutters in any given reading about two-thirds are words that were stuttered in the preceding reading. No comparable data are available for the percentage of consistency that one might expect in populations other than stutterers.

Concerning Form 7   In making out Form 7 you divide *A* by *B*— that is, you divide the percentage of words stuttered in the first reading, for example, by the percentage of words stuttered in the second reading that were also stuttered in the first reading. The value you obtain in dividing *A* by *B* provides a general comparison between the consistency of stuttering that could have occurred by chance and the consistency of stuttering that actually did occur. When this value is 1.0 or less it represents an absence of consistency; it shows that the stutterer was no more consistent, or even less consistent, in stuttering on words previously stuttered than on other words. The term "chance" as used here has the meaning suggested in the following explanation. Suppose, for example, one person stutters 10 percent of all the words in the first reading of a passage. Now, in the second reading of the passage he is no more likely by chance to stutter on one word than on any other word. Therefore, by chance 10 percent of the words he stutters in the second reading will be among the 10 percent that he stuttered in the first reading and 90 percent will be among the 90 percent he did not stutter in the first reading. If more than 10 percent of the words he stutters in the second reading are among the words that he stuttered in the first reading, he is more consistent than he would have been by chance. In that case the value you obtain in dividing *A* by *B* will be greater than 1.0.

In general, the higher the value obtained by dividing *A* by *B*, the greater the degree of consistency it represents—the more, that is, the observed consistency exceeds chance consistency. This statement needs to be duly qualified by consideration of the magnitude of *B* in each case. If, for example, 80 percent of all words in the passage were stuttered in the first reading, then even if 100 percent of the words that are stuttered in the second reading were also stuttered in the first, *A* divided by *B*—in this case, 100 divided by 80—would give a value of only 1.25. If, on the other hand, 10 percent of all words were stuttered in the first reading, and 100 percent of all words stuttered in the second reading were also stuttered in the first reading, then A divided by B would be 100 divided by 10, which would give a value of 10. The value obtained is to be evaluated, therefore, by reference to the magnitude of the B term in each case.

Procedure for Measuring the Consistency Effect

Using the procedure described on p. 259, obtain a sample of oral reading from a stutterer. When he has finished, ask him to read the passage a second time and a third time. Tape-record the readings if possible. (You may, if you prefer, use the first three readings you tape-recorded in doing Assignment 1 on p. 267.)

During the first reading of the passage, follow along on your own copy and write the numeral 1 above each word you judge to be stuttered. During the second reading write a 2 and during the third reading a 3 above each word classified by you as stuttered. You may do this while the stutterer is reading, or if you use a tape recorder you may mark the stuttered words later while listening to the tape recording.

Count the words you judged as stuttered and enter your total for the three readings in the appropriate spaces on Form 7. Then complete Form 7.

ASSIGNMENTS

Use Form 7 and the procedure described above.

1. Obtain from one stutterer a series of three consecutive readings of Oral Reading Test Passage No. 1 or No. 2.
2. Mark and tally the words judged by you as stuttered in each reading of the passage, and enter your tallies on Form 7.
3. Complete the computations called for on Form 7.
4. It is possible, also, of course, to measure the consistency of disfluency, as disfluency is defined on p. 263, by employing the procedure used here for measuring the consistency of stuttering. In measuring the consistency of disfluency, do not sort the disfluencies into those to be classified as stuttering and those not to be so classified.

MEASURES OF AMOUNT OF SPEAKING

There are two particularly meaningful ways in which you can gauge the amount of speaking someone does. You can have the person keep a speaking-time log or you can observe or measure his or her verbal output in given situations. The speaking-time log is a record made by the individual of the amount of time he or she spends in talking to specified persons or in particular situations.

Speaking-Time Log

A log of the amount of time a person spends in speaking reveals important kinds of information about him:

1. The total amount of time he spends in speaking each day for which he keeps a log, and his average speaking time per day over the period or periods sampled.
2. The specific situations in which he speaks and the persons with whom he speaks in these situations.
3. The degree of variability in the individual's speaking situations, the persons with whom he speaks, and his total speaking time, from day to day.

There are many reasons why it is important to determine the amount of speaking done each day by any stutterer, or any person with a voice disorder or any other type of communicative problem:

1. A person's speaking time is a fundamental indicator of the degree to which he or she is handicapped by the communicative difficulty. A stutterer or a cerebral palsied person who speaks less than two minutes per day, for example—and there are some who do no more speaking than this—is allowing his speech problem to affect him much more than one who speaks as much as a half-hour or more per day. The one who does very little speaking is probably the more handicapped, even though the person who talks much more may not speak as well as he does. After all, the importance of a particular individual's speech problem is felt by him in a peculiarly basic way in the extent to which it restricts or inhibits his communication with other people.
2. A person's speaking time is an indicator of his or her social adjustment. In planning therapy, you necessarily take account of the speaker's relationships with other people. You would proceed differently with someone who has no close friends and few acquaintances and who spends most of her time by herself with nonsocial hobbies and private daydreams, from the way you would work with a sociable person whose relationships with other people are generally good.
3. An individual's speaking-time log amounts to a particularly meaningful account of how he spends his time. By examining a log covering several days, you can see more clearly than you could otherwise the person's basic pattern of relationships with others. Such a record provides, in fact, information for an essentially sociometric study of the person, an identification of the individuals whom he seeks out more and less and who seeks him out often and seldom for the sorts of association that are represented by a sharing of speaking time. So far as truth lies in the old saying that a person is known by the company he keeps, it may be said that a person can become

known by the speaking-time log he or she keeps. This means that a person's speaking-time log can be of value to you in your counseling of him, and it can clarify for him much that is important about himself.

4. The speaking-time log of an individual also helps to bring into focus his needs for various kinds of speech practice and his unrealized opportunities to obtain that practice in his daily comings and goings. You can spot speaking situations that he meets more or less regularly, judge their probable degree of difficulty for him, and evaluate their suitability for particular retraining purposes. By studying the person's speaking-time logs with him you can help him recognize ways of increasing the amount of speaking he does and of expanding the number and variety of the situations in which he does it. In view of the generally valid rule that the more a person in need of speech improvement talks the better, the uses that you can make of the log in raising a speaker's verbal output to an optimal level possible can be important.

There are no adequate speaking-time norms. Data obtained informally from normally speaking students at the University of Iowa suggest that the average of them has about 45 minutes per day of what might be called solid speaking time. The average student probably spends considerably more time than that, of course, in conversational or other speech situations; the figure of 45 minutes is meant to represent actual speaking time. It has been our clinical experience that those stutterers who turn in speaking-time records of as much as one hour per day seem to be doing somewhat more speaking than is done by most other persons, stutterers or nonstutterers, of comparable age and circumstance. Such observations can provide, of course, only a rough basis for evaluating the performance of a given speaker. The major value of a speaking-time log is as a record of changes in amount of speaking from month to month, perhaps, or from one time to another, and therefore as a basis for counseling in meaningful relation to the planning of therapy and the evaluation of its effectiveness.

How to Keep a Speaking-Time Log

Since most of the log entries are for less than one minute, speaking time should always be recorded in seconds. It takes one second or less to say "Hello" or "Good-by." It takes most individuals less than four seconds to say "Now is the time for all good men to come to the aid of the party." In a 30-minute conversation between two persons who share the talking about equally, each would speak about 12 minutes or so. If one does most of the talking, the time might be split 24 and 2 minutes perhaps, or 20 and 6, but the total will never be 30 minutes. A person should practice timing himself quite accurately with a stop watch or the second hand of a wrist watch in making various common remarks and typical contributions to conversation or discussion in order to sharpen his ability to estimate his speaking time. By engaging in this sort of practice yourself you can improve your ability to judge the validity of specific entries in the speaking-time logs turned in to you by the speakers with whom you work clinically.

At first most persons are almost sure to overestimate their speaking time. What one is to record for each instance or situation is an estimate of his or her actual speaking time.

An actual speaking-time log (Form 8, completed—with real names disguised) is shown on p. 275 as a general model. The speaker should make log entries often enough during the day to insure reasonable accuracy and completeness. If one makes entries as often as three times a day—at midmorning, midafternoon, and just before bedtime—one can readily recall the persons one talked with and the situations in which one talked with them, and estimate fairly closely the times involved.

Entries should be numbered, and each one should be identified by a brief description of the situation, such as "Buying movie ticket," or the name of the listener, "Sally," for example, or both, as in "Telephoned Bob about exam."

The estimates for each day should be totaled and the total expressed in hours, minutes, and seconds. In addition to showing the total speaking time, the record should indicate:

1. The total number of speaking situations
2. The number of these that involved:
   a. One other person
   b. Two or three other persons
   c. Four or more other persons
3. The number of situations in which the other persons were:
   a. Members of the speaker's own family
   b. Close friends or associates, such as sweetheart, persons with whom he shares a car pool, landlady or house mother, close classmates, etc.
   c. Others with whom the person has previously spoken
   d. Those spoken with for the first time
4. The number of situations in which the other persons were:
   a. Members of the speaker's own sex
   b. Members of the opposite sex
   c. Members of both sexes
5. The number of situations in which the other persons were:
   a. Mostly of the same age as the speaker (generally within a couple of years or so, but with allowance for the difference between "same age" at 12 and at 45
   b. Mostly older

    c. Mostly younger
    d. Mixed
6. The number of situations in which the other persons were:
    a. Associated with the speech clinic as students or patients or staff members
    b. Not associated with the speech clinic.

Provision was made for these classifications on Form 8. You may break down the data in other ways, of course, in accordance with your particular purposes.

ASSIGNMENTS

1. Keep a speaking-time log for yourself for each of three successive days and record the results on Form 8.
2. Obtain three successive daily speaking-time logs for one of your normally speaking friends and for each of two individuals assigned to you as persons with clinically significant speech problems. Provide each person with a copy of Form 8 on which to record his or her data.

Example of a Speaking-Time Record for One Day (Names Disguised)

Speaking-Time Log

Name _____ George Doe _____   Age _19_   Sex _M_

Clinician _____ Mary Roe _____   Date _February 23, 1978_

Situations	Time (seconds)	Situations	Time (seconds)
1. Herb	180	16. Bud	12
2. Betty	18	17. Jim, returned book	12
3. Waitress	12	18. Bert	18
4. Dr. Bern for test score	180	19. Bud	24
5. Vivian, arranging date	720	20. Mary, telephone	30
6. Ralph	18	21. Bob	36
7. Vivian, telephone	24	22. Pete	12
8. Bud	30	23. Bud	30
9. Stutterers' Group	18	24. Clerk in store	6
10. Ed	18	25. Fern	18
11. Vivian, Bud, Art	18	26. Ann, compared class notes	180
12. Stranger	6	27. Waitress	6
13. Waitress	6	28. Martha	24
14. Bob, argument	120	29. Herb	24
15. Sam	24	30. Herb, bedtime snack	120

Speaking time in seconds: 1944
Speaking time in minutes = total seconds divided by 60: 32.4

Total number of situations: 30

with 1 other person	28	with others of same age	24
with 2–3 other persons	1	with others mostly older	5
with 4 or more other persons	1	with others mostly younger	0
with members of own family	0	with others both older and younger	1
with close friends or associates	14		
with others previously spoken to	14	with others associated with clinic	9
with others spoken with first time	2		
with others of own sex	18	with others not associated with clinic	21
with others of opposite sex	10		
with others of both sexes	2		

Oral Reading Test Passage No. 1

Your Rate of Oral Reading °

Your rate of speech will be adequate if it is slow enough to provide for clearness and comprehension, and rapid enough to sustain interest. Your rate is faulty if it is too slow or too rapid to accomplish these ends. The easiest way to begin work on the adjustment of your speech to an ideal rate is to measure your present rate in words per minute in a fixed situation which you can keep constant over a number of trials. The best method is to pick a page of simple, factual prose to be read. Read this page in your natural manner, timing yourself in seconds. Count the number of words, divide by the number of seconds, and multiply this result by sixty to calculate the number of words per minute. As you attempt to increase or retard your rate, repeat this procedure from time to time, using the same reading material, to enable you to check your success.

A common accompaniment of rapid rate is staccato speech, in which the duration of words and syllables is too short, whereas in slow speech the words and syllables frequently are overprolonged. When the person with too rapid rate tries to slow down, he tends to make the error of keeping the duration of his tones short, and of attempting to accomplish the slower rate solely by lengthening the pauses between phrases and by introducing new pauses. On the other hand, the person who is working to speed up his rate tends to do this by shortening the pauses alone and retaining his prolonged tones. It is impossible at the present time to set down in rules the ideal relation between the duration of tones and pauses in speech. Further research is needed before this can be done with any great accuracy.

Oral Reading Test Passage No. 2

Arthur, the Young Rat

Once, a long time ago, there was a young rat named Arthur who could never make up his flighty mind. Whenever his swell friends used to ask him to go out to play with them, he would only answer airily, "I don't know." He wouldn't try to say yes, or no either. He would always shrink from making a specific choice.

His proud Aunt Helen scolded him: "Now look here," she stated, "no one is going to aid or care for you if you carry on like this. You have no more mind than a stray blade of grass."

That very night there was a big thundering crash and in the foggy morning some zealous men—with twenty boys and girls—rode up and looked closely at the fallen barn. One of them slipped back a broken board and saw a squashed young rat, quite dead, half in and half out of his hole. Thus, in the end the poor shirker got his just dues. Oddly enough his Aunt Helen was glad. "I hate such oozy, oily sneaks," said she.

° Reprinted by permission of the publisher, from Grant Fairbanks, *Voice and Articulation Drillbook* (New York: Harper & Row, 1940) p. 144.

FORM 4
Measures of Rate of Speaking and Oral Reading

Name _____   Age _____ Sex _____

Examiner _____   Date _____

Reading passage used: No. 1 _____   No. 2 _____   Other (specify) _____

Speaking procedure used: Job Task _____   TAT Task _____

Other (describe): _____

	Passage No. 1	Passage No. 2	Other
I. Oral reading rate:			
A. Number of words	_____	_____	_____
B. Number of seconds	_____	_____	_____
C. Number of sentences	_____	_____	_____
D. Overall rate in words per minute (OR:WPM)	_____	_____	_____
E. Mean sentence rate in words per minute (MSR:WPM)	_____	_____	_____

	Job Task	TAT Task	Other
II. Speaking rate:			
A. Number of words	_____	_____	_____
B. Number of seconds	_____	_____	_____
C. Number of sentences	_____	_____	_____
D. Overall rate in words per minute (OR:WPM)	_____	_____	_____
E. Mean sentence rate in words per minute (MSR:WPM)	_____	_____	_____

To compute overall rate in words per minute: Divide the number of words by the number of seconds and multiply the result by 60, the number of seconds in one minute. Under either I or II, above, use the formula A/B × 60 = OR:WPM.

To compute mean sentence rate in words per minute: Under either I or II, above, carry out the following operations: (a) count the number of words in each sentence; (b) time the speaking of each sentence in seconds; (c) for each sentence, divide the number of seconds by the number of words to find the time in seconds consumed in speaking the average word; (d) divide 60 seconds by the result obtained in (c) and the quotient will be the rate in words per minute at which the sentence was uttered; (e) sum the rates, in words per minute, for all the sentences and divide the total by the number of sentences to determine the mean sentence rate in words per minute; enter this value in E.

FORM 5
Measures of Disfluency of Speaking and Oral Reading

Name _____ Age _____ Sex _____

Examiner _____ Date _____

Reading passage used: No. 1 _____ No. 2 _____ Other (specify) _____

Speaking procedure used: Job Task ___ TAT Task ___ Other (describe) _____

	Reading Passage			Speaking Task		
	No. 1	No. 2	Other	Job	TAT	Other
A. Number of words	___	___	___	___	___	___
B. Number of disfluencies						
a. Interjections per 100 words = a/A × 100	___	___	___	___	___	___
b. Part-word repetitions per 100 words = b/A × 100	___	___	___	___	___	___
c. Word repetitions per 100 words = c/A × 100	___	___	___	___	___	___
d. Phrase repetitions per 100 words = d/A × 100	___	___	___	___	___	___
e. Revisions per 100 words = e/A × 100	___	___	___	___	___	___
f. Incomplete phrases per 100 words = f/A × 100	___	___	___	___	___	___
g. Broken words per 100 words = g/A × 100	___	___	___	___	___	___
h. Prolonged sounds per 100 words = h/A × 100	___	___	___	___	___	___
i. Dysrhythmic phonations in words per 100 words = i/A × 100	___	___	___	___	___	___
j. Tension pauses per 100 words = j/A × 100	___	___	___	___	___	___
k. Total repetitions (b+c+d) per 100 words: i/A × 100 = Repetition Index (RI)	___	___	___	___	___	___
l. Total disfluencies=(a+b+ . . . h) per 100 words = j/A × 100 = Total Disfluency Index (TDI)	___	___	___	___	___	___

FORM 6
Measures of Adaptation of Stuttering and Oral Reading Rate

Name _____ Age _____ Sex _____

Examiner _____ Date _____

Reading passage used: _____

Adaptation of Stuttering

Reading	Number of Words Stuttered	Percentages of Adaptation	
1	a _____		
2	b _____	$(a-b)/a \times 100 =$ _____	
3	c _____	$(a-c)/a \times 100 =$ _____	$(b-c)/b \times 100 =$ _____
4	d _____	$(a-d)/a \times 100 =$ _____	$(c-d)/c \times 100 =$ _____
5	e _____	$(a-e)/a \times 100 =$ _____	$(d-e)/d \times 100 =$ _____

Adaptation of Oral Reading Rate

Reading	Time in Seconds	Percentages of Adaptation	
1	a _____		
2	b _____	$(a-b)/a \times 100 =$ _____	
3	c _____	$(a-c)/a \times 100 =$ _____	$(b-c)/b \times 100 =$ _____
4	d _____	$(a-d)/a \times 100 =$ _____	$(c-d)/c \times 100 =$ _____
5	e _____	$(a-e)/a \times 100 =$ _____	$(d-e)/d \times 100 =$ _____

FORM 7
Measures of Stuttering Consistency

Name _____ Age _____ Sex _____
Examiner _____ Date _____
Reading Passage Used: _____

Consistency Index: 2-1

Number of words stuttered in Reading No. 2   _____

A. Percent of these words that were stuttered in Reading No. 1
   (this percentage is the Consistency Index for Reading 2 relative to Reading 1, or CI:2-1)   _____
B. Percent of all words stuttered in Reading No. 1   _____
   A divided by B   _____

Consistency Index: 3-2

Number of words stuttered in Reading No. 3   _____

A. Percent of these words that were stuttered in Reading No. 2
   (this percentage is the Consistency Index for Reading 3 relative to Reading 2, or CI:3-2)   _____
B. Percent of all words stuttered in Reading No. 2   _____
   A divided by B   _____

Consistency Index: 3-1

A. Percent of the words stuttered in Reading No. 3 that were
   also stuttered in Reading No. 1 (this percentage is the Con-
   sistency Index for Reading 3 relative to Reading 1, or
   CI:3-1)   _____
B. Percent of all words stuttered in Reading No. 1   _____
   A divided by B   _____

FORM 8
Speaking-Time Log

Name _____ Age _____ Sex _____

Clinician _____ Date _____

	Situations	Time (seconds)		Situations	Time (seconds)
1.	_____	_____	26.	_____	_____
2.	_____	_____	27.	_____	_____
3.	_____	_____	28.	_____	_____
4.	_____	_____	29.	_____	_____
5.	_____	_____	30.	_____	_____
6.	_____	_____	31.	_____	_____
7.	_____	_____	32.	_____	_____
8.	_____	_____	33.	_____	_____
9.	_____	_____	34.	_____	_____
10.	_____	_____	35.	_____	_____
11.	_____	_____	36.	_____	_____
12.	_____	_____	37.	_____	_____
13.	_____	_____	38.	_____	_____
14.	_____	_____	39.	_____	_____
15.	_____	_____	40.	_____	_____
16.	_____	_____	41.	_____	_____
17.	_____	_____	42.	_____	_____
18.	_____	_____	43.	_____	_____
19.	_____	_____	44.	_____	_____
20.	_____	_____	45.	_____	_____
21.	_____	_____	46.	_____	_____
22.	_____	_____	47.	_____	_____
23.	_____	_____	48.	_____	_____
24.	_____	_____	49.	_____	_____
25.	_____	_____	50.	_____	_____

Speaking time in seconds: _____

Speaking time in minutes = total seconds divided by 60: _____

Total number of situations:

with 1 other person _____   with members of own
with 2-3 other persons _____   family _____
with 4 or more other   with close friends or
    persons _____   associates _____
                                       with others previously
                                           spoken to _____
                                       with others spoken to
                                           for first time _____

with others of own sex _____
with others of opposite
sex   _____
with others of both
sexes   _____
with others of same
age   _____
with others mostly
older   _____

with others mostly
younger   _____
with others both older
and younger   _____
with others associated
with clinic   _____
with others not asso-
ciated with clinic   _____

REFERENCES

1. Cotton, J., Syllabic rate: a new concept in the study of speech rate variation. *Speech Monographs*, 1936, *3*:112–117.
2. Darley, F. L., A normative study of oral reading rate. M.A. thesis, University of Iowa, 1940.
3. Franke, P., A preliminary study validating the measurement of oral reading rate in words per minute. M.A. thesis, University of Iowa, 1939.
4. Gilbert, J. H., A note on oral reading rate. *Journal of Speech and Hearing Research*, 1968, *11*:219–221.
5. Johnson, W., Measurements of oral reading and speaking rate and disfluency of adult male and female stutterers and nonstutterers. *Journal of Speech and Hearing Disorders*, Monograph Supplement, No. 7, 1961, 1–20.
6. Johnson, W., ed., assisted by Leutenegger, R., *Stuttering in Children and Adults: Thirty Years of Research at the University of Iowa*. Minneapolis: University of Minnesota Press, 1955.
7. Johnson, W., and Knott, J. R., The distribution of moments of stuttering in successive readings of the same material. *Journal of Speech Disorders*, 1937, *2*:17–19.
8. Kelly, J. C., and Steer, M. D., Revised concept of rate. *Journal of Speech and Hearing Disorders*, 1949, *14*:222–226.
9. Lumley, F. H., Rates of speech in radio speaking. *Quarterly Journal of Speech*, 1933, *19*:393–403.
10. Murray, H. A., *Thematic Apperception Test*. Cambridge, Mass.: Harvard University Press, 1943.
11. Skalbeck, O. M., A statistical analysis of three measures of word length. M.A. thesis, University of Iowa, 1938.
12. Tate, M. W., and Cullinan, W. L., Measurement of consistency of stuttering. *Journal of Speech and Hearing Research*, 1962, *5*:272–283.
13. Thorndike, E. L., *A Teacher's Word Book of 20,000 Words*. New York: Teachers College, Columbia University, 1932.

10
THE PROBLEM
OF STUTTERING

Dean E. Williams

Stuttering is a problem in which many factors and many persons interact in complex ways. It is a problem that involves not only a speaker but his listeners as well. Indeed, it may be said with peculiar validity that in the beginning stuttering is not so much a problem for the speaker, who is most often a small child, as it is for his most important listeners, who are usually, although not always necessarily, his parents. After the child takes on the problem, he makes it more and more a part of himself as he grows older with it; but it remains a kind of trouble that he shares with those around him who never abandon their investment in it—and each newcomer borrows from him that part of it which serves his own need to be responsive to the stutterer's distress.

In order then to evaluate the problem of stuttering, you need to give attention to how the one who is said to be the stutterer speaks, and to what he says about the way he speaks, and to the feelings he has because of it and because of what he tells himself about it. You need to find out also what his listeners say about his mode of speaking and how they feel about it. And you need to discover where and when the speaker does what he and others take to be his stuttering, and what they do because he does these things at the times and in the places where he does them, and what he does because they do what they do.

Procedures for examining the stuttering problem are appropriately selected and designed to reveal significant aspects of (1) the attitudes and reactions of listeners to the speaker and his speech, (2) the attitudes and reactions of the speaker to those of his listeners and to himself and his own speech, and (3) the speech behavior of the speaker.

The purpose of the examination, which is similar in stuttering to current trends in behavior diagnosis (11), is to develop a program of analysis which is closely related to subsequent treatment. Your task is to pursue all possible avenues open to you in order to answer as best you can the following questions: (a) What specific behavior patterns require change in their frequency of occurrence, their intensity, their duration, or in the conditions under which they occur? (b) What are the conditions under which this behavior was acquired, and what factors are currently maintaining it? (c) What are the best practical means which can produce the desired changes in this individual (manipulation of the environment, the behavior, or the self-attitude of the client.? (*11*, p. 419)

Suggested examination procedures will be discussed for the same age groups as those used in the supplementary case history on the stuttering problem (Chapter 2, pp. 65–72). However, the suggested examination procedures for the elementary-school-age child will be presented following those for the preschool child and those for the adult stutterer. This order is reasonable because stuttering is constantly developing in complexity the longer the child lives and copes with the problem. Therefore, if the child is of a lower elementary age the examination procedures may incorporate some of the same tests presented for the preschooler. On the other hand, as the client approaches junior-high age, procedures suggested for the high schooler become increasingly appropriate.

EXAMINATION OF THE PRESCHOOL-AGE CHILD

Ordinarily a child between the ages of 3 to 5 is referred to you because someone is concerned about his speech fluency. This concern may be phrased in a simple question such as "Is he stuttering?" or a statement such as "He is stuttering. What can I do about it?" The clinician's task is to analyze and evaluate the child's speaking behavior and draw some reasonable conclusions.

Over the years one of the questions that has haunted most responsible clinicians is "How do I tell if a person is 'really' stuttering or if he or she just has a great many normal disfluencies?" It's easy to become enmeshed in this trap. The trap is there only if clinicians turn their attention solely to the speaking behavior of the child and on the basis of it attempt to make a decision. By definition the word "stuttering" is an *evaluative* word, not a descriptive one. To be descriptive, one would need to report that a child repeats part of the word so many times or prolongs a sound for so long a time in one specific situation and so much in the next one, et cetera. Since most children repeat part of the word or prolong sounds occasionally, your task is to determine if this particular child is doing too much of it—for it is when a child is doing "too much" that *someone* evaluates it as "stuttering." "Too much" is a floating cork on the continuum of disfluency. "Too much" according to whom? This question of course involves the listener—the "evaluator."

There is no person alive today who can describe exactly the point on the continuum of disfluency at which a child would fall from the category of "speaking" normally" into that of "stuttering." Johnson has written on this issue extensively (7, 8). Van Riper made the following succinct statement about this point:

> All stuttering yardsticks are not of the same length. . . . Some mothers have greater tolerances for their children's broken words than other mothers. Some children seem to be able to tolerate fewer of these morphemic interruptions than other children can. Nevertheless, despite the variations in normative criteria, a speaker must keep his broken words within the frequency of the limits of his listeners or be noticed and judged as having the disorder of stuttering (21, p. 21).

The fact that parents brought their child to a speech clinician with the question "Is he stuttering?" or the statement "He is stuttering" indicates that the child's disfluency has gone beyond *their* yardstick of normal speech. Most certainly it may not go beyond the yardstick of some other person. But that isn't the point. For these parents it did. To them it represents a problem. Your task is to evaluate the various facets of this problem. You must develop a program of analysis that coincides with the purposes of an examination as described under a, b, and c above.[1]

The Case History

The supplementary case history that outlines the stuttering problem in Chapter 2 (pp. 65–72) is of fundamental importance in the investigation of the stuttering problem for a child from approximately 3 to 5 years of age. Detailed questioning and attentive listening at this time can elicit much information about the parent's perception of just what they consider the stuttering to be, their place in it, their interactions with the child, and the ways that they have reacted to the child. In short, it can bring you up to date to the time of their visit with you and set the stage for your observations of the child and his or her speaking behavior.

Speech Sample

First you will want to obtain a speech sample from the child. Consult Chapter 9 for an explanation of the procedures to follow in obtaining a 200- to 300-word speech sample in conversation and in response to pictures. Next, familiarize yourself with the system of classification of disfluency types, also explained in Chapter 9. From the disfluency analysis of the speech sample, you then can obtain a "total disfluency index," a "disfluency type index," and a "repetition index."

---

[1] Your observations and questions—and your subsequent discussions with the parents—can be sharpened by reviewing references 22 (chap. 14), 7, and 19.

Verbal Complexity   After you obtain a representative speech sample, determine the extent to which the child's frequency of total disfluency or of *any one type* of disfluency increases or decreases as you vary the verbal complexity required from the child. These levels of verbal complexity include the following:

1. *Naming objects.* The child makes a one-word response in naming objects pictured on cards.
2. *Short-phrase response.* The child makes statements about what's going on in a picture. The purpose is to elicit a two- to five-word response.
3. *Telling a story about a picture.* Use pictures that contain considerable activity or use a sequence of pictures that tell a story requiring a longer sequential speech response. Ask the child to tell the story.
4. *Relating information.* In this task the child can tell you all he can about a pet or a television program that he likes. Another meaningful task is to ask him to tell you about his house. You or he can draw the house on a piece of paper and put in the kitchen, living room, et cetera. Then the child can tell you what goes on in each room.
5. *Answering questions.* Devise a list of questions to ask the child that will require his verbal response. The types of questions can require responses of increasing length.
6. *Asking questions.* While looking at pictures or while playing games, request the child to ask as many questions as he can about the activity.
7. *Giving instructions.* While playing with toys, ask the child to tell you what you should do first, what you should do next, et cetera.

Listener Reaction Complexity   While obtaining the samples described above, you should be reacting to the child in an easy, attentive, relaxed way. It can be informative, however, if you begin to vary the ways you interact with the child. Again, careful observation should be made of the increase in frequency of total disfluency or of any one disfluency type as you vary your reaction pattern. You can vary reactions in the following ways:

1. *Begin to hurry your activities.* Increase the rate of your speech, increase your hand movements, or increase the speed of requesting answers.
2. *Interrupting.* While the child is telling you about the activities in a picture, you can interrupt him and note verbally some other activity. You can ask a question and then ask a new question before he finishes answering the first question.
3. *Loss of attention.* When the child is talking to you as you are playing together with toys or while he is relating an event, begin to do something else and indicate by your action that you're not paying attention to him.

4. *Cease following directions.* While the child is giving you directions about how to play a game with some toys or explaining how a toy works, cease following his directions and start doing things other than what he's directing you to do.
5. *Say it again.* After the child makes a verbal response, respond with the statement, "I didn't hear that; would you say it again?" or "I didn't understand that; would you tell me again?"

Social Complexity   Procedures described for evaluating the effect on the frequency of disfluency of varying language and reaction complexity are done by the examiner. If possible, arrange situations in which other people can talk with the child. These may include the following: (1) an adult enters the room to talk with the child; (2) the parents enter the room (the examiner leaves) and talk with the child; (3) the examiner takes the child out of the room to talk with the secretary or colleague, and the like.

Child's Behavior and Behavior Changes During the Speech Examination

During the course of the speech examination outlined above, you should be particularly alert to the general behavior of the child. Is he tense or relaxed? Does he speak with a loud or a soft voice? Is his speaking rate overly fast or slow? Does he appear to be spontaneous in responding to you or is he rather inhibited and cautious in his response? Using these observations as a base, begin to note any change in behavior during the occurrence of any one type of disfluency. For example, during the occurrence of an "interjection" type of disfluency, there may be no observable change in his behavior. However, during a part-word repetition you may observe a change in certain aspects of behavior. Note particularly any fixating of body behavior (hand movement, squirming) during the occurrence of a disfluency. Observe his eye movement during speech and then during the occurrence of a disfluency. Is there a fixating of eye movement on an object during the occurrence of a disfluency? Is there a change in his voice quality, pitch, or loudness during the occurrence of a disfluency from that observed during fluent speech production? Observations such as these can provide clues to the extent, if any, that the child is reacting to the way he's talking. Also valuable information can be obtained by observing any relative increase or decrease in frequency of total disfluency or of any one type of disfluency during the tasks described in the preceding sections on verbal listener reaction, and social complexity. Such frequency changes during the particular tasks can provide clues for needed changes in the behavior of the "significant others" in the child's environment.

Parent's Evaluation of Speaking Behavior

Up to this point we have been speaking about the total disfluency and different types of disfluency in the child's speech. The evaluation of the occurrence of "stuttering" has not been discussed. The parents brought the child to you because they were concerned about his "stuttering." Therefore, it is important to determine the nature of the disfluencies that they consider to be stuttering. One cannot assume that what you might indicate as "stuttering" is the same thing as they indicate by the word. Be careful! You may refer only to the part-word repetitions. They may consider to be stuttering not only part-word repetitions but also interjections, revisions, and any other type of disfluency. Or they may consider only prolongations as "something wrong" because he appears to be "stuck." They may dismiss the part-word repetitions as something that "all children do."

It is desirable to videotape part or all of the speech examination. If this is not possible, you can make an audio tape recording or you can conduct the speech examination in a room with an observation window. In the latter instance, you will need a second clinician who can be with the parents during the speech examination. On a sheet of paper list each type of disfluency. Then when the child is speaking, ask the parents to indicate upon the occurrence of any type of disfluency whether or not they consider that to be "stuttering." You can make a check (√) following the disfluency if they do not consider it to be stuttering and an (X) if they do consider it to be stuttering. You may also obtain an estimate of how sure they are that it is stuttering. It is not uncommon that the parents will report that they are "not quite sure about that one" or that "definitely that is one." This procedure can assist you in isolating and defining the type of speaking behavior that they are evaluating as "stuttering." After all, they are the critical evaluators.

Not only can you determine from the parents the types of disfluency and the nature of the speaking behavior that they consider to be "stuttering"; you can also establish the degree to which the child's speaking behavior today is representative of the speaking behavior that concerns the parents in his home environment. Every attempt should be made to get the parents to be descriptive about what the child is doing. Do not accept such words as "worse" or "not quite so bad." Be concerned about the increase in duration of repetition or prolongation and an increase or decrease in tensing behavior in certain areas of the body.

Johnson (8) has demonstrated that children who are referred to a speech clinician because of a "stuttering problem" present a wide range of frequency of disfluency. Some children exhibit disfluency at such a high frequency rate that there is little doubt about the nature of the behavior the parents are concerned about. On the other hand some children exhibit disfluency that according to the norms discussed earlier will be well within the range of normal frequency. This latter example raises the question of whether parents are just overreacting to a normal phenomenon or whether the child, through the disfluency behavior, is doing something behaviorally that is "perceptually insulting" to the parent. In other words, he can easily be doing something behaviorally as he talks that draws attention away from the content of the speech to the disfluency behavior itself. You should analyze carefully the speaking behavior *both* fluent and disfluent in order to determine the behavioral changes that are perceptually insulting to the parent.

Van Riper (*21*, pp. 21–28) discusses some of the features of speaking that may draw one's attention to the disfluency behavior. He discusses these in an attempt to answer the question of what is "abnormal" as opposed to "normal" disfluency. He attempts to define what is "normal disfluency." Professionally we are not yet at the stage of development where we are able with any validity to do this. Considerable research must be done in the area of disfluent speaking behavior before this can be done with any validity. For the present, it is nonproductive to wrestle with the point of what is "real stuttering." It is more realistic, at this time, to be concerned with what is perceptually irritating. This implies that it is "irritating to *someone*." It does not imply that it is irritating to everyone. The fact is that the parents are concerned about something in the way the child is talking and hence are reacting to it. You must be concerned about what is perceptually irritating or insulting to *them*.

Duration and Rate of Disfluency   The duration of repetition, for example, may appear superficially to be a good indicator of perceptually insulting behavior. Research findings would indicate that it is not highly reliable. Silverman (*18*) found that normal-speaking preschoolers demonstrated, at times, five to six part-word repetitions per instance of disfluency. Yet no one considered them to be stuttering. It is not unusual for a child to demonstrate three to four repetitions of a syllable per instance of disfluency. If the repetitions occur in the same tempo, with the same smoothness, at the same tensing level as the ongoing speech, they are not particularly noticeable. If, however, the part-word repetitions occur at a slower or a much faster rate than the general syllable tempo of speaking, then the listener's attention is likely to be drawn to the repetitions.

You are urged to study the "fluent" speech of the child carefully. Study it in terms of the syllable rate, tensing level, inflection, and breath flow. If any of these characteristics changes around the area of occurrence of a disfluency, it is likely to draw one's attention to the disfluency and cause the listener to begin to wonder if something is "wrong." It is

the *difference* between the forward flow (fluent) and the speaking behavior during the occurrence of a disfluency that is crucial. If you
observe only during the occurrence of disfluency and attempt to judge
whether the rate of repetition is "too fast" or "too slow" or demonstrates some indication of "tensing," you're likely to be misled. It is
entirely possible that you are observing a young child who is generally
tense as he talks. There may be considerable tensing in the chest and
oral area. Any part-word repetition that occurs in his speech will sound
rather "tense." This behavior is not unusual nor is it different from the
way he's talking all of the time in terms of "tensing." Similarly a child
who demonstrates hyperactivity and is making fast movements, squirming
and jumping around in a chair, and talking at an exceedingly rapid rate
may demonstrate a part-word repetition that is exceedingly fast. It
may sound very fast to the listener and yet it is not out of line with
his general behavior at that time. In these situations our concern is less
with changing anything about the disfluency than it is with changing
his general behavior while talking.

Articulation of Vowels   Next study the nature of the vowel produced
in conjunction with the consonant during a syllable repetition. An instance of repetition is more likely to be noticed if the child says "ma—
ma—ma" than if he says "mo—mo—mov—move—moving." That is, if
he is approximating the phoneme he wants to make and moving toward
the next phoneme, the repetitions sound much smoother and "forward
moving" and "normal" than if he interjects the "uh" or some other
phoneme after the consonant.

Total Frequency of Disfluency and Clustering   A final but critical
point must be made with regard to disfluency in children. Inasmuch as
our society considers part-word repetitions and prolongations to be
stuttering because they are breaks in the production of the word as
opposed to other types of disfluencies that usually occur between words,
it is easy to attend only to the occurrence of these types of disfluency.
Study your disfluency analysis in order to determine the degree to which
a relatively high frequency of part-word repetition is part of a picture
of high frequency of all types of disfluency. In short, is the child just
an exceedingly disfluent child? Data (5, 8, 26) indicate that children who
are considered to be "stutterers" often have high frequency of all types
of disfluency. The fact that part-word repetition is singled out by the
listener is a function of the listener and not of the child's speech. The
studies referred to found that "on the average" a child who stutters
has more disfluencies of all types, except revision, than does the average
normal-speaking child.

In the case of a highly disfluent child, observe also the degree to
which there is "clustering" of disfluencies. That is, two or three or four
different types of disfluencies may occur in a "run" as the person is

beginning to express an idea or is in the middle of expressing it. An example of this is "I th—th—think that I—I—I want um—um—um th—th—th—th—then I um wh—wh—what I um—um—um I know I want that." When these kinds of disfluency behaviors are observed, it is advisable to be alert to the possibility of a language problem. The increased disfluency may indicate nothing more than difficulty in language formulation and production.

Summary

A careful analysis of the information presented by the parents during the case history, a review of the disfluency analysis, and a study of the variability of disfluency will enable the clinician to make reasonable suggestions to the parents about what they can do to encourage an increase in forward-moving normally fluent speech.

EXAMINATION OF THE HIGH-SCHOOL-AGE OR ADULT STUTTERER

The information you receive from the adult stutterer should assist you (1) in planning therapy and (2) in serving as a "baseline" so that future improvement can be evaluated. Pertinent areas of information include (a) the case history, (b) a description of his or her speaking behavior, (c) an analysis of the variability of stuttering frequency and duration, and (d) his or her own concepts of and reactions to the stuttering.

Case History

The case history outline is contained in Chapter 2. For the adult, the case history is important because it is a means of bringing up to date information about those factors that may have influenced and are influencing the patient's concept of his or her own problem. However, remember that time is continuous. Anything that occurs, even one minute ago, is "history." Therefore, the information that one obtains in a case history should be blended into the current thinking and reactions of the stutterer. Furthermore, as therapy begins, one is constantly interested in obtaining information about the "history" of the patient's experiences from one clinical session to the next. In this manner you can assist an individual to evaluate and reevaluate not only the ways his or her attitudes and beliefs have changed up to the present time, but the ways they are changing in the present and likely to change in the future.

Description of Speaking Behavior

During the period of time in which you take the case history and indeed during the entire evaluation procedure, you will be observing the behaviors used that comprise the patient's overall "stuttering behavior." There are times, however, when it is desirable to have a uniform means of obtaining a speech sample, so that you can report the number of instances of stuttering per 100 words (or syllables) spoken, or percent of stuttered words (or syllables) per total spoken. This will be done for both conversational speech and oral reading. In Chapter 9 the procedures for obtaining a conversational speech sample and a reading speech sample are described.

Next you will need to describe the behavioral reactions associated with an instance of stuttering. Form 9 is presented to assist you in this task. It will provide a "rough" description of some of the behavior used by the speaker that interferes with talking. Obviously, this is only a partial list, so be prepared to report other kinds of behavior. It will assist you, however, in obtaining an estimate of how consistent the speaker is in employing certain behaviors during each instance of stuttering.

In addition to the two tasks described above, it is especially important for therapy planning that you observe carefully and describe in detail the sequencing of behavior during the speech process.[2] To do this, you will want to view a speaker's "nonstuttered" speech in context with his or her "stuttered" speech. Observe the rate, tensing, and rhythm of speaking during a speaker's nonstuttered elements, as well as during his or her stuttering. It is advisable to think in terms of time-space and to obtain a description of the sequence of behavior. Does she, for example, speak with an extremely rapid rate and then slow down and then begin to tense her neck muscles two or three words before she begins to "stutter"? Then what is the first behavior that interferes with speaking, then what does she do, and then what does she do? Follow this until she says the word. Then, following her saying the word, does she finish her statement on one exhalation of breath with rapid rate and considerable tensing? This example is used merely to illustrate the way a clinician can describe a behavioral sequence. You have to work at developing a "then what does she *do*, and then what does she *do*" way of observing. We are dealing with a behavioral *process*. It is helpful to learn to describe it that way.

You can describe the interrupted speech as it occurs in the above sequence in terms of various characteristics:

1. *Audible characteristics.* Included here are such behaviors as cessation of vocalization, part-word repetition, prolongation, interjections, and vocal fry.
2. *Muscle tensing.* Note particularly tensing around the oral area and neck and throughout the body.

[2] A condensed version of the following discussion of the evaluation of the stuttering problem in an adult is contained in reference 20.

3. *Changes of rate of movement.* Observe during the behavioral process increased or decreased tensing as the rate of movement of the jaw increases or decreases. The rate of tongue movement may increase or decrease, or the rate of part-word repetition or interjections may increase dramatically, or slow down and then turn into a prolongation.
4. *Nonspeech behavior.* Observe behavior that coincides with an instance of stuttering but is extraneous to the process of talking, particularly eyeblinking, head jerking, and knee slapping.

Next, describe any fairly consistent, stereotyped pattern of behavior. This may include a pattern of interjecting a sound over and over until the speaker says the following word with little or no difficulty. It may include a pattern of beginning to tense as he begins a word and then backing up and saying two or three words and then beginning to tense as he says the word and then backing up, et cetera. One fairly common behavior pattern that occurs when an adult begins to stutter is a rapid acceleration of jaw movement and tensing from the time he begins until he completes the word. Another common behavior is essentially holding the breath following the production of one word and before beginning the word on which you would judge that the speaker was "stuttering." A person may say, for example, "I see you." As she completes the word "see," she will hold her breath and will continue to hold it as she struggles in an effort to begin saying "you." Careful description of the behavioral *process* as discussed above can provide vital clues for behavior modification.[3]

Another dimension of description includes the evaluation or judgment on the part of the clinician as to the intent or purpose of certain aspects of speaking behavior. The clinician should verify through discussion with the stutterer the "intent" of certain behavior. The stutterer can be helpful in assessing this and usually can report what it is he was "trying to do." This aspect of description, in which the stutterer himself becomes involved in observing and reporting, can prove beneficial during therapy.

Such terms as avoidant behavior, postponement, disguise, timers, starters, et cetera, are judgments of the *intent* of what the stutterer is trying to do. For example, if you observe the interjecting of "ah" over and over for a period of time followed by the word being spoken with little or no difficulty, one may guess that the stutterer is using this as "avoidant behavior" or "postponement behavior." If he uses phrase repetition such as "When I, when I, when I go," one may guess that he is using the phrase to try to get a "running start and to say the word without stuttering." The stutterer, upon reflection, usually can tell you if you are correct.

---

[3] In order for beginning clinicians to learn to describe the behavioral process, we have found it helpful to videotape segments of stutterers' speaking behavior. These segments can be played and replayed for the clinicians so they can study the sequencing of behavior.

Awareness of the two different kinds of reporting described above point out the importance of describing the behaviors used in the stuttering process in time sequence. When you use *only* a "behavior checklist" of some type, it is easy to miss the importance of what you are observing. Any behavioral unit is taken out of context of time and sequence and intent. For example, if a stutterer blinks her eyes rapidly, this in itself is information that is not particularly helpful for therapy: if she blinks her eyes rapidly immediately prior to the beginning of stuttering, one may assume that she is doing this in order to try to "avoid" stuttering or to "get the word out without stuttering"; but if she has already begun stuttering and blinks her eyes rapidly in combination with a head-jerk, then she may be using this combination to help "get out of the stutter." Therefore, it becomes important not only to describe the stuttering behaviors but to determine in as great detail as possible just what a stutterer believes he is doing this behavior for. It is essential that the beginning clinician carefully evaluate "clinical reports" from other professionals in order to separate the description of what a stutterer is *doing* from the evaluation of what the clinician *thinks* he or she is trying to do.

Finally, you will want to arrive at a "rating of severity." Obtaining a rating enables the clinician not only to include such information in reports to colleagues but also to provide a baseline of "severity" so that during the course of therapy improvement on various dimensions can be noted. Different procedures for assessing severity of the overt stuttering behavior will be described later in this chapter (see pp. 309–313).

Variability of Stuttering

One of the predominant and also one of the most confusing features of stuttering is the extreme variability in frequency and duration of stuttering in different situations. You will want to assess, as carefully as you can, the conditions under which the client's stuttering frequency, duration, and emotions increase and decrease. On Form 11, at the end of this chapter, the stutterer can rate various situations on the dimensions of "avoidance," "reactions," "stuttering," and "frequency." This uniform questionnaire can provide comparable data from different stutterers. Its most important use to the clinician, however, is to provide a point of departure to begin a discussion of those situations that engender more and less difficulty in a given stutterer. We believe that in addition to using the hypothetical speaking situations presented in Form 11, it is meaningful to devise through consultation with the stutterer a list of situations which present immediate and real fear for him or her. You can ask a speaker to rate each situation she mentions on a 5-point scale with 1 representing no stuttering and 5 representing severe stuttering. From this you can devise your own clinical profile of the types of situations in which *she* has more difficulty and those in which she has less. The types of situations that you might want to explore can be categorized in five different ways:

1. *Number of listeners.* This refers to whether there is one listener, two listeners, a small group, a classroom, or a large audience.
2. *The characteristics of the listeners.* This includes whether she is speaking to a woman, a man, persons older or younger than she is, friends, strangers, the boss, her mother-in-law, et cetera.
3. *Nature of the speaking situation.* This includes situations in which she is asking questions, answering questions, telling jokes, giving short answers, explaining an event, giving directions, et cetera.
4. *The emotional setting.* This includes situations in which she is in a subservient role, a dominant role, angry, embarrassed about an event unrelated to speaking, arguing, not believed, in the wrong and obliged to explain why, et cetera.
5. *Specific situations.* This includes telephoning, making introductions, telling her name, her address, her home town, et cetera, regardless of whom she is talking to.

Not only will the frequency and duration of stuttering vary from situation to situation, but the stutterer's emotional reactions will also vary in different situations. These emotional reactions are difficult to describe systematically, yet they can be related directly to the amount that the stutterer "avoids" the situation or minimizes the amount of his or her talking in it. You can use the same list of situations enumerated for you above to learn more about a patient's emotional reactions in these situations. A 5-point scale can be used for the stutterer to rate the *degree* of emotional reaction. Ask a patient also to describe the *nature* of the emotional reaction. In some situations he may report that he is embarrassed, in others being ashamed if he stutters, in others being humiliated. In still others he may report only being frustrated or irritated at himself or at the person to whom he is talking. His differences in emotional reaction present an interesting dilemma about the concept of "severity" of the stuttering problem. It also points up the fallacy of just obtaining a frequency count of stuttering in a specified situation and considering that to represent "severity." Listener judgments of overt stuttering behavior constitute only one dimension of "severity." One must be concerned also with the severity of the problem as perceived by the stutterer.

There are certain situations, as when arguing with friends, in which the frequency and duration of stuttering may increase considerably but in which the feelings are not as intense as in other situations. In fact a stutterer may experience feelings only of being irritated or frustrated at not being able to talk as fast as he wants to. On the other hand, he may in talking to his boss avoid, substitute, and end up stuttering only one time. However, the emotional reaction associated with the one instance of stuttering to his boss was much more intense than his reaction in the other situation. He may forget soon the high frequency of stuttering exhibited while arguing with friends but remember for months the one instance of stuttering in talking with the boss. This one instance of stuttering could affect him for a great length of time by guiding and directing the talking he does and does not do. This example points up the fact that "stuttering severity" is a multidimensional concept.

Another dimension of the variability of stuttering is represented by the situations in which a speaker avoids talking or reduces tremendously the amount of talking. This dimension often represents one of the most severe forms of the "handicap" of stuttering. There are some situations in which she may volunteer a great deal of information, others in which she may volunteer some information, and others in which she will volunteer little or no information. There are other situations in which she will talk only when she has to. There are some that she will avoid entering at all costs. There are others in which she will respond only by shaking her head or by giving one-word responses.

Perceptions and Attending Behavior While Talking

Certain dimensions of the stutterer's perceptions should be probed in order for you to structure and plan a therapy program. An understanding of them can provide a perspective from which to assess the attending and the evaluating he is doing as he talks in various situations.

You can discuss with him the question: "When you are in the process of stuttering, to what are you attending? Of what are you most aware?" Is he attending to other people's reactions or is he most aware of his "own feelings" (the hotness of his face, the lead in his stomach, the tightness in his throat)? Is he overly aware of the sound of his abnormal vocalizations, or is he more aware of the "dead silence" of nonvocalization? Or is he aware only of a blur and a confusion of "feelings—sounds—faces"?

Another question is this: "While you are talking and stuttering to people, how do you perceive that they feel about you, or how do you perceive the way you are feeling about yourself at the time?" Does he think that they are feeling sorry for him? Is he feeling inferior to them? Is he feeling childish? Is he feeling that he is being evaluated as "not being too smart"? Is he feeling that as he talks they are continually being repulsed or are rejecting in their reactions to him? Is he feeling that whatever he is saying will not be considered important if he stutters while saying it? Is he feeling that the listener is increasingly contemplating ways to get away from him so that the conversation can be ended quickly? These questions and others that you may think of will assist you in determining the direction counseling will take as a patient begins to change his or her behavior and talk to more and more people.

The next dimension is one not often pursued in a diagnostic evaluation, yet it is of considerable importance. It consists of a discussion of this question: "What do you *do* when you stutter, or what are you *afraid you will do* that bothers you the most?" Clinical observation indicates that most stutterers have some aspect of their behavior that they dread much more than others. Is it jerking his head? Is it running out of breath or a feeling of "panic" that he will run out of breath before he completes the word? Is it fear of having to stop to take a breath before he completes the word? Is it fear of stuttering to the point that there will be no sound and he won't be able to move his jaw or mouth? Is it stuttering to the point that he is talking on residual air or "disintegrating" into vocal fry?

You should also explore what aspects of his or her own stuttering behavior least bother the speaker. What does he commonly do when he stutters that, if he didn't ever do any more than that, he "wouldn't mind too much?" Most stutterers will report, for example, that if they had no more than several part-word repetitions or a slight "prolongation" or an "inconspicuous tense pause," they would not mind too much. It's when stuttering behavior goes beyond that point that the stutterer begins getting scared and begins introducing more involved "tricks" of behavior. Most stutterers have a "reservoir" of behaviors that they use during the sequence of stuttering. For most stutterers, observation can help you determine what his or her "par" stuttering is like. This is the "small stutter" about which the speaker is not too concerned. It's when the stuttering gets beyond this point that stutterers go from one behavior trick to the next one, to the next one, to the next one, all the time increasing in panic because of the fear that they will run out of behavior tricks to use. As he nears the end of his behavior "tricks," a stutterer usually gets involved in the kind of behavior that he detests. By establishing a hierarchy of *behavior fears,* the clinician is guided in therapy planning.

A final dimension revolves around this question: "What in your listeners' reactions bothers you the most?" Is the stutterer afraid that they will laugh? Is he afraid that they will give him a "sick smile?" Is he afraid that they may interrupt him or look away or finish the word for him? Most stutterers, upon reflection, can report certain listener reactions that they fear much more than others. What are they?

Tests of Attitudes

The previous discussion has centered around the many different dimensions of the stutterer's emotions and reactions that can affect the manner in which you structure a therapy program. Although there is an absence of experimental data, clinical experience indicates that the higher the negative emotional feelings, the stronger the avoidance reactions. And the lower the self-esteem of the stutterer, the more difficulty he or she will experience in transferring to outside speaking situations the behavioral changes practiced during a therapy session. Moreover, until these attitudes and emotional reactions are met constructively as a part of the therapy program, the probability is reduced that the stutterer will maintain increased fluency after therapy is terminated. By contrast, a stutterer who shows little avoidant behavior and who demonstrates relatively little negative emotional reaction may respond well to a fairly direct fluency-shaping procedure.

Unfortunately there are no tests available today that will predict with reasonable certainty the degree to which each of the variables mentioned above will influence progress in therapy. There are several tests available, however, that can provide meaningful information to the thoughtful clinician.

The stutterer's response to the self-ratings of Form 11 can be helpful. Study particularly the stutterer's responses to the Avoidance and Reaction sections. Then compare them to his responses to the Stuttering and Frequency sections. The responses can provide a cohesive picture of the speaker's attitudes toward stuttering as they relate to his or her speaking performance.

Three tests have been developed relatively recently to assess the "severity" of the stutterer's problem. They were designed to "tap" the interrelation of speaking performance, attitude, avoidance, and expectancy. Every clinician involved in the area of stuttering should become familiar with them and use them appropriately in the assessment of a stutterer's problem and in the structuring of therapy.

Perceptions of Stuttering Inventory (PSI), described by Woolf (27), consists of 60 statements about stuttering. The stutterer is instructed to read each item carefully and to check all of the items that are characteristic of him or of his stuttering. The test is based on the hypothesis that expectancy is a major dimension of stuttering and that in its more advanced forms, stuttering can be conceptualized along three primary parameters: struggle, avoidance, and expectancy. The 60 test items have been classified so that 20 refer to each of the three parameters. The number of positive responses in each category can be profiled.

The Measurement of Stuttering Severity developed by Lanyon (13), consists of a 64-item inventory of behaviors and attitudes related to stuttering. Forty-six items refer to behavior experienced while talking and 18 items refer to attitudes about talking. The stutterer simply marks "True" or "False" after each statement.

Communication Inventory developed by Erickson (6), consists of two scales: Severity Scale and Adjective Checklist. The Severity Scale (S-Scale) consists of 39 items relating to attitudes about talking which differentiate stutterers from nonstutterers. The respondent marks "True" or "False" after each item. The Adjective Checklist consists of a list of adjectives which differentiated the self-descriptions of stutterers who obtained high scores on the S-Scale from self-descriptions of stutterers who obtained low scores.

Speaking-Time Log

The procedures described up to this point can be accomplished during one evaluation period. As you begin therapy with a client you can ask him to keep a log of his speaking time each day. The procedures to use and the rationale for doing it are described in Chapter 9 (see pp. 271–274). A stutterer who keeps a speaking-time log conscientiously for two or three days can provide you with a capsulized picture of his actual routine speaking performance. When compared to available information for non-stutterers, it presents an operational definition of the ways he functions during the day. When repeated at regular intervals during therapy, the changes that occur represent the most basic meaning of "improvement."

Personality Characteristics

During the evaluation process the experienced clinician is constantly asking the question, "What kind of person is this?" You must become alert to cues from the client's general behavior that will permit you to make an estimate of how the client will react to you and to therapy. Is your client the kind of person who will accept responsibility for changing what he is doing, or will he sit placidly by and wait for you to do something "for him?" It has been said often that to be helped a person has to be helpable.

Many stutterers' behavior characteristics will not become evident until they are *asked to change*. During the first interview, however, you will begin to make "guesses" about how any one client will respond to therapy. Some hints of this can be determined by assessing the ways in which the person has met problems in the past. In short, to what degree is he or she a "problem solver"?

During your taking of the case history, during the various speech tests, and during the description of her stuttering and the study of the conditions under which it varies, you can make observations about the way a client has met problems in the past. How has she met academic problems, family squabbles, dating problems? To what degree is she independent and does she shift for herself in everyday life as opposed to "waiting for people to do things for her?" As problems have arisen in the past, has she been "action" oriented or merely "talk-about-it" oriented or "hand-wringing" oriented? To what degree does she want to know what *she* can do to talk better, as opposed to what you can do for her?

Some clinicians prefer to have various personality inventories administered by persons qualified by training to give and analyze them. They use them to attempt to assess those personality characteristics that may affect therapy. There is, however, considerable disagreement and there is a lack of valid data as to just what those characteristics might be. We urge that you use discretion and the utmost caution in attempting to evaluate the results of personality inventories with regard to what they "tell you" that is helpful in planning therapy or in estimating prognosis.

During the first interview you will be making "first guesses" about those characteristics that may interfere with or facilitate the therapy process. Keep in mind that they are "first guesses" and be ready to change your own evaluation as you come to know the stutterer better.

EXAMINATION OF THE ELEMENTARY-SCHOOL-AGE CHILD

Inasmuch as a child of this age range generally considers himself to be a stutterer as well as being considered one by others in his environment, the information obtained should assist you in the same ways as that obtained for the adult stutterer described previously.

Case History

The case history outline is contained in Chapter 2. For a child of this age, special attention should be directed to the relationship between the behavioral aspects of his stuttering behavior and his beliefs as to what is wrong with his speech.[4] The behavior the child uses to cope with talking is often closely related to what he believes is wrong or what people have "told him to do to not stutter." Question him closely as to what he believes is wrong (why he stutters) and then ask him what things he does to "help" himself talk. Observe the degree to which the behavior he employs (his stuttering pattern) corresponds to his "helping" the thing he thinks is wrong; for example, he "pushes" (tenses his lip, jaw, and throat area) to produce the word "people say he can't get out." Or he talks cautiously and slowly, then suddenly with a burst of speed explodes a word or phrase. This child has been told, at times, to talk slowly so he won't stutter, and at other times while stuttering has been told to "spit it out." Now he reports that he talks slowly so he won't stutter, *and* when he does anyway (which is often) he has to hurry and "spit it out" so it won't get "stuck." Examples of the questions you may ask include "What do you think is wrong? Why do you think you cannot talk the way other youngsters talk? What do you do to help? What have people told you to do to help? Does it help? How much of the time does it help? Why don't you think it helps at other times?" Your assessment of the degree to which faulty beliefs and related behaviors exist will assist in planning therapy.

Description of Speaking Behavior

You will need to obtain samples of conversational speech and oral reading. In part, the conversational speech sample can be obtained ac-

4 This problem is discussed at length in reference 23.

cording to the instructions given in Chapter 9 (pp. 258–259). In addition, however, it is advisable to obtain the speech sample in accordance with the procedures outlined in this chapter for the examination of preschool children, which involve verbal tasks of differing language, reaction, and social complexity (see pp. 287–288). For the elementary-school-age stutterer there is often marked variation in the severity of stuttering at these different levels of speaking complexity.

The reading task should vary according to the age of the child. For the 10- to 12-year-old, the procedures outlined in Chapter 9 are appropriate. For the 6- to 8- or 9-year-old, we have found it advisable to vary the procedure. Obtain three reading passages, one a year or two below a child's reading level, the second at his reading level, and the third a year or two above his reading level. By tabulating stuttering frequency as he reads each passage, you will obtain an indication of the ways he copes with the stress involved in increased difficulty of reading. In addition, a marked breakdown in fluency with the difficult reading task may provide a hint of at least one reason for the breakdown and fragmentation of fluency for this child. This point will be discussed further in the section on variability of stuttering.

You can obtain ratings of severity using the same procedures described for the adult stutterer (pp. 309–313). Because there may be extreme variability in the severity of stuttering during the language, reaction, and social complexity tasks and during reading, it is advisable to obtain a severity rating for each different task.

You should use the same principles in describing the speaking behavior of this age group as you apply with the adult. It is helpful to think in terms of the question "What does he do *first* that interferes with talking (or, that makes talking difficult), then what does he do, then what, and so forth?" Observe carefully his speaking behavior during "nonstuttered" speech as well as during "stuttered" speech. In brief, observe his behavior during the total *process* of talking that includes an instance of stuttering. Remember: an instance of stuttering does not occur in a vacuum unrelated to anything else he does as he talks. It is merely one aspect of a total *process*. Generally there is little need to question the child about the "intent" of his behavior (as was discussed for the adult). With the exception of certain older children, most will not know.

Variability of Stuttering

Various dimensions of variability were discussed in the section on the adult stutterer. Generally these are not applicable to the elementary-school-age stutterer. There may be some older children who can provide partial information for the described dimensions; most will not. Some will be able to tell you of a few speaking situations that they "don't like" or in which they "stutter." Obviously you should obtain as much of this information as you can. For the most part, however, you can use the language, reaction, and social situation complexity tasks and the oral-reading tasks described previously to assist you in evaluating variability. Additional information should be obtained if possible by careful questioning of his parents and of his teacher.

Whereas in the case of the adult stutterer you are concerned ordinarily with those situations in which "more or less" than average stuttering occurs, with younger children (6 to 8 years of age) be prepared to explore the situations in which they either stutter or do *not* stutter. This information is often overlooked; it can provide meaningful information for nucleus situations that may need immediate attention in therapy planning.

We have found it not uncommon for a child to stutter in only one or two situations and in no others. For example, one child may stutter during "show and tell" time and while reciting orally but stutter little or not at all in other situations. Another may stutter only when she reads orally or only when talking to her parents at home. One of the developing aspects of the stuttering problem is for a child, as he gets older, to generalize to more and more situations the negative reaction patterns we label as his "stuttering."

OTHER TESTS

In the first edition of *Diagnostic Methods in Speech Pathology* (9) Johnson recommended the routine use of three measures for evaluating the stuttering problem: (1) the Iowa Scale of Attitude Toward Stuttering, (2) the adaptation effect, and (3) the consistency effect. These measures have proven to be of little value in routine clinical use for the following reasons:

The Iowa Scale of Attitude Toward Stuttering

This scale, developed by Ammons and Johnson (1), consists of a series of statements concerning where, when, or how a stutterer thinks he should or should not talk or vocations for which he should or should not prepare. The stutterer or close members of his family answer each statement in terms of the extent to which they agree or disagree with it. When it was developed, the test undoubtedly had clinical value. However, today most adult stutterers (the age group for which the scale is applicable) and their families have had sufficient exposure to the stuttering problem that they know how they "should" believe or behave and they respond to the statements accordingly. Their responses, which usually reflect an "acceptance of stuttering," bear little relationship to the way they react in actual practice. Therefore, the Iowa Scale of Attitude Toward Stuttering is not included in this edition.

The Adaptation Effect

Since the adaptation effect was first reported and named in 1937 by Johnson and Knott (10) it has been investigated in so many research studies that it is impractical to list here even a few of them. The adaptation effect refers to the fact that there is a tendency for a stutterer to stutter less frequently with each successive oral reading of the same passage to the same listener(s). Of major concern in this chapter is precisely what routine administration of this test in the clinical situation will tell you that will help in planning therapy or in predicting or assessing improvement. Research evidence suggests that it will provide little meaningful information. First, the adaptation effect is a reliable phenomenon when tabulated for groups of stutterers. That is, if the frequency of stuttering during successive oral readings of the same passage is tabulated for 10 to 12 stutterers and the average frequency for the group is computed, adaptation is a stable phenomenon. However, as Cullinan (3) reports, an individual is unreliable in his adaptation performance; he may show adaptation one day and not the next, or vice versa. Therefore, the results obtained from a client during an evaluation session are difficult if not impossible to interpret.

Second, Johnson (9) suggested that adaptation may be considered to be a miniature "model of improvement," therefore of predictive value. However, Lanyon (12) found no significant relationship between the percentage of adaptation shown by a stutterer and the amount of improvement he demonstrated after a year of therapy. In view of the fact that no data support the predictive value of an adaptation score, Lanyon's findings must be considered thoughtfully.

Third, the suggestion has been made that clinical impressions may be formed from a stutterer's adaptation score (9); whether he or she adapts or not may reflect the extent and nature of anxiety at the time of evaluation. This suggestion is difficult to reconcile with the research evidence that both stutterers and nonstutterers as groups show adaptation. Furthermore, some individuals within both groups do and do not show adaptation (24). These data suggest that one should use extreme caution in the interpretations one makes about the nature of "anxiety and stuttering" as it may be reflected by an adaptation score.

We conclude that there is no reasonable basis for obtaining adaptation scores for stutterers as a part of a routine clinical evaluation. However, because of its value for research investigations and because of its possible usefulness in the differential diagnosis of fluency problems, a discussion of adaptation and the procedures to follow in measuring it are presented in Chapter 9.

The Consistency Effect

Research has indicated that when a stutterer reads the same passage two or more times in succession, he stutters on the same words from reading to reading more than can be accounted for by chance alone. This finding was first reported by Johnson and Knott (10) who named it the consistency effect. Again, as with the adaptation effect, our task is to determine precisely what a consistency score routinely obtained will tell you that will assist in planning therapy or in predicting or assessing improvement for the next stutterer with whom you work.

Unlike the case of the adaptation effect, Cullinan (4) found that the consistency effect is stable not only for grouped data but for individuals on different days. Hence, the consistency score is likely to be a reliable indicator of the degree to which a stutterer stutters consistently on the same words. This may assist you in determining what constitutes some "hard words" or "hard sounds" for a speaker, although the information usually can be obtained by asking him or by observing the words on which he stutters and observing similarities among them.

Other than the above, the consistency effect suffers from the same problems of interpretation as the adaptation effect does. Lanyon (12) found that consistency scores obtained for an individual were not related to improvement in therapy. Williams, Silverman, and Kools (25) found that both stutterers and nonstutterers demonstrate the consistency effect. Hence, one must be cautious in interpreting the consistency effect solely as reflecting "fear of" or "anxiety about" stuttering. Undoubtedly anxiety is a factor, but the other variables involved are not at all clear.

As with the adaptation scores, there is no reasonable basis for routinely obtaining consistency scores for stutterers. However, a discussion of the consistency effect and the procedures used to measure it are presented in Chapter 9 because of its possible usefulness in research investigations and in differential diagnosis of fluency problems.

Check List of Stuttering Behavior

Since we do not classify every speech disfluency we hear as stuttering, we need, particularly in our work as diagnostic clinicians, to be clear about those disfluencies and related reactions that we do and do not classify as stuttering. By recording on Form 9 your observations of what you regard as a speaker's stutterings, you can sharpen your awareness of just what he does in speaking that you think he should change or eliminate. You can help the stutterer become aware of those things he does—and that you feel he should work on—if you use the checklist to point them up for him. He, too, can use the checklist to sharpen his own perception of his speech-disrupting behavior. By using a tape recorder or videotape or by watching himself in a mirror while speaking, he can observe his stuttering behavior and use his observations, as noted on the checklist, as a basis for analysis and discussion. They will be especially helpful as a guide for increasing his awareness of just what it is that he is doing to interfere with talking, and hence, the behavior he must change to approximate more nearly forward-moving fluent speech.

Form 9 has spaces for recording observations of six stuttered words—words that you or the stutterer himself or some other observer regards as stuttered. It is not necessary, of course, to observe six consecutive stuttered words. Indeed, this would not always be possible. Choose words separated in time so that you can be relatively thorough in noting details and in recording your observations.

Earlier in this chapter we discussed the importance of noting not only what behaviors are involved in stuttering but also the sequence of the behaviors. Form 9 requires that you place a check mark opposite each of the behaviors noted. In addition, observe the order in which he does them. What does he do first, then what does he do, and then what does he do? Place a 1, 2, 3, 4, et cetera, after each check to note the numerical order in which the behaviors occur.

FORM 9
Checklist of Stuttering Behavior

Name _____ Age _____ Sex _____
Observer _____ Date _____

Instruction to Observer

Observe the stutterer as he or she speaks or reads aloud. Focus your attention on such disfluencies and related reactions as you would classify as stuttering. Observe these reactions as they are associated with the speaking of specific words. Write each such word at the top of a column and make a check mark in the appropriate space to indicate each type of disfluency or other reaction observed. Note by the use of 1, 2, 3, et cetera, the sequencing of the behaviors. Under "Supplementary Observations" add descriptive details concerning any of the numbered items checked, and comment on apparent emotionality of the speaker, general degree of tension, relevant remarks made by the speaker, et cetera.

Types of Reaction	Word 1	Word 2	Word 3	Word 4	Word 5	Word 6
1. Repeating part of word						
2. Repeating whole monosyllabic word						
3. Repeating this and other word(s)						
4. Saying "uh—uh" or the like						
5. Prolonging sound(s)						
6. Pausing in middle of word						
7. Failing to complete the word						
8. Holding breath						
9. Gasping						
10. Inhaling irregularly						
11. Exhaling irregularly						
12. Speaking on exhausted breath						
13. Delay in starting word						
14. Pressing lips together						
15. Pressing tongue against teeth or palate						
16. Closing eyes						
17. Protruding tongue						
18. Enlarging eyes						
19. Opening mouth irrelevantly						
20. Dilating nostrils						
21. Turning head sideways						

22. Bending head downward
23. Moving head up or back
24. Moving hands or fingers
25. Moving legs or feet
26. Moving body
27. Other (specify)
28. _____
29. _____
30. _____

Supplementary Observations:

Rating of Severity of Stuttering

The rating scale is one of the most widely used means of evaluating the speech of stutterers. Such a scale and the procedure employed in using it may be simple or elaborate. The method which we present here for routine clinical use is quite simple. You will use it with a more cultivated sense of its limitations and its practical value if you first examine such discussions of scaling theory and procedure, together with research methods and findings as those of Lewis and Sherman (*14*), Sherman (*16*), and Young (*28*). Meanwhile, it will serve to clarify the problem somewhat if we consider briefly the procedure employed by Young in securing severity ratings of tape-recorded samples of the speech of 50 adult male stutterers. He employed three groups of listeners (stutterers, speech clinicians, and laymen).

> The listeners in each session attended to the 50 tape-recorded speech samples, taking four short rest periods while the experimenter changed the test tapes, and rated the severity of stuttering of each sample on the basis of a nine-point equal-appearing intervals scale. Two short samples of speech were chosen to represent the extremes on this scale and were incorporated as part of the instructions to the raters. These segments were chosen from the tape-recorded speech samples of the two speakers who exhibited the highest and lowest total numbers of disfluencies (*28*, p. 37).

Young gave the raters these instructions:

> You are about to hear some samples of speech from speakers who consider themselves to be stutterers. Your task will be to make an over-all rating of the severity of stuttering in each sample. You will do this on a nine-point scale on which a rating of 1 means no stuttering. (You may or may not judge any given sample to contain stuttering.) A rating of 2 means very mild stuttering and a rating of 9 means very severe stuttering. A rating of 5, in the middle of this scale, indicates an average severity of stuttering. The other values on the scale, 3, 4, and 6, 7, 8, represent equal intervals between these scale points. Before you start, however, you will hear a few segments of speech arbitrarily chosen to represent extremes on this nine-point scale. Now we will begin the judging procedure. Remember, a rating of 1 means no stuttering and a rating of 9 indicates very severe stuttering, while a rating of 5 is to be considered a middle point between these two extremes. Please be sure to rate every sample, giving only one rating. Each sample is numbered, and the number of each sample will be announced just before the sample is presented. Write your rating in the space provided in each case. You will be allowed a short pause after each sample to record your rating. Are there any questions? (*28*, p. 37)

"Twenty-four hundred ratings of severity of stuttering were obtained from the 48 experimental listeners. The mean rating of severity of stuttering for all 48 listeners was 3.84, with the means for G1 (stutterers), G2 (clinicians), and G3 (laymen) being 4.01, 3.88, and 3.68, respectively."

It may be that in an occasional clinical situation or, more likely, in the laboratory, you will prefer to use the relatively precise and elaborate scaling methods represented by this quotation; but probably you would not often employ them for general clinical purposes. This description of Young's procedure, however, should serve to bring into focus the question of how best to rate the severity of stuttering in routine clinical situations where procedures of the type described by Young are not feasible. In recommending the gross rating method presently to be described, we are at pains to call attention to its limitations, and to urge that you regard the ratings obtained by means of it as rough measures only. It is to be taken for granted that you and others who work with you will make judgments of the severity of the problem of every stutterer you serve clinically. The major virtue of the rating procedure here presented is that it insures a certain degree of uniformity and comparability of the judgments that you and others make of particular stutterers. For all these precautions, however, it is by no means to be overlooked or under-emphasized that the sorts of listener judgments represented by ratings, however rough and even wildly unscientific they may be, are among the most substantial facts of life that stutterers face hour after hour day in and day out. They are, therefore, extremely important—regardless of their precision or reliability as gauged by laboratory standards. It is, for all practical purposes, impossible to disregard them in working with stutterers clinically.

A scale of severity can provide for distinguishing mild from severe stuttering, or mild from moderate or severe stuttering, or for still finer distinctions. The accompanying scale, Form 10, represents a continuum from 0 (no stuttering) through 1 (very mild stuttering) to 7 (very severe stuttering). You should think of the intermediate degrees of severity between 1 and 7 as falling at equally spaced intervals, with the midpoint of the scale, or 4, representing average or moderate stuttering. The various scale values are defined for the purpose of making the ratings of different observers as comparable as possible. It is not assumed that any one of these definitions will necessarily fit exactly the speaking performance of any specific stutterer on any particular occasion; the definitions are intended simply as guide lines.

It is desirable that each stutterer be rated by more than one clinician if possible and by a number of his lay associates and friends. He should also rate himself. Discrepancies among these ratings can be analyzed and discussed to advantage.

You may base your rating of a stutterer on more than one sample of his speech, and the more samples of his speech you observe the more valid your rating is likely to be. If you base your rating on a single sample be sure to describe the sample and situation clearly enough to indicate whether or not your rating might be comparable with another one made by you or someone else. If you use the rating sheet for evaluating more than one sample of speech, or for making a general rating on the basis of all observations made on the stutterer's speech during a stated period of time, supply the information called for at the end of the rating sheet accordingly. Comparison of ratings based on oral reading and speaking can sometimes provide a basis for worthwhile analysis of factors related to variations in severity of a given speaker's stuttering. A similar use can be made of ratings made by different observers or in different situations.

Careful study of Form 10, however, reveals serious limitations for its use as a tool to estimate improvement during therapy. There is a definition accompanying each scale value. This definition includes the variables of stuttering frequency and duration, muscle tensing, and extraneous body movements. As Van Riper (21, chap. 9) points out, all behavioral variables do not increase or decrease proportionally for most stutterers for each scale value. If, for example, during the first two weeks of therapy a stutterer decreases extraneous body movements significantly but the frequency and duration of stutterings remain relatively constant, how would this effect the scale value of severity? Van Riper revised the Severity Scale so it can be used as a profile (see Figure 10.1). He suggests

Scale	Frequency Percent	Tension-Struggle	Duration	Postponement-Avoidance Percent
1.	Under 1	None	Under $\frac{1}{2}$ sec.	None
2.	1-2	Rare but present	Average $\frac{1}{2}$ sec.	Less than 5
3.	3-5	Usual but mild	Average 1 sec.	5-10
4.	6-8	Severe	Average 2 sec.	11-20
5.	9-12	Very severe	Average 3 sec.	21-31
6.	13-25	Overflow to eyes and limbs	Average 4 sec.	31-70
7.	More than 25	Overflow to trunk	Longer than 5 sec.	More than 70

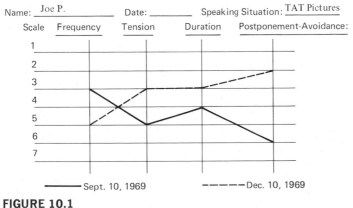

FIGURE 10.1
Profile of stuttering severity.

that the clinician chart separately each of the variables of frequency, tension, duration, and postponement-avoidance. By charting each one at regular intervals during the course of therapy, the clinician can be aided in therapy planning.

Procedures for estimating listener judgments of severity have been devised other than the ones described above. You are urged to become familiar with them. The more you become aware of those variables that affect judgments of severity, the more you will be sensitive to the behavior variables that you work to change during therapy.

Riley (15) devised an instrument which permits numerical scores for frequency, duration, and physical concomitants. These individual scores can be totaled; the total score can be converted to a percentile and then equated to "severity equivalents." These equivalents range from "very mild" to "very severe."

In 1961 Young (28) reported that frequency of stuttering and rate of speech were the two behavioral variables that correlated highest with listener judgments of stuttering. Andrews and Ingham (2) devised a rather elaborate formula to arrive at a severity "score." The formula is based on a predicted relationship between stuttering frequency and speaking rate. They utilize a percentage of syllables stuttered and the syllables spoken per minute to compute a "score." This score reportedly correlates highly with scaled judgments of severity.

FORM 10
Scale for Rating Severity of Stuttering

Speaker _____   Age _____ Sex _____ Date _____
Rater _____   Identification _____

Instructions:

Indicate your identification by some such term as "speaker's clinician," "clinical observer," "clinical student," or "friend," "mother," "classmate," et cetera. Rate the severity of the speaker's stuttering on a scale from 0 to 7, as follows:

0   No stuttering
1   Very mild—stuttering on less than 1 percent of words; very little relevant tension; disfluencies generally less than one second in duration; patterns of disfluency simple; no apparent associated movements of body, arms, legs, or head.
2   Mild—stuttering on 1 to 2 percent of words; tension scarcely perceptible; very few, if any, disfluencies last as long as a full second; patterns of disfluency simple; no conspicuous associated movements of body, arms, legs, or head.
3   Mild to moderate—stuttering on about 2 to 5 percent of words; tension noticeable but not very distracting; most disfluencies do not last longer than a full second; patterns of disfluency mostly simple; no distracting associated movements.
4   Moderate—stuttering on about 5 to 8 percent of words; tension occasionally distracting; disfluencies average about one second in duration; disfluency patterns characterized by an occasional complicating sound or facial grimace; an occasional distracting associated movement.
5   Moderate to severe—stuttering on about 8 to 12 percent of words; consistently noticeable tension; disfluencies average about 2 seconds in duration; a few distracting sounds and facial grimaces; a few distracting associated movements.
6   Severe—stuttering on about 12 to 25 percent of words; conspicuous tension; disfluencies average 3 to 4 seconds in duration; conspicuous distracting sounds and facial grimaces; conspicuous distracting associated movements.
7   Very severe—stuttering on more than 25 percent of words; very conspicuous tension; disfluencies average more than 4 seconds in duration; very conspicuous distracting sounds and facial grimaces; very conspicuous distracting associated movements.

The Stutterer's Self-Ratings of Reactions to Speech Situations

By filling out Form 11 a stutterer indicates four aspects of his adjustment to a sample of 40 common types of speech situations. The responses he makes to the rating scales are especially useful in providing indications of trouble spots and of his possible need for counseling with respect to certain aspects of the problem.

Shumak (17) analyzed the responses made to this test by 95 adult male stutterers between approximately 17 and 30 years of age in the University of Iowa Speech Clinic. By correlating the scores made on the four parts of the test, she found that to some degree (r = 0.52) the more frequently the subject stuttered in specified types of speech situations the more he tried to avoid entering these situations. She also reported that the more the stutterer disliked the speech situations the more he avoided going into situations (r = 0.84). Moreover, the more the speaker stuttered in the situations the more he disliked speaking in them (r = 0.57). As these findings suggest, you can use a stutterer's responses to this test as a means of helping him to understand some of the more important interactions among the different facets of his total problem.

In administering the test, present it to the stutterer and ask him to read the instructions. In scoring his responses, add the numbers written by him in each column and write the sum in the space designated Total. Divide this sum by the number of items answered, carry to one decimal place, and enter the quotient in the space designated Average. The lower the average the better—that is, low scores represent better reactions than high scores.

Evaluate the average for each column with reference to the values shown in Table 10.1, based on the work of Shumak (17). The values shown in Table 10.1 are for adults, mostly of college age, and for the most part stutterers who are college or university students. In the absence

TABLE 10.1
Means, Standard Deviations, Ranges, and Indicated Percentile Values for Each of the Four Modes of Response to the Stutterer's Self-Ratings of Reactions to Speech Situations for 95 Adult Male Stutterers

Mode of Response	Mean	SD	25th Percentile	50th Percentile	75th Percentile	Range of Scores
Avoidance	2.31	0.66	1.82	2.20	2.80	1.02–4.20
Reaction	2.57	0.62	2.10	2.56	2.97	1.41–3.97
Stuttering	2.54	0.60	2.08	2.53	2.98	1.20–3.92
Frequency	3.80	0.45	3.48	3.88	4.11	2.39–4.72

Source: Shumak, *17.*

of norms for younger age levels, use those given in Table 10.1 with all due caution in evaluating scores. The rating sheet can be administered to junior or senior high school stutterers, but it can hardly be used for most subjects below 14 or 15 years of age.

With these considerations in mind, then, you may use Table 10.1 in this general way: a score of 2.8 for Avoidance, for example, would place the stutterer who makes it at the 75th percentile for Shumak's college-age stutterers; this would mean that 75 percent of Shumak's subjects made lower scores than his—and low scores are good scores. A score of 2.8 for Avoidance, therefore, is not very good.

You may also interpret the average in a general way by reference to the descriptions of the five numbered responses for each column. Thus, you might fairly interpret an average of 2.8 for Avoidance as showing that the stutterer probably does not try to avoid speaking situations "on the average," though sometimes he would like to and occasionally actually does try to avoid them.

Of more importance than the average, however, which is clearly a rather abstract bit of information in this instance, is the number of items rated 1, 2, 3, 4, and 5, respectively, in each column. If, for example, 25 of the 40 items are rated 4 or 5 under Frequency, you would doubtless conclude that one of the important objectives of therapy would be to increase the frequency with which the person enters into common speech situations. In general, the more often the stutterer talks the better, and the greater the variety of situations in which he does his talking the better. After all, in a very important sense, the working time for a stutterer working on his speech is his *speaking* time. For this reason a measure of the frequency with which a stutterer meets representative speech situations such as this rating sheet lists, is of value from a clinical point of view. It is a measure that you may well make periodically during therapy. Moreover, an examination of the response made to each item will often suggest to you specific activities or goals to be attempted during remedial training.

The stutterer's responses in the Stuttering column yield practical information concerning the specific types of situations to which he needs particularly to make a better speech adjustment—and from them you may also draw possible tentative generalizations as to the common denominators in his hard and easy situations, respectively. These common denominators—which may be such things as the age or status of listeners, audience or group situations, et cetera—are helpful in suggesting specific needs for counseling and additional speaking experience and specific types of practice.

The responses made in the Reaction and Avoidance columns should be compared with those in the other two columns. They indicate motivational tendencies to be developed (such as those suggested by 1's and

2's in both the Reaction and Avoidance columns), eliminated, or reversed (such as those implied by the 4's and 5's especially).

ASSIGNMENTS

1. Do the following activities with four children in lower elementary school who *do not* stutter:
   a. Interview each in as much detail as possible with regard to the "talking questions" outlined in the problem profile from the child (pp. 69–70) for the elementary-school-age stutterer in the supplementary case history on the stuttering problem (Chapter 2). What do their responses tell you about how they view themselves as "talkers"?
   b. Obtain a tape-recorded speech sample from each child by following the instructions described in the examination of the preschool child (pp. 286–288). Then (1) vary the verbal complexity as described earlier in this chapter, (2) vary the listener reaction complexity, and (3) vary the social complexity. Do a disfluency analysis of each child's speech. Use the first speech sample as a "base score." Note the changes that occurred in both the total frequency of disfluencies and the relative proportions of the various types of disfluency as you varied the complexity of the speaking tasks.
2. Ask two adult stutterers to fill out The Stutterer's Self-Ratings of Reactions to Speech Situations, Form 11. Then ask each stutterer to construct a list of situations which create in him or her immediate and real fear. Ask each stutterer to rate each situation on a 5-point scale as described in this chapter in the analysis of variability of stuttering (pp. 295–297).
3. Ask two nonstuttering adults to do insofar as possible the same tasks described in 2 above but have them use a 5-point scale, with 1 representing "most comfortable" and 5 representing "most uncomfortable." Study the similarities and differences between the responses of the stutterers and the nonstutterers.
4. Using the same procedures described in 2 and 3 above, obtain the same information, insofar as possible, from elementary-school-age children (two who stutter and two who do not stutter). To what degree are they able to provide meaningful information on these points as compared to adults? To understand the continuously developing aspects of a problem, note the degree to which the adult stutterers are more aware than the younger stutterers of specific fears, situations, or individuals that they associate with stuttering.

FORM 11
Stutterer's Self-Ratings of Reactions to Speech Situations

Name _____ Age _____ Sex _____

Examiner _____ Date _____

After each item put a number from 1 to 5 in each of the four columns.

Start with right-hand column headed Frequency. Study the five possible answers to be made in responding to each item, and write the number of the answer that best fits the situation for you in each case. Thus, if you habitually take your meals at home and seldom eat in a restaurant, certainly not as often as once a week, write the number 5 in the Frequency column opposite item No. 1, "Ordering in a restaurant." In like manner respond to each of the other 39 items by writing the most appropriate number in the Frequency column. When you have finished with this column fold it under so you cannot see the numbers you have written. This is done to keep you from being influenced unduly by the numbers you have written in the Frequency column when you write your responses to the 40 situations in the Stuttering column.

Now, write the number of the response that best indicates how much you stutter in each situation. For example, if in ordering meals in a restaurant you stutter mildly (for you), write the number 2 in the Stuttering column after item No. 1. In like manner respond to the other 39 items. Then fold under the Stuttering column so you will not be able to see the numbers you have written in it when you make your responses in the Reaction column.

Following the same procedure, write your responses in the Reaction column, fold it under, and, finally, write your responses in the Avoidance column.

Numbers, for each of the columns, are to be interpreted as follows:

A. Avoidance:
   1. I never try to avoid this situation and have no desire to avoid it.
   2. I don't try to avoid this situation, but sometimes I would like to.
   3. More often than not I do not try to avoid this situation, but sometimes I do try to avoid it.
   4. More often than not I do try to avoid this situation.
   5. I avoid this situation every time I possibly can.
B. Reaction:
   1. I definitely enjoy speaking in this situation.
   2. I would rather speak in this situation than not.
   3. It's hard to say whether I'd rather speak in this situation or not.
   4. I would rather not speak in this situation.
   5. I very much dislike speaking in this situation.
C. Stuttering:
   1. I don't stutter at all (or only very rarely) in this situation.
   2. I stutter mildly (for me) in this situation.
   3. I stutter with average severity (for me) in this situation.
   4. I stutter more than average (for me) in this situation.
   5. I stutter severely (for me) in this situation.
D. Frequency:
   1. This is a situation I meet very often, two or three times a day, or even more, on the average.

2. I meet this situation at least once a day with rare exceptions (except Sunday, perhaps).
3. I meet this situation from three to five times a week on the average.
4. I meet this situation once a week, with few exceptions, and occasionally I meet it twice a week.
5. I rarely meet this situation—certainly not as often as once a week.

	Avoidance	Reaction	Stuttering	Frequency
1. Ordering in a restaurant				
2. Introducing myself (face to face)				
3. Telephoning to ask price, train fare, etc.				
4. Buying plane, train, or bus ticket				
5. Short class recitation (ten words or less)				
6. Telephoning for taxi				
7. Introducing one person to another				
8. Buying something from store clerk				
9. Conversation with good friend				
10. Talking with an instructor after class or in his office				
11. Long distance telephone call to someone I know				
12. Conversation with father				
13. Asking girl for date (or talking to man who asks me for a date)				
14. Making short speech (one or two minutes) in familiar class				
15. Giving my name over telephone				
16. Conversation with my mother				
17. Asking a secretary if I can see her employer				
18. Going to house and asking for someone				
19. Making a speech to unfamiliar audience				
20. Participating in committee meeting				
21. Asking instructor question in class				
22. Saying hello to a friend going by				
23. Asking for a job				
24. Telling a person a message from someone else				
25. Telling a funny story with one stranger in a crowd				
26. Parlor games requiring speech				
27. Reading aloud to friends				
28. Participating in a bull session				

29. Dinner conversation with strangers   _____ _____ _____ _____
30. Talking with my barber (or beauty
    operator)   _____ _____ _____ _____
31. Telephoning to make appointment, or
    arrange meeting place with someone   _____ _____ _____ _____
32. Answering roll call in class   _____ _____ _____ _____
33. Asking at a desk for book, or card to
    be filled out, etc.   _____ _____ _____ _____
34. Talking with someone I don't know
    well while waiting for bus or class,
    etc.   _____ _____ _____ _____
35. Talking with other players during a
    playground game   _____ _____ _____ _____
36. Taking leave of a hostess   _____ _____ _____ _____
37. Conversation with friend while walk-
    ing along the street   _____ _____ _____ _____
38. Buying stamps at post office   _____ ___   _____ _____
39. Giving directions or information to
    strangers   _____ _____ _____ _____
40. Taking leave of a girl (boy) after a
    date   _____ _____ _____ _____

                                Total   _____ _____ _____ _____

                              Average   _____
                              No. of 1's   _____
                               "   " 2's   _____
                               "   " 3's   _____
                               "   " 4's   _____
                               "   " 5's   _____

REFERENCES

1. Ammons, R., and Johnson, W., The construction and application of a test of attitude toward stuttering. *Journal of Speech and Hearing Disorders,* 1944, 9:39–49.
2. Andrews, G., and Ingham, R., Stuttering: considerations in the evaluation of treatment. *British Journal of Disorders of Communication,* 1971, 6: 129–138.
3. Cullinan, W., Stability of adaptation in the oral performance of stutterers. *Journal of Speech and Hearing Research,* 1963, 6:70–83.
4. Cullinan, W. L., Stability of consistency measures in stuttering. *Journal of Speech and Hearing Research,* 1963, 6:134–138.
5. Emrick, C., Language performance of stuttering and non-stuttering children. Ph.D. dissertation, University of Iowa, 1971.
6. Erickson, R. L., Assessing communication attitudes among stutterers. *Journal of Speech and Hearing Research,* 1969, 12:711–724.
7. Johnson, W., *Stuttering and What You Can Do About It.* Minneapolis: University of Minnesota Press, 1961.
8. Johnson, W., and Associates, *The Onset of Stuttering.* Minneapolis: University of Minnesota Press, 1959.
9. Johnson, W., Darley, F. L., and Spriestersbach, D. C., *Diagnostic Methods in Speech Pathology.* New York: Harper & Row, 1963.
10. Johnson, W., and Knott, J. R., The distribution of moments of stuttering in successive oral readings of the same material. *Journal of Speech Disorders,* 1937, 2:17–19.
11. Kanfer, F. H., and Saslow, G., Behavioral diagnosis. In Franks, C. M., ed., *Behavior Therapy: Appraisal and Status,* pp. 417–444. New York: McGraw-Hill, 1969.
12. Lanyon, R. I., The relationship of adaptation and consistency to improvement in stuttering therapy. *Journal of Speech and Hearing Research,* 1965, 8:263–269.
13. Lanyon, R. I., The measurement of stuttering severity. *Journal of Speech and Hearing Research,* 1967, 10:836–843.
14. Lewis, D., and Sherman, D., Measuring the severity of stuttering. *Journal of Speech and Hearing Disorders,* 1951, 16:320–326.
15. Riley, G. D., A stuttering severity instrument for children and adults. *Journal of Speech and Hearing Disorders,* 1972, 37:314–322.
16. Sherman, D., Clinical and experimental use of the Iowa scale of severity of stuttering. *Journal of Speech and Hearing Disorders,* 1952, 17:316–320.
17. Shumak, I. C., A speech situation rating sheet for stutterers. In Johnson, W., ed., *Stuttering in Children and Adults: Thirty Years of Research at the University of Iowa,* pp. 341–347. Minneapolis: University of Minnesota Press, 1955.
18. Silverman, E. M., Generality of disfluency data collected from preschoolers. *Journal of Speech and Hearing Research,* 1972, 15:84–92.
19. *Stuttering: Its Prevention.* Memphis, Tenn.: Speech Foundation of America, 1962.
20. *Therapy for Stutterers.* Memphis, Tenn.: Speech Foundation of America, 1974.

21. Van Riper, C., *The Nature of Stuttering*. Englewood Cliffs, N.J.: Prentice-Hall, 1971.
22. Van Riper, C., *The Treatment of Stuttering*. Englewood Cliffs, N.J.: Prentice-Hall, 1973.
23. Williams, D. E., Stuttering therapy for children. In Travis, L. E., ed., *Handbook of Speech Pathology and Audiology*, pp. 1073–1093. Englewood Cliffs, N.J.: Prentice-Hall, 1971.
24. Williams, D. E., Silverman, F. H., and Kools, J. A., Disfluency behavior of elementary school stutterers and non-stutterers: The adaptation effect. *Journal of Speech and Hearing Research*, 1968, *11*:622–630.
25. Williams, D. E., Silverman, F. H., and Kools, J. A., Disfluency behavior of elementary school stutterers: The consistency effect. *Journal of Speech and Hearing Research*, 1969, *12*:301–307.
26. Williams, D., Silverman, F., and Kools, J., Disfluency analysis of elementary school aged stuttering and non-stuttering children. Unpublished manuscript, University of Iowa.
27. Woolf, G., The assessment of stuttering as struggle, avoidance, and expectancy. *British Journal of Disorders of Communication*, 1967, *2*:158–171.
28. Young, M. A., Predicting ratings of severity of stuttering. *Journal of Speech and Hearing Disorders*, Monograph Supplement, No. 7, 1961, 31–54.

11

EXAMINATION OF THE SPEECH MECHANISM

D. C. Spriestersbach,
Hughlett L. Morris,
and Frederic L. Darley

An important step in appraisal of a speech disorder is the examination of the speech mechanism. In this chapter we consider procedures for examining the lips, teeth, tongue, palate, palatopharyngeal mechanism, and the total speech apparatus in action. Other aspects of the speech mechanism are considered in the discussions of the appraisal of respiration and phonation (Chapter 6) and resonance (Chapter 7).

Evaluation of the speech mechanism is complicated by the fact that many observations involve estimates or judgments rather than direct measurements. The range in motility, shape, and size of the structures is great. Since certain particulars of normative data on the shape, size, and motility of the structures are not available, you as a clinician must evaluate them largely on the basis of your own experience. Furthermore, the relationships among the sizes of contiguous structures and spaces are more important than the measures of size per se. Finally, the combined effect of several deviations of the speech mechanism may be cumulative and may prove to be disabling to the speaker even though the magnitude of individual deviations may be of little clinical significance; yet it is difficult to assign the weight to be given to each of the several deviations in evaluating their combined effects. For these reasons it is important that you make as many observations of oral structures as possible so that you will acquire firsthand knowledge of the usual and the exceptional as well as a practical sense regarding the significance of the effect of any given structural condition on speech.

We do not usually find dramatic deviations of the oral structures which can be conclusively related to specific deviations in speech. While unusual size and shape of these structures may contribute to a speech problem, most individuals show considerable ability to compensate for structural irregularities. Many individuals who have poorly aligned or missing teeth or short and immobile upper lips may speak quite satisfactorily, at least in certain contexts and for specific purposes. We must be careful, therefore, in relating findings from examination of the speech mechanism to the speech imperfections that we observe. As a general rule, if the speaker can produce a phoneme correctly in some contexts, particularly those involving contextual speech, any structural deviations he or she may have cannot be assumed to be highly significant in relation to misarticulations of that phoneme.

It is important that we understand clearly why we examine the oral structures. Almost always we are chiefly interested in their functional adequacy. If in our judgment the structures are not adequate for speech, we must decide whether the speaker can be helped to obtain more effective function from the deviant structures or whether physical changes must be made in them before we attempt to change their function. As a consequence, Form 12, the Speech Mechanism Examination, calls for a rating of the adequacy for speech of the oral structures in terms which are suggestive of the possible practical clinical decisions to be made. The ratings to be made are as follows:

1. Normal.
2. Slight deviation—probably no adverse effect on speech.
3. Moderate deviation—possible adverse effect on speech; remedial services may be required, particularly if other structures of the speech mechanism are also deviant.
4. Extreme deviation—sufficient to prevent normal production of speech; modification of structure is required, either with or without clinical speech services.

When you give a structure a rating of 4, you are indicating that in your judgment the speaker will not be able to produce certain sounds or qualities of voice until some changes are made in the function or potential for function of the affected structure. If you feel that physical changes must be made before function can be changed, your retraining program will likely not include efforts to change the speech behavior until the indicated changes have been made. It follows, of course, that you should be prepared to recommend that the speaker secure the services of the appropriate professional person who can accomplish the desired physical changes (usually a surgeon or dentist).

When you give a structure a rating of 3, you are indicating that you may be able to provide a retraining program which will enable the speaker to make the necessary compensations required by the deviant structure. Structural changes may not be required in this case unless several related structures are involved. In any event, a rating of 3 implies you feel that a program of experimental speech therapy is justified. You would use a rating of 2 to indicate that a structure does not fall clearly within the normal range but that the deviation has no practical clinical significance so far as speech is concerned.

The specific observations called for in the Speech Mechanism Examination may best be considered against a background of essential information about the functional contribution made by each of the structures to the speech act.

THE LIPS

Normally the lips serve to modify the breath stream in the production of the labial phonemes. In general, however, a highly precise modification of the breath stream is not essential in producing labial phonemes. Furthermore, since the lips are highly mobile, it is quite possible for the lower lip to make contact with even an unusually short upper lip. As a consequence, deviations of the lips will rarely be rated as extreme. Such a point of view is consistent with the findings of Fairbanks and Green (7). It is consistent also with data reported by Spriestersbach, Moll, and Morris (27), who concluded that deviations of the lip structure do not play a significant part in accounting for the articulation problems of speakers with cleft lip and palate. In fact, they reported that persons with only clefts of the lip had essentially normal articulation.

Nevertheless we must evaluate the lips and make judgments of their contribution to the articulation problems of the speakers we observe because, if for no other reason, professional workers from other fields frequently relate structural deviations of the lips to articulation errors. We must be prepared, therefore, to explain the lack of a relationship when such a judgment is consistent with our observations. It should also be appreciated that lip structures, particularly in the case of any speaker with a repaired cleft lip, need to be evaluated because of the important role they play in the appearance of the individual. The psychological impact of a badly scarred lip may sometimes be great enough to cause a speaker to react negatively to speaking situations.

We are interested in several aspects of lip structure and function. We need to note whether there is evidence of cleft lip or other tissue deficiency. The activities of protrusion and retraction should be observed, with special attention to laterality of movement. Many clinicians use a task of repeated /u/–/i/, /u/–/i/ to sample that kind of ability.

A different kind of lip motility is assessed by tasks which require rapid opening-closing movements, such as repetition of /pʌ/. Data reported by Blomquist (3) and Sprague (26) indicate that we may expect normal-speaking children to produce between three and six /pʌ/ sounds per second. Rates lower than three per second should probably be regarded as unusually slow. Normal-speaking adults produce six to seven repetitions of /pʌ/ per second according to Snyder (25).

We need to add another word of caution about the task in general. The activity of repeating /pʌ/ probably involves as much mandibular movement as lip movement and the results should be so interpreted. If information is sought about lip movements, it would be preferable to stabilize the mandible in either the open or occluded position.

THE TEETH

Normally the teeth play an important role in the production of labio-dental, linguadental, and postdental fricatives; if the dentition has an adverse effect on speech production, these groups of phonemes are most likely affected. However, as in the case of the lips, ample clinical and research evidence exists to support the view that many speakers are able to make major compensations for dental deviations, particularly if they are not accompanied by other relevant deviations of the speech mechanism. Consequently it is difficult with our present knowledge to generalize about the relationship between articulation proficiency and dental status. (For a review of this topic, see the paper by Starr, 28). As in the case of the lips, dental deviations are easily observed and inexperienced examiners frequently attempt to account for articulation difficulties on the basis of these deviations. In contrast to the situation with the lips, however, dental conditions may frequently be considered extreme in relation to the production of consonants, particularly the sibilants, if there is severe openbite or mesioclusion.

Eruption of Teeth

Because of the possible importance of dental deviations in accounting for certain misarticulations of children, it is important to review basic information about dental development. Tables 11.1 and 11.2 provide information about ages of eruption for the deciduous and the permanent teeth.

Dental Occlusion

The task of describing dental occlusion is not an easy one and has generated considerable discussion in the dental profession, specifically among orthodontists. The classification system of Angle is used for most purposes. However, there are limitations to that system because it includes primarily reference to the anterior-posterior relationship between the maxillary and the mandibular arches. An additional dimension, mesial-lateral, is needed and that dimension is usually expressed with reference to crossbite designation. Some good references about methods for describing dental occlusion are Moyers (22, pp. 303–323), Ackerman and Proffit (1), and Hitchcock (11, pp. 21–42).

Our purpose here is not to provide a highly technical description of dental and occlusal relationships seen in an orthodontic practice but rather to describe some of the relationships that the speech clinician may

TABLE 11.1
Ages in Months of Eruption of Deciduous Teeth of Normal Boys and Girls (Sexes Combined)

Deciduous Tooth	Age of Eruption (in Months, ± 1 SD)
Maxillary	
Central incisor	10 (8–12)
Lateral incisor	11 (9–13)
Canine	19 (16–22)
First molar	16 (13–19) boys
	(14–18) girls
Second molar	29 (25–33)
Mandibular	
Central incisor	8 (6–10)
Lateral incisor	13 (10–16)
Canine	20 (17–23)
First molar	16 (14–18)
Second molar	27 (23–31) boys
	(24–30) girls

Source: From *20.*

encounter. Our specific interest is in occlusions which may have adverse effects on speech production. Principally those are occlusions which disrupt the relationships between the incisors or those which result in a significant reduction in size of or change in shape of the oral cavity.

Following are some definitions which may be helpful.

Normal occlusion: The teeth are well aligned, and the upper and lower arches are in correct front-to-back (anteroposterior) and side-to-side (lateral) relationship to each other and to the rest of the skull anatomy. The upper jaw (maxilla) is slightly larger than the lower jaw (mandible). An important aspect of this relationship involves the occlusion of the upper and lower first permanent molars in which the anterior cusps of the upper molar fit in the "groove" between the anterior and posterior cusps of the lower molar. (See Bloomer's discussion and diagrams [2, pp. 727–728] for a clear presentation of the nature of this relationship.) In this discussion, "normal" does not mean "average." Several studies have shown that perhaps as many as 75 percent of American children have some degree of malocclusion (14).

Neutroclusion (Angle's Class I): The upper and lower dental arches are in correct anteroposterior and lateral relationship to each other and to the skull, but there is misalignment of individual teeth; for example,

TABLE 11.2
Mean Ages of Eruption of Permanent Teeth of White Children Living in the Northern Temperate Zone (N = more than 93,000)

| Order of Emergence | Tooth | | Mean Age of Emergence | | Sex Differ- ence |
	Maxilla	Mandible	Boys Yrs.	Girls Yrs.	Mos.
1		Molar 1	6.21	5.94	3.5
2	Molar 1		6.40	6.22	2.0
3		Incisor 1	6.54	6.26	3.5
4	Incisor 1		7.47	7.20	3.5
5		Incisor 2	7.70	7.34	4.5
6	Incisor 2		8.67	8.20	5.5
7 (Boys)					
		Premolar 1	10.40	10.03	4.5
8 (Girls)					
8 (Boys)					
		Cuspid	10.79	9.86	11.1
7 (Girls)					
9		Premolar 1	10.82	10.18	7.7
10	Premolar 2		11.18	10.88	3.6
11		Premolar 2	11.47	10.89	7.0
12	Cuspid		11.69	10.98	8.5
13		Molar 2	12.12	11.66	5.5
14	Molar 2		12.68	12.27	4.9

Source: Compiled from 24 published reports, after Hurme (12).

teeth may be rotated or jumbled, or teeth may be displaced toward the lips, cheeks, or tongue from their normal positions.

Distoclusion (Angle's Class II): The mandible with its superimposed dental arch is too far back (posterior) in relation to the maxilla and to the rest of the skull.

Mesioclusion (Angle's Class III): The mandible with its superimposed dental arch is too far forward (anterior) in relation to the maxilla and the rest of the skull.

Crossbite: There is misalignment in the mesial-lateral dimension. According to Moyers (21) the most common crossbite is that in which the maxillary teeth seem to fit outside (buccally) the mandibular teeth. However, the maxillary teeth may also be in crossbite toward the midline (lingually). Either type of crossbite may be observed anteriorly, posteriorly, or both.

The following terms are defined to assist in describing conditions of the anterior teeth:

Openbite: Absence of contact between the maxillary and mandibular anterior teeth resulting in open spaces between them when the posterior teeth are in occlusion.

Closebite: The maxillary anterior teeth overlap the mandibular anterior teeth excessively when the posterior teeth are in occlusion.

Edentulous spaces: Spaces resulting from the absence or loss of teeth.

Lack of proximal contact: Lack of contact between any two adjacent teeth; that is, space between the teeth.

Misalignment or malalignment: An abnormal position of a tooth in the dental arch.

Jumbling: A piling-up or crossing-over of several teeth.

Supernumerary teeth: Teeth in excess of the normal number.

Linguoversion: Deflection of a tooth toward the tongue from its normal position.

Labioversion: Deflection of a tooth toward the lips from its normal position.

Buccalversion: Deflection of a tooth toward the cheeks from its normal position.

Dental Appliances and Prostheses

In examining the speech mechanism the speech clinician needs to give special attention to any dental appliances and prostheses present since they may be detrimental to speech sound articulation. Typically, dental appliances are used by the orthodontist in the treatment of malocclusion and are not usually placed on a permanent basis. A dental prosthesis may be temporary, such as a partial denture in the instance of a young child; but it may be part of long-term management, in the instance of a denture (full or partial) worn by an adult.

Appliances and prostheses placed in the maxillary arch are more crucial to speech production than those placed in the mandibular arch. In addition, appliances which are fitted inside the arch have a greater effect on articulation than those placed on the outside of the arch. Information about how long the individual has had the appliance or prosthesis is also helpful.

Two special kinds of dental prosthesis are the obturator and the palatal lift. Both are prostheses designed for the physical management of a palatal (palatopharyngeal) problem. The obturator serves to reduce the size of the palatopharyngeal space, while the palatal lift serves to hold the soft palate in an elevated position.

THE TONGUE

Normally the tongue is a highly mobile structure, capable of moving rapidly and precisely. When it functions in conjunction with the other oral articulators, it participates in the production of phonemes by channeling, impeding, and obstructing the breath stream as it passes through the mouth. It also assists in modifying the resonance cavities used in speech. Its strength and motility may be impaired as the result of poor muscular development, paresis due to pathology of the nervous system, or disease or accident resulting in the removal of portions of the tongue. While there are reports of individuals who have developed satisfactory speech without a tongue or with a partial tongue (30), under usual conditions the tongue is one of the most important structures of the oral mechanism.

Tongues vary in size and shape. So do the oral cavities in which they function. Sometimes the two do not seem to fit together well. Unfortunately there is no easy way to quantify tongue size. Judgments concerning its size in relation to the dental arches are made largely on the basis of experience in viewing these structures.

The motility of the tongue is necessarily affected by pathologies which affect its innervation. However, individuals with articulation problems without neuropathology affecting the tongue have been found to be able to manipulate the tongue as effectively, at least when tested on unlearned nonspeech tasks, as individuals with normal speech.

On the basis of the findings of Fairbanks and Spriestersbach (8), the following scale might be used for judging the rate at which a person can touch the alveolar ridge with the tongue tip without speech: below average, less than 3.5 contacts per second; average, from 3.5 to 6.0 contacts per second; above average, more than 6.0 contacts per second. On the basis of the work of Sprague (26), the following scale might be used in judging the rate at which a child can articulate /tʌ/: below average, less than 3 per second; average, from 3.0 to 5.5 per second; above average, more than 5.5 per second. The examiner may want to stabilize the mandible during the performance of this activity as in /pʌ/; however, it may not be necessary since /tʌ/ typically requires less jaw movement than /pʌ/.

The rate at which a speaker can elevate the back of the tongue, making contact with the palate in the production of /kʌ/, is also of interest. Data reported by Blomquist (3), Irwin and Becklund (13), and Fletcher (9) indicate that we may expect normal children to repeat /kʌ/ between three and five times per second. Normal adults produce between five and six repetitions of /kʌ/ per second according to Kreul (16), Lundeen (19), Sigurd (24), and Ewanowski (6).

Another task which yields useful information about a speaker's motor control of the articulators is rapid repetition of the sequence /pʌ–tʌ–kʌ/. This activity requires the sequential production of labial closing-opening, tongue tip–alveolar contact, and back of tongue–palatal contact, a demanding programming task. You will be interested in the rate at which the series can be produced; data from Leshin (18) and Yoss and Darley (*31*) show that normal children on the average produce the series three or four times per second, while data from Snyder (*25*) indicate that normal adults produce the series an average of seven times per second. You will probably be even more interested in the efficiency of the speaker in producing the sequence: Does he maintain the correct syllable order? Does he repeat one or more of the syllables? Does he seem to make a special effort to accomplish the task by slowing down, "helping" position his articulators with his fingers, or some other maneuver? Speakers with defective articulation who are identified as displaying apraxia of speech typically have inordinate difficulty in maintaining the correct syllable sequence at a normal rate (*31*).

There are no available data to indicate the rate at which speakers can touch the corners of the mouth with the tongue. However, clinical experience indicates that the rate of performing complete cycles of contacts, touching both corners of the mouth with the tongue, is of the same order of magnitude as the rates quoted above.

It is possible that the lingual frenum (also called frenulum) may restrict the activity of the anterior portion of the tongue. When this condition is severe (so-called tongue-tie), the speaker has difficulty touching the alveolar ridge with the tip of his tongue, and the blade of the tongue will look like the top of a heart when he attempts to protrude it between his teeth. However, restriction by the frenum will typically not be marked enough to impair the functioning of the tongue for speech. If he can touch the upper gum ridge with the tip of his tongue, the restriction is probably not sufficient to affect speech production.

Finally, in the past there has been considerable attention on the part of some speech pathologists and dentists to the function of the tongue in swallowing as an important etiological factor for certain types of malocclusion. Labels such as "tongue thrust" or "reverse swallow" are frequently used to describe the phenomenon and the assumption is made that unusual swallowing patterns which are characterized by excessive forward thrust of the tongue during the swallow contribute to the malocclusion. Some clinicians maintain that in some patients there are observations about oral activity (specifically the lips) during swallow that provide diagnostic clues about the behavior.

There are indications in the literature (and we have made concurring clinical observations) that some individuals, probably few in number, do indeed demonstrate unusual swallowing movements during which there is unusual lip activity, such as lip pursing at the initial stages of swallowing. If that activity is relevant to speech production, and it may not be, it is because such swallowing patterns are associated with malocclusion and it is the malocclusion that is related to problems in articulation.

In general, then, we agree with the statement by the Joint Committee on Dentistry and Speech Pathology-Audiology (*14*), that there is insufficient information about the disorder and about the possible disruption in the communication process associated with it to warrant inclusion of observations of lingual patterns in swallowing in the examination of the speech mechanism.

THE PALATE AND THE PALATOPHARYNGEAL MECHANISM

The role of the palate and the palatopharyngeal (also called velopharyngeal) mechanism in speech production is to provide partition of the nasal cavity from the oral cavity when needed. In simple terms, separation of the two cavities is required for oral speech and coupling of the two cavities is required for nasal speech. The hard palate provides a permanent divider between the greater portion of the two cavities. The palatopharyngeal mechanism is used by normal speakers to open and close the relatively small palatopharyngeal port at the back of the mouth. The palatopharyngeal port is open for tasks requiring nasal emission of air or nasal resonance, and it is closed for tasks requiring oral emission of air and no nasal resonance. Conversational speech ordinarily is associated with relatively high levels of palatopharyngeal activity.

The Palate

The role of the hard and soft palates as a divider generally is not difficult to evaluate. Unless there are structural deficits resulting from cleft palate or surgical removal of the palate or portions of it, the assumption usually can be made that the palate is intact and adequately serves the role of partition between the two cavities.

Sometimes there is a palatal defect after cleft palate surgery either because of failure to heal properly or because the surgeon deliberately left some portion of the cleft palate unsutured. In the latter case, the defect is likely to be in the region of the alveolus (gum ridge) and is usually labeled as an alveolar cleft. Or there may be passage between the gingivolabial sulcus (the space between the alveolus and the lip) and the nasal cavity, usually referred to as a nasolabial fistula.

When there is a failure to heal, the opening usually is in the hard palate (posterior to the alveolus) and is called a palatal fistula. Obviously the palatal fistula appears along the lines of suture. Usually the fistula is at the margin between the anterior third and the posterior two-thirds of the palate but it can be at other locations along the anteroposterior dimension of the palate.

The alveolar cleft is relatively easy to detect by inspection. The palatal fistula generally also can be observed without difficulty, except for very small ones. However, a nasolabial fistula is usually difficult to discover, so difficult, in fact, that mention of it here is made only for the sake of completeness.

Estimating the effect of a palatal defect on speech production is sometimes not a simple task. Essentially the objective is to determine the degree to which the defect permits escape of oral air pressure into the nasal cavity during speech. For large defects there is probably an alteration in patterns of resonance also.

In general, there are two questions to be asked: how large is the fistula and where is it?

The importance of size is easily understood: the larger the fistula, the more likely there is to be nasal escape of oral air pressure during speech. There are no standards to be used in making such a judgment. One approach is to assume that if a palatal fistula or defect is large enough to be detected, it is a possible source of air leak until shown to the contrary.

A fistula in the anterior and middle thirds of the palate is likely to result in greater nasal escape of air pressure in speech than one at either the extreme anterior or posterior margin of the palate. Usually a nasolabial fistula will not result in loss of oral air pressure because the pressure of the lip will tend to occlude it. A cleft uvula is not expected to result in loss of oral air pressure because the important contact of the palate with the pharyngeal wall occurs at a point anterior—along the anteroposterior dimension of the palate—to the uvula.

In addition to partitioning the nasal cavity from the oral cavity, the palate also serves as the vault of the oral cavity. Consequently, position and contour of the palatal vault contribute to the size and shape of the oral cavity. In the majority of patients with communication problems, the oral cavity is of adequate size and shape for lingual activity in speech. Sometimes, however, the palatal vault may be so low and so narrow that the oral cavity seems almost too small for the tongue (or the tongue seems too large for the oral cavity). In such rare instances, the low narrow palatal vault may be a contributing factor to a communication problem.

The Palatopharyngeal Mechanism

It is a misconception to suppose that the adequacy of the palatopharyngeal mechanism can be assessed by a clinical examination of the speech mechanism. We know from a wealth of research data that palatopharyngeal function is too complex and depends on too many variables to be described adequately by simple peroral observations of palatal length or apparent palatal movement during the phonation of /ɑ/ or during elicitation of the gag reflex. Because of the complexity of the phenomenon, considerable expertise and some special equipment are frequently required for reliable diagnosis.

One special procedure used is radiography. X-ray films of various types provide visual information about the relationships among the palato-pharyngeal structures. Single-exposure still films taken from the lateral position while the subject sustains a vowel, such as /u/, or a continuant fricative, such as /s/, are commonly used in many diagnostic centers. From such films, the examiner can estimate whether appropriate contact is made between the soft palate and the posterior pharyngeal wall during that specific production of phoneme. Additional information is obtained by similar film studies made with a motion picture camera system since, with such a system, structural relationships during a short contextual speech passage can be observed.

All x-ray films taken from the lateral position have the disadvantage of showing structural relationships in the midline, however, and sometimes the examiner needs more than that. For such views, frontal and base x-ray films are sometimes obtained. These films are informative, par-ticularly with certain types of patients, but require a considerable amount of technical expertise. Consequently they are not available in many diag-nostic centers.

Another set of procedures frequently used in the diagnosis of palato-pharyngeal function are those which involve measures of air pressure and airflow rate. A number of these procedures are in current use, most of them designed to permit study of the patterns of airstream manage-ment during speech. For example, data are available to indicate that during the repetition of a consonant-vowel syllable, such as /pʌ/ or /kʌ/, the normal speaker (demonstrating palatopharyngeal function which is presumed normal) exhibits an amount of nasal airflow and oral airflow which can be specified. Measurement of airflow rate is made by means of special instrumentation in combination with a face mask in which nasal and oral airflows can be separated. Diagnosis of palato-pharyngeal function of an individual with suspected pathology can be made by comparing his or her measurements with those for the normal speaker.

A review of the radiographic and pressure flow procedures, as well as several other more recently developed procedures, is provided by Warren (29).

Almost all of these procedures are used during various types of speech and nonspeech activities, and the activity must be carefully monitored in order to obtain interpretable results. Typically, then, such definitive diagnosis of palatopharyngeal competence is performed by specialists in major health centers. However, the speech pathologist in clinical prac-tice outside such a center frequently needs to make preliminary diagnosis of palatopharyngeal function in order to decide whether to provide habili-tation services on a trial basis. It is for that purpose that we present this discussion.

Because of the complexity of palatopharyngeal function, we need to make several kinds of observations. We have already considered one type: observations of the apparent adequacy of the hard and soft palate as a partition between the nasal and oral cavities. If there are defects in the palate, such as an unoperated cleft palate, an acquired cleft resulting from ablative surgery, or a palatal fistula, the probabilities are that palatopharyngeal function is impaired.

Judgments about adequacy of structure size, spatial relationships, and structural mobility are less easily made. In making such observations, three major questions are involved: what constitutes normal variance, how reliable are the observations, and for what purposes are the observations made?

Obviously there is considerable variance among normal individuals with regard to palatal length, arch width, and palatal vault height. Beginning clinicians will need to make many such observations before they have a notion about what normal limits are. In general, the purpose is to be as descriptive as possible and with appropriate caution to make inferences about probable hazard to speech production. Spatial relationships are often more important than structure size; for example, a relatively short palate may function well in a shallow nasopharynx but might not if the nasopharynx were deeper (in anteroposterior dimension).

The problem of observer reliability in making these observations is the same as in making other clinical judgments. For example, there may be differences in observed palatal elevation or pharyngeal wall movement among a series of productions of sustained /a/. Differences may also be obtained if the observations are made from views of the mechanism taken from different perspectives. Finally, there may be differences in the standards used to make the judgments within observers (from one time to another) and between observers. Clinicians need to consider these sources of variance and to attempt to account for them as best they can in making their judgments.

A central issue is of course the purpose of the observation. Clearly the restrictions imposed by the observation technique used clinically are such that definitive conclusions about the effect of oral structures on speech production are generally difficult to make. Our concern about describing structures is relevant only to the degree that the structures influence function; for example, palatal length and pharyngeal wall movement are important only as the two variables contribute to palatopharyngeal function. Consequently in the final analysis observations about function are more crucial to the examination than observations about structure.

Articulation tests and descriptions of voice quality provide some valuable information about palatopharyngeal function. Details about the use of these diagnostic methods are presented in Chapters 6 and 8 and will not be repeated here. In essence, such observations involve the assessment of the extent to which there is nasal emission of air pressure during the articulation of fricatives, affricates, and plosives, and the extent to which the patient can be stimulated by auditory-visual means to produce these phonemes with oral emission. Assessment of voice quality is helpful but less reliable as an index to palatopharyngeal function than articulation testing because of the apparent complexity of hypernasality (4).

Traditionally a blowing task has been used as the major nonspeech procedure for assessing palatopharyngeal function. The justification for the use of a blowing task has been that palatopharyngeal closure is required to direct the airstream orally. However, there are several problems in using a blowing task for this purpose. A major one is that under certain conditions (such as those involving tongue-palate valving) palatopharyngeal closure may not be required for the oral expulsion of air. Another problem is that palatopharyngeal function during blowing (and sucking) is probably different in nature and extent from palatopharyngeal function during speech; ability to do the first may not be a good predictor of the second (10, 23). In spite of these serious limitations, observations of blowing activities can yield useful information if the observations are interpreted with caution, particularly in the case of young children.

The relevant observation to be made during the blowing task has to do with whether there is nasal emission of oral air pressure during the blowing attempt. The observation can be made auditorily, by listening for audible signs of nasal emission of the air pressure, or noting the clouding of a mirror held beneath the nares during a task such as blowing out a match. Or the observation can be made by comparing measures of oral air pressure produced with the nares open and occluded (a ratio can be obtained by dividing the former reading by the latter). For the latter task, an instrument is needed for measurement of the air pressure demonstrated under the two conditions. A number of manometers and spirometers are suitable for that purpose. For certain technical reasons, to be maximally useful such an instrument must include a "bleed valve," which provides for a constant leak of air pressure during the blowing attempt. In addition, there must be some procedure for reliable assessment of the blowing effort between attempts by the same patient. One instrument that is particularly useful in a clinical situation because of size, inexpensiveness, and ease of maintenance is the Hunter manometer.[1] An oral manometer ratio, described in some detail by Morris (21), is clearly not a highly precise measure of palatopharyngeal competence and indeed is subject to influence by a number of irrelevant variables. But to date there is no other procedure that gives information so simply about the relative ability of a patient to direct the airstream orally during a nonspeech task.

Finally, there is need for observations about consistency of performance. Appropriate questions to be asked include the following: Is there

[1] The Hunter Mfg. Co., Old Quarry Road, Coralville, Iowa 52241

nasal emission of oral air pressure during the production of all fricatives, affricates, or plosives, or at times is no emission detected? With auditory and visual stimulation, can the patient be assisted to articulate in an oral manner "pressure" consonants which he normally nasalizes? Do any of the manometer ratios taken indicate palatopharyngeal competence? Does using a slow rate of production seem to make the articulation more normally oral? Are there apparent differences in the amount of nasal emission heard among various kinds of speech activities? Is there other evidence of inconsistency in palatopharyngeal function?

THE FAUCES

We are interested in examining the area of the fauces because in some instances the faucial isthmus may be restricted to a degree that makes the free movement of air from the oropharynx into the oral cavity difficult. In some instances the tonsils may be enlarged to the degree that they touch at the midline during phonation. Such a condition may result in a muffling of the laryngeal tone and in placing an unusual requirement on the palatopharyngeal port mechanism to achieve tight closure if nasal escape of air is to be prevented.

The muscles which underlie the mucous membranes of the faucial pillars are intermeshed with the muscles of the soft palate, pharynx, and tongue. On the basis of clinical observations it is assumed that mesial movement—movement toward the midline—of the posterior pillars during phonation and gagging is an indication that the muscles of the lateral walls of the pharynx are playing some part in palatopharyngeal closure. It has also been assumed that such movements reflect a desirable type of possible compensatory activity in those instances in which adequate palatopharyngeal closure is not achieved by action of the soft palate. On the other hand, some individuals have only remnants of pillars or none at all. Their absence should not be viewed with concern since there is no evidence that such speakers have any unique problems in achieving palatopharyngeal competence.

THE NOSE AND THE NASAL CAVITIES

The nasal cavities are part of the respiratory system used in speech and consequently are generally included in an examination of the speech mechanism. Our major interest is in determining whether there is sufficient nasal airway for providing normal nasal resonance and an adequate nasal pathway for speech purposes. Information about the nose and the nasal cavities is generally obtained by observation and history, since physical examination by use of special instrumentation is conducted by the physician.

Of particular concern is nasal or nasopharyngeal obstruction which seems to interfere with the normal use of the nasal pathway. An example of an obstruction in the nasal cavity is a deviated nasal septum. In the nasopharynx hypertrophied adenoids often constitute an obstruction. Typically the adenoidal pad is hidden from view by the soft palate; sometimes, however, the inferior margin of the adenoidal pad can be seen. Nasopharyngeal tumors may occlude the airway. For patients with cleft palate (or other palatal problem) a pharyngeal flap or obturator that is very wide may result in obstruction of the airway. Mouth breathing is one symptom of nasal obstruction. Another is "noisy" breathing in which the effect of the obstruction can be "heard."

PERFORMANCE OF VOLITIONAL ORAL MOVEMENTS

In the foregoing portions of the speech mechanism examination you have asked the speaker to perform a number of tasks which permit you to make observations with regard to shape, size, position, or speed of movement of the individual components of the speech apparatus. One further set of observations will be useful: note how efficiently the speaker performs nonspeech volitional oral movements which demand his "putting it all together." When asked to do any simple or complex activity, does he perform it briskly and accurately or does he fumble, grope, or effortfully struggle to do it? Is trial and error evident in arriving at the target? Can he perform the task upon request or must he be shown what is meant and how it should be done?

Speakers who display highly inconsistent and variable articulation errors in the absence of weakness, slowness, incoordination, and altered muscle tone may be identified as displaying an apraxia of speech. They demonstrate difficulty in volitional performance of skilled acts, although under other conditions they may be able to perform the same acts involuntarily, "accidentally," or reactively. It has been shown (5) that some, though not all, adult speakers who display an apraxia of speech display an associated oral apraxia; oral apraxia is also a primary finding in children who are identified as presenting a developmental apraxia of speech (31). Therefore your examination of the speech mechanism should be extended to include the performance of tasks which may reveal the presence of an oral apraxia. Such tasks could include whistling; coughing; puffing out the cheeks; protruding, wiggling, elevating, and depressing the tongue tip; licking the lips; chattering the teeth; and the like. Scale your observations of these performances to show how accurately and promptly they were done and whether they were performed spontaneously on command or required a demonstration.

You may carry the examination one step further and ask the speaker to perform a sequence of two or three such tasks (17). The breakdown in performance may appear on the sequential performance of several tasks more prominently than on the isolated performance of single tasks.

SUMMARY

As we indicated in our introductory comments, it is frequently difficult
to attribute any single speech disorder to a particular structural deviation. A given structural deviation may be of significance only if it occurs
as one of a constellation of deviations. We suggest that you view the
deviations as constellations. We also, and most importantly, suggest that
you interpret the results of the speech mechanism examination in the
light of the findings from the speech and language examination of the
patient. It seems pointless to emphasize a finding of a space between
the upper incisors, for example, when the only problem revealed by the
speech and language examination is a substitution of /w/ for /r/.

ASSIGNMENTS

1. Examine ten normal adults and two normal children, in rapid consecutive order if possible. Follow Form 12, Speech Mechanism
   Examination, in conducting your examination. Note the range of oral
   structures in the normal individual. What variation among structures do you see? What relationships among structures are apparent?
   In the normal children, look particularly for tonsillar tissue and at
   dental development.
2. Examine three patients (both children and adults, if possible) with oral
   structure deficits which have been previously diagnosed (cleft palate,
   malocclusion, etc.) Obtain the results of a speech and language examination for each patient. Can any of the speech and language
   patterns be attributed to an oral structure deficit or a combination
   of deficits?

FORM 12
Speech Mechanism Examination

1. Lips
   a. Structure
      Touch when teeth are in occlusion: yes _____ no _____
      Upper lip length: normal _____ short _____ long _____
      (describe)
      Evidence of cleft lip or other structural deficit: yes _____ (describe)
      no _____
      Other structural deficit: (describe)
   b. Function
      Can protrude: yes _____ no _____
      Can retract unilaterally
         Left: yes _____ no _____
         Right: yes _____ no _____
      Equal retraction bilaterally: yes _____ no _____
      Number of times can produce /pʌ/ in 5 seconds: trial 1 _____
      trial 2 _____ trial 3 _____
      Does stabilizing the jaw facilitate the activity? yes _____ no _____
   c. Adequacy for speech: 1 _____ 2 _____ 3 _____
      4 _____
2. Teeth
   a. Structure
      Occlusion: normal _____ neutroclusion _____
      distoclusion _____ mesioclusion _____
      Anteroposterior relationship of incisors: normal _____ mixed (some
      in labioversion, some in linguaversion) but all upper and lower
      teeth contact; all upper incisors lingual to lower incisors but in
      contact _____ not in contact _____
      Vertical relationship of incisors: normal _____ openbite _____
      closebite _____
      Continuity of cutting edge of incisors: normal _____ ro-
      tated _____ jumbled _____ missing teeth _____ super-
      numerary teeth _____
      If lack of continuity, identify teeth involved and describe nature of
      deviation:
   b. Dental appliance or prosthesis: yes _____ (describe) no _____
   c. Adequacy for speech: 1 _____ 2 _____ 3 _____
      4 _____
3. Tongue
   a. Structure:
      Size in relation to dental arches: too large _____ appro-
      priate _____ too small _____ symmetrical _____ asym-
      metrical _____
   b. Function:
      Can curl tongue up and back: yes _____ no _____

Number of times can touch anterior alveolar ridge with tongue tip without sound in 5 seconds:

trial 1 _____ trial 2 _____ trial 3 _____

above average _____ average _____ below average _____

Number of times can touch the corners of mouth with tongue tip in 5 seconds:

trial 1 _____ trial 2 _____ trial 3 _____

above average _____ average _____ below average _____

Number of times can produce /tʌ/ in 5 seconds:

trial 1 _____ trial 2 _____ trial 3 _____

above average _____ average _____ below average _____

Number of times can produce /kʌ/ in 5 seconds:

trial 1 _____ trial 2 _____ trial 3 _____

above average _____ average _____ below average _____

Restrictiveness of lingual frenum:

not restrictive _____ somewhat restrictive _____

markedly restrictive _____

  c. Adequacy for speech: 1 _____ 2 _____ 3 _____

    4 _____

4. Hard palate

  a. Structure:

Intactness: normal _____ cleft, repaired _____ cleft, unrepaired _____

Palatal fistula: yes _____ (describe) no _____

Alveolar cleft: yes _____ (describe) no _____

Palatal contour: normal configuration _____ flat contour _____

deep and narrow contour _____

  b. Adequacy for speech: 1 _____ 2 _____ 3 _____ 4 _____

5. Palatopharyngeal mechanism

  a. Structure:

Soft palate:

Intactness: normal _____ cleft, repaired _____ cleft, unrepaired _____ symmetrical _____ asymmetrical _____

Length: satisfactory _____ short _____ very short _____

Uvula:

normal _____ bifid _____ deviated from midline to right _____ to left _____ absent _____

Oropharynx:

Depth: shallow _____ normal _____ deep _____

Width: narrow _____ normal _____ wide _____

  b. Function:

Soft palate:

Movement during prolonged phonation of /ɑ/: none _____

some _____ marked _____

Movement during short, repeated phonations of /ɑ/: none _____
some _____ marked _____

Movement during gag reflex: none _____ some _____
marked _____

If some movement, is amount:
Same for both halves _____ more for right half _____
more for left half _____

Oropharynx:
Mesial movement of lateral pharyngeal walls during phonation of
/ɑ/: none _____ some _____ marked _____
Mesial movement of lateral pharyngeal walls during gag reflex:
none _____ some _____ marked _____

Audible nasal emission while blowing out a match: yes _____
no _____

Inconsistency in nasal emission during speech or blowing tasks:
yes _____ (describe) no _____

Patient stimulable to oral productions of pressure consonants:
yes _____ (describe) no _____

Nares constriction during speech or blowing task: yes _____ (describe) no _____

Oral manometer ratio (instrument _____):
Trial 1: nostrils open _____ nostrils closed _____
ratio _____
Trial 2: nostrils open _____ nostrils closed _____
ratio _____
Trial 3: nostrils open _____ nostrils closed _____
ratio _____

c. Adequacy for speech: 1 _____ 2 _____ 3 _____
4 _____

6. Fauces
a. Structure:
Tonsils: normal _____ enlarged _____ atrophied _____
absent _____
Pillars: normal _____ scarred _____ inflamed _____
absent _____
Area of faucial isthmus: above average _____ average _____
below average _____

b. Function:
Posterior movement during phonation of /ɑ/: none _____
some _____ marked _____
Mesial movement during phonation of /ɑ/: none _____
some _____ marked _____
Restriction of velar activity by pillars: none _____ some _____
marked _____

c. Adequacy for speech: 1 _____ 2 _____ 3 _____
4 _____

7. Nasal cavities
   a. Structure:
      Septum: normal _____   deviated right _____
         deviated left _____
      Nasal obstruction:
      Right: none _____   some _____   marked _____
      Left: none _____   some _____   marked _____
   b. Function:
      Evidence of mouth breathing: yes _____ (describe)   no _____
      Adenoids visible: yes _____   no _____
      Pharyngeal flap: yes _____   no _____
      Obturator: yes _____   no _____
   c. Adequacy for speech: 1 _____   2 _____   3 _____
      4 _____

8. Volitional oral movements:

		Use this scale to evaluate:
Stick out your tongue	_____	8 Accurate, immediate, on command
Blow	_____	
Show me your teeth	_____	7 Accurate after trial and error, searching movements, on command
Pucker your lips	_____	
Touch your nose with tip of tongue	_____	
Bite your lower lip	_____	6 Crude, defective in amplitude, accuracy or speed, on command
Whistle	_____	
Lick your lips	_____	5 Partial, important part missing, on command
Clear your throat	_____	
Move your tongue in and out	_____	4 Same as 8, after demonstration
Click your teeth together once	_____	3 Same as 7, after demonstration
Smile	_____	2 Same as 6, after demonstration
Click your tongue	_____	
Chatter your teeth as if cold	_____	1 Same as 5, after demonstration
Touch your chin with tip of tongue	_____	OP Perseverative
Cough	_____	OI Irrelevant; some other oral performance including speech
Puff out your cheeks	_____	
Wiggle your tongue from side to side	_____	NO Nil. No oral performance
Show how you kiss someone	_____	
Alternately pucker and smile	_____	
Total	_____	

9. Sequential movements; indicate number of trials needed to pass or *F* for "failed":
   Show how you whistle, then smile _____

Bite lower lip, then blow _____
Stick out tongue, chatter teeth, then blow _____
Puff cheeks, wiggle tongue, then click tongue _____
10. Summary and evaluation
    a. Specify the deviations which you have rated as significant:
        Rating of 4: _____
        Rating of 3: _____
        Rating of 2: _____
    b. Relate these deviations to your findings from testing the speech of the patient. Comment on account to be taken of these deviations in planning a program of remedial speech services for the patient.

REFERENCES

1. Ackerman, J. L., and Proffit, W. R., Diagnosis and planning treatment in orthodontics. In Graber, T. M., and Swain, B. F., eds., *Current Orthodontic Concepts and Techniques*, pp. 1–110. Philadelphia: Saunders, 1975.
2. Bloomer, H. H., Speech defects associated with dental malocclusions. In Travis, L. E., ed., *Handbook of Speech Pathology and Audiology*, pp. 715–766. Englewood Cliffs, N.J.: Prentice-Hall, 1971.
3. Blomquist, B. L., Diadochokinetic movements of nine-, ten-, and eleven-year-old children. *Journal of Speech and Hearing Disorders*, 1950, *15*: 159–164.
4. Curtis, J. F., The acoustics of nasalized speech. *Cleft Palate Journal*, 1970, 7:380–396.
5. DeRenzi, E., Pieczuro, A., and Vignolo, L. A., Oral apraxia and aphasia. *Cortex*, 1966, *2*:50–73.
6. Ewanowski, S. J., Selected motor speech behavior of patients with parkinsonism. Ph.D. dissertation, University of Wisconsin, 1964.
7. Fairbanks, G., and Green, E., A study of minor organic deviations in "functional" disorders of articulation: 2. Dimensions and relationships of the lips. *Journal of Speech and Hearing Disorders*, 1950, *15*:165–168.
8. Fairbanks, G., and Spriestersbach, D. C., A study of minor organic deviations in "functional" disorders of articulation: 1. Rate of movement of oral structures. *Journal of Speech and Hearing Disorders*, 1950, *15*:60–69.
9. Fletcher, S. G., Time-by-count measurement of diadochokinetic syllable rate. *Journal of Speech and Hearing Research*, 1972, *15*:763–770.
10. Flowers, C. R., and Morris, H. L., Oral-pharyngeal movements during swallowing and speech. *Cleft Palate Journal*, 1973, *10*:181–191.
11. Hitchcock, H. P., *Orthodontics for Undergraduates*. Philadelphia: Lea & Febiger, 1974.
12. Hurme, V. O., Ranges of normalcy in the eruption of permanent teeth. *Journal of Dentistry for Children*, 1949, *16*:11–15.
13. Irwin, J. V., and Becklund, O., Norms for maximum repetitive rates for certain sounds established with the Sylrater. *Journal of Speech and Hearing Disorders*, 1953, *18*:149–160.
14. Joint Committee on Dentistry and Speech Pathology-Audiology, Position statement of tongue thrust. *Asha*, 1975, *17*:331–337.
15. Kelly, J. E., Sanchez, M., and Van Kirk, L. E., An assessment of the occlusion of teeth of children. Data from the National Health Survey. National Center for Health Statistics, U. S. Public Health Service, 1973. DHEW Publication No. (HRA) 74-1612.
16. Kreul, J. E., Neuromuscular control examination (NMC) for parkinsonism: vowel prolongation and diadochokinetic and reading rates. *Journal of Speech and Hearing Research*, 1972, *15*:72–83.
17. LaPointe, L. L., and Wertz, R. T., Oral-movement abilities and articulatory characteristics of brain-injured adults. *Perceptual and Motor Skills*, 1974, *39*:39–46.
18. Leshin, S., A study of diadochokinetic movements of lips and tongue in children. M.A. thesis, University of Michigan, 1948.

19. Lundeen, D. J., The relationship of diadochokinesis to various speech sounds. *Journal of Speech and Hearing Disorders,* 1950, *15:*54–59.

20. Lunt, R. C., and Law, D. B., A review of the chronology of eruption of deciduous teeth. *Journal of the American Dental Association,* 1974, *89:* 872–879.

21. Morris, H. L., The oral manometer as a diagnostic tool in clinical speech pathology. *Journal of Speech and Hearing Disorders,* 1966, *31:*362–369.

22. Moyers, R. E., *Handbook of Orthodontics.* 3rd ed., Chicago: Year Book Medical Publishers, 1973.

23. Shelton, R. L., Brooks, A., and Youngstrom, K. A., Patterns of swallow in cleft palate children. *Cleft Palate Journal,* 1966, *3:*200–210.

24. Sigurd, B., Maximum rate and minimal duration of repeated syllables. *Language and Speech Journal,* 1973, *16:*373–395.

25. Snyder, J., A study of diadochokinesis of lips, tongue, and palate of adults with non-defective speech. M.A. thesis, University of Michigan, 1955.

26. Sprague, A. L., The relationship between selected measures of expressive language and motor skill in eight-year-old boys. Ph.D. dissertation, University of Iowa, 1961.

27. Spriestersbach, D. C., Moll, K. L., and Morris, H. L., Subject classification and articulation of speakers with cleft palates. *Journal of Speech and Hearing Research,* 1961, *4:*362–372.

28. Starr, C. D., Dental and occlusal hazards to normal speech production. In Grabb, W. C., Rosenstein, S. W., and Bzoch, K. R., eds., *Cleft Lip and Palate: Surgical, Dental and Speech Aspects,* pp. 670–680. Boston: Little, Brown, 1971.

29. Warren, D. W., Instrumentation. In McWilliams, B. J., and Wertz, R. T., eds., *Speech, Language and Psychosocial Aspects of Cleft Lip and Cleft Palate: The State of the Art.* pp. 26–33. ASHA Reports, Number 9. Washington, D.C., American Speech and Hearing Association, 1973.

30. Weinberg, B., Christensen, R., Logan, W., Bosma, J., and Wornall, A., Severe hypoplasia of the tongue. *Journal of Speech and Hearing Disorders,* 1969, *34:*157–168.

31. Yoss, K. A., and Darley, F. L., Developmental apraxia of speech in children with defective articulation. *Journal of Speech and Hearing Research,* 1974, *17:*399–416.

12

THE APPRAISAL OF AUDITORY FUNCTIONING

**Charles V. Anderson
and Julia M. Davis**

INTRODUCTION

Auditory sensation and perception comprise one of the two major components of the process of oral communication. Although the appraisal of receptive auditory behavior is complex and broad enough to form a large portion of the professional field of audiology, it is important that the speech-language pathologist, as an evaluator of communication behavior, also became familiar with the process of auditory reception and its appraisal.

A hearing loss may be one of the many causes of speech, voice, and language disorders. In our zeal to define and describe the preponderant disorder presented by a client, we must remain cognizant that the presence of a speech, voice, or language disorder does not preclude the presence of a hearing impairment; indeed, it may increase the likelihood of a hearing disorder.

It is the intent of this chapter to create an awareness of the processes and the appraisal of auditory sensation and perception and their effect upon linguistic functioning. Accompanying this awareness must be an understanding of the effects of an auditory disorder upon communication and a sensitivity to indications that one may be present and need further evaluation. In view of the large number of procedures and concepts that need to be covered, you should not anticipate an in-depth discussion or coverage of any single item. Among the references given at the end of the chapter you will find excellent detailed presentations of each specific procedure or concept.

The complete audiologic evaluation has the basic purposes of (1) describing what the patient hears and how he hears it, (2) describing the communication ability of the patient, (3) providing information which will assist in determining the site(s) of lesion(s) within the auditory system, and (4) providing the basis from which a plan of habilitation can be developed. These purposes quite obviously dictate the evaluation of reception, processing, and use of auditory signals, including the effects of a hearing disorder upon linguistic functioning.

To accomplish these goals, the audiologist must rely upon case history information, tests and measurements, and observations of communicative behavior. The case history is discussed in Chapter 2. In this chapter we will concentrate on tests, measurements, and observations.

HOW AND WHAT WE HEAR

Although it is assumed that you have already studied acoustics and the anatomy of the auditory system, we will briefly review aspects of these two areas of knowledge necessary for the discussion which follows.

Acoustics

The three types of signals most commonly used in testing hearing are pure tones, speech, and noise. A pure tone is simply an acoustic signal consisting of a single frequency. Speech and noise are obviously more complex signals comprised of several or many frequencies, often at a variety of levels within the single signal.

The frequency of a signal is determined by the number of complete cycles of condensation and rarefaction a sound wave completes in a given unit of time. For our purposes, frequency is the number of cycles per second (cps), designated as Hertz (Hz), a term chosen to honor an eighteenth century German physicist. One Hz is equal to one cps. A pure tone is identified by its Hz. A 1000 Hz pure-tone signal is one in which the cycle is completed 1000 times per second.

The range of human hearing is often described as extending from 20 Hz to 20,000 Hz. In the clinical measurement of hearing, however, we often restrict our interest to the range from 125 Hz to 8000 Hz. This restriction is justified by the knowledge that this range encompasses the frequencies (1) contributing information in human speech, (2) to which the human being is most sensitive, and (3) most easily measured and controlled for testing purposes.

Although we may use all frequencies between 125 and 8000 Hz in hearing testing, we have specific clinical interest in the pure tones at octave frequencies based upon 125 Hz (125, 250, 500, 1000, 2000, 4000, and 8000 Hz), and certain of the half octaves, namely, 750, 1500, 3000, and 6000 Hz. As is clearly demonstrated in this series, an octave step is simply double its lower value. Half octaves, for clinical purposes, are the arithmetic midpoints of the standard octaves.

Two questions are often asked by the beginning student: (1) why use octaves? and (2) why base the scale upon 125 Hz? The basic answer to both questions is efficiency and convenience. When using individual pure tones for test signals, it is a highly inefficient use of clinical time to test each of the 7876 individual frequencies included in the range from 125 to 8000 Hz. As a result a procedure for sampling this range must be used. Clinical practice has accepted the standard convention of the octave. The use of 125 Hz has developed from the commonly used tuning fork frequencies based upon middle C = 256 Hz. The starting frequency using this system is 128 Hz and the series goes 128, 256, 512, 1024, 2048, 4096, and 8192 Hz. For the convenience of calculation and our memories, the standards now specify 125 Hz, et cetera. Thus, through time, relatively rational decision making has arrived at an efficient and convenient frequency scale for our use in clinical hearing testing.

The speech signals used in hearing testing are rarely measured individually to determine the frequency components; however, our knowledge about the frequency components of speech is of value in specifying the signal and interpreting the test results. An approximation of the frequencies and levels represented in conversational speech is shown by the shaded area in Figure 12.1

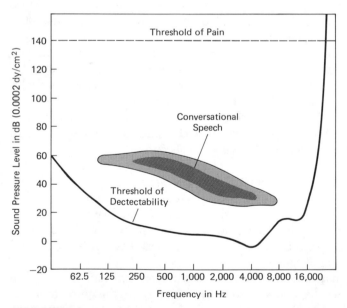

FIGURE 12.1

A graphic representation of the typical thresholds of detectability and pain for pure tones given by young adult normal-hearing listeners. The shaded area represents the typical distribution of energy in conversational speech. Modeled after a similar figure in Davis and Silverman (*16*).

Some pieces of hearing-testing equipment, especially older models, use unique noises, such as sawtooth noise, in which the frequency components have harmonic relationships. The preponderant type of noise source in modern equipment, and therefore that used in audiologic evaluation, is white noise. Analogous to white light, this noise has equal representation of all frequencies and therefore is broad band in its frequency range. Various filtering networks are used to shape the spectrum of this white noise for specific purposes. The two most common variations are (1) narrow band noise and (2) speech noise. The labels are reasonably self-explanatory in that narrow band noise is filtered so that only a small band of frequencies is produced. Each narrow band of noise is identified by its center frequency. The center frequencies are typically those of the pure tones used in hearing testing. Speech noise is shaped through filtering so that its spectrum covers the frequency range and relative amplitude of frequencies generally represented in speech signals.

As you will recall from your study of acoustics, the amplitude of an acoustic signal can be an expression of any of a number of characteristics of the sound wave (e.g., particle displacement, pressure, and power). The amplitude of signals used in clinical hearing testing is based on sound pressure. Depending on the system of units used, sound pressure is expressed in either dynes per square centimeter (dy/cm^2) or newtons per square meter (N/m^2). Currently the pascal (Pa) has been substituted for 1 N/m^2. We will use dy/cm^2, since this is traditional in audiologic literature.

The range of amplitudes of sound used by humans, that is, from the faintest sound detectable to the most intense sound which can be tolerated, is generally accepted as 0.0002 dy/cm^2 to 2000 dy/cm^2. This is an enormous range, the most intense sound being 10 million times as great as the faintest sound. In order to avoid the obligation of manipulating large numbers, it has become conventional to use the decibel notation. The decibel, abbreviated dB, is one-tenth of a bel, a unit named in honor of Alexander Graham Bell. Decibel values are based upon logarithms of ratios; therefore, the scale has no absolute zero in contrast to many of our more common measurements, such as length. Without an absolute zero value, it is imperative that a reference be given for the zero point on the scale whenever we use decibels. This designation is made either by giving the specific value or by indicating which of the several conventional dB scales is used. The conventional scales are well defined and standardized so the reference is known and implied by use of the scale designation.

Since a thorough understanding of the decibel is essential for many of the tests used in measuring hearing, we will discuss two of the dB scales, sound pressure level (SPL) and hearing level (HL), in detail.

The reference level for 0 dB SPL is 0.0002 dy/cm^2, the value generally accepted to represent the faintest sound detectable by humans. All dB

SPL values are derived from the ratio of the sound pressure in dy/cm²
of the signal in question to the reference pressure of 0.0002 dy/cm².
The specific formula for calculating dB SPL is dB SPL = 20 log p_1/p_0.
The formula reads dB SPL equals 20 times the logarithm, to the base 10,
of the ratio of the pressure of the signal in question (p_1), to the reference pressure (p_0). Of course for SPL, p_0 is always 0.0002 dy/cm². Let us
now use this formula to determine the dB SPL of the most intense sound
humans can tolerate, which we said was 2000 dy/cm². Substituting in the
formula, we proceed as follows:

$$\text{dB SPL} = 20 \log_{10} \frac{p_1}{p_0}$$

$$\text{dB SPL} = 20 \log_{10} \frac{2000 \text{ dy/cm}^2}{0.0002 \text{ dy/cm}^2}$$

dB SPL = 20 $\log_{10}$ 10,000,000
dB SPL = 20 × 7*
dB SPL = 140

Another manipulation of this formula which is often helpful in understanding the decibel is to determine the dB SPL of a signal which is
twice the amplitude of another. For experience in this aspect of measurement, let us determine the dB SPL value of a signal which has twice the
sound pressure of the faintest sound detectable. The sound pressure value
of this signal is 0.0004 dy/cm². Using the formula for SPL we find

$$\text{dB SPL} = 20 \log_{10} \frac{p_1}{p_0}$$

$$\text{dB SPL} = 20 \log_{10} \frac{0.0004 \text{ dy/cm}^2}{0.0002 \text{ dy/cm}^2}$$

dB SPL = 20 $\log_{10}$ 2
dB SPL = 20 × 0.3*
dB SPL = 6

This relation holds anywhere on the SPL scale. Thus we can see that
doubling the sound pressure brings about only a 6 dB increase in SPL.
It is important to remember this relation lest we naively begin to think
of decibels in standard arithmetic fashion, and assume, for instance,
that a 60 dB SPL signal is twice as strong as a 30 dB SPL signal when in
reality it is nearly 32 times as great in sound pressure.

The solid line marked "threshold of detectability" in Figure 12.1
demonstrates the SPL required for normal young adults to be able to
detect the presence of individual pure tones. It is clear in this figure that
these values of SPL are dependent upon frequency. We are not equally
sensitive to the presence of signals across the frequency range. If we
wish to use detectability as a measure of hearing for clinical purposes, a

* For additional training in the use of logarithms and the decibel consult reference
7.

method must be available for quick and easy comparison between the hearing sensitivity of the individual and that of some standard for human listeners. One such method is to use the information in Figure 12.1 and base our reference for zero dB upon the best of normal hearing sensitivity. Decibel notation provides an excellent means for easing the comparison. Remember, so long as we provide a reference value for zero dB, we can begin the decibel scale wherever we wish. Since the values on the line in Figure 12.1 represent the best of normal hearing sensitivity and, thus, a good base to which we can compare the hearing of individual patients, we can use these values as our reference for a clinical dB scale. This procedure is, in fact, what has been done to standardize the hearing level (HL) scale used clinically. The SPL values which fall on the line in Figure 12.1 for the pure-tone signals we wish to use clinically become our reference level for zero dB HL. Since the reference value for zero dB HL is based upon human hearing and not upon physical measurement of the signal, and since human listeners are not equally sensitive to the presence of signals of different frequencies, we must know the frequency of the pure tone before we can go to the standard and learn the SPL value and ultimately the sound pressure in dy/cm² of a given HL.

The HL scale described above is standardized by the American National Standards Institute (ANSI) and is used almost exclusively in the United States for reporting the results on the clinical audiogram discussed later in this chapter.

THE AUDITORY SYSTEM

Considering the complexity of the tasks to be accomplished and the precision with which we hear, the human auditory system is a marvel. Figure 12.2 provides a schematic of this system showing the pathways traversed by an auditory signal as we hear it. Sound may be transmitted to the sensory end organ for hearing within the cochlea either by *bone conduction* or by *air conduction*.

When sound is transmitted by *bone conduction*, the pathway is through the bones of the skull. All of us with normal or nearly normal sensory end organs for hearing experience hearing our own voices by bone conduction. The placement of the butt end of a vibrating tuning fork any place on the skull or teeth gives rise to the reception of the tone via bone conduction. The transmission and processing of signals received via bone conduction beyond the level of the cochlea are apparently the same, for practical purposes, as those received by air conduction.

The standard pathway through which we hear sound from the external environment, however, is *air conduction*. The sound arrives at our *external ear* as an airborne signal. Entering through the *external auditory meatus,* the sound traverses the *external auditory canal* at the end of which it impinges upon the *tympanic membrane*. This encounter sets

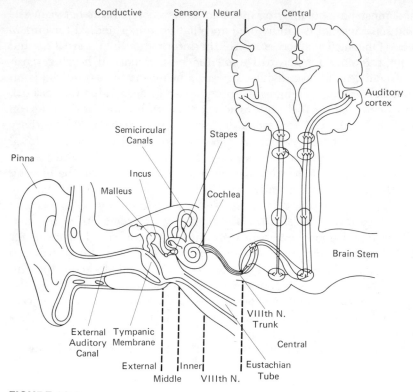

FIGURE 12.2

A schematized drawing of the afferent auditory system. The divisions marked by solid lines represent the functional divisions of the auditory system while those marked with dashed lines represent anatomical divisions of the ear and auditory system.

the tympanic membrane into motion and transmits the signal to the *ossicular chain* and through the *middle ear.*

The ossicular chain, suspended within the middle ear, is composed of the three smallest bones in the body. In sequence, these bones are identified as the *malleus, incus,* and *stapes.* The malleus is imbedded in the tympanic membrane at a point known as the umbo, and the base or footplate of the stapes abuts against the *oval window* of the cochlea. By virtue of function, the external and middle ears comprise the *conductive* portion of the auditory system.

Two muscles, the *tensor tympani* attached to the malleus and the *stapedius* attached to the stapes, are found in the middle ear. These muscles are known to contract reflexively when the auditory system is stimulated by an intense signal. The efficiency of the ossicular chain is lessened by this contraction which may serve to protect the inner ear from damage caused by intense sound. Because of the time involved in activating the reflex, however, it is probably not highly effective in this function.

Extending downward from the middle ear space is the *eustachian tube*. Through its connection with the nasopharynx in the oral cavity, this tube allows the air pressure to be equalized on either side of the tympanic membrane, another condition contributing to the maximum efficiency of the ossicular chain. Although closed when at rest, this tube opens during yawning and swallowing. Most of us have experienced at least short periods of time waiting for the eustachian tube to function following rapid descent in an airplane or elevator. Until the pressure is equalized between the external environment and the middle ear, we may experience a feeling of fullness in the ear, a change in our hearing, or pain in the ear.

The conductive mechanism is an exquisitely designed system for human hearing. It serves as described above to transmit sound, especially the frequencies most important for understanding speech, from the external environment to the sensory receptor mechanism. It does this efficiently by providing a well-designed impedance-matching device between the air of the external auditory canal and the fluid of the inner ear. As you will recall from your study of physics, impedance is the opposition offered to the flow of energy. A fluid typically offers a greater impedance to the flow of sound than does air. If it were not for the impedance-matching qualities of the conductive hearing mechanism, much of the sound energy we use would be reflected from the oval window and lost to us for hearing. For us to receive an adequate magnitude of sound at the sensory receptors, it is essential that we possess a normally functioning conductive mechanism.

At the oval window the signal leaves the middle ear and enters the *inner ear*. Within the inner ear we find two sensory end organs. The vestibular portion within the saccule, utricle, and semicircular canals has the end organ for our sense of balance. The remaining portion of the inner ear is the *cochlea*, which contains the sensory end organ for hearing. The movement of the footplate of the stapes in the oval window transmits the mechanical action of the signal to the fluids of the inner ear. This action is carried through the cochlea via a traveling wave on the *basilar membrane*, upon which the *organ of Corti* rests. The cellular structure of the organ of Corti includes the *hair cells* essential to our reception of the auditory signal by the nervous system. Our knowledge of the precision with which this change from a mechanical acoustic signal to a neural signal is accomplished is described in detail by Glattke (25). The inner ear is described as the *sensory* portion of the auditory system since it is here that the signal is ultimately transduced from a mechanical, acoustic signal into a signal to be carried to the brain by the nervous system.

The signal is transmitted into the central nervous system via the *VIIIth cranial nerve,* known as the stato-acoustic nerve. The larger portion of this nerve trunk carries the signal from the auditory receptors while the smaller branch carries information from the vestibular end organ. This nerve trunk traverses from the modiolus of the cochlea to the cochlear nucleus of the brain stem and is referred to as the *neural* portion of the auditory system.

From the brain stem on to the cortex the auditory signal traverses the *central auditory pathways.* Almost immediately upon entering the brain stem at the level of the pons and medulla, many of these neural pathways carry the auditory signals across to the opposite (contralateral) side of the system. The remaining pathways begin their ascent of the central nervous system on the same (ipsilateral) side as the entering signal. This dominant contralateral representation continues with the ascent of the central nervous system to the level of the cerebral hemispheres. The presence of both a contralateral and ipsilateral ascent, the several levels of synapse, and the crossing of fibers at more than one level provide opportunities for recoding and cross-correlation of auditory signals at various levels of the central nervous system. For the majority of humans the processing of speech signals is finalized in the left cortical hemisphere with several interhemispheric tracts.

Beginning at the cochlea, we find encoding of information for our use in processing auditory signals. Although neural units at cortical levels appear to be diffuse in representation of frequency information (19) at lower levels of the auditory system, neural fibers respond most efficiently at or near a characteristic frequency. Such frequency coding is obviously used in our judgments of pitch. Through a process of increased amplitude of the traveling wave on the basilar membrane the coding of intensity begins in the cochlea. Apparently increased stimulation of individual units and the stimulation of more units with an increase in amplitude begin the coding which we use in judging loudness (25).

Binaural functions (i.e., those involving the reception of signals from both ears), such as localization of auditory signals in space, become a reality as the independent input from either ear begins to be cross-correlated at the level of the superior olivary complex. Multilevel synapses and bilateral representation of the signal within the ascending pathways provide ample opportunity for recoding, correlation, and summation of information to be used for total auditory processing up through the cortical levels.

Our discussion of the auditory system needs to acknowledge the presence of descending auditory pathways through the central system to the cochlea. This descending system, though less well understood than the ascending system, is known to contribute to our auditory processing. Electrophysiologic studies of animals have demonstrated inhibitory effects upon the ascending system with stimulation of the descending system. Glattke suggests, "It may be most appropriate to think of the efferent [descending] system as a *regulatory* system aiding in stimulus sorting rather than as an inhibitory system which shuts out all auditory input" (25, p. 331).

Complex both in structure and function, the auditory system is remarkably orderly in the transmission and processing of auditory signals. The ultimate culmination of its function is, of course, found at the cerebral hemisphere and cortical levels as we process and use oral language.

MEASUREMENT OF HEARING AND THE AUDITORY SYSTEM

Purpose

The basic purpose of the measurement of human hearing and the auditory system is to describe as precisely as necessary and possible what the person hears and how the auditory system is functioning. Measurements and the interpretation of their significance by the audiologist are utilized not only in the diagnosis and treatment of communication disorders but also by the physician for medical diagnosis and treatment. The choice of procedures and the interpretation of the significance of the results may be dependent upon the degree to which either or both types of diagnosis and treatment are to be addressed. For instance, the immediate concern for a child with an infection in the middle ear will be medical management, while the primary objective for the individual who has a permanent hearing impairment for which no medical treatment is known will more likely be the management of the communication disorder. Audiologic and medical management are often concurrent; fortunately, many of our hearing tests serve both functions equally well.

Any test or measurement of hearing or function must meet certain general criteria: (1) the measurement is reliable; (2) any task required of the listener needs only minimal instructions; and (3) the measurement uses clinical time efficiently.

It is imperative that all our measurements be reliable. We need assurance that if the measure is repeated immediately, later in the day, or at another time by the same or a different clinician, essentially the same results can be obtained. (We are assuming that the listener and his hearing have not changed between measurements.) Our concern here is that the technique itself does not introduce measurement error. The effective clinician also learns to make observations of behavior which will permit assessment of consistency on the part of the patient or client. Listening behavior and thus response to hearing tests may change through non-auditory variables such as shifts in decision-making criteria and attention to the task, thus introducing error into the measurements.

Individuals who present themselves for evaluation cannot be assumed to have had any experience with hearing tests nor to possess any particular knowledge about the tests. In order to avoid the necessity for lengthy special training and the risk of frustrating the listener, we need simple, straightforward tasks which can be accomplished with ease by the naive listener after brief instruction.

The use of expensive equipment by highly skilled professionals contributes to the high cost of clinical time. If the public is to be able to afford our services, we must be efficient in our use of this commodity. The most elegant procedure may simply be recorded in history if ultimately it cannot be afforded by those who need the services or by the public in general.

Instrumentation

The vast majority of our measurements of the auditory system involves some measurement of a listener's experience of hearing, calling upon the listener to cooperate by providing a voluntary response. These tests and measurements are performed with the assistance of electronic devices known as *audiometers*. Audiometers allow us to specify the auditory signals to be used and to control their presentation. Numbers designating signal parameters, such as level, frequency, and duration, appear on dials, buttons, and switches which are controlled either directly or indirectly by the operator. The accuracy of these numbers is ultimately dependent upon the calibration of the equipment; that is, the values on the dials must represent accurate measures of the designated signal parameters. It is essential that the operator know the calibration status of the equipment used in order to avoid misinterpretations based solely on inaccurate measurements. Universally accepted standards for the calibration of audiometers are provided by the ANSI and should be followed rigidly. Once an audiometer is calibrated, it is necessary to monitor this calibration routinely with instrumentation and human listeners whose hearing is known.

Audiometers are classified in many ways. Several of the more common designations are discussed below. Pure-tone and speech audiometers are obviously classified according to the signals which can be presented. Portable audiometers are capable of being transported from one testing site to another. The clinical audiometer is most often a console instrument which is situated in one place in a clinic. Automatic audiometers allow the listener or a computer to control the presentation of the signal and record responses. One type of automatic audiometer in common use requires the listener to control the level of pure-tone signal by pushing a button as long as he hears a signal and releasing it when he no longer hears it. A pen attached to the listener-controlled attenuator records this action.

Regardless of the sophistication of the equipment being used or the test of hearing being administered, one must always be concerned about the environment in which the testing takes place. Sounds in the environment must not be allowed to interfere with or distract from the signal and its reception. Since the levels and frequencies of signals used in hearing testing are known through our standards, and we can measure the frequency and level of background noise in the test environment, it is possible to know if environmental sounds will interfere with specific measurements of hearing. In fact, the ANSI also has a standard for acceptable limits of background noise in audiometry (3). In order to control this environmental sound, most clinical evaluations of hearing are done within sound-treated rooms to isolate the test environment from the outside world. Even with these precautions, it is necessary to monitor the environment for sounds such as those created by ventilating and lighting systems or people talking in the immediate area.

Using the various types of audiometers, we can present signals through earphones, bone conduction vibrators, or loud speakers. The use of earphones allows for air conduction presentation to one ear at a time, *monaurally,* or to both ears, *binaurally.* The bone conduction vibrator will set the whole skull into vibration, allowing for equal signal levels at either cochlea regardless of placement of the vibrator. The two most common placements of the bone conduction vibrator are in the center of the forehead or behind either pinna on the mastoid. Earphones and vibrators are held in place by use of headbands which should be standardized for amount of pressure applied. Loud speakers are used to present signals within a sound-treated test room. Such presentation is referred to as *sound field* and allows the listener to hear binaurally. The term free field is often inappropriately used and should be avoided.

Audiometry

The techniques and procedures used to measure hearing fall under the general heading of *audiometry.* Audiometry is subclassified further by designating the type of signal used (for example, pure-tone, brief-tone, and speech audiometry), the method of obtaining a response (for instance, behavioral, manual, automatic, and EEG audiometry), or the purpose for which it is applied, such as diagnostic audiometry. The use of the term audiometry implies a measurement of the act of hearing requiring some response from the listener and should not be used to designate measurements of the auditory system, such as acoustic impedance.

Threshold Measures   Behavioral threshold measures have been at the core of audiometry throughout its development and use. A behavioral sensory threshold is generally accepted as the value of signal which, if exceeded, will elicit a response. In the case of *absolute thresholds* for hearing, the lowest level of signal which elicits a response is sought, while with *differential thresholds* it is the smallest change in the signal which elicits a response. Since, in addition to the listener's hearing ability, a host of variables (for example, method of signal presentation, instructions, listener criteria, and signal parameters other than the one in question) are known to affect the threshold value, we must not be naive in our assumptions of specificity or our interpretation of the term "absolute." As Stevens so aptly stated, "What gets recorded as threshold is then an arbitrary point within a range of variability" (54, p. 33). Remember that as an administrator of threshold tests, the clinician makes a statistical decision based upon a sample of instructed behaviors from the listener.

Pure-Tone Thresholds   The threshold of audibility for pure tones is by far the most commonly obtained measure of hearing. It is a measure of hearing sensitivity for which the listener is simply instructed to listen by either air conduction or bone conduction and indicate each time a tone is heard. In the standard procedure, the listener is asked only to detect the presence of the auditory signal, not to describe it, define it, or make any particular use of it.

Using techniques which combine our knowledge of psychophysical methods and our need to use clinical time efficiently, the clinician typically presents short bursts of tone to one ear at irregular intervals in five dB steps and requests the listener to indicate each time a signal is detected. The examiner controls the signal presentation and either approaches the eventual threshold level by increasing the level in five dB steps from one which is inaudible to one which is audible (an *ascending* series of trials) or the reverse in which the level of signal changes from audibility to inaudibility (a *descending* series of trials). A *bracketing* procedure is sometimes used in which threshold is approached and crossed by both ascending and descending series. Regardless of the approach, threshold must be crossed a sufficient number of times to arrive at a statistical determination of the level at which threshold will be identified. It is common practice to choose the lowest level at which the listener correctly detects the presence of the signal on at least 50 percent of the trials. The number of trials may vary but most often is from four to six.

A number of procedures for obtaining pure-tone thresholds are extant, each with its own cadre of supporters armed with good reasons for its use. The procedure we advocate is based upon the technique originally described by Hughson and Westlake in 1944 (31). It is the technique of choice for three reasons: (1) it meets the general criteria for hearing tests described above, (2) it has been investigated and shown to be as valid as any other regularly used method (11), and (3) it is a commonly accepted clinical practice in the United States (43). With the Hughson-Westlake method, pure-tone thresholds are obtained by presenting the signal in an ascending series of five dB steps and asking the listener either to raise a hand or push a button each time a sound is heard. When using the hand-raising response, the clinician may also request that the listener raise the right hand for sounds heard in the right ear and the left hand for signals heard in the left ear. This modification has the obvious label of the ear choice technique. In describing the Hughson-Westlake technique, Carhart and Jerger (*11*) present a convincing argument for its adoption.

The standard test frequencies for pure-tone thresholds by air conduction are 125–8000 Hz in interval steps of one octave with half-octave frequencies of 750, 1500, 3000, and 6000 Hz being available. Because of limitations of the bone conduction vibrator, the frequency range for these thresholds is restricted to the octave and half-octave frequencies between 250 and 4000 Hz. The range of HL is also restricted for bone conduction. The maximum bone conduction level typically will be 65–70 dB HL as opposed to 110 dB HL for air conduction. The frequency 250 Hz is often not used for bone conduction thresholds because of the difficulty in determining whether the response is from tactile or auditory stimulation.

Pure-Tone Audiogram   Pure-tone thresholds may be reported in tabled form as shown in Figure 12.3 or, more commonly, in the tradi-

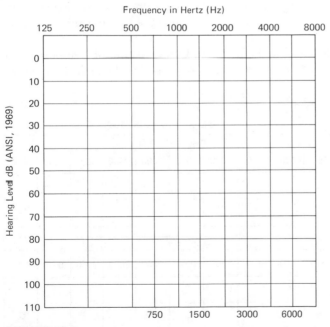

FIGURE 12.3
The form used for clinical pure-tone audiograms following the recommendations of the American Speech and Hearing Association Committee on Audiometric Evaluation (*4*).

tional pure-tone audiogram (Figure 12.4). The reference level for 0 dB in clinical audiometry is now usually that of the International Standards Organization (32) or, in the United States, of the American National Standards Institute (2). The ANSI standard was approved in 1969 but not published until 1970; thus, the standard is referenced ANSI, 1969, while the publication is referenced ANSI, 1970. These standards are derived from measures of the thresholds of audibility for young adults with no history of ear disease or exposure to damagingly high levels of sound. As pointed out earlier, these standard values represent the best of normal hearing sensitivity. Values referenced as such are expressed in dB HL.

It is now universally accepted that the level of the signal is recorded on the vertical axis of the clinical pure-tone audiogram and the frequency of the pure tones on the horizontal axis. Tradition has placed the 0 dB HL line near the top of the graph with an increase in magnitude as we progress toward the bottom of the graph. This particular quirk has caused problems with terminology since the terms lower and higher have one meaning when referring to the placement of threshold values on the graph and another when referring to the level of the signal (that is, a symbol which is lower on the graph in reality represents a signal which is higher in magnitude). Therefore, it is advisable, when referring to clinical threshold measures, to reserve the terms lower and higher for reference to signal magnitude, as is done in psychoacoustics, or to avoid the use of the terms unless accompanied with a referent. One technique often used is to discuss thresholds as poorer or better.

The clinical pure-tone audiogram and the system of symbols used with it have developed by tradition, and there has been little success-

Pure-Tone Thresholds—Hearing Level in dB (ANSI, 1969)

Ear	Right Ear										
Frequency in Hertz	125	250	500	750	1000	1500	2000	3000	4000	6000	8000
Air Conduction											
Bone Conduction											

Ear	Left Ear										
Frequency in Hertz	125	250	500	750	1000	1500	2000	3000	4000	6000	8000
Air Conduction											
Bone Conduction											

FIGURE 12.4
A typical form used to report clinical pure-tone thresholds in a table. Threshold values are written in the appropriate spaces.

ful attempt until recently to standardize the form or the symbols. We are recommending that the guidelines adopted by the American Speech and Hearing Association (4) be followed. The symbols used in these guidelines are shown in Figure 12.5. According to these standards, the graph is to be proportioned so that the distance for one octave on the horizontal axis is equal to the distance for 20 dB on the vertical axis. The horizontal axis should be labeled *Frequency in Hertz (Hz)* while the vertical axis is labeled *Hearing Level in Decibels (dB)*. In order to insure against misinterpretation, it is helpful to add the specific standard (for instance, ANSI, 1969) to the HL label. Obviously, not everyone reporting pure-tone thresholds will be following these guidelines. Even though variation in symbols will continue to exist, there are some traditional practices upon which you can rely: (1) all symbols in red refer to responses obtained while presenting signals to the right ear and all in blue are for the left ear, (2) the specific symbols for air conduction thresholds are in almost universal use while the symbols for bone conduction thresholds may vary

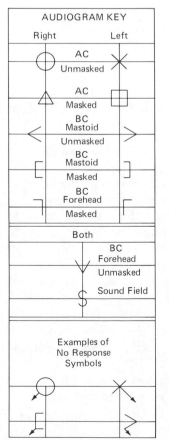

FIGURE 12.5

The symbols to be used when reporting thresholds on the clinical pure-tone audiogram following the recommendations of the American Speech and Hearing Association Committee on Audiometric Evaluation (4). AC and BC represent air conduction and bone conduction respectively.

from user to user (43), (3) a symbol legend should accompany the audiogram for reference, and (4) so long as the proportions are equal, the size of the graph will not alter the relations among symbol placements and configuration of the graphs.

In order to obtain an estimate of the level at which the listener will hear speech, we calculate a measure identified as the *pure tone average* (PTA). This measure is determined by averaging the thresholds for pure tones at 500, 1000, and 2000 Hz. Given the consistency in the development of our standards, this average will come within 10 dB of predicting the lowest level at which speech is intelligible unless there is a large difference in HL among these frequencies. In the latter situation, the average of the two better thresholds among the three should be used as the predictor.

In hopes of providing a direct prediction of receptive communication ability, several attempts have been made over the years to obtain a measure of percentage of hearing loss from the pure-tone audiogram. No one method has as yet been successful in correlating well with the degree of impairment since the exclusive use of pure-tone thresholds in the calculation of percentage of hearing loss ignores the essential ingredients of clarity of speech, oral communication needs, and individual differences among people who happen to have hearing disorders. Nevertheless, standard formulas are in use to determine percentage of hearing loss for compensation in medicolegal procedures. The two most popular currently are those of the American Academy of Ophthalmology and Otolaryngology (1) and the National Institute of Occupational Safety and Health.

Additional Threshold Measures   Thresholds of hearing sensitivity can be obtained by presenting speech, music, narrow bands of noise, noise makers, or environmental sounds through earphones or in the sound field. On occasion, these signals may be presented by bone conduction. Since there are essentially no standards for the use of such signals, the local clinic needs to do an "in-house" calibration of sorts with listeners who have known hearing losses and listeners with normal hearing sensitivity. One specific measure often used to corroborate the best pure-tone threshold or as a gross estimate of the best hearing sensitivity across the frequency range covered by speech is a threshold of audibility for speech materials, called a Speech Detection Threshold (SDT) or a Speech Awareness Threshold (SAT). The complex nature of speech sounds makes it difficult to know what portion of the frequency spectrum of each speech signal is being detected.

Of the signals other than pure tones used for measures of the threshold of audibility, narrow bands of noise, if properly calibrated, will most closely approximate the precision with which thresholds across the frequency range can be obtained with pure tones. The major difficulty with signals other than pure tones is that they are complex in their frequency spectra, and the listener may respond to only a small portion of the spectrum presented. The thresholds obtained for these complex signals may reflect only the best threshold for a single frequency within the spectrum. Since for threshold of audibility measures we ask the listener only to tell us when a signal is present, we do not know if only a portion or all of the signal is audible when the person responds. It is probably in this area of using signals with complex frequency spectra for threshold testing that most errors in clinical judgment due to reliance upon numbers are made.

The information obtained from the pure-tone audiogram is best viewed only as being applicable to the range of frequencies and levels over which the listener can detect the presence of auditory signals when presented by air conduction or bone conduction. Comparison of air and bone conduction thresholds and observations of the configuration of thresholds across the frequency range are used in interpreting the test results. Any further generalizations, such as prediction of speech discrimination ability, without additional information or test results are fraught with danger, especially if made by the naive observer.

Speech Audiometry   The speech reception threshold (SRT) and speech discrimination scores are the two most common measures of speech audiometry administered in hearing evaluations. They are typically presented by air conduction monaurally or by sound field. Although obtained routinely by some clinicians, the bone conduction SRT has not received widespread acceptance.

Test materials used in speech audiometry can be presented through monitored live voice or by either disc or tape recordings. In the monitored live-voice presentation, the clinician speaks into a microphone and controls the level at which the listener hears the message. The monitoring of presentation level is accomplished through the use of a VU meter which, if calibrated and monitored precisely, will allow the clinician to infer the accuracy of the level of each presentation. Those individual monitored live-voice presentations which do not meet the clinician's predetermined calibration criterion are ignored in determining this threshold. One advantage of using recorded materials for speech audiometry is that the calibration efforts can be invested in the original recording. Through the use of a calibration tone on the recording, a properly recorded set of materials can be used by the clinician without having to be concerned with each individual presentation. Recorded materials provide the additional advantage of standardizing the dialect, articulation patterns, and fundamental frequency of the speaker delivering the speech materials, all of which are known to affect the intelligibility of oral messages.

Speech reception threshold, unlike the pure-tone threshold and SDT, not only requires that the presence of the signal be detected but also that the listener be able to identify the word. For this reason, the SRT is defined as the threshold of intelligibility (18). In other words, the SRT is the lowest level, in dB, at which the listener can hear and understand speech signals. Although many types of speech signals can be used to obtain the SRT, it is now common practice to use two-syllable words spoken with equal stress on both syllables. These words are spondaic in stress pattern and are therefore called spondees. The Committee on Audiometric Evaluation of the American Speech and Hearing Association is currently developing guidelines for the procedures and words to be used in such measures; it is choosing to designate the measure as the Spondaic Threshold (ST). Such a guideline will be a welcome addition since there has been little standardization of procedures for this measure. For specific SRT procedures, the reader is urged to await the publication of the ASHA guidelines or to study Hopkinson (29).

If the SRT is the only measure of hearing obtained, it must be used with caution. As in the case of thresholds of audibility for complex signals such as the SDT, the listener can often identify spondees by hearing only a small portion of the frequency spectrum. By virtue of this, the listener may have hearing sensitivity at or near a specific frequency which will allow the correct identification of 50 percent of the words on the basis of a minimum amount of spectral information.

The two major contributions of the SRT to our understanding of a person's hearing are (1) to corroborate the pure-tone average and (2) to give us a base from which we can determine the appropriate levels above threshold—(*sensation level* (SL))—to present other signals used in speech audiometry. The astute clinician, as pointed out by Hopkinson (29), can also gain qualitative information about the listener's ability to handle speech materials.

The speech materials for the SRT are presented either by monitored live voice or by recorded materials. The most common procedure appears to be monitored live voice (43). As pointed out by Hopkinson (29), it is generally agreed that with proper monitoring of presentation level, the SRT obtained with monitored live voice will show results similar to those from recorded materials. The flexibility of monitored live-voice presentations is persuasive in most clinicians' choice of presentation for SRT.

Speech discrimination testing is accomplished in order to approach an evaluation of the listener's ability to understand speech once it is heard at a comfortable level. A number of messages ranging from nonsense syllables to continuous discourse have been used in the measurement of speech discrimination. Regardless of the materials used for this testing, it is common practice, except for special purposes, to present the speech at a suprathreshold level, a procedure which will eliminate level of presentation as a determinant of the score, typically near a most comfortable listening level (MCL). In most standard evaluations of hearing, lists of one-syllable words are used to make a determination of discrimination ability. The earliest standardized lists were phonetically balanced (PB) lists of 50 monosyllabic words developed at the Harvard University Psychoacoustics Laboratory (PAL) for use in evaluating communication equipment (18). The basic premise of the PAL PB 50 lists, that is, phonetic balance, has persisted in many of our attempts to measure speech discrimination ability clinically. According to Martin and Pennington's report (43) the Central Institute for the Deaf (CID) W-22 monosyllabic word lists are those most commonly in use today. These lists were derived from the original PAL PB 50's with an attempt to reduce the vocabulary to a level more likely to be common for the wide range of speakers of American English who may present themselves for clinical evaluation. Similar lists of monosyllables based upon the consonant nucleus consonant (CNC) lists of Lehiste and Peterson (40) have been developed at Northwestern University and are available as NU Auditory Test #6 (57). These discrimination tests are all typically administered by presenting the words in a carrier phrase such as "you will say . . ." and having the listener respond by repeating the word. Such a response presents an obvious problem when the listener has an articulation problem, speaks with a different American dialect, or speaks with a foreign dialect, since errors in production are used to infer errors in reception.

In an attempt to provide for a more orderly analysis of errors and a response fraught with fewer problems, the Modified Rhyme Test (MRT) (30) has been developed from the original Rhyme Test of Fairbanks (20). In this test, the listener is to choose the correct response from a set of six foils, each of which varies from the others by only the initial or final consonant.

An additional approach to testing speech discrimination used in some clinics is a list of synthetic sentences similar to those developed by Jerger, Speaks, and Trammel (36) as shown in Table 12.1. These sentences read much like standard English but are not meaningful. For each utterance, the listener chooses a response from a closed set of ten synthetic sentences.

TABLE 12.1
Five Synthetic Sentences Representative of Those Developed by Jerger

1. Small boat with a picture has become
2. Built the government with the force almost
3. Go change your car color is red
4. Forward march said the boy had a
5. March around without a care in your

Source: From Jerger et al., *36*.

Each of these discrimination tests and a host of others not covered in this discussion have attempted in their individual ways to resolve the problems of separating intelligibility of speech from other language skills such as vocabulary, comprehension, and memory. Perhaps the ideal choice of material would be nonsense syllables which carry no meaning in the language; however, no one has satisfactorily solved the problem of an appropriate response to such materials since our spelling is not phonetic and few clinical patients know and can use a standard phonetic alphabet. No single speech discrimination test has gained universal acceptance for the many purposes for which we wish to use them. In view of this state of affairs, clinicians must know the discrimination test used and the inferences which can be drawn from the scores obtained if they are to make appropriate interpretations.

Regardless of the speech discrimination test used, it is important that in standard evaluations the materials be recorded rather than presented by monitored live voice. It is known that the fundamental frequency of the speaker's voice, rate of speech, articulation patterns, and dialectical attributes can all affect the discrimination score obtained. The presentation as well as the material need to be standardized if speech discrimination scores are to be compared across clinicians administering the tests.

SPECIAL AUDIOMETRIC TESTS

Hearing tests designed to meet special purposes above and beyond those used in the basic evaluation fall into two major groups: (1) those providing additional information for inference about the site of the lesion within the auditory system, and (2) those aimed at learning more about the client who is difficult to test, that is, the person who either cannot or will not cooperate voluntarily in routine behavioral tests.

Site of Lesion Tests

Routine audiometric tests used in the basic evaluation of hearing provide helpful information in our understanding of how a person hears. More specific information, however, is needed if the audiologist is to have a thorough understanding of the functioning of the system and if the physician is to be more precise in the medical diagnosis and treatment. For these purposes, special tests have been developed which provide measures of loudness, effects of time, and the interaction of coincident or competing signals.

Loudness was one of the earliest specific aspects of suprathreshold hearing to be measured clinically. Pohlman and Kranz noted in 1924 that with some individuals who demonstrate a loss of hearing sensitivity for a frequency in one ear and a nearly normal threshold in the other ear ". . . it takes comparatively little additional energy to cause the deficiency [meaning the difference in HL of signals] to seemingly disappear quite completely" (51, p. 337). In other words, even though threshold signals differed in HL between the two ears, suprathreshold HL's were nearly equal for judgments of equal loudness.

In a discussion of the loss of hearing sensitivity for high frequency tones, Fowler in 1928 noted an apparent discrepancy in loudness judgments for tones when a listener made suprathreshold comparisons between his normal ear and the ear with the loss of hearing sensitivity. He commented that "the loudness of tones (near 4,096) of from 10 to 25 sensation units above threshold in the left (non-affected) ear appeared the same loudness as five sensation units above the threshold of the right (affected) ear" (21, p. 155).

Both of these reports are early observations of what has become known as *recruitment of loudness*, defined as an abnormal growth of loudness as the level of a tone is increased above threshold. Graphic demonstration of the phenomenon is shown in Figure 12.6, the results of the Alternate Binaural Loudness Balance Test (ABLB) described by Fowler in 1937 (22). In this test, a tone of a given frequency is presented alternatively to the better and poorer ears; the listener judges the comparative loudness of the tones. Signal levels are adjusted in the test ear until that tone and the tone in the other ear at a predetermined level are judged to be equal in loudness. These judgments are made for each test frequency at several levels in the control ear. As can be seen in Figure 12.6, if equal steps in SL bring about equal judgments of growth in loudness, then the functions are linear (solid line). Recruitment is demonstrated by nonlinear functions, an example of which is shown by the dashed line.

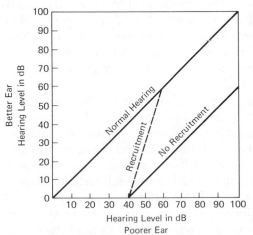

Hearing Level in dB
Poorer Ear

FIGURE 12.6
A graphic display of three functions representing the results of the loudness balancing done in the Alternate Binaural Loudness Balance Test of Fowler (21). The solid lines represent linear functions obtained when recruitment of loudness is not present; the dashed line represents a function which might be obtained from a person demonstrating recruitment of loudness.

Fowler's ABLB has proven over the years to be an excellent test. Unfortunately, only a limited number of patients present themselves with a sufficient difference in thresholds for a given pure tone between the two ears (generally accepted as 20 dB) to allow administration of the test. In an attempt to make the test applicable to more patients, Reger (52) described a Monaural Bi-frequency Loudness Balance Test. In this procedure the listener is asked to compare the loudness of two different frequencies in the same ear. The threshold for one tone is better than the other by an amount sufficient to demonstrate recruitment of loudness. Although this technique extends the number of patients for whom recruitment of loudness can be measured, the task may be confusing to the listener who must make loudness judgments of signals with pitch differences. In addition, equal loudness contours across frequencies change with level for normal-hearing listeners. These data must be taken into consideration when interpreting the results.

Under the assumptions that loudness balance tasks, especially those done monaurally, are too difficult for patients and that too many patients present hearing loss patterns inappropriate for the use of the loudness balance techniques, clinicians and researchers have developed procedures described as indirect measures of recruitment. The most popular area of endeavor has been the use of the difference limen (DL) for intensity. Hirsh, Palva, and Goodman (28) provided an excellent summary of the classical studies using DL for intensity. They reported that measures of DL for intensity did not correlate well with loudness balance measures of recruitment.

Following the early studies with the clinical use of DL for intensity, Jerger, Shedd, and Harford (35) developed the Short Increment Sensitivity Index (SISI), a variation on the same theme. The SISI test, when interpreted within the confines of its well-known limitations, has proven useful as supportive information about loudness measures. In the SISI test, the listener is asked to identify short duration (100 msec) increments of intensity (1 dB superimposed upon a constant pure-tone signal which is at 20 dB SL). Typically, a percent-correct identification score is given on the presentation of 20 increments. For reasons not totally agreed upon, the normal-hearing listener identifies only a small number of these increments.

Adaptation, the phenomenon of reduced loudness with continuous presentation of the signal, has been given considerable study by psychoacousticians and is now used regularly in audiologic evaluations. Adaptation measures have been especially helpful in the inference of the site of a lesion within the auditory system. A number of specific techniques are used clinically, the most popular of which measure threshold adaptation. There are two common approaches to this measure. (1) In the Carhart procedure, it is determined how much shift in the level of the signal must be brought about in order for the listener to hear the signal continuously for 60 seconds (*10*). (2) The technique of Rosenberg (*53*) measures the amount of shift in level of signal which can be heard at the end of 60 seconds continuous presentation. Modifications of these procedures have been described by Owens (*50*). These types of measures have been referred to as *Tone Decay Tests.*

Brief-tone audiometry uses signals of very short duration. The normal-hearing listener's threshold will improve as the duration of the signal is extended up to approximately 200 msec. Beyond this duration, the threshold appears to remain constant for recognizing the presence of tone bursts (*24*). Listeners with certain types of hearing disorders will demonstrate an inability to make full use of the added information provided by signals of longer duration. They tend to show much less or no improvement in threshold with signals of longer duration. The use of this phenomenon in clinical testing is referred to as *brief-tone audiometry.* It is accomplished by obtaining thresholds of sensitivity for pure-tone signals at several brief durations representative of the range through which normal-hearing listeners demonstrate the phenomenon.

Békésy audiometry uses a device constructed to record listener-controlled changes in signal level. Among his many contributions, Georg von Békésy, the Nobel Prize–winning scientist, first described his audiometer in 1947 (*6*). Although the Békésy audiometer can be used for the presentation of any auditory signal, it is most commonly used clinically for the measurement of pure-tone thresholds. The listener is instructed to press the switch when the tone is heard and release it when the tone is no longer heard. This hand-held switch causes the signal level to decrease when engaged and increase when disengaged. A pen attached to the attenuator mechanism records the excursions in levels which are assumed to envelope the threshold. Pure-tone thresholds can be measured from 100 to 10,000 Hz, at fixed discrete frequencies, preset frequency intervals, or as the full frequency range is swept. A Békésy audiogram showing the tracing of a normal-hearing listener's excursions about threshold as the frequency range is swept is shown in Figure 12.7.

Electrophysiological Measures of Hearing

Several electrophysiologic activities in the human are known to demonstrate measurable change correlated with the presentation of auditory signals. Among these are (1) brain wave activity as shown on the electroencephalogram (EEG), (2) resistance to the transmission of small electrical currents through the body demonstrated through electrodermal responses (EDR), (3) electrical activity within the cochlea and VIIIth cranial nerve measured through electrocochleography (ECoG), (4) basic processes such as respiration, blood flow, and heart beat. EEG, EDR, and ECoG are currently all in use clinically for patients who cannot or will not respond adequately in standard audiometric procedures. All of these techniques

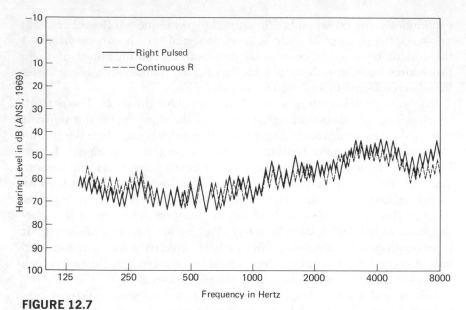

FIGURE 12.7

A representative tracing of pure-tone thresholds across frequencies by Békésy audiometry. The solid line represents threshold for a tone which is pulsed and the dashed line represents theshold for a tone which is on continuously.

require specialized training and are typically administered only in selected centers where the expertise and special equipment are available. The information gained from these tests is often helpful in understanding the hearing status of a listener but should not be expected to be definitive in all cases. They typically provide estimates of thresholds at some point within the nervous system but, of course, do not represent measures of how the signal is processed.

Tests for Nonorganic Hearing Loss

The clinician who relies on voluntary behavioral responses as indices of measurement must always be alert to the possibility that such responses are not accurate in reflecting what the person actually hears. Whether these inaccuracies are willful on the part of the patient or not is of little consequence if the test results are inaccurate. The astute clinician never relies solely on test results nor ignores test behavior which may provide insight into this accuracy. Although a listener may wish to have the examiner believe his hearing is better than it is, the most common practice is for the listener to present his hearing as poorer than it is. *Nonorganic hearing loss* is represented by that portion of the test results which suggest exaggeration of the degree of hearing loss.

A number of audiometric procedures are available for use when there is suspicion or suggestion that the patient's responses are inappropriate, even though consistent, in reflecting his or her hearing ability. Some of these techniques are simple modifications of standard procedures developed with experience by the clinician. There are also specific tests devised to mislead or trick, if you prefer, the patient into more accurate responses. Still other test procedures have been developed to avoid the need for voluntary responses.

The clinician, although suspecting inaccurate responses, must continue to appraise rather than be lured into hasty decisions about the patient's honesty or ability to cooperate in standard test procedures. The clinician must remain the objective observer of behavior and recorder of test responses and avoid a combative interaction with the patient.

Modifications of standard procedures are many. We will discuss a few of the more common useful techniques. The first action taken by the clinician should be to ascertain that the instructions are understood. Instructions may need to be restated, expanded, or demonstrated for clarity. It is always helpful to have the patient describe or demonstrate what he thinks he is to do in the particular tests. For threshold tests, it is often necessary to reassure the listener that he will hear sounds which are quiet and barely audible. We have all had the experience of overhearing a patient mutter "I can't hear that," or observing a child shake her head no while listening to a quiet tone near threshold.

Once you are sure the instructions are understood, it is often helpful to refrain from presenting any signal not to be used in the actual test. The confused listener may become more so, or the listener wishing to mislead the examiner may use the levels of the extra signals as cues for succeeding judgments.

Formal tests for nonorganic hearing loss usually are aimed at circumventing the mechanism the listener is using to establish criteria for response. In some situations, such as with the Doerfler-Stewart test, noise is introduced as a competitor to the speech signal in the hope that the listener's judgment of loudness will be distorted and cause him or her to respond to lower level speech signals.

The confusion technique in the Swinging Story Test, as described in audiology texts, is to shift information rapidly from one ear to the other with portions of the story presented below professed threshold. The listener is then requested to repeat the story and the examiner records information which should not have been heard.

In another technique, the signal parameters of Békésy audiometry are altered. Listeners with nonorganic hearing loss will often show inconsistencies in responses as parameters are adjusted.

The electrophysiologic techniques described above are also of value in assessing the hearing of individuals who are inconsistent in response or who appear to be exhibiting a nonorganic hearing loss.

Measures of Central Auditory Function

Just as the function increases in complexity as the auditory system progresses from peripheral to central portions, so must the measures used to assess these functions. The tests reviewed so far in this discussion are often of little value in measuring this function since they evaluate primarily peripheral hearing abilities. Tests designed to assess central auditory function typically place stress upon binaural listening, whether their primary purpose be aimed at identifying the site of the lesion or at describing communication ability. The presentation of signals is most often dichotic (separate signals or portions of a signal to either ear) and may involve competing messages. The listener's task is (1) to report all information received or (2) to report the specified signal despite competition for attention of another acoustic signal. Lynn and Gilroy (42) have described a battery of tests aimed at assisting in the determination of the site of a lesion. Willeford (62) has presented similar material in relation to evaluating the auditory processing abilities of children, especially those with learning disabilities.

Most test procedures used for these purposes lack standardization and are often developed for local use. One exception is the Staggered Spondaic Word (SSW) test of Katz (37). The presentation technique for the SSW is shown in Table 12.2. The response by a normal-hearing listener is to repeat both spondaic words despite the overlapping of the last syllable of one spondee and the first syllable of the second spondee. The listener is presented with a noncompeting and a competing message for each presentation to either ear. Through an intricate scoring system, Katz has developed guides to interpretation of the results.

Development of tests for central auditory function is relatively recent, and much research is needed in the area to provide more precision in their use.

ACOUSTIC IMPEDANCE

In recent years, techniques for measuring acoustic impedance have come into general clinical use and are often a part of the standard battery of

TABLE 12.2
A Schematic of the Order of Presentation of Syllables in One Item of the Staggered Spondaic Word Test of Katz

	Noncompeting 1	Competing 2	Noncompeting 3
Right ear	up	stairs	
Left ear		down	town

Source: From Katz, 37.

measurements administered in a hearing evaluation. As described by Lilly, acoustic impedance is simply the ". . . 'opposition' encountered by an acoustic wave" (41, p. 346). The auditory system presents such impedance to acoustic signals. Clinically, we use measures of acoustic impedance at the surface of the tympanic membrane when a tone is sounded in the external auditory canal. The apparatus used for these measures is schematized in Figure 12.8.

Three basic measures of impedance are obtained for clinical use: (1) static acoustic impedance, (2) tympanometry, and (3) acoustic reflex. None of these measures requires a voluntary behavioral response from the patient and, therefore, requires only his or her passive cooperation. Because of the developmental stage in which we find the instrumentation and techniques for reporting measures of acoustic impedance, the terminology and procedures are still in need of standardization. Fortunately, such standardization is in the process of being accomplished by a committee of the ANSI.

Measures of static acoustic impedance provide information about the system at rest with atmospheric pressure in the external auditory canal. Using absolute physical measures of acoustic impedance, one can compare the stiffness or looseness of the individual system to the same measures observed across subject groups. With some equipment, these measures are inferred from a measure of equivalent volume of air.

Tympanometry is the technique used to observe dynamic changes in acoustic impedance at the tympanic membrane concomitant with changes

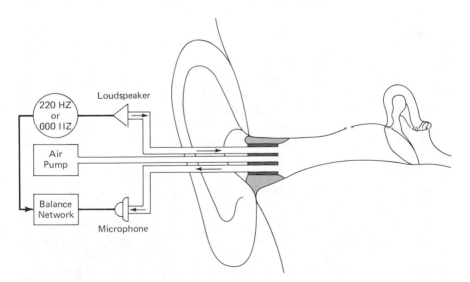

FIGURE 12.8
A schematized representation of the device used in masking clinical acoustic impedance measurements.

in air pressure within the external auditory canal. These dynamic changes are reflected in patterns shown on *tympanograms*. Maximum compliance or "flexibility" for the normal system occurs when the air pressure in the external auditory canal is at atmospheric pressure, providing a normal tympanogram. Increased or decreased air pressure within the middle ear as well as changes in middle ear structure and functioning will be reflected by characteristic patterns on the tympanogram.

Additional dynamic changes in acoustic impedance can be observed when the middle ear muscles contract as the result of reflex action or when the Eustachian tube opens. Either of the above occurrences will change the impedance offered to sound at the tympanic membrane. In the normal system the acoustic reflex is most easily elicited by sounding a high-level signal in either ear, causing a bilateral reflex. The most common signals used to elicit the acoustic reflex are pure tones, narrow bands of noise, or a broadband signal, such as white noise. Interpretations can be made in reference to the presence or absence of the reflex and at what level each of these signals elicits a reflex. Considerable use is currently being made of the reflex to predict pure-tone thresholds as originally described by Niemeyer & Sesterhenn (47) and developed further by Jerger et al. (34).

AUDITORY MASKING

When testing hearing monaurally, as is done in many of the tests discussed above, the clinician must be assured that the response is elicited via stimulation of the test ear or the results attributed to that ear may be in error. This assurance is in question whenever it is possible that the contralateral (nontest) ear is responding in addition to, or rather than, the test ear. Any signal with sufficient strength to set the skull into vibration will be present at both cochleas. If this level is sufficient to stimulate the contralateral ear in monaural testing, *crossover* has occurred and steps need to be taken to isolate the test ear.

The resistance or interference to the transmission of the signal across the head is known as *interaural* (between the ears) *attenuation* (IA). The assumed IA for bone-conducted signals is 0 dB since the signal may be at equal levels at either ear regardless of the site at which the skull is set into vibration. Fortunately, we can be assured of at least 40 dB of IA for signals presented by air conduction in clinical testing.

In audiometry, we introduce masking noise into the nontest ear in order to isolate the test ear for response. *Masking* is simply the presence of one sound causing another sound to become less audible (27). The masking noises used in clinical audiometry are typically chosen from those discussed earlier, that is, broadband, narrowband, or speech noise. We choose the noise which will accomplish our goal most efficiently. The frequencies most effective in masking a pure tone, for instance, lie within a narrow band around the frequency of that tone. Therefore, the most appropriate masking noise is dependent upon the frequencies in the test signal. By limiting the frequencies represented in the noise, we control the amount of noise heard by the listener and avoid what might be unnecessary distraction or, in some cases, discomfort for the listener.

The efficient and appropriate use of masking in audiometry requires a thorough understanding of the signals, the noises, the auditory system, and the interactions among these factors. In addition to knowing when to use masking and which masking noise to select, the clinician must also determine the minimum and maximum levels of masking to be used.

In order to determine if crossover may occur and thus whether masking is needed, the clinician must take into account (1) the level of the signal presented to the test ear, (2) the assumed amount of IA, and (3) the bone conduction threshold of the nontest ear. The choice of masker is related to the frequency spectrum of the signal. Minimum level of masking is determined by the assumed level of signal in the nontest ear and is necessary to insure that the purpose of masking is met. Maximum masking level is crucial since the masking noise can also cross over to the test ear and thus provide a new contamination of test results. Maximum masking level is determined by the level of noise in the nontest ear, the IA, and the assumed bone conduction threshold for the test ear.

Appropriate masking and its use are essential to accurate audiometry. Whenever there is a discrepancy in measures between the two ears, the possibility of cross hearing and the possible need for contralateral masking need to be considered.

TESTING THE HEARING OF CHILDREN

The standard battery of hearing tests—pure-tone thresholds by air conduction and bone conduction, SRT, and speech discrimination—can often be given to a child as young as 5 years of age. With a few modifications, even the average 4-year-old may be able to cooperate in the procedures. One need not assume, however, that the hearing of infants and preschoolers cannot be tested. On the contrary, modification in technique, careful observation, and appropriate questions of those who know the child will often provide information sufficient to make appropriate diagnostic decisions. The testing of very young children may require several testing sessions and may tax the ingenuity of the clinician. Nevertheless, the competent audiologist will compile information leading to judgments of hearing ability.

The clinician who wishes to evaluate the hearing of children should possess a thorough knowledge of the development of auditory behavior in children. This allows the clinician not only to select appropriate tasks but also to draw inferences from the individual child's behavior.

Early in a child's life, prior to 4 months of age, we use procedures which take advantage of reflex, startle, and alerting behavior in response to moderate to high levels of sound. As the child matures beyond this early developmental stage, we expect to observe search and localization behavior at slightly lower levels. Certainly by the age of 1 year we begin to expect direct localization of sound in general and even near threshold for speech signals. As the child's auditory behavior matures, we expect to get more precise responses to relatively quieter sounds until the age of 2 years when conditioning techniques can be used to elicit excellent estimates of thresholds. Through the application of principles and procedures of classical and operant conditioning, reliable results can often be obtained from an otherwise difficult-to-test child. Materials for speech audiometry can be modified to the child's vocabulary level and the response mode changed to permit reasonable estimates of SRT and discrimination ability. For example, instead of being required to repeat words, the child may be presented with an array of pictures from which he or she chooses the one representing the stimulus.

Acoustic impedance measures are often helpful in providing information and adding support to initial impressions. Electrophysiologic measures are also helpful in difficult situations. Northern and Downs (48) provide an expansion of this brief overview of audiometric procedures with children.

We would be less than honest if we left you with the impression that testing the hearing of infants and young children is done with ease and that test results are always consistent and reliable. The clinician needs to learn to approach the child with care and to evaluate those behaviors which the child is capable of exhibiting. In addition, the clinician needs to be prepared to be thwarted on occasion in his or her efforts to gather a full battery of test results. Continuing evaluation is often the rule in determining the hearing abilities of children. The young child from whom no information about hearing ability can be obtained is rare. No child should be assumed to be too young to be evaluated for hearing.

IDENTIFICATION PROCEDURES

In public health, industrial, military, and educational settings, individuals with hearing disorders or the potential for developing hearing disorders need to be identified as efficiently as possible. It may also be of value to identify those for whom a hearing loss can be ruled out. A number of procedures have been developed for these screening purposes, the most popular of which are pure-tone screening tests and impedance measures.

Pure-tone screening tests typically use the technique of presenting a series of air-conducted pure tones (500–4000 Hz) at a single level (often 20 or 25 dB HL) to either ear of each listener and noting those signals which are not detected. Individuals who fail to respond to one or more of these signals are identified for further evaluation and referral.

Since the primary concern is often to identify individuals for medical intervention, acoustic impedance measures are coming into common use in these identification programs. The combination of pure-tone screening and acoustic impedance, though slightly more time consuming, appears to provide more precise identification than either technique alone.

The discussion above provides a brief overview of two of the many procedures used for identification of hearing disorders. For a more thorough presentation of these procedures, you are referred to Anderson (5) and Studebaker and Brandy (55).

LINGUISTIC FUNCTIONING

As shown in Chapter 4, the assessment of language skills always involves multiple aspects of linguistic functioning. Basically, the examiner seeks information about how the person *receives* language produced by others and how he *produces* language of his own. These two basic forms of language are called the reception and expression of language, and all language evaluations, no matter what the population to be tested, should include an estimate of functioning in both areas. Reception and expression of messages, however, involve many different interrelated aspects of the language used as well as different sensory modalities that may be employed in the processing of linguistic items. Particularly in the case of the hearing-impaired, visual reception of messages plays a major part along with auditory reception, and both should be taken into account when considering the person's receptive skills. The message itself includes such factors as the vocabulary used, morphological information, syntactic structure, semantic relationship among words, and information-bearing factors such as pitch and inflectional patterns.

These aspects of language are usually investigated as a matter of course in children and adults who exhibit speech problems or who are suspected of having language disorders. Unfortunately, the hearing-impaired are often thought of as a group apart; since the source of their difficulty is more easily ascertained (hearing test results indicate an organic problem on which to concentrate remedial efforts), the assessment of their language skills is often postponed or neglected in favor of a hearing aid evaluation and enrollment in a program of lipreading and auditory training, designed to improve reception of speech.

For persons who have lost their hearing in adulthood, concentration on their hearing and discrimination of speech is quite appropriate. Children whose hearing losses occurred before language was learned, however, usually exhibit varying degrees of language delay. While the selection of amplification and emphasis on visual and auditory training are important aspects of remediation for hearing-impaired children and should not be delayed, we should *always* base remedial plans on the needs of the child, and these cannot be properly ascertained unless his or her linguistic skills are thoroughly investigated and understood. What are the communication problems faced by a child with hearing impairment? If he has difficulty understanding what goes on around him, which elements in the messages are causing him the difficulty? If he has difficulty discriminating speech, does this problem result in any particular pattern of language misusage? How do his language skills differ from those of his peer group, his classmates? What are the probabilities of his success in various types of educational settings, such as the normal classroom or a special class for the hearing-impaired? The answers to these and other vital questions depend upon a thorough understanding of the level of linguistic functioning demonstrated by the child. It is not pure tones to which he must listen daily, and knowledge of his ability to discriminate certain consonants and vowels simply does not offer the information necessary to plan for the habilitation of the hearing-impaired child.

LANGUAGE ASSESSMENT OF THE HEARING-IMPAIRED

At the present time there are no language tests specifically designed for use with hearing-impaired children. The use of the available language tests discussed in Chapter 4 is feasible if we keep certain important facts in mind.

Avoidance of Visual Clues

Hearing-impaired children develop keen observational skills as a matter of necessity. Because of the reduction in the amount and quality of the auditory information they receive, it becomes advantageous for them to use vision in order to monitor their environment. Facial expressions and movements of hand or eye, for example, may be observed closely and included in the total amount of information that helps the child make a decision about what is said or desired or expected. As a result, we must take special care not to transmit information to such children during testing procedures that may influence their performance on the tasks at hand. Some language tests involve point-to-the-picture responses, for example, the Peabody Picture Vocabulary Test (17) and the Test for Auditory Comprehension of Language (12), which provide an opportunity for guessing on the child's part. Visually alert children, whether hearing-impaired or not, may watch for subtle cues such as where the examiner's eyes fall on the test page or where his hand rests on the page, and then use that information as a basis for a response when they are unsure of the answer. We have known children who could be manipulated into pointing to pictures in a pattern chosen by the examiner just by allowing the hand to fall on the test page in such a way that the forefinger "pointed" toward the desired response.

Even if the child chooses a response independently, he can often be influenced to change his choice by the facial expression of the examiner or a request that he repeat his response. Such a request usually casts doubt on the original response and in the face of uncertainty the child will "try again," changing his answer in the hope of achieving success. You should avoid making such requests. Establish the rules before the test starts; for example, "You may point to only one picture." If the child then points to two pictures, accept the last one selected.

Although subtle visual clues may be used by any child, they are more likely to be observed by the hearing-impaired child who has become accustomed to depending on such information in his or her daily life. Therefore, you should practice using a neutral tone of voice and facial expression and refrain from looking at the item named or furnishing any other clues to the expected response.

Structure and Control of Testing Environment

Much formal assessment of children is done with examiner and child seated side by side or across a small table from each other. We must maximize the hearing-impaired child's opportunity to observe the examiner's face and to hear the stimulus material. Visual and auditory distractions should be held to a minimum as with other children; extra care should be taken to insure that extraneous noise sources, such as heating units, noise in the halls, and tape recorder motors are as far removed as possible from the child's hearing aid. Indeed, we must be sure the child's hearing aid is in place and working properly before testing begins. Lighting should be manipulated so that the examiner's face is well illumined. Directions or stimuli should be repeated at least twice, once with the child watching the examiner's face and once when the child is looking at the stimulus array. There is a tendency for novice examiners to raise their voices when interacting with the hearing-impaired, but this practice may be inappropriate when one is seated close to the child or when the child is wearing amplification. Therefore, be careful to use a normal tone of voice, precise but not exaggerated articulation, and a slightly slower rate of speech than normal. These precautions, coupled with good lighting and acoustic features, should provide the hearing-impaired child with a reasonable opportunity to perform as well as possible.

Inappropriate Test Procedures

Some language tests, for example, the Boehm Test of Basic Concepts (8), are designed to be given to groups of children and instructions are suggested that might be confusing to a child who has receptive problems. An excerpt from the directions for the Boehm will illustrate the problem:

> Look for the gray box like this one on your page. Put your finger on the gray box with the book in it. Now take your finger off the box and pick up your pencil. Look at the pictures of writing paper with stars. Mark the paper with the star at the top. . . . Mark the paper with the star at the top.

These instructions can be simplified when the test is given individually, since the examiner can turn pages and indicate to the child which array of pictures is to be considered for each test item. The directions could then become: "Mark the paper with the star at the top."

Individual testing is recommended for any child suspected of having a hearing problem. Since the purpose of language tests is to determine how the child responds to certain language stimuli, we must make sure he or she *receives* the stimuli as well as possible; otherwise we may be testing the child's ability to receive the stimuli under adverse conditions, an important factor which should be tested separately.

Some items on available language tests, particularly those designed to test morphemes such as " 's," "es," "ed," and "ing," are difficult for the hearing-impaired to hear or to see on the lips. This problem cannot be avoided, since these elements of our language are important and invariant; we cannot substitute other elements for them. In choosing tests to be administered to the hearing-impaired, however, we should concentrate on those which are not based solely or heavily on such items because the results of their administration may be equivocal and difficult to interpret. We will say more about that later.

With these facts in mind, we turn to a discussion of the evaluation of linguistic functioning in hearing-impaired children.

RECEPTION OF LANGUAGE

Reception of language by hearing-impaired children may involve either oral, written, or signed messages and generally involves both visual and auditory senses. We will concentrate on the reception of oral messages (speech) since this is the form most commonly encountered by persons in our culture. Hearing-impaired children are expected to learn to understand and interpret speech, and unless they are classified as deaf children and taught by other than the oral method, they are expected to learn oral language. Therefore, their ability to receive spoken speech is of primary importance to early linguistic development. Furthermore, the ability to deal with the rapid flow of oral language encountered in daily life is particularly important to the child who must attend educational classes for normally hearing children. The teacher of such a class must teach in the usual way with, one would hope, a few modifications for the benefit of the hearing-impaired member of the class. These modifications seldom involve the extensive use of written language or even the significant reduction of orally produced instructions or explanations.

Finally, hearing-impaired adults are faced with a world of rapid speech as they work, shop, attend meetings, care for children, and carry out other activities associated with normal living.

Auditory Processing of Language

The auditory processing of language involves several closely interrelated auditory "skills." These include auditory reception, auditory closure and synthesis, auditory sequencing, and auditory memory. The sophistication of the tools used to assess these skills varies sharply, and most standardized tasks for this purpose are open to some question with regard to their validity and usefulness with the hearing-impaired.

The assessment of *auditory reception* in the hearing-impaired has been limited in scope in some respects. While speech discrimination tasks are routinely employed, little effort has been made to assess more complex auditory processing of verbal messages by hearing-impaired persons for the following reasons:

1. There has been little necessity for such assessment in the population most capable of performing in this regard. We refer here to adults who have lost their hearing after having learned language. Since they are capable of using language normally, the major question in assessing reception in adults is not whether a given listener can process language auditorily, but to what extent this processing is now dependent upon information other than auditory or modified auditory input. For this purpose, standardized speech reception and discrimination tasks described earlier in this chapter are most appropriate.
2. Persons who have been hearing-impaired from birth or prelinguistically often exhibit language processing difficulties which are more accurately considered *language* disorders, rather than *hearing* disorders per se. In this event, we attempt to maximize the individual's chances of understanding the message presented to him and therefore present it in a form in which he has the greatest opportunity of performing well—the written or perhaps the signed form. At the very least, visual clues in the form of speechreading are made available to the person being tested, and auditory reception alone is seldom investigated beyond the level of speech reception and speech discrimination tests. While it is logical to assume that auditory reception in the hearing-impaired will be poor, some assessment of *how poor* is important, especially if other tests of auditory processing are to be employed, since performance on any auditory task will be influenced by the reception of the stimuli involved in the task.

Auditory reception is often tested by the use of standardized word lists or sentences which are repeated or written down by the listener. In some instances environmental sounds are to be identified or matched to a source. Since this activity requries immediate processing and repetition, it is perhaps the purest of the tests employed, requiring only that listeners "hear" and imitate what they hear. Obviously the task will be influenced by the person's knowledge and understanding of the words or other stimuli used, and the score will be influenced by the listener's ability to match what he or she hears to some store of auditory knowledge. If the auditory input is distorted, then *partial* auditory information may be matched to possible patterns already known. The decision about which word was spoken or which sound was produced will thus use prior knowledge of the stimulus. In effect, both auditory closure (the use of partial information to determine the whole) and auditory memory may influence responses to a task of auditory reception by the hearing-impaired. A simpler task than repetition is provided in other auditory discrimination tasks in which the listener is required only to decide whether two words or syllables are the same or different (60). The necessity of being familiar with the stimuli spoken is reduced and persons being tested rely solely on their ability to recognize differences between the sounds that they hear. This type of auditory discrimination test is used primarily with young children. The norms are restrictive and weighted toward the recognition of different pairs rather than similar ones.

There are tests described as auditory perceptual tests which are designed to measure central auditory abilities by reducing the redundancy of the speech signal presented in order to make reception and understanding of the message more difficult. Redundancy is reduced by filtering out some of the frequencies in the message spectrum or by presenting a competing stimulus such as speech or noise at the same time as the stimuli to be perceived. These tests have not been used extensively with hearing-impaired children, since perception of a message is dependent upon its reception; if reception is impaired, perception is also likely to be impaired, and the original purpose of the test (to determine central auditory function) is precluded because of faulty peripheral (receptive) function.

Auditory closure tasks generally require that the subject listen to partial information and utilize the information given to identify an auditory "whole" or gestalt. This is a constant, daily task for the hearing-impaired listener. Because all the phonemes of English are not of equal intensity, frequency, or duration, any reduction in hearing sensitivity or acuity is likely to render some phonemes less audible than others. The result is that the hearing-impaired listener must rely on partial auditory information in order to make judgments concerning identification of auditory input. Additional distortion of the auditory message by omitting some portions of it, as is the case in tests of auditory closure, may result in the delivery of far less information than intended when the test was designed. Therefore, the hearing-impaired listener's reception of auditory input will influence his ability to achieve closure; we cannot assume that the task is the same for him as for the normal listener, who can be presumed to receive the auditory information given in an undistorted manner.

Auditory sequencing requires that the listener be able to receive sequentially presented information and either repeat it back in the proper order or arrange test items in an order that corresponds to the presentation array. The task usually proceeds from lengths of two units to longer and longer sequences to be remembered and reproduced in order. The test may involve nonverbal items, such as block-tapping patterns or sequences of environmental sounds. In order to sequence heard items the listener must be able to receive them, hold them in memory, then reproduce them in the proper order. This type of task is identical in many respects to *auditory memory* tasks.

Auditory memory is poorly understood. That it plays an important role in the processing of language is obvious, but the testing and training of it are only grossly understood. Activities usually associated with both memory and sequencing involve the use of series of digits, word strings, and phrases which are repeated by the subject after being spoken by the examiner. In some cases, informal test stimuli consist of a series of instructions to be followed, such as "Put the pencil on the table, stand up, and come here." Norms have been established for normal listeners for certain types of stimuli, such as digits and word strings (Auditory Memory Span Test, [61]; Auditory Memory subtest, ITPA [39]). When stimuli involve language units, the performance of the listener will be influenced by the degree of his or her familiarity with the items used. A string of known words would constitute quite a different array than a string of unknown words, which might involve processing on a phonetic rather than a semantic basis. Thus the listener could be expected to perform more poorly on unfamiliar material which could not be "chunked" easily into larger perceptual units or classified by a well-established categorizing system, resulting in a greater number of bits of information to be processed, stored, and recalled. On the other hand, even if the material is familiar but not perceived (received accurately), its ambiguity could affect its recall (49). For example, if the sequence to be remembered consists of similar sounding words or letters that can easily be confused by hearing-impaired listeners, the task is likely to be confounded by auditory reception, auditory closure, and knowledge of the stimuli to be used.

It becomes difficult, then, to separate out and assess the various facets of auditory processing when the listener is hearing-impaired. The most commonly used tests do not attempt to do this. For example, subtests of the Illinois Test of Psycholinguistic Abilities (Auditory Closure, Auditory Memory, Auditory Reception) all utilize language of a fairly sophisticated nature, the processing of which involves the interrelation of all of these auditory subskills. In the case of normally hearing children auditory reception does not refer to quite the same activity as in the case of the hearing-impaired, since it is assumed to be a representational-level task and to involve the attaching of meaning to the auditory signal. The signal is assumed to be clear to the listener, and this is an assumption that cannot be made with the hearing-impaired. If a child has a severe hearing loss, can discriminate speech stimuli only if a closed set of response items is made available, and has great difficulty participating in conversational speech, results of tests of auditory closure or auditory memory may be so biased by these limitations as to be useless, at least as far as their original purpose is concerned. On the other hand, if the child has a relatively mild hearing loss, participates in conversational speech easily, and scores well on tests of speech discrimination, results of a test of auditory memory or closure are likely to be more meaningful and should be included in the battery of tests to be administered.

Visual Processing of Language

The reliance on visual information as a means of understanding and monitoring the environment leads naturally to the use of visual clues in the comprehension of speech and language. There is considerable controversy about the use of vision in this regard. Some authorities maintain that the use of visual clues combined with auditory information will enhance the reception of messages by approximately 20 percent (56, 46), but at least one investigator suggests that the simultaneous use of visual and auditory sensory channels actually interferes with the learning of new material (23). Methods of teaching deaf children are based on differing philosophies regarding the use of visual and auditory information simultaneously and will be discussed further in Chapter 16.

Most hearing-impaired persons make extensive use of visual information in communication, primarily through the use of *speechreading* or *lipreading*. These terms are used interchangeably and refer to the observation of oral and facial movements that lead to the comprehension of a spoken message. The measurement of speechreading skill is usually accomplished by means of a formal test of lipreading. Most such tests utilize words, sentences, and paragraphs which must be comprehended on the basis of visual information only. No voice is used during the presentation of the stimuli, which may be on film or presented live by the examiner. Stimuli are frequently presented only once, at most twice, and the viewer is required to write down what he or she observed or to choose the observed item from a multiple-choice array. Tests for young children often employ a point-to-the-picture task. Scoring of the tests is usually accomplished by counting the number of words or sentences understood correctly.

Speechreading is a linguistic skill, not a visual skill, although vision obviously plays an important part in it. Although some methods of teaching speechreading emphasize training in visual perception—speed of visual processing, visual closure, and visual memory—there is little or no evidence to support the theory that such training enhances one's ability to comprehend spoken messages through lipreading. A speech-reader may interpret a certain mouth movement as one of lip rounding, but unless she is familiar with the word spoken (for example, shoe), the information is of little value to her. Consequently, the greater her facility with language, its rules, and the probability of occurrence of words, phrases, and morphological affixes, the more likely she is to be able to speech-read successfully. Because of its dependence on linguistic facility, lipreading can more easily be measured in a population of persons whose hearing losses occurred after language was learned than in a prelinguistically hearing-impaired population, at least insofar as the validity of the tests is concerned, since it can be assumed that the person being tested is familiar with the words and sentence structures used in the test. Failure to receive the message can be attributed to an inability to comprehend what was said on the basis of the visual clues provided rather than to an inability to understand the message in any form.

Tests of speechreading, therefore, must take into consideration the probable language level of the person to be tested. For these reasons, speechreading tests are generally controlled with respect to vocabulary and syntactic complexity; all standard tests currently in use avoid complex sentence structure (relative clauses, compound sentences) and utilize vocabulary most likely to be understood by the general population.

In choosing a test of speechreading several factors should be considered. First is the vocabulary level of the test. Young children who are hearing-impaired have reduced vocabulary as well as delayed syntactic skills, and attempts to assess the lipreading skills of persons with delayed language development should concentrate on vocabulary and sentence structure that they are likely to know. Otherwise the test becomes a test of language rather than of lipreading. For these reasons, lipreading tests for children usually include vocabulary suitable for kindergarten and first-grade students or younger. Conversely, speechreading tests for adults use more difficult vocabulary and more varied sentence structure.

The second factor involves the nature of the response required of the examinee. If persons to be tested can read and write at an adult level, they can respond to test stimuli by writing down what they saw or by choosing one of several written words or sentences presented to them as possible responses. If their academic skills are of third-grade level or below, best results will be obtained with the use of a test requiring a simpler response, such as pointing to an item in a picture display or repeating the word or sentence presented. If a patient's speech is very poor and he cannot write well, a point-to-the-picture task is most appropriate. Table 12.3 provides a list of commonly used tests of lipreading and some identifying information about each.

Informal tests of speechreading ability can also be helpful in assess-

TABLE 12.3
Commonly Used Tests of Lipreading

Test	Age Level	Stimuli	Presentation Method	Method of Response	Scoring	Comments
Children's Speechreading Test (9)	3–9 yrs.*	Words, few simple sentences	Live, inaudible voice	Points to picture	1 point for each item. Total = 70	Test includes identification of objects, numbers, pictures, colors, actions, foods, clothing, body parts, animals, and simple directions
Craig Lipreading Inventory (15)	Grades 1–10 Ages 6–15	Words and sentences	Live, with or without voice	Points to picture (stimulus word or sentence is written under the picture)	1 point for each item. Total: words = 33 sentences = 24	Vocabulary consists of words from kindergarten and first-grade materials. Sentences are all present or present progressive tense, declarative, active, simple.
Costello Test of Speechreading (14)	No age given	Words and sentences	Live, without voice	Word or sentence repetition	1 point for each item. Total: words = 50 sentences = 50	Vocabulary taken from simple concepts from kindergarten lists. Sentences vary in length and type (question, statement), verb tense (present, past), and complexity.
Cavender Test of Lipreading Ability (13)	School children, no ages given	Sentences	Live, without voice	Multiple choice; subject underlines one word of five pos-	1 point for each word correctly underlined.	Vocabulary from first three grades of school (Gates). Sentences vary in length, type, verb tense, and complexity.

Barley Speechreading Test-CID Everyday Sentences (33)	Age 8–9 to adulthood	Sentences	Live, without voice	Writes what was spoken	1 point for each word. Total: Form A = 125 and Form B = 117	Vocabulary is appropriate for adults, but of high frequency usage. Sentences vary in length, type, and grammatical structure. Many contractions are used.
Diagnostic Test of Speechreading (45)	Age 4–9 years	Words, phrases sentences	Film	Points to picture	1 point for each word, phrase, and sentence correct. Total = 64	Vocabulary represents that found in educational curriculum for deaf children aged 4 to 9. Parts of speech occur in proportion to their use in spoken language.
Keaster Film Test of Lipreading (38)	Adults	Sentences	Film, no voice	Writes what was spoken	1 point for each word correct. Total = 188	Vocabulary unspecified; sentences vary in length, type, and grammatical structure.
Utley Film ** Test "How Well Can You Read Lips" (58)	Age 10 to adult	Words, sentences, story	Film,** no voice	Writes what was spoken	1 point for each word. Total = 125 or 1 point for each sentence whose meaning is perceived with reasonable accuracy.	Vocabulary is at least third-grade level and taken from the 1000 most common words (Thorndike). Sentences involve colloquial and idiomatic expressions and vary in length, type, and structure.

* A simple checklist is included for infants 0–3 years.
** The Utley Film Test appears to be a difficult test. When the same stimuli are delivered live, test scores are significantly higher.

ment of a person's ability to use visual information for purposes of communication. Simple conversation or questions in a relaxed interview or play situation will often indicate the amount of difficulty the person has in understanding speech, although the difficulty may lie in comprehension of the language employed and not just the *speech* to be lip-read. In conducting informal assessment of speechreading skill, be careful to use language that you can reasonably expect the person to know. Also you must be careful not to ask questions all of which can be answered by yes or no responses, since many hearing-impaired people, especially children, will base yes or no answers on the facial expression of the examiner or some other extraneous clue, without any real comprehension of the question. If you suspect that a child is giving "agreeable" answers with no comprehension, and yes and no responses are all you can obtain from him, ask nonsense questions in a reasonable way. For example, ask "Did you ride an elephant to the clinic today?" or "Do you have apples on your feet?" Look pleasant and expectant for some sentences, doubtful for others. A few such questions may serve to corroborate other findings that are open to question. If the child seems to choose answers on the basis of facial expression or at random, considerable skepticism should govern your interpretation of test results involving the processing of spoken language for whatever purpose.

The third factor to be considered in choosing a speechreading test is the mode of presentation of stimuli. Filmed tests allow for greater standardization of presentation, as we can be sure that the stimuli are spoken exactly the same for each test and variables such as speaker intelligibility, rate of presentation, lighting, distance from the speaker, facial expression, and gestures are held constant for each presentation. These variables cannot be easily controlled in live presentations, especially if different speakers are used, but there are advantages to live testing of speechreading ability, especially when testing young children. Attention to the speaker is more easily maintained, or at least monitored, so that items are presented only when the examinee is ready and watching. For poor lip-readers live presentation may be less frustrating; as the examiner you can encourage the person, but you must be careful not to change significantly the way the test words are spoken, such as slowing down or exaggerating lip movements excessively.

Finally, the intended use of the test results is a factor in choosing a test. Whether lipreading test results can be generalized to actual ability to use visual information in communicative situations is not certain. There is some evidence that teacher ratings of lipreading ability correlate with lipreading test results, but this conclusion generally applies only to deaf children in classes for the deaf, since other persons being tested may not have a readily accessible "judge" of lipreading ability. Teacher ratings may be based on general linguistic ability, which in turn may be reflected in speechreading scores. This relationship may not hold for adults who are adventitiously hearing-impaired.

There are several uses for speechreading test results. They may form the basis for a training program in speechreading, they may be used to assess the success of lipreading training, or they may be used to compare a person's ability to communicate with and without amplification. If before- and after-training tests are planned, filmed tests which provide alternate forms of the test stimuli should be administered where possible. If used for the purpose of grossly estimating speechreading ability, live presentation of any test that utilizes language of an appropriate level is a good choice. We must remember at all times that speaker, rate of presentation, and linguistic level differences influence test results. As if that does not provide enough difficulty in assessing lipreading skill, remember that there are no true norms for lipreading ability in existence. People vary so widely in their speechreading skills and the ability to lip-read appears to correlate so poorly with other factors involved in hearing loss that assessment of the lipreading skill of an individual is a gross measure at best. Tests should be chosen with care and results should be interpreted with caution.

The majority of individuals classified as deaf make use of some form of *manual communication*. These individuals usually possess little residual hearing and cannot rely on auditory information for purposes of communication. Speechreading alone, without auditory input to accompany it, is a poor means of learning and processing spoken language. Even though they may have been educated by methods which stressed speechreading as a receptive tool, deaf adults tend to learn and use signs and fingerspelling in order to communicate, particularly among themselves (59). Until quite recently speech and hearing personnel have seldom learned any form of manual communication and have found it difficult to communicate with and assess the language skills of deaf children or adults. This inability and unwillingness on the part of many to use the language form most meaningful to the deaf has influenced our assessment of linguistic functioning of this population. Either we have ignored the problem entirely or we have assumed that we were assessing language skills when in reality we may have been only assessing the person's ability to receive language auditorily and visually through speechreading (26). Unless the deaf person has good lipreading, reading, or writing skills, it is almost impossible to assess his or her language. Our limitations must be considered when evaluating young children prior to making educational, amplification, and habilitative recommendations. We recommend, therefore, that whenever possible speech and hearing personnel, especially audiologists, learn fingerspelling and some basic manual signs.

Several of the tests designed to assess receptive language can be administered with sign and speech. This procedure is especially appropriate for children who are being educated in programs that make use of one of the newly developed forms of signed English. We have found that such children exhibit much better language *reception* when this procedure is used than when speech alone is used as a stimulus. If knowledge of language concepts is the ability to be tested, the use of sign and speech simultaneously yields a more accurate estimate of this ability. If reception of *oral speech* is the ability to be tested, the use of sign would contaminate the results. A word of caution here: many signs are quite graphic and obvious in their meaning. The presentation of such a sign may cause the child to give the correct response to the test item without actually having knowledge of the concept represented. For example, the sign for "ball" is made by placing the fingertips of both hands together to form the shape of a ball. It would be difficult to miss the meaning even if one had never been exposed to the sign or word before, especially if the response is to be given by pointing to one of three or four pictures, only one of which looks like the hand-shape shown. This ideographic nature of sign does not hold for the majority of test items on language inventories and should not preclude its use as long as care is exercised in interpreting test results.

EXPRESSION OF LANGUAGE

Although assessment of reception of language is filled with problems, assessment of expressive language skills in hearing-impaired children is even more difficult. Tests designed to measure expressive language were not developed with the hearing-impaired in mind. The most common means of assessing expression involve articulation tests, linguistic analysis of spontaneous speech or written output, and repetition of sentence stimuli previously provided by the examiner. Each of these approaches presents difficulties when the person to be examined is significantly hearing-impaired.

Articulation

Articulation testing usually involves the naming of pictures or the reading of words or sentences. In some instances words or phrases are repeated after the examiner. These test procedures are appropriate for hard-of-hearing children as long as (1) the pictures represent vocabulary known by the child, (2) the child can read the words or phrases presented, and (3) the child can understand the examiner's production of items to be repeated. Even if all these requirements are met, there is still likely to be difficulty with intelligibility that may make phonemic analysis of the child's production difficult to accomplish.

Investigations of the speech of the hearing-impaired have identified the following as its major characteristics:

1. Apparent omission of initial and final consonants, due to improper closure of articulators or failure to complete the phoneme.
2. Substitution of consonants, primarily voiced-voiceless confusions.
3. Addition of a neutral vowel between abutting elements of a consonant cluster.
4. Hypernasality which may result in substitution of /m/ for /b/, /n/ for /t/, et cetera.
5. Substitution of vowels, with neutral vowels being used most often.
6. Omission of the final vowel of a diphthong or division of diphthongs into two separate vowels.
7. Poor production of fricative and affricative phonemes.
8. Reduced rate of speaking.
9. Abnormal vocal pitch (too high or too low).
10. Poor rhythm, intonation, and stress patterns (all syllables may be stressed equally or stress may be applied to the wrong syllable).

Articulation testing should, therefore, provide an opportunity to examine these aspects of speech production; for this reason, spontaneous speech should be elicited in order to estimate rate, rhythm, inflection, and other prosodic features, as well as phonemic usage during contextual speech. In addition, a standard articulation test should be employed.

Because of the high probability of speech of reduced intelligibility in this population, it is a good idea to record the child's responses with a high-fidelity recording system for later analysis and comparison to the transcription made by the examiner during the examination. In this way you can avoid asking the child to repeat his production many times as you try to classify his utterances. Being asked to repeat items several times tends to be frustrating to the hearing-impaired child (or any child, for that matter) and may result in reluctance to continue the task. The fidelity of the recording is important if it is to be useful, so precautions should be taken to control ambient noise in the examination room and the distance of the patient from the microphone. It is also a good idea to observe the child closely during his production of the stimuli, making note of any articulatory postures that are consistently substituted for correct production of phonemes under test (such as bringing the tongue tip forward to the teeth whenever /s/ appears in the stimuli, even though no audible speech sound accompanies the gesture). Otherwise, standard procedures for articulation testing as discussed in Chapter 8 are appropriate.

Syntax

The grammatical aspects of linguistic output are tested in two major ways: (1) by use of a screening test which requires the child to repeat an appropriate syntactic pattern after having been exposed to it, and

(2) by use of one of several approaches to the linguistic analysis of spontaneous speech samples collected from the child. Chapter 4 provides a detailed description of both types of tests.

The screening tests are the simpler tools to use, as the child is required only to attend to certain specific stimuli and apply them to the appropriate picture or repeat them after the examiner. We must remember, however, that these tests were not developed with the hearing-impaired in mind, and no attempt has been made to control phonemic content with regard to its audibility or visibility to the listener with hearing loss. Since most children with permanent hearing impairment have hearing losses in the high frequencies, they are not likely to hear high-frequency phonemes clearly (such as /s/, /θ/, /ʃ/, /z/, /t/, /tʃ/), since these phonemes tend also to be of relatively low amplitude in normal speech. In addition, many high-frequency phonemes are also difficult to lip-read (/s/, /t/, /k/) so that the child may not perceive them in the examiner's production. The poor visibility and audibility of certain phonemes becomes an important factor in testing such items as "The cat sits; the cats sit" (Northwestern Syntax Screening Test), because the difference between the two sentences consists solely of the location of the "s" denoting plurality for the noun (cats) or singular person for the verb (sits). All tests of morphological rules and grammar involve items such as these which are unstressed and difficult to hear and lip-read (-ed, -ing, -s) and which, therefore, may not be perceived by the hearing-impaired. Failure on such items may indicate a lack of knowledge of the rule being tested, but failure can also occur simply because the item is not correctly perceived by the subject. The failure to hear a certain phoneme is less likely to contaminate test results when pictured stimuli are used, since presumably children will use the plural form for the noun if it is within their repertoire when they see two items (for example, cats) in the picture to be described.

On the other hand, even if the item is correctly perceived, the child's production of the required sentence may be devoid of word endings (-ed, -ing, -s) necessary for a correct production of the sentence involved. The question then remains as to whether the child knows the rule but cannot produce the phonemes necessary to demonstrate his knowledge, or whether he does not have knowledge of the rule. Since the high-frequency, low-amplitude, unstressed phonemes are the most difficult for the hearing-impaired to perceive, they are also the most difficult for him to produce consistently as a result of poor auditory feedback for these phonemes. In order to determine the child's probable knowledge of these grammatical elements, we need to employ a combination of procedures. If, for example, articulation test results indicate that the child consistently substitutes some phoneme or articulatory posture for the phoneme under investigation and fails to produce this posture or phoneme during the screening test for syntax, it probably can be assumed that he does not have control over the use of the rule under investigation. If he does produce a consistent substitution, even though it is not a phoneme that can be clearly identified, he should be given credit for accurate usage of the rule under test. In addition, linguistic analysis of spontaneous speech should be employed to determine further the child's use of grammatical rules and relationships. This type of assessment is probably the most meaningful way of evaluating linguistic output, particularly if the results are to be used as a basis for remediation.

Spontaneous expression of language can be spoken or written, and guidelines for the analysis of both types of output are available. If the child is 8 years of age or older, he may be able to write well enough to express himself in writing. The Myklebust Picture Story Language Test (44) is designed to elicit a written story about a standard picture, a black-and-white photograph of a child playing with family figures, furniture, and toys. The child's story is then analyzed according to its grammatical usage, abstraction, and total output. The picture can be used to elicit spoken as well as written responses without seriously changing the linguistic characteristics of the responses obtained.

Unfortunately the picture on which the test is standardized is somewhat dated and appears to be uninteresting to most children. Hearing-impaired children in particular have difficulty writing a story about the picture, listing instead either items seen or actions implied by the picture (for example, the boy is sitting, the boy is playing, the boy is looking). This is not, however, a function of the picture as such naming and listing behavior is common in hard-of-hearing children when they are asked to describe a picture or an event. For this reason, linguistic analysis of spontaneous output (oral or written) of hearing-impaired children is quite difficult to obtain, since most methods require at least 50 utterances for meaningful analysis. Obtaining that many spontaneous utterances from most young hearing-impaired children, especially during a single evaluation session, is unlikely. Chances of obtaining a 50-item sample are greater if several stimuli are used to elicit the sample. It is often necessary to encourage output by asking questions in order to get the child started. Care must be taken to ask questions that cannot easily be answered by one word or yes-no answers. Questions such as "What is this?" or "What are they doing?" will encourage one-word answers; queries like "What is happening?" or "How do you think he feels?" or "Tell me about this" may encourage longer responses. Even with these precautions an adequate sample may not be obtained during the evaluation session. It is frequently necessary to make arrangements to record the child at home, at school, or in therapy in order to increase the size of the sample to be used for analysis. Remember that clarity of the recording is vital, so take precautions to insure good recording conditions whenever possible.

All language samples to be used for analysis, whether obtained in the clinic, home, or school, should be recorded and transcribed for later analysis. Videotape recordings should be made whenever possible, since it is sometimes easier to understand unclear speech if you can observe the speaker as you listen. Any analysis of expressive language depends largely on the intelligibility of the samples to be analyzed, since decisions about the appropriateness of grammatical structures, morphological endings, and semantic relationships employed by the child are dependent upon being able to identify the words used with some degree of certainty. While receptive language may be assessed even though the child never speaks intelligibly, expressive language by definition requires spoken or written output that can be examined and which therefore must be intelligible or legible. These requirements may frequently preclude accurate assessment of linguistic skills in the young hearing-impaired child, necessitating a period of diagnostic teaching before assessment can be completed. (Diagnostic teaching refers to the use of regular sessions with a clinician during which the child is observed carefully as various stimuli and methods of presentation are tried, in an effort to assess the child's level of functioning over a period of time and in a more relaxed situation than that of a formal evaluation session with a strange examiner). Visits to the child's home, if possible, may offer valuable information regarding his ability to manipulate and interact with his environment, linguistically and in other ways. Every piece of information obtained, both formally and informally, should be combined and used in the final assessment of the child's linguistic abilities. The term "final" as used here does not mean that a single assessment is appropriate, but only that decisions concerning the child's therapy or educational placement should be based on the maximum amount of information that can be obtained from all sources.

In the case of children whose expressive language is limited to gestures or formal signs, an attempt should be made to analyze these with regard to their variety, appropriateness, structure, and usefulness. An analysis is best achieved by systematic observation of the child when he or she is interacting with parents, siblings, or teachers. If you are not able to read sign, you will have to rely on analysis by someone who is. In this case, videotape recordings of the child are especially helpful.

Assessment of the hearing-impaired, particularly hearing-impaired children, should not be considered complete without as comprehensive an evaluation of their language skills as it is possible to obtain. The earlier in the child's life this is accomplished, the more useful the results may be in planning a program of remediation. The fact that these children may be difficult to communicate with or may give little evidence of any linguistic skills should not be used as an excuse for failing to look closely at their ability to communicate in a variety of settings. Since hearing-impaired children present a relatively pure form of language disorder, language assessment should be considered a major portion of any attempt at diagnosis and appraisal of this population.

SUMMARY

The complete appraisal of auditory functioning involves evaluation of the person's hearing sensitivity, acuity, and processing as well as linguistic functioning. The choice of procedures for this appraisal will depend upon the purposes of the appraisal as well as the needs and abilities of the person being evaluated. Recognition of the importance of auditory functioning in the communication process demands an alertness to a potential disorder and a sensitivity to its effect upon the process. Speech pathologists should learn to recognize the need for appraisal of auditory function and to make appropriate referrals for evaluation.

ASSIGNMENTS

1. Draw a form for the pure-tone audiogram which meets the guidelines of the American Speech and Hearing Association, label the form appropriately, and give the symbols to be used.
2. Upon what do we base our expectations for the type of hearing test that can be administered to young children?
3. Observe a group of children under 5 years of age and a group of adults over 65 years of age for at least 30 minutes each. During the observations note each instance when one individual appeared *not* to hear another. For each instance recorded (1) note the specific behavior of the speaker and the listener, (2) describe the background noise and distraction, (3) describe how clearly the listener could see the face of the speaker, (4) indicate how likely the listener knew the topic of conversation, and (5) make a judgment as to the cause of the error in hearing. How often did it appear to be an environmental cause and how often because the listener had a hearing problem? Did one or two people appear to have more difficulty than the others?
4. Practice administering a language comprehension test (Peabody Picture Vocabulary Test, Test for Auditory Comprehension of Language, or others) to a child in a room filled with noise. Take care that the child can see and hear you. Note the child's behavior as he tries to understand in the presence of competing noise.
5. Obtain well-fitting earplugs and wear them to classes for an entire day. Make notes about your behavior and feelings throughout the day.

REFERENCES

1. American Academy of Ophthalmology and Otolaryngology (AAOO), Guide for the Evaluation of Hearing Impairment. *Transactions of the American*

Academy of Ophthalmology and Otolaryngology, 1959, *64*:235–238.

2. American National Standards Institute, Specifications for Audiometers. ANSI S3.6–1969. New York: American National Standards Institute, 1970.

3. American Standards Association, Criteria for background noise in audiometric rooms. ASA S3.1–1960.

4. ASHA Committee on Audiometric Evaluation, Guidelines for Audiometric Symbols. *Asha*, 1974, *16*:260–264.

5. Anderson, C. V., Screening the hearing of preschool and school-age children. In Katz, J., ed., *Handbook of Clinical Audiology*, pp. 520–539. Baltimore: Williams & Wilkins, 1972.

6. Békésy, Georg von, A new audiometer. *Acta Otaloryngologica*, 1947, *35*: 411.

7. Berlin, C. I., Programmed instruction in the decibel. In Northern, J. L., ed., *Hearing Disorders*, Appendix, pp. 279–296. Boston: Little, Brown, 1976.

8. Boehm, A., *Boehm Test of Basic Concepts*. New York: The Psychological Corporation, 1971.

9. Butt, D. S., and Chreist, F. M., A speechreading test for young children. *Volta Review*, 1968, *70*:225–239.

10. Carhart, R., Clinical determination of abnormal auditory adaptation. *Archives of Otolaryngology*, 1957, *65*:32–39.

11. Carhart, R., and Jerger, J. F., Preferred method for clinical determination of pure-tone thresholds. *Journal of Speech and Hearing Disorders*, 1959, *24*:330–345.

12. Carrow, E., *Test for Auditory Comprehension of Language*. Austin, Tex.: Urban Research Group, 1973.

13. Cavender, B. J., The construction and investigation of a test of lip reading ability and a study of factors assumed to affect the results. M.A. thesis, Indiana University, 1949.

14. Costello, M. R., A study of speechreading as a developing language process in deaf and hard of hearing children. Ph.D. dissertation, Northwestern University, 1957.

15. Craig, W. H., Effects of preschool training in the development of reading and lipreading skills of deaf children. *American Annals of the Deaf*, 1964, *109*:280–296.

16. Davis, H., and Silverman, S. R., eds., *Hearing and Deafness*. 3rd ed. New York: Holt, Rinehart and Winston, 1970.

17. Dunn, L. M., *Peabody Picture Vocabulary Test*. Circle Pines, Minn.: American Guidance Service, 1965.

18. Egan, J. P., Articulation testing methods. *Laryngoscope*, 1948, *58*:955–991.

19. Evans, E. F., Ross, H. F., and Whitfield, I. C., The spatial distribution of unit characteristic frequency in the primary auditory cortex of the cat. *Journal of Physiology*, 1965, *179*:238–247.

20. Fairbanks, G., Test of phonemic differentiation: the rhyme test. *Journal of the Acoustical Society of America*, 1958, *30*:596–601.

21. Fowler, E. P., Marked deafened areas in normal ears. *Archives of Otolaryngology*, 1928, *8*:151–155.

22. Fowler, E. P., Measuring the sensation of loudness. *Archives of Otolaryngology*, 1937, *26*:514–521.
23. Gaeth, J., Deafness in children. In Freeman, M., and Ward, P., eds., *National Symposium of Deafness in Childhood*, Nashville, Tenn.: Vanderbilt University Press, 1967.
24. Garner, W. R., and Miller, G. A., The masked threshold of pure tones as a function of duration. *Journal of Experimental Psychology*, 1947, *37*:292–303.
25. Glattke, T. J., Elements of auditory physiology. In Minifie, F. D., Hixon, T. J., and Williams, F., eds., *Normal Aspects of Speech, Hearing, and Language*, pp. 285–341. Englewood Cliffs, N.J.: Prentice-Hall, 1973.
26. Gochnour, E. A., Evaluating the communication skills of the adult deaf. *Asha*, 1973, *15*:687–691.
27. Hirsh, I. J., *The Measurement of Hearing*. New York: McGraw-Hill, 1952.
28. Hirsh, I. J., Palva, T., and Goodman, A., Difference limen and recruitment. *Archives of Otolaryngology*, 1954, *60*:525–540.
29. Hopkinson, N. T., Speech reception threshold. In Katz, J., ed., *Handbook of Clinical Audiology*, pp. 143–156. Baltimore: Williams & Wilkins, 1972.
30. House, A. S., Williams, C. E., Hecker, M. H. L., and Kryter, K. D., Articulation testing methods: Consonantal differentiation with a closed-response set. *Journal of the Acoustical Society of America*, 1965, *37*: 158–166.
31. Hughson, W., and Westlake, H., Manual for program outline for rehabilitation of aural casualties both military and civilian. *Transactions of the American Academy of Ophthalmology and Otolaryngology*, 1944, *48*:1–15.
32. International Standards Organization, Technical Committee 43-Acoustics, No. 554, A standard reference zero for the calibration of pure-tone audiometers. New York: American Standards Association, 1964.
33. Jeffers, J., and Barley, M., The Barley speechreading test—C.I.D. "Everyday Speech Sentences." *California Journal of Communication Disorders*, 1971, *1*:43–45.
34. Jerger, J. F., Burney, P., Mauldin, L., and Crump, B., Predicting hearing loss from the acoustic reflex. *Journal of Speech and Hearing Disorders*, 1974, *39*:11–22.
35. Jerger, J. F., Shedd, E., and Harford, R., On the direction of extremely small changes in sound intensity. *Archives of Otolaryngology*, 1959, *69*: 200–211.
36. Jerger, J. F., Speaks, C., and Trammel, J. L., A new approach to speech audiometry. *Journal of Speech and Hearing Disorders*, 1968, *33*:318–328.
37. Katz, J., The SSW test: an interim report. *Journal of Speech and Hearing Disorders*, 1968, *33*:132–146.
38. Keaster, J., An inquiry into current concepts of visual speech reception. *Laryngoscope*, 1949, *65*:80–84.
39. Kirk, S. A., McCarthy, J. J., and Kirk, W. D., *Illinois Test of Psycholinguistic Abilities*. Rev. Ed. Urbana: University of Illinois Press, 1969.
40. Lehiste, I., and Peterson, G. E., Linguistic considerations in the study of

speech intelligibility. *Journal of the Acoustical Society of America,* 1959, *31:*280–286.

41. Lilly, D. J., Acoustic impedance at the tympanic membrane. In Jerger, J. F., ed., *Modern Developments in Audiology.* 2nd ed., pp. 345–406. New York: Academic Press, 1973.

42. Lynn, G. E., and Gilroy, J., Central aspects of audition. In Northern, J., ed., *Hearing Disorders,* pp. 102–116. Boston: Little, Brown, 1976.

43. Martin, F. N., and Pennington, C. D., Current trends in audiometric practices. *Asha,* 1971, *13:*671–677.

44. Myklebust, H., *Picture Story Language Test.* New York: Grune & Stratton, 1965.

45. Myklebust, H., and Neyhus, A., *Diagnostic Test of Speechreading.* New York: Grune & Stratton, 1971.

46. Neely, K. K., Effect of visual factors on the intelligibility of speech. *Journal of the Acoustical Society of America,* 1956, 28:1272–1277.

47. Niemeyer, W., and Sesterhenn, G., Calculating the hearing threshold from the stapedius reflex threshold for different stimuli. *Audiology,* 1974, *13:* 421–428.

48. Northern, J. L., and Downs, M., *Hearing in Children.* Baltimore: Williams & Wilkins, 1974.

49. Novak, R., and Davis, J., Effects of low-pass filtering on the rate of learning and retrieval from memory of speech-like stimuli. *Journal of Speech and Hearing Research,* 1974, 17:279–285.

50. Owens, E., Tone decay in eighth nerve and cochlear lesions. *Journal of Speech and Hearing Disorders,* 1964, 29:14–22.

51. Pohlman, A. G., and Kranz, F. W., Binaural minimum audition in a subject with ranges of deficient acuity. *Proceedings of the Society for Experimental Biology,* 1924, *21:*335–337.

52. Reger, S. N., Differences in loudness response of normal and hard-of-hearing ears at intensity levels slightly above threshold. *Annals of Otology, Rhinology, and Laryngology,* 1936, 45:1029–1039.

53. Rosenberg, P. E., Tone decay. *Maico Audiologic Library Series,* VII, Report No. 6, 1969.

54. Stevens, S. S., *Handbook of Experimental Psychology.* New York: Wiley, 1951.

55. Studebaker, G. A., and Brandy, W. T., Industrial and military audiology. In Rose, D. E., ed., *Audiological Assessment,* pp. 423–470. Englewood Cliffs, N.J.: Prentice-Hall, 1971.

56. Sumby, W. H., and Pollack, I., Visual contributions to speech intelligibility in noise. *Journal of the Acoustical Society of America,* 1954, *26:* 212–215.

57. Tillman, T. W., and Carhart, R., An expanded test for speech discrimination utilizing CNC monosyllabic words. Tech. Report, SAM-TR-66-55. Brooks Air Force Base, Tex.: USAF School of Aerospace Medicine, 1966.

58. Utley, J. A., A test of lipreading ability. *Journal of Speech and Hearing Disorders,* 1946, *11:*109–116.

59. Vernon, M., Sociological and psychological factors associated with pro-

found hearing loss. *Journal of Speech and Hearing Research,* 1969, *12:* 541–563.

60. Wepman, J., *Wepman Auditory Discrimination Test.* Los Angeles: Western Psychological Services, 1975.

61. Wepman, J., and Morency, A., *Auditory Memory Span Test.* Los Angeles: Western Psychological Services, 1975.

62. Willeford, J. A., Central auditory function in children with learning disabilities. *Audiology and Hearing Education,* 1976, *2:*12–20.

13
THE EXAMINATION REPORT

Frederic L. Darley

In this chapter we present an outline for the examination report, together with a number of suggestions about its preparation and the uses to be made of it.

The examination report serves two major purposes: it is a record and it is a communication. As a record it serves as a baseline against which to compare future reports and to evaluate future developments; it may be used in the preparation of annual or other periodic reports of the clinical program; it may be shared, ethically and judiciously, with students in professional training courses; it may be utilized in research. As a communication, the examination report is addressed to appropriate professional persons or agencies, on request and with approval of either the person being served or the parents or others responsible for him or her. Both as a record and as a communication it should be clear, valid, and no longer than necessary.

Here are a few suggestions to guide you in writing the examination report:

1. Use the fewest possible words to give a serious-minded reader the information he or she needs. Avoid personal comments that are beside the point, and forego cleverness. Include the more important facts and omit needless detail. Go to the point without unneeded howevers and neverthelesses. Write short and simple sentences. Use common words. If you must use a technical term put it in a context that makes it meaning clear, or else define it; your reader may not be a speech-language pathologist. Keep the tone of your report basically impersonal, but if you can make a statement more clear and simple by using a personal pronoun, use it.

2. Don't include comments which are critical of other professional specialists or agencies.
3. Don't reveal information given to you in unmistakable confidence. Let the person, or those responsible for him or her, give any strictly confidential information they may have to other examiners or agencies themselves. In describing especially significant aspects of the problem, however, such as parent-child relationships, be as clear as possible, and in case of doubt ask permission to pass along specific details that you consider essential to adequate understanding of the problem.

Follow the basic rule of releasing the examination report only with permission or on request of the person served. If a copy of the report, or of some part of it, is requested by someone other than the person served, obtain his or her permission before complying with the request. When you refer a person to another specialist or agency for an examination, it is understood that the person served consents to the exchange of information between you and the other specialist or agency. In case of doubt, obtain explicit consent. Also, it is understood that when a person is referred to you for examination or consultation, you are free to report your findings to the referring practitioner or agency. Again, in case of doubt, because of the nature of your findings perhaps, obtain permission.

Some clinicians routinely ask all persons they serve to sign a general form giving them permission to make certain uses of the information obtained from them or about them. Without regard to the question of the legal status of this or any other form of release or permission employed in clinical relationships, we present an example of such a release form (p. 402).

The following is a suggested outline for the examination report. In using it you will, of course, adapt it to the particulars of each specific case.

EXAMINATION REPORT

Start the report with the name, sex, birth date, age (years and months), and address of the examinee; and the full name(s) of the informant(s), stating the relationship of each to the person whose history is under review.

Problem

Briefly and clearly indicate the type of communication problem. Describe it in the informant's own words, if possible. Be specific. A statement such as "He does not make his *s*'s well and he does not sound his *r*'s" is

The Examination Report

Authorization of Use of Clinical and Scientific Material

Date _____

I hereby authorize _____ (name of clinic) to make customary and constructive use, exercising due discretion, for educational, scientific, and professional purposes, and in the public interest, of information, photographs, sound recordings, films, and other records or materials pertaining to, and in consideration of, my enrollment, examination, instruction, and scientific participation, or that of my minor child(ren), _____ (name or names), or that of _____ (name or names), for whom I am legally responsible, in _____ (name of clinic).

I further consent to the release of relevant confidential material to qualified professional personnel in furtherance of clinical services in behalf of me, or any other person(s) named above, as deemed necessary by _____ (name of clinic).

Witness:

_____

Name: _____
Address: _____
_____

Relationship, if not the
person(s) in question: _____

---

more clear and specific than "He doesn't talk plainly," and more understandable to some readers than "He presents a functional articulatory disorder with lateral /s/ and omission of /r/."

Referral

Give the full name and the relationship or title of the individual or agency who referred the person to your clinic.

History

If it is the policy of your clinic to include the complete case history in the examination report, write it, unless otherwise directed by your supervisor, in accordance with the case history outline presented in Chapter 2. Organize it under the major headings of History of Problem, Developmental History, Medical History, School History, Social History, Family History, and Comments on the Interview.

If it is your clinic policy to include a summary of the case history in the examination report, write it as an abstract without divisions and headings. Make the abstract no longer than a page to a page and a half, typed single-spaced. Include only the most important relevant findings, both positive and negative (noncontributory), from each part of the history.

Examinations

Speech, Voice, and Language Examinations   Summarize the results of each test or set of observations of speech, voice, or language. Name each test and explain it briefly so the reader may visualize what was done. State concisely the significance of the findings.

For example, in a report of the testing of a 5-year-old child with an articulation problem, begin with the results of the General Speech Behavior Rating; then continue with the results of the articulation test. In reviewing the articulation test, explain how the speech responses were elicited; list the scores earned and the comparable normative values; list omissions, substitutions, and distortions of phonemes, indicating the positions in the word in which the errors were made; summarize the information about the consistency of these errors and the child's response to auditory stimulation. Clarify the meaning of phonetic symbols, which a layman or a specialist in another field may not understand, in some such way as this: "She substituted *t* for *th,* saying *t*umb for *th*umb." Also indicate the general intelligibility of the person's speech.

Follow a similar procedure in reporting tests of language development, aphasia, vocal function, and stuttering. Name or briefly describe each procedure, and summarize and explain the results.

Examination of Oral Speech Mechanism   Report pertinent information, listing deviations noted and their possible significance in relation to the person's speech problem.

Audiological Examination   Summarize essential findings of the audiological examination. On the basis of the audiologist's report, indicate the results obtained, and the probable validity of the test. Following are typical entries:

Case A: On a sweep-check test with a pure-tone audiometer set at 10 decibels above zero, hearing was found to be essentially normal.

Case B: As the child's responses to the pure tones of an audiometer were judged to be unreliable, other testing methods were employed. He responded correctly (by dropping a marble into a box) to whispered commands given behind his back at a distance of 8 feet. It is believed that his hearing is essentially normal. If there is a hearing loss, it is probably of minor significance in relationship to his speech problem. Retesting in six months is recommended.

If a test of hearing threshold was administered with a pure-tone audiometer and some hearing loss was discovered, summarize the results in a simple table such as the one below. The figures in the top line represent the frequencies tested (125 to 8000 Hz), R and L indicate the right and left ears, and the numbers in the columns refer to hearing loss in decibels for each ear at the various frequencies tested:

	125	250	500	1000	2000	4000	8000
R	10	10	15	15	20	25	30
L	5	5	10	15	20	20	40

Other information may be extracted from the audiogram, such as the person's "average pure-tone loss for speech" (the average of the values in decibels for the three speech frequencies, 500, 1000, and 2000 Hz) in the better ear. If speech audiometry was used, state the type of stimulus (phonetically balanced word lists or spondees) and report and evaluate in practical terms the speech reception threshold in decibels. Enclose all direct quotations from the audiologist's report in quotation marks and credit them to the audiological examiner.

Psychological Evaluation

Quoting the psychologist's report, give the full name of each test administered. Report the results of intelligence testing by stating the obtained mental age (MA) and intelligence quotient (I.Q.). Indicate the general level of intelligence of the person tested. In addition, quote verbatim those portions of the psychologist's report that describe details of the person's behavior during the test which bear on the question of the probable validity of the results obtained. Enclose all extracts in quotation marks and credit the remarks to the examiner. The findings from personality tests should be summarized largely in the examiner's own words, with quotation marks.

Impression

Make a brief statement of the conclusions about the nature of the communication problem, its probable etiology, and the degree of its severity. Identify the person or persons responsible for this conclusion. Examples of such entries are the following:

Stuttering, severe

Functional articulatory problem, mild

Articulatory problem, moderately severe; whether its basis is primarily functional or organic has not yet been determined

Speech retardation, severe, secondary to general mental retardation

Recommendations

Summarize the decisions reached by the clinic staff on the basis of the findings of the examination. Indicate whether there should be referral to other specialists or agencies for further examinations, referral to a speech-language pathologist near the speaker's home, counseling of the parents, a particular program of therapy for the speaker, or some other form of help. Indicate the nature of any counseling done after the examination with the person served or his or her parents or other responsible individuals. Make clear the present status of the problem, and the disposition made of it following examination. State all recommendations in clear and specific terms.

Note: If entries for the *Impression* and *Recommendations* sections are prepared for you by one or more other members of the clinic staff, copy them verbatim but without quotation marks.)

PART TWO

Differential Diagnosis

14
DIFFERENTIAL DIAGNOSIS OF DISORDERS OF FLUENCY

Dean E. Williams

The label *fluent* applied to a speaker means different things to different people. Perceptually, "fluency" encompasses a fluid summation of the processes of respiration, phonation, articulation, resonance, and prosody. Few speakers, however, accomplish excellence in all dimensions of "fluidity." Hence, a generally wide range of normal overall fluency is observed. It is when a speaker exceeds the "normal" limits on one or more of the dimensions that the speech-language pathologist becomes involved.

In speech pathology the term "fluency of speech" has come to mean the continuous smooth ongoingness of articulation. When there are breaks in the "temporal ongoingness," the person is said to be speaking "disfluently." The different types of speech disfluencies that can be identified are listed in Chapter 9. Obviously there can be many reasons for the occurrence of such disruptions in the temporal process of articulating. Unfortunately only limited research has been done to investigate the reasons for increases or decreases in disfluency, let alone the reasons why specific types of disfluency vary. Most of the work reported has been done within the framework of studying stuttering. As discussed in Chapter 10, the label "stuttering" is an evaluative word which refers to a person's opinion of the way someone is speaking. It is not a descriptive term for a definitive entity within the speech behavior of the speaker. To restrict investigations to a study of the "real" disfluencies that constitute "stuttering" limits the investigation of all aspects of disfluent behavior that would further our knowledge of various fluency problems that may develop at any age.

Wingate (30) attempted to provide a "standard definition of stuttering." He believed that such a definition "can serve as a stable and veridical frame of reference, to reorient and perhaps reduce some amount of the controversy in the area of stuttering, and to provide a basis for a more systematic and efficient approach in the study of stuttering." In his attempt to differentiate "stuttering" from "normal disfluency" he decided that the "kernel" characteristics of stuttering speech are repetitions (audible or silent) of single-unit speech elements and prolongations (audible or silent). "One or the other, or both of these kernel characteristics are found in *all* cases of stuttering; in effect, it is by virtue of these characteristics that certain types of disfluent speech are called 'stuttering.'" On the surface this "definition" may look clear-cut. Many researchers have adopted it and now include only phoneme or one-syllable repetition and prolongation in their analysis of "stuttering."

If one takes a second look at the definition, however, it makes sense only if stutterers can be differentiated from nonstutterers on the basis of that definition. Much research is available which indicates that most children have some part-word repetition and prolongation in their speech. Therefore, by his definition, most children stutter. Later in the presentation of his definition he states that "these disruptions usually occur frequently or are marked in character and are not readily controllable." The term "frequently" and the expression "marked in character" require an *evaluation* by the listener. The term "readily controllable" is also an *evaluation* that should be quantitatively determined. Therefore, we are left with the declaration that most children stutter and that it is only when they do too much "stuttering" that people decide they have a "problem of stuttering." His definition can easily be interpreted as saying that when a child has too much disfluency (particularly part-word repetition and prolongation) and his listeners evaluate that he is doing too much of it, then they consider this to be "stuttering."

The evaluative label of "stuttering" is applied to varying amounts of disfluency, "breaks in fluency," "fluency failure," "fragmentation of fluency," or whatever one wants to call it. More descriptively, we are referring to interruptions in the fluent flow of speech. These consist of prolongations, repetitions, interjections, revisions, broken words, et cetera. They can be observed and measured reliably. The need in the area of fluency disorders is to cease arguing about and attempting to "validate" the term stutter. We should recognize it for what it is—an evaluation. The need is to attempt differential diagnosis on the basis of factors that contribute to increased disfluency in speech, recognizing that the higher persons move on the continuum of disfluency, the more likely it is that the important listeners in their environment—and they themselves—will begin to react to these disfluencies as "stuttering." Therefore, we are attempting to make a distinction between the behavior of disfluency and the reaction on the part of a speaker that results in his tensing, struggling to "control" or minimize, or in a more general sense coping constructively with the breakdown in fluency. It is this reaction and his resulting attempts to cope with it that result in the problem of stuttering. Having made this distinction, it becomes increasingly possible to investigate the many variables that may contribute to increased or decreased disfluency. Within this framework there is no ambiguity about the fact that a child may have difficulty with language formulation—to be disfluent as he or she struggles to cope with language—and begin to react negatively to the disfluencies. Clinically, the result can be a problem of stuttering. But the research question that needs to be asked is, "What aspects of language development are likely to promote increased—or decreased—disfluency?" Likewise an adult may suffer a stroke after which her total frequency of disfluency—or of certain types of disfluency—may increase dramatically. She may react to these emotionally and behaviorally and within this context begin a "stuttererlike" reaction to them. A clinician needs to do more than conclude, "Golly, she's beginning to stutter." The clinician needs to obtain and evaluate information about the relative change in all types of disfluency, in rate, in prosody, et cetera; the available information about localization of the neurological damage; the resulting motor impairment; and her emotional well-being.

From the viewpoint just proposed one can open up new areas of research that are sorely needed and have been sadly neglected. These consist of investigations of the factors that can contribute to breaking up the forward flow of speaking behavior. The assumption that "stuttering" is a definable entity within the person promotes researchers to try to find within the person *the cause* for the stuttering. From our present perspective it amounts to erroneously asking, "What is the *one* cause for increased disfluency in speech?"

In this chapter we will discuss, insofar as information is available, fluency problems of children and of adults. They will be discussed with reference to the clinical problem of stuttering because it is from this perspective that most have been studied.

FLUENCY PROBLEMS OF CHILDREN

In this section we will discuss fairly common factors that can result in a relative increase in children's speech disfluencies. These include environmental variables, language development, and cluttering.

Environmental Variables

Most clinicians investigate this area in the case of a child from 3 to 5 years of age who is brought to them because of increased disfluency thought to be stuttering. One investigates aspects of verbal interaction and personal relationship that may have an inhibiting or disrupting influence on the temporal ongoingness of speech production. Much has been written about such factors. (See, for example, discussions by Bloodstein [2] and by Van Riper [26]. Also study carefully the questions suggested in the basic clinical case history outline and the supplementary case history outline on the stuttering problem, pp. 65–72). As discussed in Chapter 2, the clinician tries to determine what in the child's verbal interactions may be responsible for the increased disfluency in order to suggest to the significant persons in the child's environment ways to change their interacting with the child and thus promote increased fluency of speech. This, then, is a form of differential diagnosis.

Language Development

As important as the verbal interaction variables have proven to be, there are other variables that affect the frequency, duration, and type of disfluency. One that is receiving increased attention is language dysfunction. Westby (29), Johnston (16), and Muma (18) have found a positive relationship between increased disfluency and certain language variables. Pratt (19) found significant differences between preschool stutterers and nonstutterers with regard to both perceptual and production aspects of probes that examined phonological and syntactic-semantic abilities. The data presented in these studies are not sufficiently definitive to permit their use by a diagnostic clinician. However, the findings should encourage an increased alertness to the possibility of language dysfunction in some young children who experience increase in disfluencies of speech.

Hall (13) has reported on two language-disordered school-age children who suddenly became excessively disfluent during the course of articulation and language remediation. She proposes that increase in disfluent speech behavior is exhibited by some children as a result of their struggle to acquire language skills.

Riley and Riley (20), responding to the proposed positive relationship between language skills and increased disfluency, have developed a diagnostic model which combines various components of language with those of interpersonal relationship. They refer to "specific components" and to "general components" of the problem. Under "specific components" they list "(1) auditory monitoring, (2) auditory cognition, (3) syntax planning, and (4) motor planning." The "general components" consist of "(1) attending disorder in the child which parallels a disruptive family environment affecting the child's attempts to communicate, (2) unrealistic expectations or standards imposed on the child by himself or by his parents, and (3) the child's need to stutter because it has become useful to him in some way or his parents need for him to stutter because his disorder satisfies some need in them." Currently they are developing procedures for assessing each component and are collecting data to test the model. Even though the model is based on sound clinical observations, it is too early to assess its validity. The important point to be made is that research is being done which one hopes will eventually enable diagnostic clinicians to do a better job than they are now able to do in assessing the role of language acquisition in increased disfluency—particularly part-word repetition and prolongation—which is likely to result in the reactions of stuttering.

Cluttering

The syndrome called cluttering is accompanied by considerable disfluency. Bloodstein (2, p. 44) describes cluttering as "a disorder of fluency marked by monotonous, rapid, jerky, repetitive, indistinct utterance with frequent telescoping of words, unaccompanied by fear, anticipation, any sense of difficulty with specific words or sounds or even a detailed awareness of speaking abnormality." This description represents a compendium of observations made by many investigators over the years. Most have directed their attention toward describing differences and similarities between the behaviors of cluttering and stuttering. This task has proven to be difficult because a child may begin displaying a relatively "pure" form of cluttering and then because of pressures to "talk better" may develop stuttering reactions. Then, of course, one is able to observe components of both disorders. Bloodstein (2, p. 293) gives an example of a boy who showed definite characteristics of cluttering; following pressures by his "parents, sister, aunt, and even a few of his friends" to "slow down," he developed a problem of stuttering at age 14.

Nonetheless, Freund (12) in 1934 undertook to tabulate the behaviors that he thought differentiated the two disorders. He reported further on his observations and theoretical considerations of the two disorders in 1952 and 1966 (10, 11).

Other authors, notably Arnold (1), Luchsinger and Arnold (17), and Weiss (28) have also listed behavioral features that distinguish cluttering from stuttering. Van Riper (27) has provided an excellent summary of their observations reproduced in Table 14.1. From this table it may appear easy to differentiate the two disorders. "However," as Van Riper states, "in actual practice we find many patients who are very difficult to categorize. In part this is due to human variability which always defies nice, tight classification especially into dichotomies but it may also be due to the criteria used. Specifically, the pairs of distinctive features appear clear and reasonable. In practice, they present great difficulties in precise assessment" (27, p. 349). He further points out that one seldom finds a speaker who demonstrates *all* of the characteristics of either disorder and that no one can specify how many characteristics of each a speaker must display before he can be placed unequivocally into that category. We would like to suggest for consideration several other reasons why the categories are not discrete.

TABLE 14.1
Differentiation Between Stuttering and Cluttering

	Clutterers	Stutterers
Freund [1952]		
(personality traits)	Aggressive	Timid
	Extroverted	Introspective
	Uncontrolled	Overinhibited
Arnold [1960]		
Handwriting	Disintegrated and incoordinated	Seemingly normal
Speaking to superiors	Better	Worse
Having to repeat	Improves	Aggravates
Calling attention to speech	Improves	Aggravates
Luchsinger and Arnold [1965]		
Onset	Gradual	Sudden
Handedness	Familial laterality disorders	Normal
Silent reading	Dyslectic or slow	Not disturbed
Language development	Severely delayed	Normal or early
Weiss [1964]		
Speaking in relaxed situation	Worse	Better
Attitude toward own speech	Careless	Fearful
Short answers	Better	Worse
EEG	Often diffuse dysrhythmia	Usually normal

Source: From Van Riper, *27;* by permission of S. Karger A. G., Basel.

We mentioned earlier that it is entirely possible for a person to begin stuttering as a result of negative reactions to cluttering. Such a person would show characteristics of both disorders. Also the suggested response to each behavioral category in Table 14.1 is not *necessarily* true. For example, Luchsinger and Arnold state that "onset" is "gradual" for clutterers and "sudden" for stutterers. In his extensive study of the onset of stuttering, Johnson (*15*) found, on the contrary, that on the average five to six months elapsed between the time parents reported they first noticed disfluencies and the time they considered that the child had a problem of stuttering.

There are exceptions to other behavioral characteristics that may "generally" characterize adults who stutter; even more important, however, are the exceptions in the behavior of children. For example, Freund states that stutterers are "timid, introspective, and overinhibited." These characteristics do not apply at all to many children who stutter. With due awareness of the limitations of the conclusions presented in Table 14.1, we believe that they provide helpful guidelines for the clinician faced with the problem of differentially diagnosing cluttering and stuttering. Currently they are the best we have.

FLUENCY PROBLEMS OF ADULTS

Some problems of fluency begin in adulthood. Ordinarily the onset is sudden and occurs in conjunction with some form of neurologic or psychiatric problem. The neuropathology is usually the result of brain damage caused by disease, a stroke, or head injuries. The psychiatric problems may be many and varied and often are identified by such terms as "anxiety tension state" and "conversion hysteria." The temporal dimension of the person's speaking behavior is affected. Speech disfluencies may increase dramatically. Speech prosody (rate, rhythm, inflection and stress patterns) may change noticeably, in certain instances to a degree that the speech sounds quite bizarre. There may be varying degrees of muscular tensing and "struggling" accompanying the person's efforts to talk. It is not surprising that when these problems occur, and especially if there is a relative increase in part-word or word repetition or in prolongations, the label "stuttering" is frequently applied. This use of the term has introduced into the literature such terms as "cortical stuttering," "neurogenic stuttering," "aphasic stuttering," and "neurotic stuttering." The use of these terms can be confusing to a clinician because it is easy to assume from them that there are different *types* of stuttering.

We must place the fluency problems that begin in adulthood into a perspective that provides a consistent base from which to assess the different behaviors. As with the fluency problems of children, there are many reasons known—and undoubtedly many unknown—why an increase in disfluency may occur in adults. Simply because certain persons lump these behaviors together into the category of "stuttering" does not mean that they are *necessarily* synonymous with the stuttering problem discussed in Chapter 10. They are not. To consider them to be synonymous creates confusion for the clinician in diagnosis and in planning therapy. This was brought forcibly to our attention by a recent phone call from a speech clinician who was planning a therapy program for a patient previously labeled a "stuttering aphasic." The clinician inquired as to whether she should work first with the problem of stuttering or with the problem of aphasia. This example raises a fundamental question: is a speech-language pathologist justified in making the diagnosis of "stuttering" on the basis of a single variable, namely, speech disfluencies—most often repetitions and prolongations of sounds—in disregard of other variables? We reiterate: "stuttering" is an evaluative not a descriptive term. No data exist that permit us to differentiate stuttering from nonstuttering with the presence of speech disfluencies as the sole criterion.

Sander (25) has reported that nonclinicians often use the terms "stuttering" and "syllable repetitions" synonymously. They reserve the word "stutterer" for a child whom they consider has a "problem of stuttering," that is, who is doing *too much* repeating. Yet if we consider the problem from a different direction, we see a different meaning of the word "stuttering." When parents bring their child to a clinic or when a classroom teacher consults a speech clinician, they often ask the question, "Is Johnny stuttering?" They are not asking if you can hear any speech disfluencies. They can hear them; they consulted the clinician because of them. They want to know if the clinician, upon assessing variables *in addition* to the fact that there are speech disfluencies, considers that the child has a problem.

Now let us return to fluency problems of adult onset. We must guard against reacting unprofessionally and arriving at a diagnosis of "stuttering" based upon a single variable, namely, the presence of syllable repetitions or sound prolongations. If a medical practitioner made a diagnosis based on the same logic, the results would be absurd. For example, if a person sprains a wrist, swelling occurs at the joint. Swelling also often occurs in an arthritic joint. If the doctor's next patient has swelling in the area of the mandibular joint, the diagnosis, if based on a single symptom, could be "sprained arthritic mumps."

Now let us reassess the logic of the diagnosis mentioned earlier of "stuttering aphasic." The diagnosis of "aphasia" was based on the conditions surrounding the onset, observations of the client's behavior, and his performance during specially designed language tasks. The diagnosis of "stuttering" was based on the observation that there were "noticeable" part-word and word repetitions during speech, or, in other words, on a single behavior variable. We suggest that before you make a diagnosis of stuttering in the case of adult fluency problems, in addition to obtaining information about the onset and development of the problem, you study in detail the patient's disfluent behavior and how it varies.

Behavioral Analysis of Stuttering

Probably the single most distinctive aspect of stuttering is its variability under different speaking conditions. The main thrust of the appraisal of the stuttering problem discussed in Chapter 10 is toward determining the variability of various dimensions of the problem for each stutterer. Even though there may be, and usually are, large differences among stutterers with regard to conditions under which their stuttering varies, there are also certain conditions under which most stutterers respond similarly.[1] Understanding of the conditions under which most stutterers

[1] The literature on stuttering is liberally sprinkled with documentation of such conditions. See Bloodstein (2) or Van Riper (26) for discussion and documentation of these conditions.

behave similarly provides a foundation for procedures that will help us differentiate the clinical problem of stuttering from other adult fluency problems. Therefore, when faced with the task of evaluating the fluency problem of an adult whose problem is recent in onset, observe his or her behavior and compare it with what we know about the behavior of stutterers:

1. Listeners affect stuttering. People are important factors in stuttering. A person's stuttering is greatly reduced or absent when talking to a horse, a dog, or himself. It takes other people as listeners to produce stuttering. Moreover, it varies in amount and severity depending on the speaker's evaluations of the person with whom he or she is communicating.
2. Manner of speaking affects stuttering. Stuttering is greatly reduced or absent under the following conditions:
   a. When talking or reading in rhythm to a stimulus, including timing each syllable with the beat of a metronome or rhythmic finger tapping.
   b. When singing.
   c. When reading aloud in unison with another person.
   d. When dramatically slowing down speaking rate (talking at approximately 25–30 words per minute) but with continuous vocalization and prolongation ("dragging out") of each vowel.
   e. When whispering or just mouthing the words in the absence of air flow.
   f. When talking in the presence of a loud masking noise (approximately 90 dB) fed into both ears.
3. Speaking task affects stuttering. There usually is a reduction in stuttering with repeated oral reading of the same passage. Moreover, when the person stutters during successive readings of the passage, the stutterings tend to occur on the same words. These are called the adaptation and consistency effects and are discussed in Chapter 9.
4. The words spoken and their location in the sentence affect stuttering (loci of stuttering).
   a. Adults stutter more often on words which begin a sentence (the first three words) than on the later words.
   b. They stutter more often on nouns, verbs, adjectives, and adverbs (lexical words) than on other parts of speech (function words).
   c. They stutter more often on longer words (five or more letters) than on shorter words.
   d. They stutter more often on words beginning with consonants than on those beginning with vowels.[2]

---

[2] The fact that stuttering occurs more often on words beginning with consonants than on those beginning with vowels may be associated more with the nature of the English language than with the nature of stuttering. Sasanuma (24) found that the

5. Miscellaneous factors affect the characteristics of stuttering.
   a. Most often a person stutters on the first syllable of the word. Stuttering may occur, however, on any syllable production but *not* after the completion of the final syllable of a word that completes the person's verbal *message* (I'm going—ing—ing—ing"; "I'm going outside—ide—ide—ide") or in a single-word answer to a question, such as, "No—o—o."
   b. Stutterers can predict words on which they will and will not stutter and people to whom they will or will not stutter. As a result, they report that they avoid the use of certain words, often substituting other words for them.
   c. Not only does each stutterer have a unique stuttering pattern, but the stuttering pattern of each stutterer varies. The severity (amount of tensing, duration of stuttering, and associated behavior) varies during a single conversation. Each speaker stutters relatively more severely on some words than on others.
   d. There is emotional reaction associated with the anticipation of stuttering and during an instance of stuttering. The reaction is more than just one of frustration. It includes embarrassment, shame, and humiliation. The intensity of these feelings usually is related to the severity of stuttering at a given time.

During the evaluation of a person with a stuttering problem, the experienced clinician usually looks for the variations of behavior described above. However, seldom does one record them systematically. No data are available which permit us to predict the percentage of time that each behavioral characteristic will obtain for each stutterer. Nor can we explain the significance of the absence of one or two of the characteristics. However, we are reasonably certain that a sufficiently high percentage of them will be present with any given stutterer to enable us to piece together a composite of the behavioral syndrome of stuttering.

Likewise there is a dearth of information available about the behavioral characteristics of fluency problems other than stuttering, including those associated with neurologic and psychiatric disorders. Seldom are the fluency behavior patterns described. They are merely "explained" as "neurogenic stuttering." This practice does little to further our understanding of the problem. It does, however, provide a professional-sounding label under which to umbrella our ignorance.

Three case reports will be presented of adults referred to the University of Iowa Speech and Hearing Clinic for evaluation of fluency problems

---

Japanese perform similarly to Americans with regard to (a), (b), and (c) but not with regard to (d). For the Japanese, more stuttering occurs on words beginning with vowels than on those beginning with consonants. However, she reported that in the Japanese language, nouns, verbs, adjectives, and adverbs (which, incidentally, are also the longer words) more often begin with vowels than with consonants whereas in English the opposite is true.

that had been diagnosed by the referring physician as "sudden onset of stuttering." They are reported in fair detail so that you can become aware of the complexities involved in assessing problems of people. As you read them, keep asking yourself the question, "What is *the cause* for the fluency problem?" After you read the neurological report are you ready to make a diagnosis? Does it change after you read the psychiatric report? Does the speech report provide "the answer"?

Case 1

LK,[3] a 53-year-old woman, reported the onset of a severe headache. "I passed out or blacked out—or at least I went to sleep. . . . When I came to, I couldn't get my words out right—just like I can't now." She was referred to the University of Iowa Hospitals.

Neurological Report   X-ray films of the skull, cerebrospinal fluid, electroencephalograms, and one-hour and five-hour brain scans were normal. A rapid-sequence brain scan demonstrated a mildly decreased blood flow through the left internal carotid and left middle cerebral arteries. There was no reduction in disfluency after intravenous amobarbital. *Diagnosis:* Stuttering associated with mild cerebral ischemia.

Psychiatric Report   Approximately 15 years prior to her hospital admission her oldest daughter's husband attempted to rape her. She and her husband pressed charges against him and at the time of the trial he did not deny his attempt. Ever since, the patient has been in great fear that her son-in-law would return and attack her. This fear increased when her husband died six years ago. (Her complaint of frequent headaches began approximately six years ago.) Quite frequently after that she has kept a hammer by her bed so that she could fight off her son-in-law should he come. She has many locks on her house, but she does not feel that they would stop him. She states that she has never accepted her husband's death, that she has had a sleep disturbance and poor appetite ever since. (Two members of her husband's immediate family stuttered.) She occasionally gets suicidal thoughts: "What is the need to go on? There is nothing to live for"; but she reports that she would not act on these thoughts. One year ago her 25-year-old son moved out of her home and she was completely alone at night. Her fear of being attacked by her son-in-law increased. She had not seen him for over a year until one week before her admission to the hospital. She was taken by her 25-year-old son to her eldest daughter's home for dinner. Her son-in-law was there. She did not speak to him nor did he speak to

---

[3] Case LK is the same patient about whom Rosenfield (23) wrote a "Letter to the Editor" entitled "Stuttering and cerebral ischemia." In his letter the speech evaluation report was abstracted to such an extent that a reader might easily misinterpret the nature of her speech behavior.

her, but she was terrified of him and she did not leave the sight of her son or daughter for fear of him. When she returned home, she felt "weak and sick." Five days later her severe headache began in connection with which she "passed out." Upon reaching consciousness, she reports that the difficulty with speaking (something like stuttering) began. She has no idea of the source of her symptoms, but she states that she is in terrible fear of her son-in-law.

Impression   Anxiety state in a depressive neurosis. The patient suffered a traumatic event with the attempted rape by her son-in-law. She made a neurotic adjustment to this conflict which was further weakened by the loss of her husband and then by her son moving from her home. Soon before the beginning of her symptoms, she was again confronted with her son-in-law which reintensified her anxiety which has now, we believe, led to her speech symptomatology. The patient has a chronic depression.

Speech Evaluation   The speech evaluation revealed no evidence of dysarthria or oral apraxia. If speech apraxia was present, it was a much milder form of difficulty than the speech deficit usually associated with that condition. She controlled phonation quite well and her prime speech errors were distortions (not substitutions) and repetitions or prolongations of correct phonemes.

The frequency of speech disfluencies remained relatively constant (range 27–31 disfluencies per 100 words spoken) during speaking or reading orally under a variety of conditions. She reported that while talking alone in her hospital room she talked the same way. On one occasion she was left alone in a clinical room (although she was observed through a one-way window as she practiced reading aloud). There was no change in frequency of disfluency. Her disfluencies did not decrease when she spoke to a rhythmic beat, sang, read orally in unison with the examiner, slowed down her rate of speech by using continuous vocalizations and "dragging out" the vowels, whispered, or just mouthed the words.

There was no adaptation effect during repeated readings of the same passage either in frequency, duration, or behavioral characteristics. The consistency effect was minimal: she was disfluent more often on the first three words of a sentence than on the other words, but there was no predictable pattern with regard to the other three factors usually associated with the loci of stuttering.

Her disfluency types consisted of part-word repetition and prolongation. Part-word repetition occurred for the most part at the beginning of a word but the prolongations never did. She consistently prolonged sounds in the following way: "go—iiinng," "fu—nnnny." The only repetitions that occurred other than at the beginning of words appeared following a prolongation, for example: "goiii—i—i—ng." Repetitions ranged from two to four per instance. Prolongations lasted approximately one to two seconds, never longer.

There was general increase in tension throughout her whole body when she began to talk. On the first day that she was seen there was no increase in tensing associated with any disfluency. By the third day tensing increased in the oral area during the repetitions that followed a prolongation (pattern described previously); this was followed by a slight head jerk timed with the completion of the word. Occasionally she would stop in the middle of the repetition, shake her head, frown, and start over again. This behavior never occurred if she spoke *only* with a part-word repetition or a prolongation. She never repeated a whole word, even a monosyllabic word.

She expressed some apprehension about talking because of the trouble she was having, but she reported that she did not anticipate difficulty on any particular word. In fact, as she stated, "That's what is so frustrating. I think I'm talking all right and then I hear my speech repeating itself. I can't believe it's me." She did not avoid or substitute words.

She reported that her main emotional reaction while talking was that of frustration because she did not know what to do about her difficulty. She said that it worried her because if she did not stop doing it before she returned home, she did not know whether she could "hold her job" as a waitress. If she lost that job, she did not know what she would do. She was "too old for any one else to hire her."

Conclusions   On the single variable of speech disfluencies, she sounded as if she "stuttered." However, her speech behavior was highly consistent. There was no condition found in which the disfluency pattern was not present and in which the behavioral characteristics were not consistent. This consistency is directly opposite to the variability observed in stuttering. Therefore, it was concluded that her fluency problem was not the clinical problem of stuttering. The only behavior similar to that of stuttering (other than the disfluencies) was the increased tensing and slight head jerk first observed the third day after admission to the hospital.

LK was seen by a speech pathologist for one hour a day for three successive days. She was informed that she was not beginning to "stutter" as she had feared. Since it was likely that the way she talked related to the condition that brought her to the hospital, it was unlikely that her "bobbles" would become worse. She was informed that it would not help to "fight" her bobbles by tensing or by trying to stop them. Instead she was encouraged to talk all she could and to read the newspaper aloud for approximately an hour a day. She followed the instructions diligently. She almost immediately ceased tensing and jerking her head. During the three-day period her disfluencies decreased in frequency to 15 percent of words spoken.

LK returned to the hospital eight weeks later. Her speech was normal from the standpoint of both fluency and phoneme accuracy. She reported that she had read aloud daily and that within a week her speech had "returned" to normal.

There is no way of knowing whether the clinical suggestions had any direct effect on her speech or whether she would have improved anyway. However, the clinical suggestions are reported here to show that they were devised in consideration of her specific fluency problem, not from the framework of a "stuttering therapy program."

Case 2

DW, a 55-year-old patient in a Veterans Administration Hospital, presented on admission complaint of "frequent spells of dizziness with several instances of passing out." *Diagnosis:* Cerebrovascular accident probably as a result of arteriosclerosis. Brain scan indicated damage to the posterior portion of the frontal cortex. The psychiatric evaluation indicated an essentially healthy individual. "Currently, the patient is in a mild depressive state but one that is appropriate for his recent medical problems." He was referred to the University of Iowa Speech and Hearing Clinic for evaluation of "stuttering."

Speech Evaluation

The speech evaluation indicated no dysarthria but mild to moderate apraxia of speech. He spoke slowly, often groping toward the target phoneme. There was little variation in pitch or loudness. He gave the appearance of "talking carefully." His disfluency pattern consisted of sound and syllable repetitions and prolongation and interjection of sounds. More disfluencies occurred on longer words and longer sentences. During regular conversation and oral reading, they occurred on 14–18 percent of the words. When he read sentences "loaded" with long words, the frequency of disfluency increased to 26 percent of the words spoken. When he read a list of monosyllabic words (no more than four letters in length), frequency decreased to 9 percent. The proportion of disfluencies remained relatively constant from situation to situation (while talking to different people, to a group, in front of a TV camera, etc.). There was no reduction in disfluency when manner of speaking was varied, for example, singing, reading in unison, speaking to a rhythmic beat. There was one exception, however: when he was asked to mouth words in the absence of airflow, he experienced considerable difficulty in producing any movement sequence that corresponded to that requested of him.

There was no adaptation effect during repeated readings of the same passage either in frequency, duration, or behavioral characteristics. In fact, frequency increased 10 percent from the first to the third reading.

Some consistency effect was noted for the longer words in the reading passage. As to the loci of disfluencies, he was more disfluent on longer words (those that contained five letters or more, particularly polysyllabic words). He was more disfluent on words beginning with consonants than on those beginning with vowels. He was more disfluent on lexical words than on function words. However, he was no more disfluent on the first words of the sentence than he was on any others.

As noted earlier, the disfluency types were prolongations and interjections of sounds and sound and syllable repetitions. One sentence was spoken thus: "I bu—b—b—bi—l———eave in goo———d k—k—gu—gover———m———ent. Repetitions lasted from two to four seconds per instance of repetition. Sound prolongations lasted one second or less and consisted mostly of a "dragging out" of the vowel more than one usually associates with prolongation; they suggested dysrhythmic phonation. In the opinion of the examiner and other observers, he appeared to be concentrating intently on how he was talking. Nevertheless, there was no noticeable increase of tension during any instance of disfluency. Occasionally he would frown during a syllable repetition on which he was changing vowels (e.g., bu—bo—boy) from one repetition to the next.

He reported no feeling of anticipation of trouble as he was talking. He said, "I never know it until I start saying it. . . . What I'm thinking and what I'm doing aren't always the same thing." He reported no particular emotional feelings associated with being disfluent. He commented, "I just want to be understood. With what's happening to me, I'm just lucky to be this well off." When asked if he would be interested in practicing some each day in an effort to improve the way he talked, he responded, "No, people can understand me. What more do I need?"

DW's speech remained relatively constant over the four-month period until he was dismissed from the hospital. There has been no contact with him since that time.

Conclusions   DW demonstrated part-word repetition and prolongation (dysrhythmic phonation) types of disfluencies. However, these disfluencies were different from those usually associated with stuttering. He frequently changed the vowel phoneme within a repeated syllable, at times a consonant phoneme. Instead of being rapid in rate, his repetitions were slow and measured. The only variability of disfluency observed during different speech tasks that corresponded to that found in stuttering is also characteristic of speech apraxia. Therefore, we concluded that the temporal dimension of speech was affected by apraxia of speech and a diagnosis of stuttering was contraindicated.

Case 3

CV, a 41-year-old woman, was admitted to the University of Iowa Hospital with the following story. On the day prior to admission, she took a nap in the afternoon. Upon awakening, she developed "numbness" of the left side of her body. Soon after there was swelling of the left side of her face and neck, her left arm, and her left leg. She complained of "weakness" in the left arm, unverified at the time because of the extreme pain she experienced if she moved her arm or hand. She reported an occipital headache. During the first hospital day she was observed to speak with "repetitive stuttering of first syllables."

On the second day the numbness, swelling, and headache subsided but the frequent speech disfluencies persisted. Examination revealed no weakness of the left arm or hand. On the third day she developed swelling and itching of the palms of both hands, the soles of both feet, and in the chest area. These were diagnosed as chronic urticaria (hives), a problem she had had at irregular intervals for several years. This condition improved steadily throughout her hospitalization.

EEG Report   Abnormal EEG with predominant left anterior temporal-midtemporal 4–5 per second slow waves. Sharp waves occurred from this same region. The findings are compatible with a focal left anterior temporal-midtemporal lesion.

Neurology Report   All neurologic signs unilateral and bilateral were normal. Reflexes were normal. There were no motor or sensory deficits. Due to the EEG report of a possible lesion in the left temporal lobe, a left carotid angiogram and a brain scan were performed. Results were "normal."

Conclusions   Although there were symptoms similar to those that occur with a "mild stroke," no definitive signs of neurological impairment could be found. Only definite diagnosis: chronic urticaria (hives).

Psychiatric Report   CV has a humble education. She became pregnant at 16, was then married, and was divorced in six months. She remarried, had two children. After the birth of the last child, she had a tubal ligation. Later she divorced her second husband and remarried. At that time she had corrective tubal surgery in order to have a fourth child. Following a normal pregnancy and birth, she had a hysterectomy. For approximately ten years prior to present hospital admission, she had a history of "collapsing," "severe depression," "fainting and dizzy spells." Previous medical reports found no reasons for these "episodes." *Dynamics:* She no longer has an "ace in the hole," that is she cannot have a baby to strengthen a marriage. She feels extremely inadequate and "lost." A beloved uncle died recently. He always functioned as a major source of strength in times of stress (her father divorced her mother when CV was a child). She has limited emotional outlets so she escapes into somatic reactions. *Secondary Gain:* Her husband is more attentive, affectionate, and stops drinking during any period when she has a "spell" or other "health problems." *Diagnosis:* Psychoneurosis; somatization (functional) reaction.

Speech Evaluation   The speech evaluation was done during the second hospital day. There was no evidence of dysarthria or speech apraxia. Her articulation was normal.

The frequency of occurrence of speech disfluencies varied from 40–50 per 100 words spoken. The frequency remained relatively constant while speaking or reading orally under a variety of conditions. There was no significant change while speaking to one or more listeners or while speaking in her room alone. There was no adaptation or consistency effect during repeated readings of the same passage. Her disfluencies did not occur in any predictable way in relation to the four factors associated with the loci of stuttering. There was no change in frequency of disfluency when she slowed down speaking rate and used continuous vocalization and prolonged vowels. There was no change when she whispered. There was no evidence of "disfluent movements" when she just "mouthed" the words. She sang fluently. During unison reading and while speaking to a rhythmic beat she remained disfluent but the frequency of disfluencies decreased from the usual 40 to 50 per 100 words spoken to approximately 20 per 100.

Her disfluency pattern was remarkably constant. It consisted of one or two quick sound or syllable repetitions followed by a prolongation (one second in duration) of the vowel being repeated, for example, "wa—wa—waaant." There was little pitch or loudness variation when she was speaking either disfluently or fluently; essentially, she spoke in a monotone. However, when she was asked to prolong a vowel, she could vary the pitch and loudness normally. There was no discernible tensing in any areas associated with talking. She reported that she anticipated no difficulty saying any particular word. Furthermore, she stated that she was "totally unconcerned" about the way she talked.

CV was seen again on the third hospital day. Frequency of disfluency had increased from 40–50 percent to approximately 80–90 percent of words spoken. She was tensing, jerking her head forward, and closing her eyes in conjunction with a disfluency. Often she would repeat a syllable once, stop, shake her head, and refuse to finish the word or the statement. When asked about the change in the way she talked, she burst into tears and exclaimed, "I don't want to stutter! I don't want to stutter!" Then she reported (she had not done so previously) that her husband stuttered, particularly when he drank, and that her best girl friend stuttered. She stated, "I couldn't stand it if I sounded as bad as they do."

CV was informed about the nature of stuttering, how it ordinarily begins, and its extreme variability in frequency and severity in different speaking tasks. Her speech behavior was contrasted to that ordinarily found with stutterers. She readily understood because of her acquaintance with the problem. We then concluded that her frequent disfluencies at the time of hospital admission probably were related to the conditions which brought her to the hospital. She was informed that tensing and generally trying to "stop" them would not help. Instead, she was encouraged to "bobble" as easily as she could and to increase rather than to decrease the amount she talked. She was seen on four successive days. The major purpose was to provide encouragement, support, and strong suggestion that "everything would be all right." In addition, two student clinicians volunteered to spend an hour each with her per day in order to provide her an opportunity to talk.

One day after clinical intervention all tensing and struggling had ceased. By the fourth day frequency of disfluency was 8–10 percent of the words spoken. She was cheerful and talked freely and spontaneously, using normal pitch and loudness variations. The next day she was dismissed from the hospital. CV was readmitted to the hospital seven weeks later for severe chronic "hives." Her speech fluency was normal. After this admission she was seen on an outpatient basis in the hospital at eight-week intervals for one year. Her speech remained normal. When asked what she believed helped her most to regain normal speech, she replied, "I have so many health problems that I just panicked when I thought that now I was a stutterer! After I found out that I wasn't, I just worked at talking again."

Conclusions Based on the single variable of speech disfluency, CV sounded as though she "stuttered." Although a few characteristics were similar to those found with the clinical problem of stuttering (fluent when she sang and when she mouthed words), for the most part her speech behavior varied little during different speaking tasks. Perhaps the most remarkable aspect of her speech was the duplication of an almost identical disfluency pattern each time she spoke. On the basis of the initial speech evaluation, it was concluded that this was a fluency problem different from that of the clinical problem of stuttering. However, in one day's time her overt emotional and behavioral reactions to the disfluency became highly similar to the reaction patterns observed with "stuttering."

As in the case of LK, there is no way of knowing whether CV would have regained normal fluency without clinical intervention. It is interesting to note, however, that tensing and struggling ceased within 24 hours after intervention, and within three days the frequency of disfluency had reduced from 80–90 percent to 8–10 percent of the words spoken.

Although only three cases are presented, they serve to alert you to the need for as much information as possible about a person before you "jump" at a conclusion about a causal relationship between variables. Case LK is an excellent example. Rosenfield (23) briefly presented her case study from the standpoint of the neurological findings. In his discussion he strongly implied that cerebral ischemia was *the cause* of increased disfluencies. A psychiatrist could have taken LK's psychiatric report and published an article in a psychiatric journal reporting that *the cause* was an "anxiety state in a depressive neurosis." An energetic speech-language pathologist might have read both articles and reported on one case of "neurogenic stuttering" and one of "neurotic stuttering" —not realizing that he was reporting on the same person.

Case DW presents a picture that suggests a fairly clear relationship between neurological impairment and increased disfluency. At least the phenomena occurred concomitantly. Moreover, the disfluent speech behavior appears to fit the syndrome of apraxia of speech more closely than it does that of stuttering.

Case CV, although presenting no hard evidence of neurological involvement, demonstrated symptoms suggestive of such involvement. But there is relatively more evidence of a positive relationship between her sudden increase in disfluencies and her emotional problems.

So far we have not touched on the fact that for certain people neurological pathologies may precipitate emotional reactions; for others, a psychoneurosis may, in time, be a contributing factor to certain neurological impairments. Because of our culture's basically dualistic philosophy (i.e., problems have to be *either* in the body *or* in the mind), we are prone to overlook the probable relationship between the two. This philosophy also encourages us to posit *the cause* for a certain behavior pattern immediately upon our observing a malfunction in *either* the neurological *or* the psychiatric system.

If we insist on proceeding in this manner, we must be able to answer the question: specifically *what* "causes" specifically *what?* Unfortunately we lack specific data concerning the "what" of the neurologic or psychiatric system that *causes* the specific "what" of the speech (i.e., disfluencies and their variability or alterations of prosody). There is value in adopting a language that does not carry with it the implication that we know more than we actually do. A more responsible language is one in which we state that "it appears that there is a relationship between two or more factors" or "one factor appears to be some function of another one." At least this type of language serves to remind us of areas where research is sorely needed. It should also prompt the diagnostic clinician (1) to read the literature carefully, analyzing the facts presented as well as cataloguing diligently relevant facts that are omitted, and (2) to gather all available information about a client and sift it thoughtfully before arriving at tentative conclusions that serve as bases for clinical intervention procedures.

Review of Reports of Differential Diagnosis of Adult Onset of "Stuttering"

There are relatively few published reports concerning the differential diagnosis of stuttering. Even these few are not consistent in what they are attempting to differentiate from what. Even so, you should become aware of the information available because it can stimulate your thinking and your future research.

Canter (5) has discussed the differential diagnosis of "neurogenic stuttering" in adults. He assumes that "neurogenic stuttering" exists in an individual whose "abnormal disfluency derives from damage to the central nervous system." There are questions that need to be asked. For example, what is the type, frequency, and duration of disfluency? How does it vary and under what conditions? What is the nature of the "damage" to the CNS? None of these questions are answered. Apparently Canter assumes that "abnormal" breaks in fluency constitute "stuttering"; he is defining "stuttering" on a single dimension much as nonprofessionals do. Then he attempts to differentiate dysarthric, apraxic, and dysnomic stuttering. He describes the syndromes of dysarthria, apraxia, and dysnomia and notes that breaks in fluency may occur within each syndrome. He does not differentiate the clinical problem of stuttering from other fluency problems that may exist as part of a different behavior syndrome. This is demonstrated clearly by his conclusion that there is "little basis for not considering" the repetitious speech observed in *palilalia* as "moments of stuttering." (The disorder of speech called palilalia will be discussed later. It should be evident at that time that it is quite different from the behavior most speech-language pathologists consider to be stuttering.)

Canter offers several general observations about the nature of the disfluent speech behavior of his "neurogenic stutterers." Although he does not relate them in any particular type of disorder, for example, dysarthria, apraxia, or dysphonia, his observations highlight the need for systematic study in these areas to help us develop meaningful guidelines for differential diagnosis. He notes that repetitions and prolongations occur on final consonants. The loci of disfluency are different from those of stuttering. Speakers may have more difficulty during unison reading than they have during self-formulated speech. The adaptation effect is not observed. A speaker may be "annoyed" by his or her disfluencies but not anxious about them. Secondary symptomatology does not develop.

Caplan (6) has compared the occurrence of "stutterlike" disfluencies of five adult dysphasic patients with the disfluency usually observed in stuttering. All subjects were classified as "predominantly expressive aphasics who were able to communicate spontaneously and meaningfully." All manifested "some degree of non-fluency in their speech." They also "showed a variety of specific language disturbances, the most notable being anomia and apraxia." No other information was provided about the subjects. Therefore, we lack specific information about each subject's neurological condition and his concomitant behavioral syndrome. The description of the subjects' disfluent speech must be evaluated with that in mind.

The subjects were disfluent on 16 to 39 percent of the words spoken.

However, interjections, revisions, and word repetitions (interjections occurring most frequently) were the high-frequency disfluencies with part-word repetitions representing the low frequency. The "majority of subjects" experienced more difficulty on the functional words of language than on the content or lexical words, contrary to the usual finding for stutterers. The subjects experienced relatively more disfluency on the initial words of a sentence, on longer words, and on words beginning with consonants, behaviors similar to those observed in stutterers. (As was discussed earlier in this chapter with respect to case DW, these behaviors are likely to occur with apraxic patients also.) The adaptation task yielded "divergent results." On the basis of the foregoing analysis Caplan concluded that the frequency of disfluency justified the label of "stuttering" but that the "nature of the dysfluencies was much like that observed in normal speakers."

Caplan pointed out that "the disorder of stuttering encompasses much more than moments of dysfluency and that dysfluency *per se* does not constitute the whole of the problem known as stuttering." He then determined the degree to which each subject's speech "sounded" like stuttering. He asked three clinicians to listen to tape-recorded samples of speech and to comment upon them. Their comments referred as much to the "intent" of the speaker as they did to a description of the speaking behavior. The implications of this outcome are important to you as a clinician concerned with differential diagnosis. If you *assume* that a person is "stuttering" and therefore evaluate all behavior from that perspective, it is deceptively easy (1) to *evaluate* hesitancy and false starts as "avoidance of a feared word," (2) to *evaluate* interjections as "antiexpectancy devices," (3) to *evaluate* revisions as "circumlocutions," and (4) to *evaluate* labored articulatory movements and a slow uneven rate as "tension and anxiety about stuttering." The degree to which you, as a clinician, fall into this evaluative trap will be the degree to which you are a victim of your own perceptual limitations surely as much as your patient is a victim of his or her own motor performance limitations imposed by neurological or psychiatric deficits. Not to recognize this is to ensure the perpetuation of confusion between fact and fiction in the differential diagnosis of fluency problems.

One of the most complete descriptions in the literature of the neurological, speech, and language findings pertaining to a single case was reported by Rosenbek, McNeil, Lemme, and Alfrey (21). The patient, a 36-year-old male, was hospitalized for severe uremia and was placed on chronic intermittent hemodialysis therapy. The subsequent physiological and neurological deterioration is described. Seven years later "a speech disturbance" described as "stuttering or stammering was first noticed and the patient also related he had some deterioration of memory." He was referred to a speech pathologist for his "stuttering." It is interesting to note that the first signs of deterioration of speech and language were sound and syllable repetitions. They were followed by problems of language and speech too numerous to mention here but described in detail in the report. Of interest for our purposes is the fact that the authors describe the patient's disfluent speech behavior in the context of other impairments of language and speech. In this perspective the disfluencies fit into a cohesive picture of a person whose neurological system is deteriorating. It is not remarkable that fluency disintegrated along with other parameters of speech production. The authors mention that the condition is terminal and that psychotic behavior is common as the condition progresses. The finding, possibly disturbing to those interested in the site of brain lesion and its specific relation to various speech disturbances, is that after the patient's death a brain autopsy revealed "no gross or microscopic changes of any significance."

In discussing the disfluent speech and the possible reasons for it, the authors conclude:

> The sound and syllable repetitions that in part characterized the patient's speech may have resulted from dysarthria, apraxia, aphasia, or one of the possible combinations of these conditions. They may have been in whole or in part secondary reactions to the communication difficulty. Their exact nature and relationship to site of lesion remain to be determined. (21)

This conclusion is especially thought provoking because it summarizes to a large extent our present knowledge concerning the causes of increased disfluency in the speech of adults.

In another report, Rosenbek, Messert, Collins, and Wertz (22) describe the disfluent speech behavior of seven patients who demonstrated what they labeled as "cortical stuttering." They restricted their disfluency analysis to selected disfluency types, namely, sound, syllable, word, and phrase repetitions, and prolongations. As one might expect, the frequency and severity of disfluency varied considerably from subject to subject. Inasmuch as information about other types of disfluency, rate, and prosody was not provided, one cannot draw any conclusions about how the selected types of disfluencies described fit into a composite picture of fluency disintegration. Also little information is presented about the variability of disfluency under different speaking conditions. They mentioned only that three subjects "had more" disfluencies during a spontaneous speech task than during an imitative speech task, two "had more" during the imitative speech task, and two showed "essentially no difference" between the two tasks. One subject whispered the words fluently during the imitative speech task but was disfluent when asked to say them aloud. No mention is made of the other six subjects on this point. They report that the subjects demonstrated a variety of disorders: four were aphasic, two had spastic dysarthria, and for one there was no diagnosis except for the statement "no language deficit." Although they did not collect their data with the goal of determining site of lesion, they state that no single cortical area was unequivocally implicated in their cases. Their review of pertinent literature revealed references to different sites in many areas of either hemisphere. They concluded that the only innocent area at this time appears to be occipital.

Clifford, Aronson, and Peterson (7) approached the problem of "adult onset of stuttering" differently. They studied 34 patients all of whom had been referred to the Mayo Clinic Section of Neurology because of a variety of *neurologic* complaints, including disorders of gait, vertigo, seizures, sensory changes, paralysis, and memory loss. All patients were judged to show "stuttering symptoms." The average age at onset of the "stuttering symptoms" was 44 years. These speech behaviors included "repetitions, hesitations, and/or prolongations of speech." All patients were given neurologic and speech evaluations. In addition they had psychiatric interviews; some were administered the Minnesota Multiphasic Personality Inventory (MMPI).

One of the major purposes of the investigation was to obtain agreement through testing and discussion among the neurologist, psychiatrist, and speech pathologist as to the conditions probably responsible for the increased disfluency of speech. They concluded that the disfluent speech of only 5 of 35 patients could be attributed mainly to neurological deficits; 2 demonstrated dysarthria, 1 was dysphasic, 1 was apraxic, and one had a neurological condition resembling the accelerated speech of Parkinson's disease. The increased disfluency of the remaining 30 patients was attributed primarily to psychiatric problems. Eighteen of these patients were diagnosed as primarily psychoneurotic. The remaining 12 are of particular interest to our discussion. Even though they were diagnosed as having a variety of problems of neurologic origin ("neurological disease," "dysphonia," "apraxia," "CNS disorder," "dysarthria," "diffuse brain damage") the major contributors to the "stuttering symptoms" were judged to be psychogenic. The labels assigned to them included "conversion hysteria," "anxiety tension," "psychoneurotic," "obsessive-compulsive," and "schizoid personality."

The speech behavior of the five patients in the neurologic group was not described. However, for the psychoneurotic group

> stuttering was of sudden or rapid onset immediately following emotionally and physically traumatic events such as automobile accidents, death of a close relative, 'spells,' financial reverses, and anxiety over suspected illness. Speech symptoms for most of them were characterized by abnormally slow rate and repetitions, prolongations, and hesitations on final syllables of words. Several patients in this group were tested for the adaptation effect and were reported to show increase or extremely rapid decrease [in frequency of occurrence with repeated reading of a passage.] There was considerable variability in severity of symptoms throughout the course of the examination. Patients made

little effort to avoid their disfluencies and lack of real concern about their speech was common.[4] (7)

In personal correspondence with the writer, Clifford expanded on the observations reported above. Nineteen of the diagnosed "psychoneurotic group" were administered the MMPI. The MMPI's yielded essentially two patterns: one was consistent with a diagnosis of hysteria (about half of the MMPI's); the other was consistent with high anxiety or psychosis. (The Mayo Clinic has added two scales to the MMPI that fit the "high anxiety" pattern: "The Worried Breadwinner" and "The Tired Housewife." These scales indicated a prevalence of feelings of being overburdened, unrewarded, financially distressed, and emotionally and sexually unfulfilled.) Clifford added a statement that is particularly relevant for a diagnostic clinician: "Although stuttering symptoms were reported to have appeared suddenly or abruptly in the psychoneurotic group, there often was a long history of other symptoms, e.g., spells, dizziness, suspected neurological diseases, etc. One patient seemed to develop the symptoms from examination to examination." In fact, such histories were reported by 21 of the 30 patients.

Even though much specific information was not reported for each patient, the study causes one to question the assumption adopted in the other studies reviewed that a sudden increase in repetitions and prolongations in adult speech must be of neurologic origin. Furthermore, the few general comments made about the speech performance of the patients suggest that much of their disfluent behavior did not correspond to the behavioral syndrome of the clinical problem of stuttering.

Discussion

From the review of the studies concerned with "adult onset of stuttering," one might draw the conclusion that there are different "types" of stuttering. It appears more logical, however, to conclude that there are different reasons for breakdowns in fluency and that the label "stuttering" has been loosely assigned as an umbrella term to encompass all of them. Such labeling does not stimulate new questions that can promote increased understanding of speaking behavior; it can only stifle them because of the implied conclusion that the speaker's increased disfluency is due to the fact that he is "stuttering."

There has been little systematic study of this so-called "stuttering" to determine the degree to which it corresponds to the behavioral syndrome observed in the clinical problem of stuttering, or, for that matter, whether it follows any predictable pattern that may help us diagnose the nature of the fluency problem. In certain neurological disorders disfluencies may

[4] It is interesting to note that "variability in severity of symptoms throughout the course of the examination" is the only behavior that appears to be consistent with the behavior associated with the clinical problem of stuttering discussed previously.

follow a predictable pattern; in others, they may not. The point is that few have thought to ask the question as to whether they do. When a person assumes that he has provided the *answer* by assigning the label "stuttering," it negates the need for any more *questions*. This situation is illustrated by the rather general uncritical acceptance of Wingate's (30) statement that the "kernel" of stuttering is sound and one-syllable repetitions and prolongations. For the general public this is unfortunately generally true. One cannot assume, however, that the reverse is *necessarily* true. That is, it does not follow logically that the "kernel" of repetitions and prolongation *is* stuttering. This is an important point for a clinician concerned with differential diagnosis to keep clearly in mind. A further example may clarify the issue.

An intoxicated person talks with "slurred speech." Therefore, one might conclude that the "kernel" characteristic of intoxication is slurred speech, particularly if the slurring is "marked in character" and is not "readily controllable." It is when one assumes the reverse of the statement to be true that the person engages in irresponsible thinking. Few persons would accept the conclusions that the kernel characteristic of "slurred speech" *is* intoxication. One has only to observe the "slurred speech" characteristics of patients with various types of dysarthria to recognize the fallacy of such reasoning.

With the preceding discussion as a background, we will next consider problems of fluency that may occur concomitantly with various neurogenic disorders in adults. Fluency problems that may accompany psychogenic disorders will not be discussed because little systematic research has been done on the type, frequency, or patterning of disfluency that might occur concomitantly with them.

Adult Fluency Problems

Neurological disorders can produce a profound effect on motor speech, as reviewed in Chapter 18. We will limit our discussion to the fluency problems that may accompany such disorders.

Dysarthria   As discussed previously, there are numerous references in the literature concerning dysarthria and stuttering. Since "dysarthria" and "stuttering" have seldom been adequately defined, such references are, for the most part, difficult to interpret meaningfully.

Darley, Aronson, and Brown (8) have described variations in 38 different dimensions of speech observed in different types of dysarthria. Two of the behavior dimensions were "phonemes repeated" and "phonemes prolonged." Fourteen of 32 patients with the parkinsonism group (hypokinetic dysarthria) "repeated phonemes." The only other patients to do so were 5 of 30 in the dystonia group (hyperkinetic dysarthria). The data reported refer only to the speech samples obtained from the patients under specified conditions. There is no implication that patients in the other dysarthric groups may not show "phoneme repetitions" at times under certain conditions.

On the other hand, many patients in all the dysarthric groups except spastic dysarthria (in pseudobulbar palsy) "prolonged phonemes." Of equal importance, however, are other dimensions of behavior described, behaviors that, if they occurred in a speaker who had relatively frequent phoneme repetitions or prolongations, could be interpreted by an unwary clinician as "secondary reactions" to his stuttering. These behaviors include "transient breathy voice," "strained-strangled voice," "voice stoppages," "audible inspiration," "variable rate," "intervals prolonged," and "short rushes of speech." We see again the need for the diagnostician to consider all possible aspects of a problem—the gestalt—and not to "jump" at a diagnostic conclusion by concentrating on one aspect of defective speech.

Consider a further example: the characteristics of parkinsonism. In parkinsonism there may be rigidity of muscles and tremor. Facies are masked. Movements may be initiated with difficulty and may become arrested; several trials may be necessary to get started. Though slow at times, alternating movements may be limited in range and very fast. Although there is no true paralysis, there is marked loss of the automatic aspect of movement. These problems may affect speech performance as they do any other motor performance. Hence, along with phoneme repetitions reported earlier, you may observe inappropriate silences, false starts, short rushes of speech, tension, and variable rate (both fast and slow).

Palilalia   The disorder of speech called palilalia is characterized by compulsive repetition of a word, phrase, or sentence. It occurs typically in patients with postencephalitic parkinsonism and with pseudobulbar palsy (4). We will discuss it separately because persons may mistakenly confuse it with stuttering. As was discussed earlier in this chapter, Canter (5) considers palilalia to be a neurogenic type of stuttering. Boller, Albert, and Denes (3) state that along with the compulsive repetition of word or phrase there is an increase in rate of speech as the reiteration takes its course. Also the "volume of voice decreases until no sound can be heard, although the patient keeps moving his lips so well, that the word may at times be recognized." They make an interesting contrast between stuttering and palilalia: they contrast the difficulty the stutterer has in attempting to start speaking with the fluent output of the palilalic who appears to be unable to stop speaking. They present a case report of a 36-year-old palilalic patient:

> He would repeat compulsively either an entire sentence or its last part and rarely, only one word, unless it was a one-word answer. When asked, for example, why he had stopped working a year before

admission, he answered, "I was tired, I was tired, Yes, sir, Yes, sir, Yes, sir." Asked what he did all day, his answer was, "I stay home all the time, all the time, all the time." . . . He was able to sing common tunes with poor melody but without palilalia. He could recite the alphabet, the days of the week and the months of the year without articulatory defect or palilalia. At the end of the series, however, he often started the whole series over again. With the months of the year, for example, when he reached "December," he began again with "January, February, etc." (3)

He could read aloud normally. When he wrote, however, he would at times repeat a phrase in a manner similar to his behavior in speaking. He appeared to be aware of his disability "but did not appear to be very worried about it." From this description of the behavior pattern of the palilalic there should be little reason for the clinician to confuse it with the problem of stuttering.

Apraxia of Speech   The fluency problems related to apraxia of speech are due to an impairment of motor speech programming. As the temporal aspect of speaking is affected, apraxic speech errors are often referred to as "stutterlike" in character. Moreover, the errors occur in the absence of the weakness, slowness, incoordination, or alteration of tone of the speech musculature which cause dysarthria. The problems in programming motor movements by speech apraxics are described by Darley, Aronson, and Brown (9):

> As they speak, they struggle to position their articulators correctly. They visibly and audibly grope as they struggle to produce correct articulatory postures and to accomplish a sequence of these postures in forming words. Their articulation is frequently off target. They often recognize that they are off target and effortfully try to correct the error. Their errors recur, nonetheless, but they are not always the same; the errors on a series of trials are highly variable. As patients struggle to avoid articulatory error by careful programming of muscle movements, they slow down, space their words and syllables evenly, and stress them equally. Thus the prosody of their speech is altered as well as their articulation. (p. 250)

As one might suspect, repetitions of sounds and syllables are quite common. Johns and Darley (14) analyzed the errors of patients with apraxia of speech: in addition to many articulatory errors of phoneme substitution, omission, and addition, the patients produced many repetitions of sounds and syllables. Examples of these errors can be found in examples presented on pp. 505–506 of Chapter 18 and in Darley, Aronson, and Brown (9, p. 250). Note that one of the characteristics of the sound and syllable repetitions is the change in the phoneme during the repetition. This represents the patient's attempt more nearly to approximate the articulatory target.

Johns and Darley (14) report that certain of their apraxic subjects anticipated difficulty. They "tiptoed" through their words, approached articulatory adjustments "cautiously." Their speech was often effortful. They "made false starts, repeated and blocked. They perseverated on phonemes, syllables, words, and phrases." They circumlocuted. In summary, they "did a creditable job of miming secondary stutterers, both acoustically and behaviorally."

In view of the nature of their neurological impairment it is not surprising that some patients with apraxia of speech react as Johns and Darley describe. After all, rather suddenly their speech is fragmenting and sounds strange to them. They want to "stop it" when they become aware that they are not "talking right"; they attempt to "keep it from happening" by taking preventive action in the only ways they know how when they anticipate they may "do it again." This "stutterlike reaction" of coping with disfluency is similar to that reported earlier in this chapter for cases LK and CV.

Darley, Aronson, and Brown (9, p. 264–266) discuss factors that do and do not influence apraxic speech behavior. Generally, speech apraxics are similar to stutterers with regard to the loci of their disfluencies. However, other conditions in which stuttering is either greatly reduced or absent either are known not to obtain for speech apraxics or no information is available with which to evaluate them.

Discussion and Suggestions

You as a diagnostic clinician, faced with the problem of differentiating among fluency problems and understanding their causes, have been cautioned throughout this chapter to obtain as much information about the patient as possible before you draw conclusions about relationships between variables.

Obtain a detailed case history of the physical, environmental, and emotional conditions that preceded, occurred concomitantly with, and followed the onset of the fluency problem. Be prepared to apply the appraisal procedures described in various chapters in this book.

Try to obtain neurological examinations and psychiatric evaluations for any adult onset of a fluency problem. In many instances a "staffing" of the patient with the neurologist and the psychiatrist in attendance may be needed in order to arrive at a reasonable diagnosis.

Assess the variability of every fluency problem under a variety of conditions in order to delineate the behavioral syndrome presented by the patient.

Beware of categorical labels assigned by other persons to a patient when there is no evidence available to justify such labels. By so doing, you will avoid finding yourself in the position of the young clinician mentioned earlier, who, when she saw the label, "stuttering aphasic" wondered whether she should work first with the "stuttering" or with the "aphasia."

ASSIGNMENTS

1. Obtain a spontaneous speech sample from two children who have been diagnosed as demonstrating problems in language development. Do a disfluency analysis of each speech sample according to the classification of disfluencies described in Chapter 9. Note differences and similarities in the total frequency of disfluencies and in the proportions of the various types of disfluency. Then study the disfluency profile of each child in relation to the nature of the language problem.

2. Compare the behavior of two children who stutter on the dimensions listed as differentiating stutterers from clutterers described in this chapter (Table 14.1). Note how many characteristics they have and do not have that accord with "description of stutterers."

3. Have four stutterers (two adults and two children) perform the tasks described on pp. 417–418 which relate to conditions under which stuttering varies. Develop a behavior profile for each one. Describe similarities and differences in the ways they perform.

4. Ask two persons with neurogenic speech problems (apraxia of speech or dysarthria) to perform as many as possible of the tasks that you asked the stutterers to perform in question 3 above. Develop a behavior profile for each and compare it to those of the stutterers.

REFERENCES

1. Arnold, G. E., Signs and symptoms. In *Studies in Tachyphemia*, pp. 33–46. New York: Speech Rehabilitation Institute, 1960.
2. Bloodstein, O., *A Handbook on Stuttering*. Chicago: The National Easter Seal Society for Crippled Children and Adults, 1975.
3. Boller, F., Albert, M., and Denes, F., Palilalia. *British Journal of Disorders of Communication*, 1975, *10*:92–97.
4. Brain, R., *Speech Disorders: Aphasia, Apraxia, and Agnosia*. Washington, D.C.: Butterworth, 1961.
5. Canter, G. J., Observations on neurogenic stuttering: a contribution to differential diagnosis. *British Journal of Disorders of Communication*, 1971, *6*:139–143.
6. Caplan, L., An investigation of some aspects of stuttering-like speech in adult dysphasic subjects. *Journal of the South African Speech and Hearing Association*, 1972, *19*:52–66.
7. Clifford, S., Aronson, A. E., and Peterson, J. S., Adult onset of stuttering: A review of thirty-five cases. Paper presented to the American Speech and Hearing Association Regional Convention, Minneapolis, Minnesota, May 1975.
8. Darley, F. L., Aronson, A. E., and Brown, J. R., Differential diagnostic patterns of dysarthria. *Journal of Speech and Hearing Research*, 1969, *12*:246–269.
9. Darley, F. L., Aronson, A. E., and Brown, J. R., *Motor Speech Disorders*. Philadelphia: Saunders, 1975.

10. Freund, H., Studies in the inter-relationship between stuttering and cluttering. *Folia Phoniatrica,* 1962, *4:*146–168.
11. Freund, H., *Psychopathology and the Problems of Stuttering.* Springfield, Ill.: Thomas, 1966.
12. Freund, H., Au den Beziehugen Zwischen Stottern und Poltern. *Mschr. Ohrenheilk,* 1934, *68:*1450.
13. Hall, P. K., The occurrence of disfluencies in language-disordered school-age children. *Journal of Speech and Hearing Disorders,* 1977, *42:*364–369.
14. Johns, D. F., and Darley, F. L., Phonemic variability in apraxia of speech. *Journal of Speech and Hearing Research,* 1970, *13:*556–583.
15. Johnson, W., and Associates, *The Onset of Stuttering.* Minneapolis: University of Minnesota Press, 1959.
16. Johnston, F. J., Disfluency Behavior and Language Performance in Four-year-old Children. Ph.D. dissertation, University of Iowa, 1973.
17. Luchsinger, R., and Arnold, G. E., *Voice-Speech-Language.* Belmont, Calif: Wadsworth, 1965.
18. Muma, J. R., Syntax of preschool fluent and disfluent speech: a transformational analysis. *Journal of Speech and Hearing Research,* 1971, *14:*428–441.
19. Pratt, J. E., An examination of linguistic perception-production in preschool stutterers and non stutterers. Ph.D. dissertation, University of Illinois, 1972.
20. Riley, G. D., and Riley, J., Component diagnostic model based on the component theory. Paper presented at the American Speech and Hearing Association Regional Convention, Portland, Oregon, 1976.
21. Rosenbek, J. C., McNeil, M. R., Lemme, M. L., Prescott, T. E., and Alfrey, A. C., Speech and language findings in a chronic hemodialysis patient: a case report. *Journal of Speech and Hearing Disorders,* 1975, *40:*245–252.
22. Rosenbek, J. C., Messert, B., Collins, M., and Wertz, R. T., Cortical stuttering. Paper presented at the Fiftieth Annual American Speech and Hearing Association Convention, Washington, D.C., November 1975.
23. Rosenfield, D. B., Letter to the Editor: Stuttering and cerebral ischemia, *New England Journal of Medicine,* 1972, *287:*991.
24. Sasanuma, S., A description of the disfluent speech behavior of stuttering and non stuttering Japanese children. Ph.D. dissertation, University of Iowa, 1968.
25. Sander, E. K., Frequency of syllable repetition and "stutterer" judgments. *Journal of Speech and Hearing Disorders,* 1963, *28:*19–30.
26. Van Riper, C., *The Nature of Stuttering.* Englewood Cliffs, N.J.: Prentice-Hall, 1971.
27. Van Riper, C., Stuttering and cluttering: the differential diagnosis. *Folia Phoniatrica,* 1970, *22:*347–353.
28. Weiss, D. A., *Cluttering.* Englewood Cliffs, N.J.: Prentice-Hall, 1964.
29. Westby, C. E., Language performance of stuttering and non stuttering children. Ph.D. dissertation, University of Iowa, 1971.
30. Wingate, M. E., A standard definition of stuttering. *Journal of Speech and Hearing Disorders,* 1964, *29:*484–489.

15

DIFFERENTIAL DIAGNOSIS OF DISORDERS OF THE OROFACIAL COMPLEX

**D. C. Spriestersbach
and Hughlett L. Morris**

Our purpose here is to describe some of the diagnostic categories used by the clinical speech pathologist which are based primarily on structural disorders of the speech mechanism. We exclude disorders which are primarily neurologic since they are discussed in Chapter 18. We also exclude structural disorders of the larynx since they are discussed in Chapter 20. The disorders considered in this discussion involve the palate and the palatopharyngeal mechanism, the teeth and their occlusion, the tongue, and the lips.

CLEFT PALATE

Congenital cleft palate, with or without cleft lip, is a good example of a physical disorder which results in defects of the speech mechanism. The disorder is a birth defect, occurring in the general population with an approximate frequency of one in 650 births. While the etiology of the cleft defect is not yet well understood, some clefts are clearly genetic in origin while others are probably developmental. Whatever the etiology, the normal pattern of growth and development of the lip and palate appears to have been interrupted at some time during the period from 6 to 12 weeks of fetal life. In many instances there may be no single etiologic factor; rather the developmental disruption may be the result of a combination of several etiologic factors. Information about the birth defect, associated problems, and contemporary treatment is provided in the comprehensive textbook edited by Grabb, Rosenstein, and Bzoch (4).

With regard to speech production, the main result of cleft palate is that the individual is not able to separate the nasal cavity from the oral cavity and so speech is characterized by excessive nasal resonance (hyper-

439

nasality). For many individuals, perhaps one in four (6), this kind of speech disorder persists even after cleft palate surgery or treatment by dental prosthesis because the treatment was not sufficient in the physiologic sense for the separation of the cavities. If that is the case, additional surgical or prosthodontic treatment is needed.

In general the structural anomaly of cleft lip appears not to affect speech production adversely (12) although it may in certain individuals.

If the cleft extends through the alveolus, the resulting changes in dentition and occlusion may be disruptive to speech production. The relationship between dentition occlusion and speech production for the cleft palate individual is the same as for the individual without a cleft; that discussion is presented later in this chapter. Individuals with cleft palate frequently demonstrate dental and occlusal defects, and the effect of the defect and of treatment appliances for the defect on speech production must always be considered in the clinical examination.

There has been considerable discussion in the literature about the degree to which cleft palate individuals have other structural defects that have adverse effects on speech production. Of particular concern in this regard are such variables as the size of the oral cavity, the width and height of the palatal vault, and the size and motility of the tongue. Clearly there is variability among cleft palate patients in palatal width and height, but such variability does not appear systematically to be a hindrance to speech production. Tongue size and motility are more difficult to evaluate, but there is no evidence to indicate that the cleft palate patient typically has a structural or neurologic deficiency of the tongue. It seems likely that these factors are important in speech production only if there are several in number, working in combination.

OTHER DISORDERS OF THE PALATOPHARYNGEAL MECHANISM

A number of disorders in addition to cleft palate have adverse effects on speech production, primarily for reasons of dysfunction of the palatopharyngeal mechanism.

Submucous Cleft Palate

Individuals with this defect typically have an intact soft palate or only the uvula is cleft, yet their speech production patterns are similar to those of patients with cleft palate. Careful examination indicates that, beneath the intact mucous membrane, there is a tissue deficiency in either the palatal musculature or the bony palatal shelf. If the palatal shelf is involved, there is usually a notch at the posterior margin of the hard palate where the posterior nasal spine is ordinarily found. The notch is detected by manual palpation. Deficiencies of musculature are more difficult to detect and frequently require special procedures.

Data are insufficient to allow a reliable estimate of the incidence of submucous cleft palate. Clinical experience indicates that the disorder is relatively rare.

The impact of the disorder on speech production is not the result of the submucous cleft or the bifid uvula per se. Rather the impact results from the fact that in patients with submucous cleft palate the palate is also deficient in length or in motility so that palatopharyngeal dysfunction results. The diagnostic picture for these patients is much like that presented by cleft palate patients with palatopharyngeal incompetence following palatal surgery, except that there is no history of clefting.

Frequently the disorder is not discovered until after the patient has undergone adenoidectomy.[1] The reason is that the adenoidal pad compensates for the deficiency in palatal length and motility; when the adenoids are removed, any such structural deficit of the palate suddenly becomes apparent. Unfortunately no methods are presently available by which predictions of postsurgical palatopharyngeal dysfunction can be made reliably (7).

Congenital Palatal Incompetence

The patient with congenital palatal incompetence displays symptoms and presents physical findings very much like those just described for submucous cleft palate, except that there is no clefting of any kind. Rather it is apparently the result of any of several abnormalities of cavity relationships. The soft palate may be congenitally short while the hard palate and the pharynx are of normal dimension. Possibly both the hard and soft palates are short while the nasopharynx is of normal depth. Or the hard and soft palates may be of normal length but are associated with an excessively deep pharynx (8).

Like the submucous cleft defect, congenital incompetence is relatively rare and is often first discovered following adenoidectomy. Frequently, the palatopharyngeal disorder is part of a syndrome which means that such patients may require the diagnostic services of specialists in birth defects.

Acquired Palatal Defects

Probably the most common acquired palatal defect is that which results from surgery for oral cancer. It is difficult to generalize about the nature of such defects and their effect on speech production because there is

---

[1] Judging by the reported clinical experience of many specialists, normal atrophy of the adenoidal pad does not seem to result in palatopharyngeal incompetence in patients with submucous cleft palate and related palatal disorders. Apparently the mechanism can compensate for the gradual small decrements in adenoidal size which result from normal atrophy.

such variety in the extent of disease and surgical treatment. If the defect is extensive, reconstructive surgery and facial prosthesis are frequently needed, so the speech pathologist needs to have good information about planned physical treatment before proceeding with therapy.

Other acquired palatal defects may be palatal paresis or paralysis resulting from head and neck trauma. In such instances the structures are intact but neurologic function is impaired.

Bradley (3) provides additional information about both congenital and acquired palatal defects.

MALOCCLUSION

Malocclusion is sometimes found as a part of certain syndromes but the disorder also may appear in isolation unrelated to other disorders. Some types of malocclusion appear to be related to genetic factors, while others may be due primarily to unusual patterns of behavior, such as vigorous thumb sucking over a relatively long period of time. Abnormal swallowing patterns are considered by some authorities to be of etiologic significance but that position is controversial.

Bloomer (2) provides a thorough discussion of occlusion and malocclusion for use by speech pathologists. From his discussion it is clear that there is great variety in type and extent of malocclusion. Consequently, as we have seen in our discussion of other structural defects of the oral mechanism, it is difficult to generalize about the impact on patterns of speech production. Some speakers appear able to compensate effectively for relatively severe dental and occlusal anomalies; others do not. For additional information see (13).

In this regard, we need to remember that sometimes orthodontic treatment appliances may also have an adverse effect on speech production, particularly if the appliance interferes with tongue placement in articulation.

DEFECTS OF THE TONGUE

On rare occasion the speech pathologist examines a patient with a deficiency in tongue size. The deficiency may be congenital (microglossia) or as the result of surgery (for example, cancer surgery). If the deficiency is the result of surgery, there will be confirmation from the surgical history. If it is a congenital disorder, diagnosis is more difficult and should be confirmed by a specialist or team of specialists in orofacial disorders. See the discussion by Bloomer (2) for additional information.

Perhaps equally rare is unusual enlargement of the tongue (macroglossia). This may be extreme enough to prevent tongue movements necessary for rapid, precise articulation. Surgical reduction of an oversize tongue is sometimes performed.

CRANIOFACIAL ANOMALIES

A number of congenital anomalies of the craniofacial complex involve deformities of the oral mechanism structures. We have most comprehensive information about the oral structures of patients with Apert's syndrome and Crouzon's disease (5, 9, 10). Again, there is great variety in type and extent of anomaly among patients with these syndromes. In general, however, the major factors which adversely effect speech production are malocclusion and palatal defects. Patients with craniofacial anomalies should be referred to special management teams for evaluation and planning as soon as possible after birth.

TONGUE THRUST

There is considerable controversy about the disorder designated tongue thrust or reverse swallow. The consensus seems to be that some individuals present certain types of malocclusions related to swallowing patterns considered by some to be abnormal (1, 11). It also seems reasonable that in some individuals the malocclusion is causally related to misarticulations, particularly of the sibilants (2, 13). However, as indicated earlier (Chapter 11), it seems unlikely that there is direct relationship between lingual patterns during swallow and speech production problems.

There is also controversy about treatment for the disorder. Our position is that the beginning clinician would do well to refer any patients considered to demonstrate this type of disorder to a specialty diagnostic clinic that includes services of a variety of disciplines, particularly speech pathology and dentistry.

ASSIGNMENTS

1. What kinds of communication disorders might be demonstrated by individuals with structural anomalies of the orofacial complex?
2. In addition to the problems in speech production that such individuals might demonstrate, what additional hazard might there be to normal patterns of speech and language learning?
3. What psychosocial problems might be associated with what types of orofacial anomalies? How might they affect speech and language?
4. What other professionals may be involved in providing treatment for such patients?

REFERENCES

1. Ackerman, J. L., and Proffit, W. R., Diagnosis and planning treatment in orthodontics. In Graber, T. M., and Swain, B. F., eds., Current Orthodontic Concepts and Techniques, pp. 1–110. Philadelphia: Saunders, 1975.

2. Bloomer, H. H., Speech defects associated with dental malocclusions and related abnormalities. In Travis, L. E., ed., *Handbook of Speech Pathology and Audiology*, pp. 715–766. Englewood Cliffs, N.J.: Prentice-Hall, 1971.

3. Bradley, D. P., Congenital and acquired palatopharyngeal insufficiency. In Grabb, W. C., Rosenstein, S. W., and Bzoch, K. R., eds., *Cleft Lip and Palate: Surgical, Dental, and Speech Aspects*, pp. 658–699. Boston: Little, Brown, 1971.

4. Grabb, W. C., Rosenstein, S. W., and Bzoch, K. R., eds., *Cleft Lip and Palate: Surgical, Dental, and Speech Aspects*. Boston: Little, Brown, 1971.

5. Elfenbein, J. L., An investigation of the verbal communication skills and the related physical structures of six individuals with Apert's and Crouzon's syndromes. M.A. thesis, University of Iowa, 1975.

6. Morris, H. L., Velopharyngeal competence and primary cleft palate surgery, 1960–1971: A critical review. *Cleft Palate Journal*, 1973, *10*: 62–71.

7. Morris, H. L., The speech pathologist looks at the tonsils and the adenoids. *Annals of Otology, Rhinology, and Laryngology*, Supplement, 1975, 84:63–66.

8. Owsley, J. Q., Chierici, G., Miller, E. R., Lawson, R. I., and Blackfield, H. M., Cephalometric evaluation of palatal dysfunction in patients without cleft palate. *Plastic and Reconstructive Surgery*, 1967, 39:562–568.

9. Peterson, S., Speech pathology in craniofacial malformations other than cleft lip and palate. In *Orofacial Anomalies: Clinical and Research Implications*, ASHA Reports No. 8, pp. 111–131. Washington, D.C.: American Speech and Hearing Association, 1973.

10. Peterson, S., and Pruzansky, S., Palatal anomalies in the syndromes of Apert and Crouzon. *Cleft Palate Journal*, 1974, *11*:394–403.

11. Proffit, W. R., and Norton, L. A., Influences of tongue activity during speech and swallowing. In Wertz, R. T., ed., *Speech and the Dentofacial Complex: The State of the Art*, ASHA Reports No. 5, pp. 106–115. Washington, D.C.: American Speech and Hearing Association, 1970.

12. Spriestersbach, D. C., Moll, K. L., and Morris, H. L., Subject classification and articulation of speakers with cleft palates. *Journal of Speech and Hearing Research*, 1964, *4*:364–379.

13. Starr, C. D., Dental and occlusal hazards to normal speech production. In Grabb, W. C., Rosenstein, S. W., and Bzoch, K. R., eds., *Cleft Lip and Palate: Surgical, Dental, and Speech Aspects*, pp. 670–680. Boston: Little, Brown, 1971.

16

DIFFERENTIAL DIAGNOSIS OF HEARING DISORDERS

Charles V. Anderson
and Julia M. Davis

INTRODUCTION

As stated earlier in Chapter 12, the four primary purposes of any audiologic evaluation are (1) to describe what the patient hears and how he or she hears it, (2) to describe the communication ability of the patient, (3) to provide information which will assist in determining the site(s) of lesion(s) within the auditory system, and (4) to provide the basis on which a plan of habilation can be developed. Fulfillment of the first two purposes leads directly to the differential diagnosis provided by the audiologist. The diagnosis of the site of a lesion is, of course, medical and is made by a physician, usually an otolaryngologist. The physician arrives at the medical diagnosis on the basis of medical case history, physical examination, and laboratory tests, in addition to the interpretation of audiometric test results provided by the audiologist. The fourth goal can be accomplished by coordination and interpretation of all information. The diagnosis, treatment, and management of hearing disorders require interdisciplinary cooperation and continuing professional interaction.

Knowledge of the medical diagnosis and scheme of treatment is essential to the diagnosis and management of the communication disorder. It is standard practice to obtain medical assessment prior to determining audiologic diagnosis and making long-range habilitative plans for the person with a hearing impairment. Information from and participation by the physician in the diagnostic and treatment process of communication disorders related to hearing loss are dictated by (1) the need for medical and surgical treatment appropriate to the physical condition and (2) the need to have a prognosis about the permanence of the hearing disorder. Knowledge of the possibility that medical treatment can be expected to stabilize a progressive hearing loss or improve the hearing ability of the patient is crucial to the description of and habilitation plan for the communication disorder. Audiologic habilitation plans for the person who has a permanent, stable hearing loss will obviously differ from those for an individual who has a progressive problem or one whose hearing can be expected to improve.

The hearing test results and the audiologist's interpretation of these results provide essential information for the physician's diagnosis and treatment plan and vice versa for the audiologist's diagnosis and treatment plan. It is in the sharing of interpretations and diagnoses that all participants in the interdisciplinary process must use care in restricting themselves to professional judgments for which they are competent and for which they are prepared to take responsibility.

The audiologist determines through measurement and observation whether a hearing loss exists, and if it does, the type, degree, and pattern of the loss. The effects of the hearing loss on the individual's ability to communicate, to learn and use language, to achieve academically, and to function in a vocation must be investigated and taken into consideration in planning appropriate habilitative measures. Information relative to these effects is gleaned from case history, measurement, observation, and multidisciplinary evaluation. This chapter will deal with some of the common difficulties that arise in fulfilling these purposes.

DETERMINATION OF THE HEARING LOSS

Basic information for both audiologic and medical diagnoses is obtained through a generally accepted standard battery of monaural hearing tests: (1) pure-tone air and bone conduction thresholds, (2) speech reception threshold (SRT), and (3) speech discrimination. Tympanometry and acoustic reflex measures are now often included in this standard battery. From these measurements the audiologist can determine whether a hearing loss exists, and if so, the type, degree, and pattern or configuration of the hearing loss.

Types of Hearing Loss

Hearing disorders are typed, in a pure sense, as *conductive, sensory, neural,* or *central.* Conductive, sensory, and neural types are grouped under the heading of *peripheral* hearing loss. The audiologic diagnosis of type is derived from assumptions about the hearing function, while medical diagnoses, using the same terminology, refer to the site and cause of the lesion within the auditory system. This categorical system which allows us to discuss normal function, anatomical location, site of lesion, and loss of function with the same terminology is convenient and meaningful; but, at the same time, it provides confusion as to which type of diagnosis is being made. It is advisable for speech-language pathologists and audiologists to help clarify the situation by including the word "type" with these terms when stating diagnoses. A summary of these terms is shown in Table 16.1.

Using the standard audiometric battery, it is rare that a central auditory disorder is identified or that sensory and neural types of hearing loss can be differentiated. The primary use of these tests in typing hearing loss is to differentiate between conductive and the combined category of *sensori-neural.* Since both conductive and sensori-neural types of hearing loss may be exhibited simultaneously, we also use the category of *mixed* hearing loss.

The differentiation of conductive from other types of hearing loss is most often arrived at from comparing pure-tone thresholds by bone conduction with those by air conduction. If such differentiation is not readily apparent, tympanometry, acoustic reflex, and other special tests can be used to contribute information or may be used to confirm or refute the initial interpretation of the audiogram. Further differentiation typically requires use of the special tests described in Chapter 12. A conductive type of hearing loss is most easily recognized by an audiogram demonstrating pure-tone thresholds for bone-conducted signals within normal limits while those for air-conducted signals are at least 10 dB poorer. The term "air-bone gap" describes the difference in thresholds for a conductive hearing loss. A sensorineural hearing loss, on the other hand, will be exhibited by air and bone conduction thresholds which are essentially equal (an air-bone gap of less than 10 dB).

Degrees of Hearing Loss

Many systems, often with divergent purposes, have been devised for the description of degree of hearing loss. Although criteria may vary some-

TABLE 16.1
Explanation of Terms Used to Designate Types of Hearing Loss

Type of Hearing Loss	Functional Loss	Anatomical Site
Conductive	Mechanical transmission of acoustic signal	External and middle ears
Sensory	Peripheral reception of signal by nervous system	Inner ear
Neural	Transmission of neural signal to central nervous system	VIIIth Nerve trunk
Central	Transmission and processing of signal within the central nervous system	Brain stem through cortex

what from clinician to clinician, the most common system describes (1) hearing within normal limits and (2) mild, (3) moderate, (4) severe, and (5) profound losses of hearing sensitivity for air-conducted sound measured by the pure-tone average (PTA) or SRT. These designations imply the degree of difficulty the person will have in hearing speech at conversational levels or the degree to which speech will have to be increased in level (usually through amplification by a hearing aid) in order to be heard. Although educational inferences are sometimes drawn from these descriptions of degree of hearing loss, they are almost always so general as to be of no value. These statements are generalizations and ignore individual differences among people. With such a broad categorization, little can be said about the individual's specific communication problems. A capsulization of this system is shown in Table 16.2.

Configuration of Hearing Loss

The configuration of the hearing loss is a description of the pattern formed by the pure-tone thresholds on the audiogram. Unless specified otherwise, configuration refers to thresholds for air conduction signals. The terminology used in these descriptions is even further from stan-

TABLE 16.2
Conversational Speech Problems Associated with Different Degrees of Hearing Loss

Degree of Hearing Loss	PTA-AC	Implied Difficulty Hearing Conversational Speech
Within normal limits	20 dB HL or less	None
Mild	20–45 dB HL	Occasional difficulty when softly spoken or when background interferes. Probably can hear over telephone. May or may not find amplification of help.
Moderate	45–65 dB HL	Difficulty with most conversational speech. Probably cannot hear over telephone. Amplification usually helpful.
Severe	65–85 dB HL	Cannot hear conversational speech without amplification.
Profound	85 dB HL or more	Usually cannot rely exclusively on auditory system for communication purposes.

dardization than our other descriptive systems. Some of the more common descriptors are summarized in Table 16.3.

Speech Discrimination

The description of speech discrimination scores is important in understanding how a person hears speech and provides data to be used in differential diagnosis. Unfortunately, as discussed in Chapter 12, the variety of speech discrimination tests and the variety of purposes for which we use discrimination scores make it difficult to develop a commonly used descriptive system. The terms used as descriptors are often the same but the meaning of these terms appears to vary from clinician to clinician. Most often you will see speech discrimination ability described as excellent, good, fair, poor, or very poor. Certainly we anticipate that the person with speech discrimination abilities described as good or excellent will understand conversational speech in quiet without difficulty, while the person with very poor discrimination will have a great deal of difficulty understanding speech. The specific scores which lead clinicians to these statements, however, are far from standardized at this time. It is important that a specific description of discrimination ability accompany speech discrimination scores.

TABLE 16.3
Descriptions of Audiogram Configurations

Configuration of Audiogram	Description of Audiogram
Flat	Thresholds across the frequencies are within 15 dB of one another.
Rising	Thresholds improve as frequency increases.
Gently falling	Thresholds become poorer by approximately 10 dB per octave as frequency increases.
Steeply falling	Thresholds become poorer by 20–30 dB per octave as frequency increases.
Precipitous	Thresholds become poorer by 30 dB or more per octave as frequency increases. Often hearing levels for tones at or below the mid-frequencies are essentially equal.
High-frequency	Configuration across lower and mid-frequencies is flat with poorer thresholds at 2000 Hz and above.

Summarizing Hearing Test Results

Hearing test results and our descriptive statements about type, degree, and configuration of hearing loss combine to form an overall impression of measured hearing ability. The more compatible and consistent these

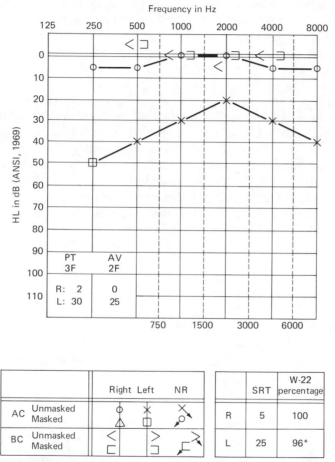

		Right Left NR				SRT	W-22 percentage
AC	Unmasked Masked				R	5	100
BC	Unmasked Masked				L	25	96*

*with contralateral masking

FIGURE 16.1

Compatible hearing test results which can be described as hearing within normal limits with no significant air-bone gap and excellent speech discrimination. In the left ear the patient demonstrates a mild conductive-type hearing loss with good speech discrimination. The configuration of the air conduction thresholds for the left ear is gently rising through 2000 Hz with poorer thresholds again in the higher frequencies.

results, the more confidence we place in our judgments. Examples of compatible test results and their descriptions are shown in Figures 16.1 through 16.4. We will use these examples to apply our previous discussion of determination of hearing loss. Remember that the hearing test results and their descriptions form only a portion of the overall diagnosis.

Each set of test results in Figures 16.1 through 16.4 presents a situation quite unlike the others. In Figure 16.1 the test results are typical of a

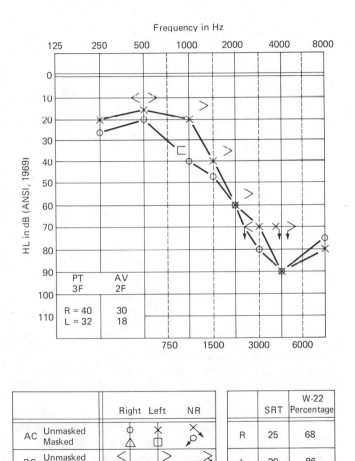

		Right	Left	NR			SRT	W-22 Percentage
AC	Unmasked				R	25	68	
	Masked							
BC	Unmasked				L	20	86	
	Masked							

FIGURE 16.2

Compatible hearing test results which can be described as follows: the patient appears to have a bilateral, sensorineural type of hearing loss demonstrating a steeply falling configuration ranging from mild at 1000 Hz and below to severe at higher frequencies. Speech discrimination scores are fair in the left ear and poor in the right ear.

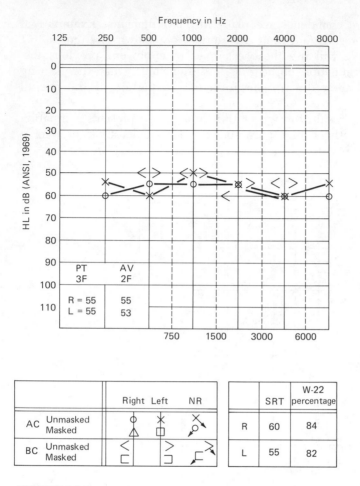

FIGURE 16.3
Hearing test results which can be interpreted as representing a bilateral, moderate, flat, sensorineural type of hearing loss with fair speech discrimination scores.

mild unilateral conductive type of hearing loss. Hearing is apparently normal in the right ear while in the left ear there is a reduction in sensitivity for air-conducted signals. Speech discrimination scores, presented at comfortable listening levels, demonstrate that once speech is loud enough this person has no difficulty understanding it. Since it is assumed that the primary hearing function with which a conductive hearing loss interferes is mechanical transmission of the signal by air conduction, we do not expect to measure any loss other than in the level of signal which reaches the sensory end organ via air conduction.

The test results in Figures 16.2 and 16.3, on the other hand, demonstrate rather clearly the common finding that sensorineural types of

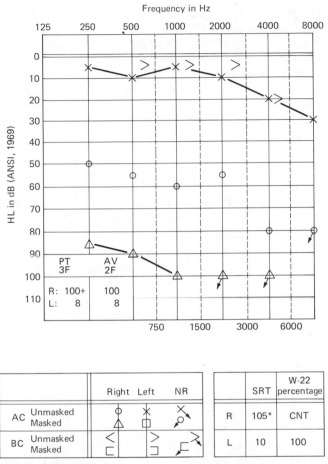

	Right	Left	NR			SRT	W-22 percentage
AC Unmasked					R	105*	CNT
AC Masked							
BC Unmasked					L	10	100
BC Masked							

*with contralateral masking

FIGURE 16.4

Standard hearing test results reported as hearing within normal limits in the left ear with no air-bone gap and excellent speech discrimination scores. There is a profound loss of hearing in the right ear. No responses to air-conducted signals at frequencies above 1000 Hz nor to any bone-conducted signals could be elicited for the right ear at the limits of the audiometer. Speech discrimination, marked CNT, could not be tested.

hearing loss not only show a reduction in sensitivity of the receptors but also a disruption in speech discrimination ability. Although reduced speech discrimination ability is typical of sensorineural hearing loss, it is not always demonstrated in our measurements. Especially with the Central Institute for the Deaf (CID) W-22 word lists, people with sensorineural hearing losses may demonstrate good speech discrimination scores. Figure 16.2 demonstrates a situation in which the sole use of the PTA or especially the SRT is of little value in understanding how this person hears. Comparison of two-frequency and three-frequency PTA provides some insight into the precipitous configuration. The speech discrimination scores demonstrate differences between the ears for purposes of understanding speech. Relying solely upon the SRT scores, however, would leave one with the impression of a mild hearing loss. This is truly a case where several types of information must be combined for any meaningful description to be made.

The hearing sensitivity for the right ear in Figure 16.4 is so poor that we are unable to complete the threshold measures and cannot even attempt a meaningful measure of speech discrimination. Although this ear is undoubtedly of no value to this person for hearing, it is important to note the degree of residual hearing.

You should take special note of the contralateral masking used in Figures 16.1, 16.2, and 16.4. In each case it was applied appropriately to avoid the possible occurrence of cross hearing. In Figure 16.4 the symbols for thresholds obtained while presenting pure tones to the right ear by air conduction without contralateral masking are presented to demonstrate the necessity for masking. Assuming that these unmasked thresholds represented responses from the right ear would obviously lead to a totally erroneous impression of the hearing in that ear.

The test results in Figures 16.1 through 16.4 are just that and do not present a total description of the person's communication disorder. Additional information such as the person's age, language abilities, socialization, educational needs, vocational needs, and medical status are essential and must be incorporated. The impact of the hearing loss represented by Figure 16.3 would be quite different for a 3-year-old child who is still in the process of acquiring language and has his educational career ahead of him than it would be for a 50-year-old adult in the middle of his vocational career. By the same token, a 50-year-old adult who is a practicing trial lawyer and quite active socially would find this hearing loss to present quite different problems to him than it would to a 50-year-old adult who works on an assembly line in a noisy factory and rarely socializes outside his family. We cannot say that the impact will be greater or less without knowing the people but obviously it will be different. The following discussion, organized by age level when appropriate, elaborates on this presentation. As will be evident in the succeeding discussion, not all of the test results and information desired or discussed earlier will be available or needed in all cases.

INFANTS AND PRESCHOOLERS

The most common symptom of hearing loss in children under the age of 3 is failure to learn to speak at the appropriate time. This failure is not always recognized as evidence of possible hearing loss, since there are several conditions that can result in the same delay of speech development. These conditions are often not easily distinguishable from each other, but hearing loss needs to be ruled out or confirmed in all cases of delayed speech and language development. It is sometimes quite difficult to accomplish this, since the conditions known to contribute to speech and language delay often result in behavior that interferes with hearing testing procedures. Patience, careful instruction and demonstration, repeated testing sessions, and skill on the part of the audiologist will result in eventual success with most children.

The conditions known to be associated with delayed development of speech and language, as reviewed in Chapter 17, are peripheral hearing loss, mental retardation, emotional disturbance, and specific language disability (also referred to as central auditory disorder, dysacusis, perceptual disturbance, minimal brain damage, and developmental or congenital aphasia).

Peripheral Hearing Loss

Young children who have peripheral hearing loss usually respond well to skillful attempts to condition them to attend and respond to sound as discussed in Chapter 12. As soon as they feel comfortable with the examiners and the procedures, children with peripheral hearing loss exhibit no unusual difficulty in attending to auditory input or responding consistently to it in a manner appropriate to their age, provided that they have sufficient hearing to allow for association between the auditory event and the expected response. These children are visually alert; they respond quickly to changes in visual input such as movement or light. They are also alert to tactile stimuli and usually react quickly to an unexpected touch. Therefore, if a child fails to condition to respond to auditory stimuli within a reasonable period of time, we should attempt conditioning with visual (light) or tactile (vibration) stimuli. If a child learns to respond quickly to such stimuli, his failure to respond to auditory events may be interpreted as evidence of auditory disorder; either he is so severely impaired that he cannot hear well enough to associate sound with the task at hand, or he is unable to use the auditory information effectively even though it is received. In either event, hearing is "impaired" for practical and useful purposes.

On the other hand, if the child cannot condition to respond to other sensory stimuli, his failure to respond to sound cannot be interpreted as hard evidence of hearing loss until and unless other conditions can be ruled out.

Case history information is often helpful. If family history reveals a pattern of hearing loss or evidence that the child falls into a high-risk category for hearing loss because of prenatal (maternal illness or genetic syndrome), perinatal (anoxia or Rh factor), or postnatal (jaundice, illness in the child) factors, hearing loss should be suspected even if initial test results are not definitive. High-risk children should be followed closely until they give normal responses to sound or until their hearing loss is confirmed and habilitative procedures instituted.

Mental Retardation

This is the most common cause of delayed speech and may be confused with hearing loss. Many cases are on record in which mentally retarded children have been classified as deaf and vice versa. Such misdiagnosis results in a waste of time, money, energy, and human potential if it persists for several years and leads to improper training and educational procedures.

Mentally retarded children often fail to condition to respond to auditory stimuli in appropriate ways. They may be quite distractible and attention span may be short. It is important to remember that behavioral responses such as localization of sound or participation in play audiometric games is likely to be more closely related to the child's mental age than to his or her chronological age. Therefore, procedures appropriate for younger children should be introduced any time a child is unable to participate in activities designed for his age level.

If all attempts to obtain auditory thresholds fail and gross reaction to sound is the only response obtainable, be careful in interpreting the responses given. For example, if the child responds to sounds at a moderate intensity level of 45 dB hearing level (HL), compare this reduced response to auditory stimuli to the child's response to other sensory events. Does he turn when touched lightly on the shoulder, or does he ignore tactile stimuli until they reach an insistent level? Does he appear to notice visual events, such as sudden movements of other persons, changes in lighting patterns, and the introduction of objects or pictures into his visual field? If the child ignores visual and tactile events until they, too, are moderately "strong," the failure to respond to soft auditory stimuli probably cannot safely be assumed to represent a moderate degree of hearing loss.

The most easily discernible difference between hearing-impaired and mentally retarded infants is their physical and motor development. The retarded child is usually delayed in developmental milestones such as sitting alone, crawling, walking, and toilet training. Careful questioning regarding these aspects of the child's development may be of great help in distinguishing between retarded and hearing-impaired babies. A word of caution, however: infants who have central nervous system disorders that affect motor functioning (such as cerebral palsy) may exhibit significant delays in development milestones in the absence of mental retardation. The same may be true of infants who have visual and auditory handicaps (i.e., "deaf-blind"). While it is difficult to assess the mental abilities of multiply handicapped children and thus to rule out mental retardation, a child who cannot see *or* hear well will be hesitant to venture forth independently because of reduced ability to monitor his environment and his relation to it. Additional evaluations by neurologists and psychologists are necessary in determining possible causes for such delay.

Emotional Disturbance (Autism)

Emotional disturbance in young children that is severe enough to interfere with speech and language development is often difficult to diagnose even by a multidisciplinary team. In some cases arrested motor as well as language development occurs; in others the child develops normally in every way except in his affective reactions to others. This child's ability to ignore sensory stimuli often interferes with diagnosis. His most outstanding characteristic is his inability to relate well to other human beings, sometimes ignoring their presence completely and effectively. He may engage in repetitive behavior such as rocking or other stereotyped movements. Attempts to engage the child's attention may appear to be partially successful, but attention is short lived. Eye contact may be minimal. Emotional affect may be inappropriate and widely variable within a short period of time. A smiling face may change abruptly to crying; the crying may cease just as abruptly, giving way to some other behavior. In less extreme cases the child tolerates the testing situation well but without really reacting to it in any consistent way. The overall impression of the child's behavior is that it is not directed toward the situation at all; rather the child is detached from you and the situation and is responding to internal stimuli exclusively. In some cases the child may ignore all sound; in others he may give a negative reaction, especially to the human voice, for example, crying, moving away from the sound source, or covering his ears.

It is exceptionally difficult to establish hearing threshold levels in such children. Repeated testing and use of behavior modification techniques are sometimes helpful. Observation of the child in other situations may furnish clues to his use or nonuse of auditory stimuli. Toys that produce sounds, especially soft sounds, may be introduced and the child's reactions noted. It should be stressed that the ambient, detached behavior described above is not typical of children with hearing impairment. However, it is certainly possible for an emotionally disturbed child to have a hearing loss and every possible attempt should be made to establish hearing levels. Since the child's behavior is not conducive to successful use of conventional hearing testing procedures, electrophysiological or acoustic reflex measurements may offer the best means of investigating reception of sound, even though these methods do not yield direct threshold values or information about the usefulness of the auditory input received.

Specific Language Disability

Considerable controversy has existed in the past regarding hearing testing in language-disordered children, whatever label is applied to them. They are reported to give inconsistent responses to auditory stimuli, and many clinicians have ignored hearing-testing data when planning for these children. Kleffner (17) discussed these factors and concluded that the pure-tone threshold may offer the best piece of evidence available in the case of difficult-to-test children. He cautions against ignoring reduced sensitivity to auditory stimuli in children suspected of language disorders other than those associated solely with hearing loss.

The language-disordered child may exhibit normal reception of sound but a decreased ability to associate sound with its source or its meaning. The disability appears to involve difficulty with associations and with sequencing and memory for auditory events. Therefore, conditioning may be more difficult to achieve than with other children. It is not unusual for these children to be able to repeat words or sounds in an echoic fashion without being able to associate them with the appropriate referent. The repetitions may be accurate with regard to inflection and articulation, indicating accurate reception of the information-bearing aspects of the words. Series of sounds or words are usually imitated less well. Although the child gives evidence of hearing much of what is said, he may give no evidence of comprehending the message to any degree.

Since hearing loss is a common occurrence in children with severe language disorders, testing should be repeated until consistent results are obtained. Amplification should be provided when appropriate, and a period of diagnostic teaching employed in order to determine further the child's habilitative needs.

When attempting differential diagnosis with young children we must be careful not to build our own biases and prejudices into the evaluation procedures. Bias is especially difficult to avoid when we have access to another examiner's test results and comments. If a child has been described as "difficult," "hyperactive," or "dull," we may unconsciously develop a perceptual set for similar behavior. Avoid such statements and labels in your own descriptions. Instead of "unresponsive," specify the stimuli presented and the conditions that prevailed, indicating those to which the child responded. Describe behavior accurately; for example, "Johnny moved around the test room constantly, touching the walls and furniture, spending a maximum of 20 seconds on any toy or object. Attempts to restrain him were met with struggles and tears."

We would like to caution you especially against the use of terms such as "deaf voice." Deaf children are often described in the literature as having "monotonous" voices, restricted in pitch and inflection. Experience indicates, however, that many young deaf children produce spontaneous vocalizations, especially laughter and crying, that sound perfectly normal with regard to pitch, inflection, and vocal quality. They may even babble with normal voice quality. When the same children are required to imitate sounds, however, they often begin to exhibit reduced or inappropriate inflection, strained voice quality, abnormal pitch, and other characteristics of the "deaf voice." Due to these inconsistencies we caution against using vocal quality during a limited observation period as evidence of either presence or absence of hearing impairment. The same warning holds true for other items, such as failure to condition easily and other characteristics discussed in the paragraphs above. A careful evaluation of all information obtained is necessary before a diagnosis can be made.

Once the presence of hearing loss is established, it must be classified as to type (conductive or sensorineural) before further steps are taken. If the child responds consistently to presentation of pure tones, determination of the type of loss is no problem. Responses by air and bone conduction are compared as described earlier in this chapter. If the child does not give consistent responses to pure tones because of age or other reasons, impedance measures or electrophysiologic measures may furnish the necessary information.

LANGUAGE DEVELOPMENT AND EDUCATIONAL NEEDS

Measures of language development in very young hearing-impaired children are difficult to accomplish, unless the child is mildly impaired. Severe hearing impairment induces a delay in language development to such an extent that the child may appear to be without language of any description until special educational procedures are initiated. Children in between the extremes usually develop language more slowly than normal, but in a similar sequence (30). For mildly and moderately hearing-impaired children, the language tests discussed in Chapter 4, with the modifications suggested in Chapter 12, are appropriate. Research indicates that hearing-impaired children exhibit delayed language development rather than deviant development (5, 6). Although few data currently exist concerning the processing strategies employed by the hearing-impaired, the information available indicates that these strategies generally vary in quantity but not in quality (10, 29) from those employed by normally hearing children. The similarity in language strategies employed by normally hearing and hearing-impaired children implies that the language deficits of the hearing-impaired may be a result of the ambiguity of the message received by them and the resulting uncertainty, rather than differences in processing strategies that may have developed as a result of reduced auditory input. Novak and Davis (25) have shown that filtering of unfamiliar auditory stimuli results in a slower rate of learning and a reduced memory span for those stimuli in normal listeners that corresponds to the learning rates and memory span deficits reported for hearing-impaired persons.

If we hypothesize that (1) language is best learned by means of the auditory system, (2) hearing-impaired children experience reduced reception of auditory events, (3) the reduced reception causes errors in the processing of language input, (4) these errors are reflected in the child's linguistic output, and (5) both reception and expression in the hearing-impaired represent delayed rather than deviant language processing, then plans for habilitation and remediation should be based on reduction of uncertainty and ambiguity in the language input. Theoretically, at least, a reduction in ambiguity should result in more accurate perception and more rapid learning of language. There are at least two sensory modalities through which *spoken* language can be channeled to the hearing-impaired: visual by means of speechreading and auditory by means of the use of residual hearing and amplification. Further visual information can be furnished through manual signals such as cued speech, fingerspelling, or signs.

Obviously, the most natural means of learning and processing language is through auditory experience with it. For this reason many educators insist that all hearing-impaired children should be taught to rely on the auditory channel for language input, often to the exclusion of other input systems (26, 28), even though intensive auditory stimulation for long periods of time may be necessary before effectiveness of the method with a given child may be assessed. Other educators, while recognizing the importance of the auditory system, focus on the fact that language is learned best at a very early age, and they advocate the use of auditory and visual information (including manual signs) from the time the hearing loss is identified, particularly in the case of children whose responses to sound are minimal and whose successful dependence upon hearing is questionable (12, 19).

It should be obvious to everyone who is knowledgeable about children, learning, and hearing impairment that no two persons are identical or even very similar. Normal children approach learning in different ways; hearing-impaired children cannot be assumed to be homogeneous in their abilities to use information presented to them. In addition, many hearing-impaired children exhibit virtually no measurable hearing. Black et al. (2) have described children who have no functional cochleas and who cannot experience sound as we conventionally think of it. A single method of teaching hearing-impaired children cannot possibly meet the needs of all such children, and insistence upon the superiority of a single method over any and all other methods reflects a bias and a refusal to recognize the realities that exist in the lives of deaf children and adults.

The problem becomes a diagnostic one: how do we identify, early in life before the optimal age for learning language is past, which children will be able to use auditory input successfully enough to maximize their language learning and which children will require visual information in addition to auditory input in order to reduce ambiguity successfully enough to allow for maximum learning? One of the most frustrating problems facing the clinician who deals with young hearing-impaired children is the lack of a diagnostic tool sophisticated enough to identify at an early age which children will be able to learn most efficiently through which channels. Unfortunately the decision as to how the child should be "taught" language must often be made before he or she has exhibited any real proclivity toward any sensory channel. Parent training, enrollment in language therapy or classes, and "preenrollment" in educational programs for the hearing-impaired must be accomplished as soon as the child is identified. Although virtually all professionals advocate reassessment and changes in the program to be followed when indicated, most early decisions about training prevail for years, until success is achieved or failure is too evident to ignore. Therefore, it is essential that early decisions be based on as much objective information as is available.

Downs (24) offers one of the few sets of guidelines available for choosing between programs that use oral-aural (emphasis on the auditory channel) and total communication (use of auditory, visual, and tactile channels, including the simultaneous presentation of sign or fingerspelling with speech). The criteria suggested by Downs include degree of residual hearing, measured intelligence, integrity of the central nervous system, and family characteristics. Although Downs' criteria represent an excellent step in the direction of quantification of factors important to future success, some of the measures (for example, intelligence quotients and central auditory processing) are not readily obtainable in very young children for whom decisions must be made. We are badly in need of some means of assessing the *probable* sensory channel of choice for each young child. In the absence of such a tool we must make decisions about a child's future with little definitive diagnostic information as a guideline.

This situation, which unfortunately prevails at the present time, makes it imperative that clinicians assess carefully and critically the information available about the success or failure of the methods of education of the hearing-impaired currently in vogue: the oral-aural method and total communication. Both of these methods have evolved from and represent improvements over earlier methods involved in the centuries-old controversy over "oral versus manual" methods of teaching. The traditional "oral" method originally emphasized the use of speechreading as the major means of speech reception. While it was successful with some children, speechreading is generally recognized to be a highly inefficient way of receiving language. The so-called "manual" method utilized speech to which were added signs for key words or concepts. The sign system used was American Sign Language, an efficient and colorful means of communication that differed significantly, however, from the spoken message, which was phrased in English.

The oral-aural method makes use of much more sophisticated amplification systems than those available even 20 years ago and advocates early introduction of amplified sound to infants. Much greater emphasis is placed on the use of auditory information than on the use of speechreading.

Total communication involves the use of all sensory channels, including excellent amplification devices, also introduced as early as possible. The major difference between this and the oral-aural method is the *addition* of manual communication. In many of the most promising programs some form of signed English is used. Seeing Essential English (1), Signing Exact English (15), Linguistics of Visible English (34), and Signed English (4) are recently developed (since 1962) and published (since 1971) systems of manual signs that correspond to the English language on a one-to-one basis. Instead of representing concepts, the signs represent morphemes of the English language, allowing for the building of words (beauty→ beautiful→ beautifully), the signing of verb tense and inflection (-s, ing, -ed, and -en), as well as other integral components of the English language. Proponents of the use of these systems suggest that they represent an easily discernible means of reducing ambiguity since the difficult-to-hear-or-see elements of the language (unstressed word endings, prepositions, auxiliary verbs) are equally as visible as the content and stressed words.

Neither of these improved methods (oral-aural or total communication) has been investigated extensively to date. Although literature in deaf education abounds with testimonials to various teaching strategies, most of them are based on individual cases, which are, naturally, success stories. Assertions are often made with no empirical data to support them. For example, we are told that children who learn to sign will not learn to speak. Conversely, we are told that children from whom signs are withheld fail to develop adequate interpersonal relations because of their communication handicap; the result is poor mental health. Neither of these claims has been substantiated adequately to date. In fact, considerable evidence now exists that the first assertion, at least, is invalid.

Recently attempts have been made to provide data that compare children who have been trained by different methods on several variables. Quigley (27) has investigated the differences in deaf children's speech, speechreading, and academic achievement when one group was trained using fingerspelling and speech and the other group was trained by oral methods. Vernon and Koh (33) investigated linguistic abilities (speech, speechreading, reading) in three groups of teenage deaf children: those who had hearing parents and attended oral preschools, those who had hearing parents and attended no preschool, and those whose parents were deaf and attended no preschool but used manual communication early in life. Moores has completed a five-year evaluation of preschools for the hearing-impaired, which utilize oral-aural, total communication, and Rochester methods [1] (35). Various linguistic measures are reported. All of the studies mentioned above as well as others present similar results: the use of early manual communication does not result in poorer speech or speechreading skills and appears to result in better reading and academic achievement than that exhibited by students taught by oral methods. With the exception of the Moores study, the oral method described did not emphasize auditory input to the extent that today's oral-aural or auditory methods do; the manual communication described utilized American Sign Language rather than Signed English. Consequently, the predominant methods in use today have still not been adequately investigated, particularly with regard to the characteristics of the children who experience the greatest success with each. Moores' data indicate the same trend, however, toward superior performance of children who use manual signs early in life.

How do the controversy over methods and the lack of data leave the clinician feeling who must make decisions about educational procedures now? Uncomfortable, in most cases. The factors discussed below appear to us to be important diagnostic considerations.

Responses to Auditory Stimuli, Unaided and Aided

Generally speaking, children who respond to frequencies through 2000 or 4000 Hz experience greater success in the use of amplification than children with so-called "corner audiograms," which reflect hearing only at frequencies of 500 Hz and below. There are exceptions to this generalization, of course. Some children who exhibit little residual hearing make excellent use of it; others who have considerable hearing fail to make good use of it even after intensive training. Erber (11) has shown a relationship between spondee discrimination and pure-tone averages in deaf children that indicates a high probability of success in the use of auditory information by children whose hearing losses do not exceed 85 dB HL. Children whose losses are greater than 100 dB HL exhibit poor auditory discrimination of spondees, while children whose thresholds are between 85 dB and 100 dB represent a "gray" area. The latter group represent one for which other diagnostic information is badly needed.

Aided thresholds for speech signals probably are of greater prognostic value than unaided ones. The child whose *aided* responses to sound are

---

[1] The Rochester method refers to the simultaneous presentation of speech and fingerspelling.

questionable at 80 to 90 dB HL seems to us to be an unlikely candidate for the oral-aural method and an appropriate candidate for total communication. Conversely, the child who responds to amplified sound at intensities within or slightly below the normal range seems to us an excellent candidate for the oral-aural method, a less appropriate candidate for total communication. In other words, we must consider the residual hearing carefully, particularly hearing for amplified sound. In addition, language activities such as babbling, ability to imitate sound, ability to lip-read words, ability to produce words, and ability to discriminate sounds should be observed and recorded. The more of these activities within the child's repertory, the better the chances are that he or she will be able to use auditory input effectively.

Intelligence

When it is possible to evaluate it before educational decisions must be made, the child's intelligence is an important indicator for educational treatment. While language development is not always related to I.Q. in normally hearing children, it is an important factor in severely hearing-impaired children. The sensory deficit is such that its effect is difficult to overcome under the best of circumstances, but far worse under circumstances of poor intelligence. The more intelligent the child, the greater the likelihood that he or she will respond well to language training. The most outstanding success stories reported by proponents of all methods generally involve highly intelligent children; children with lower mental abilities are less likely to achieve well in programs unless they are designed to provide maximum stimulation and alternatives for perception. In other words, ambiguity must be maximally reduced for children of low intelligence. Manual cues are less likely to be confused with each other than are auditory cues, particularly those of highest frequency and weakest intensity.

Parental and Home Environment

The family's commitment to providing optimal language stimulation for the child is vital to the child's success. No matter what training method is selected, it must be accepted and understood by the child's family. We cannot overemphasize the role that must be played in the child's development by the parents, especially the mother, who must become a teacher as well as a parent. Hearing-impaired children require diligent, almost constant effort on the part of the family, in order that they experience language in its natural and most useful forms. The willingness of the family to provide sustained effort over a long period of time can make the difference between success and failure for the child, regardless of the method by which he or she is taught.

If the parents have serious reservations about the teaching method being employed, they will probably be less effective in the use of the method at home. Inconsistencies in the way language is made available may result in confusion to the child. In addition, parental conflict, whether spoken or not, may contribute to feelings of guilt, particularly if the method is not immediately successful. The last thing the parents of a hearing-impaired child need is more guilt about anything.

Availability of Educational Programs

The problem as to which method to apply to a given preschool child is often solved by the availability or nonavailability of programs in the locality of the child's home. If there is only one type of educational program available, it may be necessary to enroll the child in that program, whether or not it seems most appropriate. In this event we do the parents no favor when we derogate the existing facility regardless of our feelings about the method being used there. Parents often have no choice but to enroll the child, and negative remarks by us may serve to make them feel hostile or guilty or both. Familiarize yourself with local services available for the hearing-impaired children with whom you come in contact. If in your professional view, based on evidence rather than prejudice, you feel strongly that the program is totally inappropriate for the child in question, you may have to suggest alternatives to the parents that involve serious changes in the life pattern of the family. (This course of action often occurs when no programs exist in a given area, necessitating a move on the family's part.) Recommendations in such cases must be based on objective consideration of the child's needs and the family's ability to meet them. Programs should be described as "better" or "not as appropriate" for the child under consideration, rather than as "good" or "bad" in absolute terms; furthermore, we must be prepared to justify such statements based on the individual case. It is unprofessional to make value judgments about programs or methodologies that are not based on objective evidence, experience with the method under question, and careful assessment of the procedures *as they relate to each child* and his or her individual abilities and characteristics. Furthermore, the skills, training, and effectiveness of the teacher are important. No method will succeed if the teacher is poor or the curriculum is haphazard.

These factors are also relevant when parents must make choices between residential and local programs. This decision should always be made on the basis of current assessment of the child's hearing, language, social, and educational status as they relate to the programs involved. Parents should be encouraged to investigate all programs under consideration with regard to their suitability for the child involved. Our job is not to decide or to prejudice but to provide relevant information and advice based on the diagnostic information we possess coupled with our professional knowledge of language learning and educational procedures.

SCHOOL-AGE CHILDREN

Most deaf children this age or older have been identified earlier in life and enrolled in available educational programs or therapy with a speech and hearing clinician. There is another, much larger, group of hearing-impaired children who present themselves to us for evaluation and habilitation; they constitute a heterogeneous group known as "hard-of-hearing." As a general rule these children are identified somewhat later in life than deaf children, since many of them have sufficient hearing to respond to many sounds in their environments, as well as to develop some language skills. The hearing loss is less obvious and may escape detection for several years. Assessment of the type, degree, and pattern of the hearing loss does not present a problem, as the children are usually old enough to participate in play audiometric or standard behavioral hearing test procedures as described in Chapter 12.

Educational Needs of Hard-of-Hearing Children

Although assessment of hearing status in older children is not as difficult a task as for young children, the problem of determining their linguistic and educational status is challenging and important. While the term "diagnosis" does not usually carry a connotation that includes consideration of educational placement as a diagnostic parameter, the inferences typically drawn from diagnostic statements make it dangerous to ignore the educational implications when "diagnosing" hearing loss. The literature is filled with brief descriptive statements of the speech, language, and educational "characteristics" associated with certain degrees of hearing loss, based on pure-tone thresholds, which offer too little information for generalizing (8). It is necessary to go beyond audiometric designations and describe the child in terms of what he knows about language and general knowledge and what he needs to learn in order to function in his own particular environment. When we shift to this type of assessment, we are likely to find that the "lipreading, auditory training, and preferential seating" so often recommended for hearing-impaired children encountered in our public schools has little or no relationship to the needs exhibited by the child.

It is difficult to deal with a population of hard-of-hearing children in any systematic way as individuals exhibit such a broad array of symptoms and characteristics. The term "hard-of-hearing" refers to children having hearing losses ranging from 25 dB to 85 dB HL, or even greater, depending upon the author's viewpoint. A more accurate description could probably be based on an estimate of the functional use the child has of his or her residual hearing, no matter what its degree in dB. Formal assessment of academic achievement and linguistic knowledge will lead to more accurate descriptions and prognoses for educational success.

A recent study by Davis (9) reveals the disparity that may exist between a child's academic placement, degree of hearing loss, and performance on a formal assessment of an area of knowledge considered necessary for academic achievement. Twenty-four 6- to 8-year-old children with hearing losses ranging from 35 to 70 dB HL were administered the Boehm Test of Basic Concepts (3), a test of 50 concepts of time, quantity, and space which are considered necessary for academic achievement in kindergarten through second grade. Although the children were enrolled in those grades in public schools and spent at least half of their days in classrooms for the normally hearing, 75 percent scored at or below the 10th percentile on the test. Generally speaking, the greater the hearing loss the poorer the score on the test, but this relationship did not hold for all children. With the exception of three children who exhibited high frequency losses with normal hearing in the lower frequencies and who scored above the 80th percentile, the children appeared to be seriously deficient in knowledge of concepts which form the basis for the vocabulary of instruction and workbooks in the first three grades of school. Lipreading training and preferential seating are hardly adequate as interventive steps designed to improve these children's chances of achieving academically or of communicating adequately with their peers. Concentration on lipreading and auditory training as habilitative goals presumes that being able to *receive* the stimuli will ensure their comprehension and use and ignores the underlying deficit and its effect on concept development.

Speech and hearing personnel are often charged with the responsibility of making educational placement recommendations for hearing-impaired children in public schools, based on diagnosis of their hearing losses. Generally speaking, these children may be placed in self-contained classrooms, in regular classrooms with access to a resource teacher of the hearing-impaired part of each school day, or in regular classrooms with or without remedial help from a speech clinician, reading specialist, or other professional several times a week. Thousands of hearing-impaired children scattered throughout the country receive no special help of any kind. Their speech, language, and academic problems are not well defined, but the information that exists indicates that mildly hearing-impaired children are retarded academically from one to three years (13, 18) and present speech and language difficulties, such as reduced vocabulary and reading skills, which can be expected to affect their ability to achieve academically. More severely impaired children may be as much as three to four years retarded in grade level and many drop out of school altogether.

While children who live in localities which do not provide special services for the hearing-impaired must of necessity attend classes for normal children, there is a tendency for educators to insist on such placement for hearing-impaired children even when teachers of the hearing-impaired are available. This tendency reflects a national trend in special education which recommends integration of children with varying impairments into classes of normal children. Several advantages are suggested for this type of placement, including the opportunity for better socialization of handicapped children with their peers. If a handicapped child is capable of communicating well with normal children, socialization may be successfully accomplished. A word of caution seems wise, however: self-esteem in preadolescent children has been shown to be related to academic achievement, so that children who achieve poorly in school are likely to have damaged self-esteem, which may affect their interaction with their peers. It would seem unwise, therefore, to recommend total integration of a hearing-impaired child before language skills are sufficiently developed to allow for reasonable academic and social success. Descriptions of the characteristics of hearing-impaired children who are suitable candidates for integration stress the need for language, social, and academic skills *within the normal range* for the class into which they will be placed (*14, 23*). Unfortunately, many local decisions are made on the basis of little or no assessment and considerable emotion.

Children whose language test scores reflect 4-year-old vocabulary and syntax levels can hardly be expected to achieve academically in a regular second-grade classroom for 7-year-olds, *whether they are 7, 8, or 10 years old and regardless of their audiometric scores.* The type of language to which a child can respond will inevitably determine how well he or she can understand and follow classroom instruction and materials. Concepts of time (before, after, next), space (beside, middle, next to, around), quantity (more than, less than, equal to) and other abstract ideas (skip one, take away, imagine), abound in first-grade curriculum materials and form the basis for much early learning which must then serve as the foundation for future, more advanced areas of information. Poor understanding of this basic academic vocabulary coupled with difficulty comprehending sentences, understanding verb tense, using plural and possessive markers, or distinguishing proper use of pronouns should certainly be considered important diagnostic information to be included in any decision concerning school placement or remedial activities deemed appropriate for any given child at any given point in the educational process. If thorough investigation of the child's language and academic skills reveals a pattern of language usage totally inadequate for regular classroom purposes, we, as the professionals most qualified to assess the impact of hearing loss on the child's future, must be willing to voice our concerns and urge school placement that will better suit the child's abilities, even if it means bucking the tide of popular opinion concerning mainstreaming of such children.

Hearing-impaired children must master basic skills of reading before they can be expected to move through the academic process with any degree of success. Since for normal children reading involves learning to associate visual symbols with language already learned through the auditory system, the hearing-impaired child is at a disadvantage from the outset as a result of reduced language knowledge that accompanies hearing loss. A hearing-impaired child whose hearing loss exceeds 40 dB HL and who does not exhibit some reduction in language knowledge is probably rare. This child's deficit may not be apparent until he or she is expected to deal with more abstract or difficult terms and concepts associated with higher grade levels, but eventually the auditory deficit and its effect on language become evident. For hearing-impaired children early concentration on reading *comprehension* is essential. They usually have little difficulty learning to sound out words and may be able to read aloud easily and well. Unless reading comprehension is thoroughly investigated, however, a child's reading ability may be judged as spuriously high. Even standard achievement tests of reading may overestimate a hearing-impaired child's level of functioning, as shown by Moores in his investigation of normal and deaf readers at the fifth-grade level (20). Although the two groups in his study had identical reading achievement scores, they differed significantly in their ability to process the language involved in the reading task when every fifth word was deleted and they were required to fill in the missing word.

Reading instruction for the hearing-impaired child therefore involves language instruction as well as conventional activities. The classroom teacher may have a poor understanding of the language deficit involved in hearing loss, since the majority of public school teachers have had little or no training in the area of speech, hearing, and language, and cannot be expected to know how to approach the learning problems involved. Even if the teacher thoroughly understood the language deficit, she would hardly have the time necessary to devote to individual instruction of the hearing-impaired child who must struggle to keep up, completing worksheets daily which make little sense because the instructions are not understood. When he falls helplessly behind in his ability to comprehend what he is reading, the teacher can do little to help him and he must be promoted or held back to repeat earlier failures.

Because of the great importance of an early foundation in basic academic skills, resource room assistance, tutoring, or placement in a self-contained classroom *early* in the child's academic life *before* he has failed seems advisable, rather than the more common policy of early integration and later failure that seems to be the current practice in far too many cases. It seems appropriate, therefore, that diagnosis and appraisal of a hearing-impaired child should be oriented toward the identification of much more than the status of his hearing, aided and unaided. The diagnostic procedure must include thorough investigation of the child's abilities as they relate to his needs—what he is expected to be able to achieve in the situation in which he finds himself. Furthermore, we have a responsibility to look ahead when appraising these children. We know that abstract concepts are more difficult for the hearing-impaired to learn and we also know that academic materials and subjects become more abstract as children progress through grades and subject matter. If we are to serve the hearing-impaired adequately, we must learn to anticipate their needs and to recommend and design preventive therapy where it is possible and appropriate. This action will involve earlier concern about children with mild to moderate hearing losses. It will also involve a better understanding on the part of speech and hearing clinicians of academic procedures, materials, and expectations to be encountered in today's schools. We may be surprised to find that first graders are expected to complete English worksheet pages which ask "What do pigs dream?" (21) and to progress through modern arithmetic workbooks which provide only one worksheet page per concept (32). Use of abstractions and imagination abound in modern curricula, and the hearing-impaired child's ability to deal with such materials is an important aspect of his or her functioning. It cannot be ignored by those of us who are expected to diagnose hearing impairment and to be able to plan for children who exhibit it.

DIAGNOSIS AND PLANNING FOR ADULTS

In addition to determining the presence, type, degree, and configuration of hearing loss, the audiologic diagnosis for adults should include a description of the present and potential impact of the loss on the person and his or her life-style. Some relatively common types of diagnostic decisions for adults are discussed below.

Interpretation for Site of Lesion

Although audiologists do not make diagnoses of sites and causes of lesions within the auditory system, their professional interpretations of audiologic information are relied upon by the physician. Indeed, many physicians prefer that an audiologist express the likelihood of a particular set of test results being obtained from patients with given medical diagnoses. In order to be maximally effective in medical and surgical treatment, the physician needs to be more specific than simple categorization of conductive, sensory, neural, or central. The audiologist's interpretation of the results of standard and special hearing test results often can assist in arriving at greater specificity. Although a complete coverage of interpretations of audiometric test results is beyond the scope of this chapter, we will discuss briefly some of the more general interpretations made.

A conductive type of hearing loss is described primarily on the basis of the air-bone gap. Conductive hearing disorders of medical significance may or may not demonstrate such a loss. Hearing sensitivity may be within normal limits and not even show an air-bone gap. Tympanometry, however, may demonstrate a pressure below that of the atmosphere at which the system is most compliant or a compliance which is abnormal— measures which if repeated over time suggest the need for medical intervention. Conductive hearing disorders often exhibit configurations of hearing loss, tympanograms, and reflex measures specific to the type of lesion. Otosclerosis, a progressive disease of adults, typically demonstrates a progressive loss of hearing and increasing stiffness, while a disarticulated ossicular chain will show a more stable loss of hearing with a highly compliant system.

An abnormal growth of loudness, as demonstrated by recruitment on the Alternate Binaural Loudness Balance Test or in the pattern of threshold tracings on the Békésy audiogram, is most often associated with sensory disorders. Patients with Meniere's disease, a disorder associated with dizziness and tinnitus (noises in the ear), will show hearing loss and recruitment at several or all frequencies, while patients with sensory hearing losses as the result of exposure to high levels of noise typically show these test results only at higher frequencies (especially 3000 to 6000 Hz), lack the complaint of dizziness, and report a high-pitched tinnitus. Speech discrimination with sensory disorders is often reduced but not to the extreme sometimes seen with more central lesions.

Patients with neural disorders may show a number of configurations, often unilateral and if identified early perhaps with only a mild loss of sensitivity. Unlike sensory and conductive disorders, they often demonstrate extreme threshold adaptation (in excess of 30 dB) on the tone decay tests. Speech discrimination abilities may also be extremely poor. Although tympanometry is expected to be normal for sensory and neural disorders, acoustic reflex results will relate to the type and site of the lesion.

Central auditory disorders will rarely be demonstrated on monaural tests of hearing but will show dramatic differences in performance on the dichotic listening tasks described in Chapter 12. Although little is available in the way of standardized tests, the literature consistently reports performance on different types of dichotic listening tasks to vary with the site of the lesion within the central nervous system. As data become available these tests become more and more useful clinically.

One diagnostic category which provides special problems of interpretation is that of presbycusis—literally old hearing. People who acquire a hearing loss gradually as they grow older without readily identified causes other than aging are said to have presbycusis. Historically these people have been grouped together and described stereotypically as having high-frequency sensorineural type hearing losses with poor speech discrimination. The hearing test data and communication abilities of these people have often defied categorization, however, probably because they are not a homogeneous group in relation to their lesions or hearing abilities. The hearing test measures for groups of "presbycusics" typically are scattered over the gamut of possible results. Evidence of such findings occurs repeatedly in the literature and supports the need to approach each person individually. The effects of aging on hearing and performance in oral-aural communication should be expected to be scattered as should individual performance correlating with these effects. Schuknecht (31) has described at least four separate types of presbycusis on the basis of temporal bone studies. Further research is needed to apply information on these types in clinical diagnosis of communication disorders.

Determination of Communication Disorder

The diagnosis of communication disorders in adults with hearing losses typically depends as much upon information about the person and his or her life-style as it does upon the hearing loss. Decisions which lead to recommendations and habilitative plans ultimately revolve around the human interactions of the individual. For the most part, language and educational development are established and the clinician must determine what the communication disorder means to the person who lives with it. Does it require changes in the basic social and vocational interactions? If so, have these already been acknowledged by the person with the hearing impairment? What has the person done so far to accommodate? If amplification and training were to be applied, what is the prognosis for alleviation of the problems? How do the patient, his family, close associates, employer or employees, and acquaintances react to the communication problems presented by the hearing loss? What are their expectations for the patient's performance with training in speechreading or with the use of a hearing aid? What effects of the hearing loss have already been shown in the person's behavior? Is he withdrawing from situations requiring spoken communication? Does he deny problems in hearing and understanding speech? Have his own speech patterns (voice level and articulation patterns, for instance) begun to change?

All of the above questions and many more need to be answered for the complete diagnosis of hearing impairment in adults. Attempts have been made in the past to develop instruments which will combine hearing test data and life-style information into a meaningful measure of communication abilities. Unfortunately, none has proved to be satisfactory in meeting the needs of routine clinical diagnosis. Davis (7) used speech audiometry scores in his Social Adequacy Index, while the hearing handicap scales of High, Fairbanks, and Glorig (16) and of Noble and Atherley (22) gather information about hearing experiences. These measures contribute to our understanding of communication abilities but as yet fall short in prognosis for the individual.

Indications of general communication ability can also be obtained through measures of the person's ability to use auditory input only, visual (speechreading) input only, and combined auditory and visual input. Although the results of such measures, summarized in Chapter 12, may not provide standardized interpretations, it is often possible for the clinician to gain an impression of the person's strengths and weaknesses in face-to-face communication. Such measures done with and without the assistance of a hearing aid may be quite helpful in determining communication abilities, developing habilitative plans, and providing a prognosis of success in communication.

The audiologist must apply his or her knowledge, skill, and experience to the interpretation of information for each individual. The diagnostic process continues through hearing testing, hearing aid selection and use, and habilitative planning. Referrals to (1) the physician for medical diagnosis and treatment, (2) the psychologist for intellectual and emotional assessment and counseling, (3) the social worker for assistance in social adjustment, and (4) the vocational counselor for assistance in choice and acquisition of a livelihood are important for gathering information, reaching diagnoses, and providing habilitation.

NONORGANIC HEARING LOSS

Hearing test results which lead to the impression of a more severe hearing loss than actually exists are interpreted as demonstrating *nonorganic* hearing loss. Such test results may be recognized through inconsistent test responses or test results which are not compatible with case history or general communication behavior. Inconsistent test response may occur upon repetition of the same test but more often occurs between different tests. The most common diagnostic clue to nonorganic hearing loss is an SRT level which is significantly better (by more than 10 dB) than the PTA. This is especially apparent when the SRT is better than any single pure-tone threshold.

The clinician encountering a patient demonstrating nonorganic hearing loss must not be too quick to draw conclusions concerning the reasons for such behavior. The range of reasons for exhibiting nonorganic hearing loss is wide. It may be that the patient is deliberately attempting to deceive the examiner for personal gain through compensation, release from unpleasant duties, or an excuse for poor performance. On the other hand, such test performance may be less deliberate, possibly a symptom of a more pervasive psychological disorder.

Regardless of the patient's reasons for demonstrating a nonorganic hearing loss, it is the audiologist's duty to determine the organic hearing loss, to diagnose any existing communication disorder, and to make the appropriate referrals for further evaluation. The simple diagnosis of nonorganic hearing loss is insufficient. Such a diagnosis is valuable in guiding the audiologist in his or her evaluation and interpretation of test results but must be followed up with a more definitive determination of the patient's needs.

SUMMARY

You may feel that this chapter has provided you with more information about the diagnostic process in audiology than it has about how to diagnose auditory disorders, and you would be right. It has been our purpose to alert you to the need for audiologic diagnosis and provide you with an introduction to its application.

As can be readily observed, referral to an audiologist is appropriate when a complaint or suspicion of hearing loss exists. The speech-language pathologist needs to become alert to indications that hearing loss may be a possibility. Knowledge of hearing ability provides important information about receptive communication abilities and should be an integral part of the diagnosis of disorders of communication.

ASSIGNMENTS

1. Discuss the several ways in which the terms conductive, sensorineural, and central are used in the diagnosis of hearing impairment.
2. List the guidelines and reasons which you as a speech-language pathologist would use for referring a patient to an audiologist for evaluation.
3. Why must the diagnosis of the communication disorder accompanying a hearing loss include more than audiometric test data?
4. Obtain first-grade reading, language arts, and arithmetic workbooks. Analyze the sentence structures found within them. List specialized vocabulary and rate it as "concrete" or "abstract."
5. Choose a task from one of the workbooks mentioned in question 4 and analyze it with regard to what the child must (1) understand and (2) be able to do to complete the task.

REFERENCES

1. Anthony, D. A., and Associates, *Seeing Essential English*. Greeley: University of Northern Colorado, 1971.

2. Black, F. O., Sando, I., Wagner, J. A., and Hemenway, W. G., Middle and inner ear abnormalities, 13–15, (D_1) Trisomy, *Archives of Otolaryngology*, 1971, *93*:615–619.

3. Boehm, A., *Boehm Test of Basic Concepts*. New York: Psychological Corporation, 1971.

4. Bornstein, H., A description of some current sign systems designed to represent English. *American Annals of the Deaf*, 1973, *118*:454–463.

5. Brannon, J., Linguistic word classes in the spoken language of normal, hard of hearing, and deaf children. *Journal of Speech and Hearing Research*, 1968, *11*:279–297.

6. Brannon, J., and Murry, T., The spoken syntax of normal, hard of hearing and deaf children. *Journal of Speech and Hearing Research*, 1966, *9*: 604–610.

7. Davis, H., The articulation area and the social adequacy index for hearing. *Laryngoscope*, 1948, *58*:761–768.

8. Davis, H., and Silverman, S. R., *Hearing and Deafness*. New York: Holt, Rinehart and Winston, 1970.

9. Davis, J., Performance of young hearing-impaired children on a test of basic concepts. *Journal of Speech and Hearing Research*, 1974, *17*:342–351.

10. Davis, J., and Blasdell, R., Perceptual strategies employed by normal-hearing and hearing-impaired children in the comprehension of sentences containing relative clauses. *Journal of Speech and Hearing Research*, 1975, *18*:281–295.

11. Erber, N. P., Pure-tone thresholds and word recognition abilities of hearing impaired children. *Journal of Speech and Hearing Research*, 1974, *17*:194–202.

12. Furth, H. G., *Thinking Without Language*. New York: Free Press, 1966.

13. Goetzinger, C., Harrison, C., and Baer, C., Small perceptive hearing loss: Its effect in school-age children. *The Volta Review*, 1964, *66*:124–131.

14. Griffing, B. L., Planning educational programs and services for hard-of-hearing children. In Berg, F. S., and Fletcher, S. G., eds., *The Hard of Hearing Child*, pp. 233–244. New York: Grune & Stratton, 1970.

15. Gustason, G., Pfetzing, D., and Zawolkow, E., *Signing Exact English*. Rossmoor, Calif.: Modern Signs Press, 1972.

16. High, W., Fairbanks, G., and Glorig, A., A scale for self-assessment of hearing handicap. *Journal of Speech and Hearing Disorders*, 1964, *29*: 215–230.

17. Kleffner, F. R., Hearing losses, hearing aids, and children with language disorders. *Journal of Speech and Hearing Disorders*, 1973, *38*:232–239.

18. Kodman, F., Educational status of hard of hearing children in the classroom. *Journal of Speech and Hearing Disorders*, 1963, *28*:297–299.

19. Mindel, E., and Vernon, M., *They Grow in Silence*. Silver Spring, Md.: National Association of the Deaf, 1971.

20. Moores, D. F., An investigation of the psycholinguistic functioning of deaf adolescents. *Exceptional Children*, 1970, *36*:645–652.

21. *New Directions in English*. New York: Harper & Row, 1969.

22. Noble, W. G., and Atherley, G. R. C., The hearing measurement scale:

A questionnaire for the assessment of auditory disability. *Journal of Auditory Research*, 1970, *10*:299–350.

23. Northcott, W. H., ed., *The Hearing Impaired Child in a Regular Classroom*. Washington, D.C.: The Alexander Graham Bell Association for the Deaf, 1973.

24. Northern, J. L., and Downs, M. P., *Hearing in Children*. Baltimore: Williams & Wilkins, 1974.

25. Novak, R., and Davis, J., Effects of low-pass filtering on the rate of learning and retrieval from memory of speech-like stimuli. *Journal of Speech and Hearing Research*, 1974, *17*:279–285.

26. Pollack, D., *Educational Audiology for the Limited Hearing Infant*. Springfield, Ill.: Thomas, 1970.

27. Quigley, S. P., *The Influence of Fingerspelling on the Development of Language, Communication, and Educational Achievement in Deaf Children*. Champaign, Urbana: Institute for Research on Exceptional Children, University of Illinios, 1968.

28. Rupp, R. R., An approach to the communicative needs of the very young hearing impaired child. *Journal of the Academy of Rehabilitative Audiology*, 1971, *4*:11–12.

29. Russell, W. L., Quigley, S. P., and Power, D. J., *Linguistics and Deaf Children*. Washington, D.C.: The Alexander Graham Bell Association for the Deaf, 1976.

30. Schlesinger, H., and Meadow, K., *Sound and Sign*. Berkeley: University of California Press, 1972.

31. Schuknecht, H., Further observations on the pathology of presbycusis. *Archives of Otolaryngology*, 1964, *80*:369–382.

32. *Silver Burdett Mathematics*. Palo Alto, Calif.: General Learning Corporation, 1973.

33. Vernon, M., and Koh, S., Early manual communication and deaf children's achievement. *American Annals of the Deaf*, 1970, *115*:527–536.

34. Wampler, D. W., *Linguistics of Visual English*. Santa Rosa, Calif.: 2322 Maher Drive, 1971.

35. Weiss, K. L., Goodwin, M. W., and Moores, D. F., *Characteristics of Young Deaf Children and Early Intervention Programs*, Research Report No. 91. Minneapolis, Minn.: Research, Development and Demonstration Center in Education of Handicapped Children, 1975.

17

DIFFERENTIAL DIAGNOSIS OF LANGUAGE DISORDERS

Frederic L. Darley

Most of us manage during childhood to acquire a mastery of the symbol system by means of which we communicate, and most of us manage to maintain those skills through adulthood in a functionally adequate way with varying degrees of imperfection. But some of us for various reasons fail to develop this initial mastery or develop it over a more prolonged time period than others, and some of us for various reasons experience significant degrees of impairment of these skills once mastered, even their total loss. One of our responsibilities as speech-language pathologists is to describe the language status of such children and adults, to identify different patterns of impaired acquisition or acquired dysfunction of language skills, and by analysis of antecedent events and current information about associated behavior arrive at a differential diagnosis of the language disorder.

In order to describe the patient's language status we will make use of the kinds of observations detailed in Chapters 4 and 5 of this book dealing with appraisal of language development and acquired language disorders. The overall description of the patient's oral communication (Chapter 3) will help put his or her language behavior in perspective. Information derived through systematic observations of the patient's auditory functioning (Chapter 12) will be of crucial importance. Information from the case history (Chapter 2) is essential in establishing the temporal pattern of the disorder, its characteristics, and associated behaviors.

When we have gathered all this appraisal information we should be in a position to specify not only how the patient engages in symbolic behavior but also the probable reason or reasons for his or her condition. For each patient we will delineate the temporal features of the development or dissolution of his or her language prowess, know the features of his or her past and current communicative behavior, and relate to it any distinctive associated behaviors. Thus we will have teased out a syndrome to which we can assign a name and an etiology, and for which we will hope to develop a plan of remediation. Even if we don't arrive at a final differential diagnosis, we may at least learn enough to develop some working hypotheses that can be tested during a period of experimental therapy.

PATTERNS OF DEVELOPMENTALLY DELAYED AND DISORDERED LANGUAGE

Mental Retardation

The most common cause of delayed language development is mental retardation. Most mentally retarded children acquire a language system and functional speech. Only in cases of extreme retardation in which the I.Q. obtained in psychometric testing is below 25 would we expect complete speechlessness (11). Mutism is more usually attributable to severe emotional disturbance, congenitally present in cases of autism, due to hysteria in an older child who once spoke but has stopped speaking.

The rate of language acquisition is typically slowed in cases of mental retardation in proportion to the severity of the retardation. Mentally retarded children produce single words on the average two years later than children of normal intelligence, and they demonstrate a similar lag in production of developmental sentence types. These children's vocabularies are more limited and their sentences shorter and structurally less complex than average, and they tend to use speech more for demand than for conveying ideas. They are slow as well in mastery of articulation, probably not presenting articulation problems that are different in kind from individuals not mentally retarded except possibly in a greater incidence of phoneme omission errors and the use of some bizarre substitutions (see Chapter 19, p. 525).

Mentally retarded children will not, then, be distinctively different from normal children in their comprehension and use of language but will rather be slower in developing language skills and will likely attain a lower level of achievement in most language areas than normal children. But their slowness is not confined to symbolic functioning. They are typically slow in other aspects of development—acquiring motor and self-help skills, acquiring a store of general information, learning school subjects, and demonstrating ability to do abstract thinking. Theirs is not a specific language disability, disproportionate to other areas of mental functioning, but rather part of a general picture of decelerated learning of all kinds. They do not respond to sound or to symbolic stimuli in an unusual way. They may be somewhat slow in responding to strangers and they may show a lack of understanding of social situations, but they are usually able to relate to people easily and maintain warm interpersonal relationships. They demonstrate that they can learn, though slowly. Enrichment and prolongation of language stimulation, if clinicians and parents are patient enough to sustain their efforts, result in gradual improvement of language skills within the limits defined by the child's intellectual potential.

Hearing Loss

Children with significant hearing losses will demonstrate degrees of delay of language acquisition and impairment which depend upon the degree of their hearing loss and the time in life when they occurred, whether prior to the development of language or after language had at least been partially developed. Children without hearing from early in life do a certain amount of babbling during early months, but they gradually reduce the amount, fail to echo the speech around them, and do not develop understandable words at the usual time. Although their speech development may be colossally impaired, they demonstrate symbolic behavior in other functions that do not require sound. They do not improvise vocally as other children do, humming or singing or amusing themselves by imitating the noises of their toys. They may vocalize in order to attract attention and express emotions. They learn to watch other people closely and may be especially sensitive to their facial expressions. They resort to communicating by gesture in order to compensate for their lack of verbal ability.

Hard-of-hearing children whose partial loss occurred after the acquisition of language are likely to present speech problems rather than language problems. They have some grasp of our symbol system but their reduced input and impaired monitoring system may result in unusual patterns of vocal melody and defective phoneme production. As they grow older, hard-of-hearing children will likely have more limited vocabularies than other children and their sentences may be shorter and syntactically imperfect. Their degree of doubt as to what is going on around them linguistically may be reflected in restriction of communication and reduced spontaneity of speech, smiling, and laughter. Neither the hard-of-hearing nor the deaf are different from normal children in their ability to make friends and establish and maintain close personal relationships; however, they may tend to remain on the periphery of social situations, perhaps engaging themselves with objects, though not in the compulsive manner observed in severely emotionally disturbed children.

Children with hearing losses, if they can hear sound at all, will respond reasonably consistently to it. We do not expect these children to tune in and out, to respond erratically, to fluctuate widely in their ability to hear and make sense out of the language around them; such behavior is more typical of children with auditory processing problems (specific language disability).

Autism

Children diagnosed as manifesting the clinical syndrome of infantile autism (sometimes called childhood schizophrenia) present varied histories of early language development, but they invariably have severe restriction of communication skills. Some show a period of normal language development followed by regression. Others from the beginning show no interest in the speech about them and make no attempt to imitate it. At times it may be evident that autistic children are aware of sound, but their typical response is to ignore it. But they seemingly ignore everything else that goes on around them. From the beginning of life they fail to relate in ordinary ways to people and situations. Seemingly more interested in things than in people, they hold themselves aloof from others, physically as well as linguistically. They do not engage with parents, siblings, or friends either with eyes or words. Probably a third of autistic children remain mute. The remainder develop meager communication skills; their spontaneous speech is largely egocentric and is not used to convey information or to influence the behavior of others.

In addition to impairment of communication, a number of behaviors have been designated as criteria for identification of the autistic child (18, 22), including the following: (1) gross and sustained impairment of emotional relationships with people, including aloofness, impersonal response to individuals, and difficulty in associating with other children; (2) apparent unawareness of personal identity, including abnormal exploration of parts of the body and self-directed aggression; (3) pathological preoccupation with particular objects or certain characteristics of them; (4) sustained resistance to change in the environment and a striving to maintain or restore sameness; (5) abnormal perceptual experience manifested as excessive, diminished, or unpredictable response to sensory stimuli; (6) acute, excessive, and seemingly illogical anxiety, often precipitated by change; (7) distortion in movement patterns such as hyperkinesis, immobility, toe walking, bizarre postures, or intractable ritualistic mannerisms such as rocking, spinning, and hand flapping; and (8) a background of serious retardation in which islands of normal, near normal, or exceptional intellectual function or skill may appear.

Specific Language Disability

Another group of children are significantly retarded in acquisition of communication skills even though careful appraisal reveals that they have no significant hearing loss, no neuromotor defect, normal or above normal intelligence, and no evidence of emotional disturbance. These children display an impaired ability to comprehend and use language which is disproportionate to their other cognitive abilities. They have been variously identified as displaying a developmental aphasia, congenital aphasia, central auditory disorder, dysacusis, congenital word deafness, or a specific language disability.

A wide spectrum of severity of communication impairment is found in these children. Some are so severely handicapped that they behave as though deaf. As Wood (26, p. 30) has said, such a child is "surrounded by language which he cannot understand but, equally important, few people recognize that he does not understand speech and cannot comprehend words. He has no interpreters, no way to make his wants known." Children with milder degrees of difficulty show restriction of auditory retention span, awkwardness in the use of syntactic structures, and specific difficulties in reading, writing, spelling, and arithmetic. They may seem to mishear words, pay poor attention when instructions are given, and fail to carry out orders properly.

The pattern of these children's development of language may not be distinctive. They may do little babbling; some children do none. They early demonstrate that they can hear and respond appropriately to non-language sounds. Unlike the mentally retarded their general behavior is usually more adequate, proportionately better than their language performance. They are able to relate to others and their efforts of communication through gesture differentiate them from autistic children.

The central problem in these children is a difficulty in processing auditory stimuli. They have special trouble giving their attention to the language around them and selecting from out of that noise the sounds which most warrant attention, that is, foreground speech. They are often inconsistent in their response to sound, displaying variable thresholds of responsiveness. Although they can hear, they have trouble listening, that is, using their hearing functionally. They may display problems in auditory discrimination; although they may give evidence of being able to discriminate between similar phonemes like /s/ and /z/ in isolation, when phonemes are blended into words and come at them rapidly, they cannot tell them apart and cannot reproduce them. Their storage system for speech signals is apparently defective; although they may be able to imitate speech models immediately, following a brief delay they lose what they have heard and cannot reproduce it; having been taught a lesson, they may act a few hours later as though they never heard of it. They have trouble with the sequencing of auditory input; they cannot seem to keep track of the order in which sounds come; they cannot retain and recall sequences of phonemes or numbers or other word strings. They seemingly cannot listen fast enough and process auditory signals at the rate at which they normally arrive (7, 8). They have difficulty making a whole out of a series of disconnected phonemes, for example, synthesizing "dog" out of d–o–g. They may display equal difficulty in taking a word apart and identifying its components or guessing at a missing component in a word fragment.

Associated with these evidences of impaired auditory perception and processing, other behavioral differences may appear (21). These children are frequently reported to be hyperactive and extremely distractible. They may be emotionally labile, easily frustrated, inconsistent in their behavior. The frustration of trying to cope with input that they cannot readily comprehend and process and the frequent failure of adults around them to understand their auditory handicap may lead to exacerbation of nonadaptive behavior; they may come to be considered stubborn or lazy, children who refuse to try. But rarely would we make the mistake of confusing these children with autistic children. They do try to communicate, by gesture if not by speech, and when they use speech, it is purposeful—to convey information and to influence behavior. When their auditory surroundings are simplified and when input is structured, they demonstrate that they can listen and learn and perhaps achieve to the level of the potential they were demonstrated to have on psychometric testing.

Other Groups

Many children who do not fit into any of the aforementioned categories demonstrate some retardation of language acquisition or a level of linguistic performance not commensurate with their intelligence. Some of these children are victims of psychosocial deprivation. We can find examples of all degrees from the truly isolated child devoid of stimulation through the institutionalized child without parental ties and family experiences to children in "normal homes" where the circumstances of the family situation and the family constellation have failed to provide the child with optimum opportunity to learn.

The number of people in the family, the child's position in the family group, the family socioeconomic status all have some effect on speech acquisition. Research studies have documented the existence of a kind of hierarchy with regard to rate of language acquisition within families: children without siblings are usually more accelerated, children of single births who have siblings are somewhat less so, and children of multiple births are even slower (3, 4, 14). Children in orphanages, where the adult-child ratio is highly different from that in most homes, are even slower in acquiring language skills and present more speech problems than do children who live at home (2, 16). Children from homes of lower socioeconomic status are usually linguistically delayed in comparison with children from higher social levels. The concept of socioeconomic status implies several influences including the family's economic stability, the level of the parents' education, the amount of leisure time they have, the variety of recreational activities they enjoy, the kinds of stimulating materials and experiences to which the child is exposed, the parents' sophistication regarding child-rearing practices, and the quality of the speech models provided for the children. Children from homes markedly depressed socioeconomically may well suffer from relative impoverishment of stimulation in terms of all of these variables.

In our society girls appear to have some linguistic advantage over boys, perhaps because they often enjoy a closer and more prolonged relationship with the mother and are encouraged more than boys to engage in activities involving verbal communication (13).

Parental characteristics may influence the children's language development. Parents of speech-retarded and articulatory-impaired children have been shown as a group to display excessive anxiety concerning their children, perfectionistic tendencies, emotional reactions to their speech problems, severe disciplinary methods, ignorance of behavioral problems, major marital incompatibility, unequal affection for their children, and higher than normal incidence of long illness, acute episodes, or tragedy during the child's life (1, 15, 18, 24).

Children who have an impairment of communication for some anatomic or physiological reason may display a retardation and acquisition of language skills as well. Many cerebral palsied children are retarded in language acquisition. Several studies have shown that as a group children with palatal clefts also show a higher incidence than normal of language retardation (17, 20, 24). These groups of children highlight a fact that we must always remember: retardation in acquisition of language skills may be due to more than one cause. The cerebral palsied child may be mentally retarded as well as have a neuromotor handicap. The child with a palatal cleft may have a significant hearing loss. Children may be both hard-of-hearing and mentally retarded. Any child may show the summated effects of emotional disturbance, hearing loss, and mental retardation. Specific language disability is no respector of persons; we can expect it to turn up among children who have hearing losses, mental retardation, emotional disturbances, and anatomic and neuromotor handicaps.

PATTERNS OF ACQUIRED LANGUAGE DYSFUNCTION

Aphasia

Although aphasic patients differ widely in the severity of their language impairment, they have in common a loss of efficiency in processing the symbols by which we communicate. This inefficiency is manifested in all language modalities—listening, reading, speaking, writing—although not necessarily to the same degree in all (6, 23). By definition aphasia involves difficulties both in the understanding of language and in its formulation and expression.

The aphasic patient's inefficiency in listening may make him behave at times as if he were hard of hearing. Familiar words seem to go by too rapidly for him to grasp and retain them. He clutches at fragments and nods so knowingly that his relatives and associates may believe that he "understands everything we say." If he is severely aphasic, he may not be able to recognize even single words; he will be unable to select the appropriate object or picture when told the name of it. If he is less severely impaired, his problem in listening may be more evident in the restriction of auditory retention span. He may be able to hang on to one or more words but will lose track of a series of three or four. He tells us that he cannot "listen fast enough." He may be able to repeat after us a word or two but not a longer phrase or sentence. Details of what he hears will escape him so that he only partially executes a two- or three-step command and misses parts of questions, conversation, and stories read to him.

Reading may present similarly puzzling problems. Even single words may look unfamiliar to him and somehow "wrong." He may struggle through a sentence word by word, misreading words and not appreciating his mistakes. When he has finished his word-by-word struggle, the meaning may have evaporated and he must struggle through it again. If he is capable of reading longer materials, he may overlook and fail to retain some details.

When he tries to speak, words elude him. He gropes awkwardly to retrieve them or perhaps he misspeaks. If his aphasia is severe, he may manage no more than a telegraphic kind of speech. Some patients with severe receptive difficulty produce a continuous flow of meaningless jargon or fluent speech full of neologisms, seemingly unaware that they are not communicating. Most aphasic patients asked to name common pictures and objects will respond slowly; some will fail to evoke the correct word; sometimes they will substitute a word related to the target word in any of several ways ("pencil" for "pen," "talk" for "telephone," "sharp" for "knife") or they may simply indicate that they don't know the word. When asked to express ideas, they may verbally beat around the bush without coming to the point satisfactorily. In some patients the words produced are primarily substantive words with omission of the connective words; other patients are relatively unable to produce the substantive words. Patients with less severe expressive problems may settle for an abbreviated statement which lacks details and precision, or they may produce overly long, redundant responses.

When they try to write, aphasic patients may forget how a word should look and may be confused as to how to form certain letters. In writing to dictation they misspell some words, omit others. They may make numerous efforts at self-correction, often unsuccessfully. A severely impaired patient may be unable to communicate any message in writing. A less impaired patient's spontaneous writing will be sparse, produced more slowly than average, with evidence of self-corrected errors.

These behaviors, embraced in the term aphasia, result from damage to the brain, usually to the language-dominant left hemisphere. Onset of the problem may be gradual or sudden, depending upon the etiology. The most common etiology of aphasia is a cerebrovascular accident; in the case of transient ischemic attacks or a series of small strokes the onset of the aphasia may be stepwise, but in the case of a massive stroke the onset is sudden. Aphasia due to cerebral neoplasms will ordinarily be insidious in onset, as will be aphasia due to an infectious process. Traumatically incurred aphasia will, of course, be of sudden onset.

Aphasic language behavior per se is not characterized by a significant amount of articulation difficulty, but often in association with aphasia one encounters a primary articulation difficulty identified as apraxia of speech (see Chapter 18, pp. 510–511 for a discussion of the differentiation of apraxia of speech and aphasia). Aphasic language behavior is not usually characterized by confabulation or the production of irrelevant responses to stimuli presented by the examiner. Phonatory and resonatory changes are not an integral part of aphasia, but dysarthria can coexist with aphasia. Important in making the diagnostic distinction between aphasia and other disorders with which it might be confused is the fact that in aphasic patients the language impairment is disproportionate to impairment of other intellective functions. Appraisal of the patient's performance reveals that the language problem is not attributable to dementia, sensory loss, motor dysfunction, or emotional disturbance.

Confused Language

Neurologists identify a specific impairment of mental function as a "confused state" or "confusion." In confusion the patient's responses demonstrate that he fails to comprehend his surroundings. He may think he is at home rather than in the hospital and he may misidentify people. He is likely to be disoriented in time. He tends to misinterpret events. His clarity of thinking and his memory of recent events are impaired (12, p. 206).

Several features characterize the altered communication of confused patients. They typically have difficulty maintaining interaction and tracking conversation. They may respond well to specific questions, giving exact and accurate answers when asked to name objects, read words and sentences, and do simple arithmetic. But on less structured tasks where they have more freedom in response, as when they are asked open-ended questions or are required to explain proverbs or the functions of objects, they will "wander away," produce irrelevant responses, and perhaps confabulate. (A dictionary definition: to confabulate is to "give answers and recite experiences without regard to truth.") For example, a patient asked to list three things that he had done that day replied, "I stayed away above time, and I tried to grasp things that were un-

heralded before me, and I tried to reminisce, which was impossible."
Another patient answered, "I don't know if I tried any desserts; I
suppose I did. You'd have to figure them out. I gave friends new models
of things to go by, I suppose." A patient asked to define the word
"motor" replied, "Motor is a measure of installment, I presume. It behaves in accordance with a measure of philosophy." A patient who was
asked to list three things that every good citizen should do responded,
"You should go to the store and enter inside, and then you should get
shoes started—and you should help to have the Volkswagen go and
you should help the Volkswagens with your store."

Confused patients are usually unaware of the inappropriateness of
their responses, usually less aware of their errors than are aphasic
patients. They think they are making sense even when their responses
are inadequate and irrelevant. A hospitalized patient who was asked to
list three things he had done that day replied, "First I drove the car.
Two, I made somebody happy that wasn't, and I made the United
Press Paper real happy." When he was challenged as to the veracity of his
statement, he stoutly defended its correctness.

The structure of the responses made by confused patients is typically
quite different from the structure of the responses of aphasic patients.
Confused patients usually demonstrate normal syntactic structure although the content of the sentence is inappropriate. Speech is typically
fluent and without articulatory or phonatory distortion. For example, the
voice, articulation, prosody, and syntax of a college student who had
incurred a head injury in an automobile accident were within normal
limits when he listed three things that every good citizen should do:
"He should watch out for mailboxes. He should watch out for people.
He should watch out for papers." Another patient with fluent speech
and good syntax bizarrely replied, "He should build on the right side,
he should build on the left side, and he should build on the west side."
It is the pattern of a high degree of irrelevance of content coupled with
paradoxically adequate syntax, word choice, and fluency that differentiates the language performance of confused patients from that of
aphasic and demented patients (9).

The disorder is often but not necessarily traumatically induced.
Unlike most other acquired language disorders, it is often transient
although not always. Brain lesions in these cases are usually found to be
disseminated, either multiple focal lesions or a combination of focal and
diffuse pathology.

Dementia

Patients suffering from a progressive degeneration of the brain, sometimes called organic brain syndrome, display insidious onset and gradual
progression of generalized intellectual impairment. These patients are

identified as demented. One feature of their dementia will be at least mild across-the-board language difficulty.

Ordinarily demented patients have little or no difficulty recognizing single words spoken to them or read by them, matching words and pictures, and naming pictures and objects. They ordinarily display some difficulty in auditory retention, but it usually is not severe, at least in the early stages of the disease; for example, they can repeat sentences until they become very long, and they can repeat several digits forward and perhaps backward but not so many as normal adults. On expressive language tasks they display little or no difficulty with syntax. Their sentences are well constructed and their vocabulary is not unusual. However, the more abstract the verbal task, the more trouble they will have. They may have difficulty defining words adequately and usually will have difficulty explaining proverbs, sometimes failing to see the difference between proverbs. (" 'Don't count your chickens before they are hatched.' Well, that's the same as 'Don't put all your eggs in one basket.' ") They often explain proverbs in concrete terms rather than develop a generalization ("You might break all your eggs"). A demented patient responded to the question about what every good citizen should do by saying, "He should be neighborly. He should help his neighbor—but that goes back into the same idea. He should be kind to his neighbor; say hello to his neighbor—things like that." He recognized that he was not accomplishing the task of listing separate things, but he was unable to improve his performance.

Demented patients tend to be slow in responding to all stimuli, ramble in their answers, forget what they are doing or talking about, become easily mixed up on how to mark written responses, wander in their attention, give up on tasks easily, be unsure of their answers, and repeatedly offer expressions of inadequacy and bewilderment. They do not typically make significant syntactic errors in their responses, nor in word retrieval do they come up with bizarre choices. Their speech is generally free of phonetic errors. They do not generally confabulate.

Whereas aphasic patients display a language disorder disproportionate to their overall level of cognitive function, demented patients demonstrate comparable difficulty on all mental tasks. Arithmetic is often hard for them; many patients will seem to have forgotten the basic operations involved in arithmetic, and most will be unable to perform two- and three-digit multiplication and division problems. They will be poor in recalling general information.

It is often difficult to determine whether the patient has a language-specific problem (aphasia) or whether his or her language difficulty is part of a more comprehensive "thinking" problem. Ultimately the differentiation will depend upon the total pattern of results obtained in psychometric testing. This differentiation by means of language and psychometric testing is important to the neurologist: aphasia connotes a focal lesion whereas dementia suggests a more diffuse, probably degenerative process.

Akinetic Mutism

Some patients with neurologic lesions present what has been called an akinetic or trancelike mutism. The clinical picture is one of the patient lying motionless and atonic in bed, sleeping more than normally but being easily aroused, making no spontaneous movement and no sound. In extreme forms of the disorder the patient will lie inert, mute, and immobile except that his open eyes follow events in the environment, indicating consciousness and seeming to "give promise of speech." Some observers have described lesser degrees of the disorder; in less complete manifestations of the disease the patient responds imperfectly after long latency with monosyllabic words or brief sentences, sometimes in a whisper, often in a monotone.

This disorder has been related to the existence of tumors in the region of the third ventricle, metastatic tumors in the midline of the midbrain, ischemia in the area of supply of the basilar artery, encephalitis, and traumatic lesions of frontal lobes. Through some mechanism these patients are inhibited in their cortical motor functions even though the lesions may be in the brain stem. Follow-up studies indicate that patients may improve although they may display residual mental and speech defects (10).

Emotional Disturbance

In Chapter 20 patients are described who develop a variety of dysphonias and aphonias or become mute in response to life's problems and interpersonal conflicts. Such conversion reactions are defined as "specific, relatively persistent physical symptoms or syndromes which exist in the absence of sufficiently causative, physiological pathology. They constitute an unconscious simulation of illness by the patient who is convinced of their somatic origins; and they enable the patient to remain relatively unaware of conflict, stress, or inadequacies which would otherwise be emotionally disturbing" (27, p. 308). Varieties of aphonia and dysphonia are described in that chapter.

Some patients become not only aphonic, resorting to whispering, but totally mute. Such patients, interestingly, make no pretense of not understanding speech. They demonstrate a wide discrepancy between their receptive and expressive abilities. Furthermore, they do not appear to be worried about their silence, blandly accept their inability to express themselves, and display no drive to communicate vocally. Such patients are thus quite different from patients in other categories described in this chapter. Aphasic patients for example, demonstrate impairment of both reception and expression. Aphasic and demented patients typically indicate that they want to communicate even though communication may be a struggle and what they produce is fragmentary at best.

Patients have been seen who in their apparent effort to protect themselves have retreated from psychogenic aphonia in connection with which they were at least willing to whisper, to a mute state in which they neither phonated nor whispered, resorting to writing, to a condition in which they seemingly were unwilling to communicate even by writing.

Another type of psychiatric patient is the chronic schizophrenic. The behavior of these patients is characterized by disturbance in reality relationships and concept formation, with associated affective, behavioral, and intellectual disturbances in varying degrees and mixtures. They show tendencies to withdraw from reality, inappropriate moods, unpredictable disturbances in the stream of thought, regressive tendencies, sometimes hallucinations.

The language of a chronic schizophrenic patient does not consistently fulfill normal communicative function because it is often not used primarily for informational purposes. There may be perseveration of ideas and preoccupation with certain themes. Patients may demonstrate structurally incomplete or stylized constructions and telescope their ideas.

The profile of behavior of schizophrenic patients on a language battery is different from profiles of aphasic, demented, and confused patients (5). Schizophrenic patients usually communicate readily and have no difficulty making their wishes known, but they often introduce extraneous conversation reflecting their preoccupations. Their responses are typically well worded and syntactically complete. The features that most clearly distinguish them from aphasic patients are a high degree of general communicative adequacy, in contrast to aphasic patients' general inadequacy of expression, and a high incidence of irrelevance in their comments, in contrast to a high degree of relevance in aphasic patients. In addition, listening, reading, and writing functions are relatively unimpaired in schizophrenic patients whereas they are typically impaired to a degree comparable to speaking impairment in aphasic patients. It appears that as the duration of their illness increases, schizophrenic patients deteriorate in language performance first in the direction of the profile shown by confused patients and ultimately toward the profile characteristic of demented patients.

ASSIGNMENTS

1. A child of 10 years of age is mute. What are some possible explanations for his condition?
2. Compare and contrast the deaf child, the moderately severely mentally retarded child, the autistic child, and the child with severe

specific language disability with regard to their mode of interaction with others; their response to gross sounds; their mastery of syntactic structures.

3. Why is age at onset of severe hearing loss such a crucial variable with regard to language development?
4. What terminology has been used in reference to autism? See Reference 18.
5. How do deprived children compare with autistic children with regard to delay in acquisition of motor and communication skills? See Reference 18.
6. What are some possible reasons why girls tend to excel over boys in communication skills in our society? See Reference 13.
7. What are some possible reasons why children with palatal clefts demonstrate as a group a higher than normal incidence of language retardation? Consider references 17, 20, and 24.
8. Distinguish between the terms "aphasia" and "dysphasia."
9. How is the determination made as to which cerebral hemisphere is dominant for language? Read Blume, W. T., Grabow, J. D., Darley, F. L., and Aronson, A. E., Intracarotid amobarbital test of language and memory before temporal lobectomy for seizure control. *Neurology*, 1973, 23:812–819.
10. Contrast the characteristics of aphasia, dementia, and confusion as reported in Reference 9. Which characteristics are particularly useful in distinguishing each disorder from the others?

REFERENCES

1. Becky, R. E., A study of certain factors related to retardation of speech. *Journal of Speech Disorders*, 1942, 7:223–249.
2. Brodbeck, A. J., Irwin, O. C., The speech behavior of infants without families. *Child Development*, 1946, 17:145–156.
3. Davis, E. A., *The Development of Linguistic Skill in Twins, Singletons with Siblings and Only Children from Age Five to Ten Years*. Child Welfare Monograph, No. 14. Minneapolis: University of Minnesota Press, 1937.
4. Day, E. J., The development of language in twins. I. A comparison of twins and single children. *Child Development*, 1932, 3:179–199.
5. DiSimoni, F. G., Darley, F. L., and Aronson, A. E., Patterns of dysfunction in schizophrenic patients on an aphasia test battery. *Journal of Speech and Hearing Disorders*, in press.
6. Duffy, R. J., and Ulrich, S. R., A comparison of impairments in verbal comprehension, speech, reading, and writing in adult aphasics. *Journal of Speech and Hearing Disorders*, 1976, 41:110–119.
7. Eisenson, J., *Aphasia in Children*. New York: Harper & Row, 1972.
8. Eisenson, J., Developmental aphasia: a speculative view with therapeutic implications. *Journal of Speech and Hearing Disorders*, 1968, 33:3–13.
9. Halpern, H., Darley, F. L., and Brown, J. R., Differential language and

neurologic characteristics in cerebral involvement. *Journal of Speech and Disorders*, 1973, *38*:162–173.

10. Klee, A., Akinetic mutism: review of the literature and report of a case. *Journal of Nervous and Mental Disease*, 1961. *133*:536–553.

11. Matthews, J., Communication disorders in the mentally retarded. In Travis, L. E., ed., *Handbook of Speech Pathology and Audiology*, pp. 801–818. Englewood Cliffs, N. J.: Prentice-Hall, 1971.

12. Mayo Clinic Department of Neurology, *Clinical Examinations in Neurology*. 4th ed. Philadelphia: Saunders, 1976.

13. McCarthy, D., Some possible explanations of sex differences in language development and disorders. *Journal of Psychology*, 1953, *35*:155–160.

14. McCarthy, D., *The Language Development of the Preschool Child*. Child Welfare Monographs, No. 4. Minneapolis: University of Minnesota Press, 1930.

15. Moll, K. L., and Darley, F. L., Attitudes of mothers of articulatory-impaired and speech-retarded children. *Journal of Speech and Hearing Disorders*, 1960, *25*:377–384.

16. Moore, J. K., Speech content of selected groups of orphanage and non-orphanage preschool children. *Journal of Experimental Education*, 1947, *16*:122–133.

17. Morris, H. L., Communication skills of children with cleft lips and palates. *Journal of Speech and Hearing Research*, 1962, *5*:79–90.

18. Ornitz, E. M., and Ritvo, E. R., The syndrome of autism: a critical review. *American Journal of Psychiatry*, 1976, *133*:609–621.

19. Peckarsky, A., Maternal attitudes toward children with psychogenically delayed speech. Ph.D. dissertation, New York University, 1952.

20. Phillips, B. J., and Harrison, R. J., Language skills of preschool cleft palate children. *Cleft Palate Journal*, 1969, *6*:108–119.

21. Rampp, D. L., Auditory perceptual disturbances. In Weston, A. J., ed., *Communicative Disorders: An Appraisal*, pp. 297–330. Springfield, Ill.: Thomas, 1972.

22. Schizophrenia syndrome in childhood. *British Medical Journal*, 1961, *2*:889–890.

23. Smith, A., Objective indices of severity of chronic aphasia in stroke patients. *Journal of Speech and Hearing Disorders*, 1971, *36*:167–207.

24. Smith, R. M. and McWilliams, B. J., Psycholinguistic considerations in the management of children with cleft palate. *Cleft Palate Journal*, 1968, *5*:238–249.

25. Wood, K. S., Parental maladjustment and functional articulatory defects in children. *Journal of Speech Disorders*, 1946, *11*:255–275.

26. Wood, N., *Delayed Speech and Language Development*. Englewood Cliffs, N.J.: Prentice-Hall, 1964.

27. Ziegler, F. J., Imboden, J. B., and Rodgers, D. A., Contemporary conversion reactions: III. Diagnostic considerations. *Journal of the American Medical Association*, 1963, *186*:307–311.

18
DIFFERENTIAL DIAGNOSIS OF ACQUIRED MOTOR SPEECH DISORDERS

Frederic L. Darley

Certain disorders of communication are the direct result of impairment of the innervation or the programming of those parts of the central nervous system responsible for the execution of the speech act. These expressive disorders can be divided into two types: those attributable to impairments of innervation of the speech musculature—the dysarthrias—and those attributable to an impairment of a higher-level mechanism, the motor speech programmer—apraxia of speech.

In differentiating one from the other and both of these from other disorders with which they might be confused, you will want to make use of certain observations which have been described in the appraisal portion of this book. Those which will be most useful are the following:

The general evaluation of oral communication, which provides a global look at the total speech process and identifies those areas which are readily observed to be defective (Chapter 3).
Evaluation of respiration and phonation (Chapter 6).
Evaluation of resonance (Chapter 7).
Evaluation of articulation (Chapter 8).
Evaluation of prosodic features (Chapter 9).
Evaluation of the speech mechanism (Chapter 11).

Both these families of communication disorders involve distinctive gestalts of impairment of the various basic motor processes of speech but do not involve impairment of language as an integral feature. However, in order to rule out aphasia or in order to determine the relative prominence of the components of a combined aphasic and motor speech disturbance, the clinician may make use of techniques for appraisal of acquired language disorders (Chapter 5).

IDENTIFICATION OF MOTOR SPEECH DISORDERS

Dysarthrias

Dysarthria is a generic term which embraces a large family of expressive speech problems resulting from a lesion of some motor portion of the central or peripheral nervous systems. Because of the lesion, muscles innervated by the affected nerves operate inefficiently, displaying a degree of weakness (a severe degree would be called paralysis), slowness of movement, lack of coordination, alteration of muscle tone, or some combination of these changes. These alterations of function may be manifested in any or all of the basic processes involved in the execution of speech—respiration, phonation, resonance, articulation, and prosody. A severe degree of impairment of motor function which renders the patient essentially speechless is called anarthria.

There are many causes of such lesions; the nature of the etiology may be vascular, neoplastic, traumatic, infectious, toxic, metabolic, or degenerative. The nature of the cause does not result in the distinctiveness of certain patterns of dysarthria. Rather the different patterns result from the fact that different parts or levels of the motor system are impaired. The level of impairment may be the lower motor neuron, the vestibular-reticular level in the brain stem, the extrapyramidal level, the upper motor neuron level, or the cerebellum. The site of the lesion and its extent will determine what aberrations of movement occur in what sets of muscles implicated in speech.

As previously stated, impairment of expressive speech can result from interference with execution of any of the basic processes. Some dictionary and textbook definitions and a good deal of everyday clinical usage might lead one to believe that dysarthria refers only to problems in articulation, commonly referred to as "slurred speech." Such a conception of the term is much too narrow for, as we shall see, the patterns of motor speech disturbance which we should learn to recognize all involve multiple motor processes in various combinations. It is the uniqueness of combinations of disordered speech dimensions which allows the clinician after a reasonable exposure to them to appreciate that the various types of dysarthria sound different, are recognizable, and indeed reflect the neurophysiological changes wrought in the nervous system by the etiologic agent.

In the following paragraphs the various dysarthrias, classified according to the site of lesion and the neurophysiological result, will be described. The most distinctive speech and voice phenomena in contextual speech will be listed in what have been found to be characteristic clumpings (3). Characteristics of the patients' distinctive execution of syllable repetition in oral diadochokinetic rate testing will be described. Likely findings on the oral speech mechanism examination will be mentioned. The prominent associated neurologic signs are also briefly presented. For a more complete description of the dysarthrias and their neurophysiologic substrate see reference 4.

A clinician's ear may tell him that a given patient presents a dysarthria of a certain type; a neurologist in her report of the salient features and the confirmatory signs of the syndrome presented by the patient will supply the necessary documentation that the dysarthria is indeed of the type identified. As Grewel (6) has pointed out, dysarthrias may be of localizing value, sometimes suggesting a tentative diagnosis when no other neurological signs are yet evident. But ordinarily the observations of the speech clinician will need the support of a neurological examination in accomplishing a secure diagnosis of the condition.

It is difficult to convey through the medium of words alone the "sound" of each dysarthria. The words that follow will summarize some of the main observable characteristics of each type of dysarthria, but it must be remembered that each patient is unique with regard to site and extent of lesion and the severity of his or her speech disturbance; patients who bear the same diagnostic label may not sound identical even though they share the same neurologic features. The clinician needs to listen to a spectrum of samples of each dysarthria in order to appreciate the nature of the gestalts of disordered speech-voice dimensions and the range of variability and severity which one may encounter in a series of patients. In lieu of a series of live patients, one may resort to a set of tape recordings which furnishes such a range of speech samples in each of the dysarthrias; these are available in the form of the Audiotape Seminars which accompany the text *Motor Speech Disorders* (4).

Flaccid Dysarthria   Four of the cranial nerves—V, trigeminal; VII, facial; X, vagus; XII, hypoglossal—are directly involved in the execution of speech. A lesion of the motor nucleus of any of these nerves, or of the peripheral nerves running from the nucleus to the muscles, will result in weakness of the muscles innervated by them, a condition known as flaccidity. The term *flaccid dysarthria* designates the speech consequences of lesions of the lower motor neuron in each case. The resulting speech aberrations will sound different from each other depending upon which cranial nerve is involved or whether several of them are simultaneously involved.

If nerve V is impaired, the muscles of mastication will be weakened. There may be difficulty on the part of a patient in elevating his mandible to close his mouth and keep it closed. The patient may not be able to move his mandible voluntarily to either side. If you exert some pressure on his lower teeth with a tongue depressor, he may not be able to close his teeth together.

If nerve VII is impaired, the patient may have difficulty pursing and retracting his lips and firming his cheek and mouth muscles to permit impounding of air for phonemes requiring intraoral pressure. On the speech mechanism examination you will observe a droop of the weak side of the face in the case of a unilateral lesion, the unaffected side pulling upward and outward during a smile. The nasolabial fold will appear flatter on the weak side. With a bilateral lesion the lips may not be closed at rest; the smile you elicit will be transverse; lip rounding and protrusion will be inadequate; when the patient puffs out his cheeks, you can readily break the labial seal by pressing his cheeks.

If nerve X is impaired, the patient may show palatopharyngeal weakness or laryngeal weakness or both. With unilateral paralysis of the levator muscle of the soft palate, you will note that the weak side will hang lower than the intact side at rest; on phonation, the intact side will rise, the weak side will not. With bilateral paralysis the entire palate will elevate little or not at all on phonation. The gag reflex will be absent or diminished. When laryngeal muscles are affected, unilaterally or bilaterally, laryngoscopic viewing will reveal failure of adduction to the midline or the vocal folds may appear bowed.

If nerve XII is impaired, the tongue will be weak, may appear smaller than average, may display atrophy of the borders or look shrunken and furrowed, and may demonstrate fasciculations (small visible transient contractions of parts of a muscle). Protrusion and elevation of the tip of the tongue may be difficult. In the case of a unilateral lesion the tongue on protrusion deviates to the weak side; in bilateral weakness protrusion is symmetrical but limited in extent. Lateral weakness may be evident in failure of the lateralized tongue to resist pressure you exert on the cheek.

In a particular form of lower motor neuron disease, myasthenia gravis, in which the impairment is an electrochemical one at the myoneural junction, any or all of these functions may be impaired. Their impairment will be manifested in increasing degree as the patient prolongs his speaking effort.

Following are the most deviant aspects of speech and voice observed in a series of patients unequivocally diagnosed as presenting lower motor neuron impairment:

1. A cluster of deviations indicative of *Resonatory Incompetence: hypernasality,* often of severe degree; the audible *nasal emission of air* in production of consonant phonemes which require some buildup of intraoral breath pressure; and *abnormally short phrases* during contextual speech attributable at least in part to air wastage at the palatopharyngeal port.

2. A cluster of speech and voice changes indicative of *Phonatory Incompetence: breathy voice quality* resulting from poor vocal fold adduction and air escape; *audible inhalation of air* (inspiratory stridor) due to inadequate abduction of vocal folds during inhalation; and *abnormally short phrases* during contextual speech, attributable

at least in part to inefficient laryngeal valving and the patient's in-
haling more often than normal because he or she runs out of air.

3. A cluster of deviations indicative of *Phonatory-Prosodic Insufficiency,*
probably due to hypotonia (reduced tonus) of the laryngeal muscles:
monotony of pitch, monotony of loudness, and *harshness of voice.*

4. *Imprecise articulation of consonants,* due in some cases to impaired
movements of the tongue, in other cases to bilateral weakness of the
lips, and in other cases to inadequate buildup of intraoral breath
pressure.

The various speech and voice dimensions which were studied in detail in the Mayo Clinic study of dysarthria (2, 3) are listed in Table 18.1.
At a glance one can see the relative prominence of each dimension in
the various neurologic groups studied. Examination of that table reveals
that breathiness of voice, hypernasality, nasal emission of air, and audible
inspirations were more noticeable in flaccid dysarthria than in any of
the other types. The clinician hearing these phenomena in the speech of a
patient might think first, then, of lower motor neuron impairment as a
likely explanation for these phenomena individually or when clustered
together.

Patients with flaccid paralysis will be found on neurologic examination
to have impairment of all types of movement, whether voluntary, automatic, or reflex. The most prominent signs are weakness and hypotonia,
that is, reduction of muscle tone; in myasthenia gravis the most prominent feature is progression of weakness with continued use of muscles.
Other signs noted by the neurologist are hyporeflexia (absent or reduced
muscle stretch reflexes), muscle atrophy, fasciculations visible to the
eye, and fibrillations evident on electromyography.

Spastic Dysarthria   The cranial nerves involved in speech receive
upper motor neuron supply from both cerebral hemispheres. The term
pseudobulbar palsy is used to designate paresis or paralysis of the musculature supplied by these cranial nerves when the cause is bilateral upper
motor neuron lesions. Since the bilateral nerve supply to tongue and lips
is inadequate, even a one-sided lesion can produce a speech problem.
The final common pathways to the speech muscles are not impaired, so
the muscles are not flaccid. Rather, the distorted signals from upper
motor neurons lead to changes in the muscle stretch reflexes and muscle
tone that we identify as spasticity, and the resulting speech changes are
called *spastic dysarthria.*

The characteristic clusters of disorders of speech and voice dimensions
that commonly appear in spastic dysarthria are the following:

1. A cluster of phonatory signs indicating *Phonatory Stenosis,* that is,
a narrowing of the glottis: *harsh voice quality, excessively low pitch,*
a *strained-strangled sound* indicative of effortful voice production, the

production of an *effortful grunt* at the end of an exhalation, and *pitch breaks*.

2. A cluster of features designated *Prosodic Insufficiency*, probably resulting from restricted range of movements: *monotony of pitch, monotony of loudness, reduction of the usual patterns of syllable and word stress*, and *shortness of phrases*.

3. A cluster of three speech characteristics—*imprecision of consonant articulation, distortion of vowels*, and *hypernasality*—designated *Articulatory-Resonatory Incompetence* to indicate that muscle contractions are reduced in speed, force, and range of movement, leaving the palatopharyngeal port unable to close efficiently and the articulators unable adequately to impede the breath stream.

4. Two features which constitute a portion of a larger cluster designated *Prosodic Excess: equalization of stress with excessive stress* on words and syllables usually unstressed, and *slower than normal rate*.

5. *Breathiness of voice*, the result either of slowed movements of the vocal cords on adduction thus allowing wastage of air, or possibly a compensatory phenomenon adopted by a patient in trying to produce a less effortful phonation in the face of phonatory stenosis.

Certain of these deviations are more prominent in spastic dysarthria than in any other type: low pitch level, the occurrence of pitch breaks, harshness of voice, the strained-strangled sound of phonatory stenosis, slowed rate, and shortness of phrases. The clinician hearing these in a patient might think first of spastic dysarthria as the likely presenting entity, although as Table 18.1 shows, they occur with lesser severity in other dysarthrias as well.

On the oral speech mechanism examination you will note that lip, tongue, and palatal movements are consistently executed more slowly than average, and the extent of the sluggish movements will be restricted. Oral diadochokinetic rates will be slowed but they will be rhythmical.

The neurologic picture is one of paresis of the lower face and of the extremities of the opposite side in unilateral lesions of the brain, bilateral symptoms in the case of bilateral lesions; movement patterns rather than individual muscles are impaired. The most prominent features reported by the neurologist are increased muscle tone (spasticity); weakness, particularly of distal muscles; slowness of movement; and reduced range of movement. Other signs are hyperreflexia, absent superficial abdominal reflexes, and the appearance of certain abnormal reflexes including the Babinski sign (extension of the great toe and fanning of the other toes when the sole of the foot is scratched) and the sucking reflex.

Ataxic Dysarthria   Cerebellar dysfunction results in impairment of the coordination of skilled movements, including those of speech when the lesions are generalized or occur bilaterally. The timing of the component parts of movements is off, the force with which a movement is

TABLE 18.1
Dysarthric Groups Ranked According to Degree of Impairment on Speech-Voice Dimensions (1 Represents Most Impaired)

	Groups					
Dimensions	*1*	*2*	*3*	*4*	*5*	*6*
Phonatory-Respiratory						
1. Low pitch level	Spastic	Hypokinetic	Flaccid	Hyperkinetic, dystonia	Hyperkinetic, chorea	Ataxic
2. Pitch breaks	Spastic	Ataxic	Flaccid	Hyperkinetic, dystonia	Hyperkinetic, chorea	—
3. Harshness	Spastic	Hyperkinetic, dystonia	Hyperkinetic, chorea	Ataxic	Hypokinetic	Flaccid
4. Breathiness	Flaccid	Hypokinetic	Spastic	Hyperkinetic, dystonia	Hypokinetic	—
5. Hoarseness	Flaccid	—	—	—	—	—
6. Strained-strangled sound	Spastic	Hyperkinetic, dystonia	Hyperkinetic, chorea	Ataxic	—	—
7. Voice stoppages	Hyperkinetic, dystonia	Spastic	Hyperkinetic, chorea	—	—	—
8. Audible inhalations	Flaccid	Hyperkinetic, dystonia	Spastic	Hyperkinetic, chorea	—	—
9. Forced inhalation-exhalation	Hyperkinetic, chorea	—	—	—	—	—
Articulatory						
1. Imprecise consonants	Spastic	Hyperkinetic, dystonia	Hypokinetic	Ataxic	Hyperkinetic, chorea	Flaccid
2. Vowels distorted	Hyperkinetic, dystonia	Ataxic	Hyperkinetic, chorea	Spastic	Flaccid	—
3. Irregular breakdowns	Ataxic	Hyperkinetic, dystonia	Hyperkinetic, chorea	Spastic	—	—
4. Phonemes prolonged	Ataxic	Hyperkinetic, chorea	Hyperkinetic, dystonia	Spastic	Hypokinetic	—

	C1	C2	C3	C4	C5	C6	C7	C8
5. Phonemes repeated	Hypokinetic	Hyperkinetic, dystonia	—	—	—	—	—	—
Resonatory								
1. Hypernasality	Flaccid	Spastic	Hyperkinetic, chorea	Hyperkinetic, chorea	Hyperkinetic, dystonia	Flaccid	Ataxic	Hypokinetic
2. Nasal emission of air	Flaccid	Spastic	Hyperkinetic, chorea	Hyperkinetic, chorea	Ataxic	Flaccid	Ataxic	—
Prosodic								
1. Monopitch	Hypokinetic	Spastic	Hyperkinetic, chorea	Hyperkinetic, chorea	Flaccid	Ataxic	—	Ataxic
2. Monoloudness	Hypokinetic	Spastic	Hyperkinetic, chorea	Hyperkinetic, dystonia	Flaccid	Hyperkinetic, chorea	—	Ataxic
3. Excessive loudness variations	Hyperkinetic, chorea	Hyperkinetic, dystonia	Ataxic	Spastic	—	—	—	—
4. Loudness decay	Hypokinetic	Flaccid	—	—	—	—	—	—
5. Slowed rate	Spastic	Ataxic	Hyperkinetic, dystonia	Hyperkinetic, chorea	Flaccid	—	—	—
6. Rapid rate	Hypokinetic	Hypokinetic	—	—	—	—	—	—
7. Variable rate	Hyperkinetic, chorea	Hyperkinetic, chorea	Hyperkinetic, dystonia	Ataxic	Ataxic	—	—	—
8. Short rushes of speech	Hypokinetic	Hyperkinetic, chorea	Hyperkinetic, dystonia	—	—	—	—	—
9. Reduced stress	Hypokinetic	Spastic	Hyperkinetic, dystonia	Hyperkinetic, chorea	—	—	—	—
10. Excess and equalized stress	Ataxic	Spastic	Spastic	Hyperkinetic, chorea	Hyperkinetic, dystonia	—	—	—
11. Intervals prolonged	Hyperkinetic, chorea	Ataxic	Hyperkinetic, dystonia	Hyperkinetic, dystonia	Ataxic	—	—	—
12. Inappropriate silences	Hypokinetic	Hyperkinetic, chorea	Ataxic	Hyperkinetic, dystonia	—	—	—	—

Source: From Darley et al., [2, 3].

executed may be too strong or too weak, the amplitude or range of the movement may be poorly regulated, and the direction of each movement may be poorly controlled. The result is a breakdown in the smooth, rhythmic, efficient production of speech; the resulting pattern of uncoordinated speech performance is labeled *ataxic dysarthria.*

Following are the commonly occurring disorders of speech and voice heard in groups of patients with cerebellar disease:

1. A cluster of three articulatory characteristics constituting a cluster entitled *Articulatory Inaccuracy: imprecise production of consonants, distortion of vowels,* and *irregular articulatory breakdowns.*
2. A grouping of four deviations constituting the cluster *Prosodic Excess: equalization of stress and excess stress* on usually unstressed words and syllables, *prolongation of phonemes, prolongation of intervals,* and *slow rate.* The speech sounds too deliberately paced or "measured"; the term "scanning speech" has been applied to this set of features heard frequently, but not exclusively, in ataxic dysarthria.
3. Three signs of laryngeal involvement constituting the cluster *Phonatory-Prosodic Insufficiency: harsh voice quality, monotony of pitch, monotony of loudness.*

Four of the deviations mentioned above are more common in patients with ataxic dysarthria than in any other dysarthric group, namely, equalization of stress and excess stress on usually unstressed words and syllables, irregular breakdowns of articulation, prolongation of phonemes, and prolongation of intervals between words. When a clinician hears these as prominent presenting signs, he or she may think first of ataxic dysarthria as the entity into which they most likely fit.

On the oral speech mechanism examination you may observe that any specific oral movement will be performed jerkily, erratically, without fine control of direction or timing or extent. The performance may be quite variable from trial to trial, differing from the consistently slow and limited performance of the spastic dysarthric. Oral diadochokinetic repetitions may be normally rapid but are often remarkably dysrhythmic, accompanied by irregularities of pitch and loudness.

The usual neurologic findings in patients with cerebellar disease are flabbiness of muscles and reduction of muscle tone (hypotonia); jerkiness of muscle movement; wide-based, staggering gait; jerky, irregular arm movements; clumsy, slow finger movements; tremor in the use of a limb; and increase of that tremor toward the termination of the movement.

Hypokinetic Dysarthria   In the disease of the extrapyramidal system called parkinsonism there is a general reduction of movement. This shows itself in motor speech, so the resulting dysarthria is labelled *hypokinetic dysarthria.*

Following are the most frequent characteristics of hypokinetic dysarthria identified in a series of parkinsonian patients:

1. The three most prominent characteristics are all alterations of the prosody of speech: *monotony of pitch, reduced stress,* and *monotony of loudness.*
2. *Imprecision of consonant articulation* is often prominent with a marked reduction in the excursion of the articulators so that speech is often simply a blur.
3. Speech is sometimes *arrested* resulting in *inappropriate silences* and sometimes in *repetitions* of phonemes or syllables.
4. Speech is produced in *short rushes,* the rate at times seeming to *accelerate* within a phrase. Whereas all other dysarthrias are charterized by a slower than normal rate, many parkinsonian patients speak at a rate judged to be faster than normal. The rate is often *variable.*
5. Voice quality is often *breathy,* and *loudness level is often reduced.* Inadequate audibility is the presenting complaint of some parkinsonian patients.

Some of these observed phenomena occur only in parkinsonism and so may be considered truly pathognomonic: short rushes of speech, rapid rate, and increase of rate during the speech sample. Other features are not unique to parkinsonism but are typically present to such a marked degree that they would suggest to the clinician the likelihood of the disorder being parkinsonism when they are heard; these include monopitch, monoloudness, reduced stress, inappropriate silences, repetition of phonemes, and reduced loudness.

On the oral speech mechanism examination you will probably note that repetitive tongue and lip movements are performed rapidly, sometimes inordinately rapidly, but with reduced excursion, so that the performance is incomplete and the sounds produced are lacking in precision. The face is often expressionless, unsmiling, the eyes often unblinking.

In his analysis of the parkinsonian patient's problems the neurologist will report as salient features rigidity (increased tone) that often has a cogwheel character; restriction of range of movement; accomplishment of repetitive movements rapidly but with small amplitude; slowness of individual movements; and an alternating tremor at rest which subsides with movement. Lesser signs of a confirmatory nature include loss of automatic associated movements (for example, rotation of the body and swinging of the arms in walking), paucity of movement, and hesitation and false starts in initiating movement.

Hyperkinetic Dysarthria Patients with certain lesions of the extrapyramidal system will present involuntary movements which interrupt ongoing purposeful movements. The term hyperkinesia is applied to all such occurrences of involuntary movement. Some of the movement disorders are characterized by quick, random, unpatterned movements of relatively short duration; among the quick hyperkinesias are myoclonic jerks, tics, and chorea. Other involuntary movements tend to be slower, of more gradual onset, prolonged for variable periods of time, waxing and waning; these slow hyperkinesias include athetosis, tardive dyskinesia (drug-induced movement disorder), and dystonia. The impairments of speech which result from these movement disorders are known collectively as *hyperkinetic dysarthrias*. They are of several types, as described below.

1. *Hyperkinetic dysarthria in chorea:* In the ongoing speech performance of the patient with chorea one may observe sudden brief interruption of any of the basic motor processes of speech production.

    a. Respiration may be interrupted by a sudden forced inspiration or expiration.

    b. Phonation may be altered by sudden excessive loudness variations, voice stoppages, or voice breaks. Many subjects also present the signs of phonatory stenosis in harshness of voice and the strained-strangled sound of effortful phonation against resistance.

    c. Hypernasality frequently occurs, and because of the air wastage resulting from moments of palatopharyngeal incompetence phrases may be shortened.

    d. Interference with the muscular adjustments of articulation are evident in impreciseness of consonant articulation and frequent vowel distortion.

    e. Disturbances of prosody are prominent as momentary breakdowns of speech occur, as the patient tries to complete units of speech between these breakdowns and cautiously proceeds as though to avoid anticipated breakdowns. Among the alterations of prosody that have been observed are monopitch, monoloudness, reduction of stress, prolongation of intervals, prolongation of phonemes, equalization of stress and excessive stress on usually unstressed words and syllables, and variable rate.

2. *Palatopharyngeolaryngeal myoclonus:* Some patients display a repetitive rhythmical jerking of parts of the speech musculature. Sometimes these myoclonic jerks involve only the palate, often the palate and pharynx, often the larynx as well. The myoclonic movements occur at a rate of from one to two beats per minute and are often impossible to detect during contextual speech. During vowel prolongation they are usually audible as regular momentary interruptions in phonation. Myoclonic movements of the diaphragm can be detected in regular interruptions of respiration and outflow of air.

3. *Organic voice tremor.* A tremor of laryngeal muscles may occur in association with tremor of other parts of the body, known as essential or heredofamilial tremor, or it may occur in isolation. A mild voice

tremor may not be noticeable in contextual speech but can be noted if the patient prolongs /ɑ/. The tremulous tone results from rhythmic alterations in pitch and loudness. In more severe form the tremor may be noticeable during contextual speech, particularly on certain stressed syllables where vowels are prolonged, and on prolonged phonation the tremor will be very marked, the amplitude of the oscillation sometimes being so great as to result in a voice arrest at the peak of each oscillation. In very severe form the voice tremor may resemble the laryngospasms of spastic dysphonia.

4. *Hyperkinetic dysarthria of dystonia:* In the slowest of the movement disorders, dystonia, muscular contractions develop slowly, result in a distorted posture which is prolonged for a time, and then subside. When these movements affect laryngeal musculature, phonation may be interrupted or the tone may become strained and strangled or harsh, and the voice may resemble that of spastic dysphonia. There may be excessive loudness variations and voice stoppages. If dystonic movements occur in the articulators, we can expect imprecision of consonant articulation and distortion of vowels; articulatory break-downs will occur irregularly, much as they do in cerebellar disorders, but more gradually. As the patient tries to cope with alterations in ongoing speech, prosodic changes inevitably occur, including mono-loudness, monopitch, prolongation of intervals, inappropriate silences, equalization of stress, and usually a slowing of rate.

Among the speech deviations which occur more frequently in dystonia than in any other of the neurologic groups are distortion of vowels, excessive loudness variations, alterations in loudness from very soft to very loud, and voice stoppages. Although these phenomena may be heard in other dysarthrias, their prominence in the hyperkinetic dysarthria of dystonia should give clinicians a clue to suspect dystonia when they hear them in a patient's speech.

In their description of movement disorders, neurologists will specify the nature of the onset and course of the movement disorder as these are determining factors in diagnosis. They will comment on the suddenness of myoclonic jerks, the abrupt muscle contractions in chorea which are slower than myoclonic jerks and may be momentarily sustained. They will probably also report on general slowing of voluntary movement and variable muscle tone in the quick hyperkinesias. They will identify the distinctive patterns of sustained, distorted movements and postures in the slow hyperkinesias, as well as a typical slowness of movement and variable hypertonus of the muscles.

Mixed Dysarthrias The types of dysarthria described above represent the "pure" types that have been described, those involving impairment of only one level of motor function. In many patients these dysarthrias appear in a combined form, their central nervous system lesions implicating more than one motor system. The resulting dysarthrias will display the features distinctive of each neurologic type, although the cooccurrence of certain deviations may obscure the distinctive aspect of the "pure" dysarthrias.

1. *Amyotrophic lateral sclerosis:* In this degenerative disease there is impairment of both lower and upper motor neurons. The speech result is a mixed flaccid-spastic dysarthria, although one component or the other may be more prominent in the early stages of the disease. Eventually all of the features of both types of dysarthria will become evident, and to a severe degree, rendering speech typically unintelligible and leaving the patient eventually anarthric.

2. *Multiple sclerosis:* The cerebellar and upper motor neuron systems are particularly susceptible in this inflammatory disease, so the dysarthria that occurs is often of ataxic or spastic type or a mixture of both. Many patients with multiple sclerosis present no speech problem, at least for many years after onset, and those who eventually do present a speech problem present no stereotype which can be described as "multiple sclerosis speech." The most frequent speech deviations that have been reported in multiple sclerosis are impaired control of loudness, harshness, and defective articulation. Less frequently observed are reduced stress, impaired pitch control, hypernasality, and breathiness.

3. *Wilson's disease:* Dysarthria is a common sign in this genetic, metabolic disorder resulting from inadequate processing of the dietary intake of copper. Most patients with a dysarthria display a mixed ataxic-spastic-hypokinetic dysarthria, although in certain patients one or another of the components may appear in isolation or may predominate.

Apraxia of Speech

Certain patients with lesions of the left cerebral hemisphere display another type of aberration in speech execution. Their difficulty is specifically with articulation. They seem uncertain as to where to place their tongue and lips to accomplish the articulation of certain phonemes or the sequencing of phonemes to form words. They seem actually to struggle to find the right articulation points; they audibly grope in their search for the correct sounds and sound sequences. Meaning to form a bilabial phoneme, a patient may protrude the tongue, then make a lingua-alveolar contact, and finally attain closure of the lips. Or meaning to produce a linguavelar sound, in attaining it the patient may first produce a lingua-alveolar or a linguadental or a bilabial sound. As these patients try and try again they produce variable errors. Yet at times their speech is fluent and well articulated and it quickly becomes clear that their problem is not due to the inadequacy of innervation of any specific muscle group. Although it may appear in isolation, this difficulty with articulation typically occurs in association with some impairment of language function (aphasia); yet the problem in adopting the correct mouth postures to produce words is not an integral part of the language disorder but can be identified separately from it and must be treated as an independent problem.

This difficulty in the programming of the articulation of phonemes and sequences of them has carried many labels. Some of these have emphasized the frequent cooccurrence of the disorder with aphasia and have even implied that it is an integral part of an aphasic syndrome: Broca's aphasia, motor aphasia, subcortical motor aphasia, afferent motor aphasia, efferent motor aphasia, phonematic aphasia, phonemic paraphasia, literal paraphasia, and conduction aphasia. Other terms have related this disorder more to the dysarthrias, suggesting some degree of specific muscle impairment as the cause of the problem: cortical dysarthria, anarthria. Other terms have emphasized the uniqueness of the disorder and have endeavored to separate it from any of the above: aphemia, syndrome of phonetic disintegration, articulatory dyspraxia, apraxia of vocal expression. The term we prefer to use is *apraxia of speech*, making use of the term devised by Leipmann to cover many disorders of skilled movement despite the intactness of muscle strength. It is conceived as resulting from impairment of a specific part of the brain believed to serve as a motor speech programmer. Normally this programmer receives information from a central language processor and activates the appropriate preprogrammed chains of neural output to accomplish the articulation of words. When the function of the motor speech programmer is impaired, the patient behaves as though he has "forgotten" how to perform certain movements with his articulators, for example, protruding his tongue for /θ/, although he can readily demonstrate in other activities that there is no impairment of movement of these organs, for example, licking crumbs off his lips.

Following are the hallmarks of apraxia of speech, the prominent behaviors that identify this as a separate motor speech disorder:

1. The patient, seemingly uncertain of where his articulators are or how he can make them perform, will attack given words uncertainly, will make repeated trials to articulate the phonemes, will adopt clearly mistaken articulatory postures at times, and may try to use his fingers to assist in finding the right posture. Thus he presents a continuing off-target performance. By way of illustration, here are samples of the errors made by three patients in reading the identical "My Grandfather" passage:

    You wish to know all about my grandfather. Well, he is nearly ninety-three years n—old, yet he still th—thinks as ssssswiftly as ever. He dresses himself in an old black frock c—cl—cl—uh-coat, *u*—usually *sevel*—*sevelar* buttons missing. A long beard *clearing*—clings to his *k*—*ch*—chin, giving those who *ob*—*obs*—*er*—*ob*—*serve* him a pronounced feeling of the *up*most respect. When he speaks, his voice is just a bit cracked and *quiggle*—quivers a bit. Twice*d* each day he plays *kear*—*skear*—skill—fully and with zest upon a small organ. *Excekt*—*expect* in the *wintle* when the *so*—*sss*—*sp*—*sp*—*snow* or *outses* prevents, he *suh*—*lowly* takes a *s*—short *wark* in the *o*—open air each day. We have often urged him to walk*ed* more and smoke less, but he always *anses*, "Banan*y or*!" *Gwaing*—grandfather likes to be *uh* mode*m* in his language.

You wish to know all about my *mad*—, my grandfather. Well, he is nearly *twenty-three, ninety-four,* ninety-three year*uls*—years old, yet he still thinks as *sweer*—*swivly*—swiftly as ever. He *drisses*—dresses himself in an old *bla*—*back*—black *fronk cla*—coat, usually *severable*—*severable*—several buttons *breck*—*mix*—*mince*—*mincing.* A long *bing climps*—*simps*—*climps* to his chin, *bliving* those who *deserved*—*uh*—*his*—*his*—*observed* him a *pro*—*uh*—*profound* feeling of the utm*ust respenct*—respect. When he speaks, his voice is just a bit cracked and *qui*—*quidivers*—quivers a bit. Twice each d*way* he *spell*—he plays *uh* skillfully and with *z*em*t* upon a small *orjun*—organ. *Evysempt*—*essempt*—except in the winter when the *so*—snow or ice*d refents*—*revents*—*re*—*re*—*pre*—*prevents,* he *slah*—slowly takes a *slawt waw* a short *wep*—walk in the *o*— in the *ople day*—air each *dare*—day. We have often *wurged*—*uh*—urged him to *sss*—to *sssmah*—to walk more and *sss*—*uh*—smoke less, but he always answers, "*Balawla*—banana oil!" *Grand*—*fa*—grandfather likes to be modern in his language.

You wi*ss* to know all about my *gw*andfather. Well, he is nearly ninety-three years *h*old, yet he still thinks as *chw*iftly as ever. He dresses himself in an old black *fl*ock *co*—coat, usually se*v*rial buttons *mit*—missing. A long *beers kins* to his *to*—chin, giving *who*—those who *obser*—*uh*—observe him a pronounced feeling of the *n*—utmost *ref*—*feh*—respect. When he *spuh*—*eaks,* his *v*—voice is just a bit cra*t*ch*ed* and *t*—quivers a bi*ck.* Twice *ea*—each day he plays *still*—*ful*—*ly* and with *t*—zest upon a *muh*—small organ. Exce*p* in the winter when the snow or ice pre—vents, he slowly takes *an s*—short walk in the open air each day. We have often *h*urged him to walk more and smoke less, but he always *huh*—answers, "Banana oil!" Grandfather like to be *m*—modern in his *l*aind*r*icks—*nush*—lang*w*ush—lang–*gwiss*—lang–*chuh*—lang–*druss*—It won't come out—lang*w*ish—lang*w*icks. I don't think I can say it any better.

It is apparent that these errors are highly variable, inconsistent from trial to trial, and do not reflect impairment of any specific muscle group. They show the rightness of the conclusion arrived at by Shankweiler and Harris (9) when they stated that "it is almost inconceivable that residual spasticity or weakness could give rise to errors of this kind. . . . No particular structure or region can be implicated to the exclusion of other parts of the articulatory apparatus."

2. The articulatory errors that are made appear to be complications of the act of articulation rather than simplifications. Thus we see the frequent occurrence of substitutions, additions, repetitions, and prolongations, with relatively less frequent occurrence of phoneme distortions and omissions.

3. One may detect that a given error is perseverative, the patient repeating a phoneme he recently articulated. At other times the error appears to be anticipatory, the patient introducing a phoneme prematurely.

4. Articulatory errors occur more often on consonant phonemes than on vowel phonemes, and the consonants in error are likely to be those requiring greater nicety of motor adjustment, such as the fricatives, affricates, and consonant clusters. These consonants are misarticulated more often in the initial position than in the final position.

5. As the patient experiences difficulty in articulation, he proceeds tentatively, anticipating more difficulty, thereby usually slowing his speech, spacing his words and syllables more evenly than normal, equalizing the stress. In working his way through a difficult consonant cluster he may introduce a schwa between the parts of the cluster, pronouncing "screen" as skuh—reen and "play" as puh—lay. Thus we observe some alterations in the prosody of his speech, usually compensation for the difficulty he experiences.

6. The patient's difficulty in articulating certain "target" words contrasts sharply with his fluent production of other words and even whole phrases and sentences (note samples above in this regard). The patient's volitional or purposive speech performance is much poorer than his performance in "automatic speech" or in producing reactive speech, such as uttering greetings, repeating overmemorized series such as numbers and days of the week, swearing, or reciting well-known lyrics, jingles, or prayers.

7. Longer words tend to elicit more articulatory struggle as can be demonstrated by having the patient repeat words of increasing length which share a common syllable such as "door, doorman, doorkeeper, dormitory."

8. Responses in imitation of the examiner seem to be especially hard for the patient, harder than spontaneous speech production, regardless of the length of the word.

9. Patients ordinarily display difficulty in performing the repetition of changing syllable sequences in tests of oral diadochokinetic rate.

Once they get a given sound started, they ordinarily repeat it as rapidly as average without evident dysrhythmia or other irregularity. Thus they demonstrate, as indeed they do throughout the rest of their performance, no evidence of slowness, weakness, incoordination, or alteration of muscle tone in the speech apparatus. They will, however, usually demonstrate significant difficulty in performing a sequential motion rate task, repeating the overlapping series /pʌ — tʌ — kʌ/. They have trouble keeping the correct sequence of syllables and keeping the whole series going, for example, producing /pʌ — kʌ — kʌ — tʌ — kʌ — pʌ — pʌ — kʌ — tʌ — kʌ/.

10. Unless they have some associated dysarthria, they will ordinarily give no evidence of impairment of the processes of respiration, phonation, or resonance. Disturbance is restricted to articulation and, sometimes, to prosody, usually in a compensatory effort to avoid or correct articulation difficulties.

Some, but not all, patients with apraxia of speech will demonstrate some apraxia of the speech mechanism for nonspeech activities, an impairment identified as oral apraxia. Immediately following onset of the problem patients may be unable to phonate voluntarily, protrude their tongue on command, or perform other of the volitional oral acts listed for testing in Chapter 11. After these initial major difficulties, patients may still have difficulty in performing certain skilled acts with their speech muscles, such as whistling, alternately puckering and retracting their lips, puffing out their cheeks, et cetera. In examining the patient the neurologist, as well as the speech clinician, will look for the existence of these associated oral apraxic problems and for evidence of other apraxic disturbance in the body. Oral apraxia is a fairly common accompaniment of apraxia of speech, but limb apraxia is rather infrequently associated with oral apraxia and apraxia of speech (5).

DIFFERENTIATION OF DISORDERS

Differentiating Dysarthria from Apraxia of Speech

The following are the main features which should be considered in differentiating a true dysarthria from apraxia of speech:

1. Some impairment of innervation of specific muscle groups is the hallmark of dysarthria, while evidence of such impairment is missing in the case of apraxia of speech. In the dysarthrias the neurologic examination and the oral speech mechanism examination will reveal evidence of slowness, weakness, incoordination, or change of muscle tone of the musculature involved in respiration, phonation, resonance, articulation, or prosody. A direct relationship between the type of impairment of innervation and the quality of speech aberrations can be drawn. In apraxia of speech, on the other hand, no impairment of

muscle function can usually be found. If some degree of impairment of function is discovered, one would be hard pressed to relate it to the kinds of articulatory errors that characterize the disorder.

2. The various dysarthrias that have been delineated involve in varying combination the complete array of basic motor processes—respiration, phonation, resonance, articulation, and prosody. All the dysarthrias are clusters of disturbances of multiple motor processes. On the other hand, the predominant difficulty in apraxia of speech is articulatory with only minor prosodic alterations sometimes entering the picture as probably compensatory phenomena.

3. The degree of consistency with which errors occur differentiates dysarthria from apraxia of speech. In several of the dysarthrias, most especially flaccid, spastic, and hypokinetic, the difficulties that are heard in speech production recur consistently. Even in those dysarthrias where the interruption of speech is more irregular, as in the ataxic and hyperkinetic dysarthrias, the pattern if not the timing of the disturbance can be discerned and one can predict the recurrence of specific kinds of errors as speech proceeds. In all of the dysarthrias one would expect that all the parts of a speech sample would demonstrate approximately the same degree of defectiveness. On the contrary, in apraxia of speech inconsistency is the rule. Phonemes produced correctly at one time are produced incorrectly another time. Some speech is completely free of error, particularly automatic and reactive speech, whereas other more volitional or purposive speech is likely to be more laboriously produced and spotted with error. Islands of error-free speech characterize apraxia of speech in contrast to the dysarthrias.

4. The errors typically made in articulation by dysarthric patients are in the direction of simplification of the task, usually an imprecise production in the form of distortions and omissions. In apraxia of speech, in contrast, relatively few simplifications of articulation such as distortions and omissions are observed to occur, but one can observe considerable complication of the speech act, manifested as substitutions of one phoneme for another, many of these unrelated substitutions, additions of phonemes (such as the use of a consonant cluster instead of a consonant singleton), repetitions of phonemes, and prolongations of phonemes.

5. Performance on oral diadochokinetic rate tasks will differentiate the two disorders. In the various dysarthrias repetition of the individual syllables /pʌ/, /tʌ/, and /kʌ/ and of the sequence /pʌ — tʌ — kʌ/ will likely be all of a pattern—slowed and imprecise but rhythmic in spastic dysarthria, rapid but blurred because of incomplete excursion of the articulators in hypokinetic dysarthria, markedly dysrhythmic and irregular with regard to pitch and loudness in ataxic dysarthria, et cetera. A pattern evident in production of the

individual syllables will be repeated in the sequential task. But in apraxia of speech repetition of the individual syllables will typically be normal once the patient gets the phoneme train started, and the rate, rhythm, and control of loudness and pitch will be normal; however, in producing the sequential motion rate pattern of /pʌ—tʌ—kʌ/ the apraxic patient typically demonstrates a remarkable breakdown in initiating the sequence and sustaining it.

Differentiating Apraxia of Speech from Aphasia

Following are some distinctions which will help to differentiate the programming problem of apraxia of speech from the linguistic processing problems of aphasia:

1. The "word-finding" difficulties of aphasic and apraxic patients are quite different. In groping for a given word or repeating a word in search for its meaning the aphasic patient will demonstrate that the word eludes him or that although he can say it, its meaning eludes him. The apraxic patient, on the other hand, shows that he has the target word clearly in mind and that he is not uncertain of its meaning; rather he is searching for the way to execute its phonemic constituents. He may be able to write the word that he cannot say. If asked whether he is trying to say a given word, he will answer correctly. The apraxic patient differs from the aphasic patient in that his recognition of words is much better than his ability to speak those same words. We may use a task like the following to differentiate the two groups of patients: with multiple pictures or objects in front of the patient, say a series of three words and ask the patient to point in that same sequence at the pictures or objects named. The aphasic patient through his performance will likely give evidence of inadequate recognition and comprehension of the words or retention of sequences of them, whereas the apraxic patient will ordinarily be able to respond correctly and demonstrate no impairment in perception of the signal.

2. A comparison must be made of the total performance of the patient on a battery of language tasks. Aphasia is a multimodality disorder with relatively comparable impairment in listening, reading, speaking, and writing. Apraxic patients, on the other hand, are much poorer in their speaking performance than they are in listening, reading, or writing. Studies of groups of patients with apraxia of speech (1, 7, 8, 9) have demonstrated their relative freedom from input disorders contrasted with disproportionate difficulty in speech expression. Even when apraxia is associated with an aphasic disorder, it is possible to tease out the fact that on given words on which the patient demonstrates difficulty, his difficulty speaking is inordinately greater than

his difficulty understanding that word, reading it with discernment, or writing it.

Differentiation from Psychogenic Disorders

The clinician must keep in mind the fact that every organic disorder of communication can be skillfully mimicked by a psychogenic disorder. The laryngospasm in a focal dystonia may sound almost identical to the laryngospasm of a patient with spastic (spasmodic) dysphonia. The breathiness of flaccid dysarthria may closely resemble the dysphonia of hysterical conversion. The hypernasality and nasal emission of flaccid or spastic dysarthria has even been mimicked by a spasmodic hypernasality of psychogenic origin. Articulatory imprecision of dysarthria may be distinguished only with difficulty from a lifelong idiosyncratic articulation problem.

In the final analysis the clinician will need all the help he or she can get from other professional personnel who can clarify the nature of the presenting disorder. Sometimes only periods of treatment will finally clarify the true nature of the disorder.

DEVELOPMENTAL FORMS OF MOTOR SPEECH DISORDERS

This chapter has dealt exclusively with acquired dysarthrias and apraxia of speech. Analogous problems which are congenital or of early onset are found in children. In cerebral palsied children faulty innervation of speech is frequently part of the total picture of neurologic impairment, with resulting dysarthria. Children have also been found to present a developmental form of apraxia of speech (10). These problems are discussed in Chapter 19, which deals with distinctive signs the clinician must use in arriving at a differential diagnosis of articulation problems in children.

ASSIGNMENTS

1. Distinguish between "dysarthria" and "apraxia of speech." Why is it appropriate to refer to "the dysarthrias" rather than simply to "dysarthria"?
2. One medical dictionary has defined dysarthria as "defective articulation in speech." In what ways is this definition inadequate?
3. Which cranial nerves are involved in motor speech function? What function does each cranial nerve control?
4. If the tongue deviates to the right on protrusion, which side of the tongue is weak? What is the explanation for this phenomenon?
5. Distinguish between the terms "hypokinetic" and "hyperkinetic."
6. What is a "mixed" dysarthria?

7. What is meant by a cluster of speech deviations in dysarthria? By what process were the dysarthria clusters described in this chapter first identified and named? See reference 3.

8. How has laboratory research confirmed and amplified our understanding of the dysarthrias gained from perceptual studies? Consider the following reports: Kent, R. D., Netsell, R., and Bauer, L. L., Cineradiographic assessment of articulatory mobility in the dysarthrias. *Journal of Speech and Hearing Disorders,* 1975, *40*: 467–480. Kent, R. D., and Netsell, R., A case study of an ataxic dysarthric: cineradiographic and spectrographic observations. *Journal of Speech and Hearing Disorders,* 1975, *40*:115–134. Netsell, R., Daniel, B., and Celesia, G. G., Acceleration and weakness in Parkinsonian dysarthria. *Journal of Speech and Hearing Disorders,* 1975, *40*:170–178.

9. If you note a significant degree of harshness in a patient's voice, which dysarthric group might you consider first in your attempt to determine the type of dysarthria? That is, of which dysarthric group is it most likely a component? Consider Table 18.1. Make a similar judgment in a case of rapid rate; a case of distortion of vowels; a case of reduced stress; a case of hypernasality.

10. Consult a neurology text and determine the rationale for use of the term "pseudobulbar palsy."

11. Consult several neurology texts: What information do they provide concerning patterns of dysarthric speech?

12. How prominent in dysarthric speech are repetitions and prolongations? See Table 18.1 and Reference 2.

13. How do neurologists define apraxia? What is an apraxia of speech? Why does Geschwind advise against use of the term? See Geschwind, N., The apraxias: neural mechanisms of disorders of learned movement. *American Scientist,* 1975, *63*:188–195. Why does Martin object to use of the term? See Martin, A. D., Some objections to the term apraxia of speech. *Journal of Speech and Hearing Disorders,* 1974, *39*:53–64. Why do we recommend use of the term? See Aten, J. L., Darley, F. L., Deal, J. L., and Johns, D. F., Comment on A. D. Martin's "Some objections to the term apraxia of speech." *Journal of Speech and Hearing Disorders,* 1975, *40*:416–420.

14. Analyze the errors found in the three examples of apraxic speech on pp. 505–506 of this chapter. Develop a classification system comprehensive enough to encompass them.

15. What might we expect the characteristics of oral diadochokinetic rate to be in each of the dysarthrias and apraxia of speech?

16. How are the articulatory errors characteristic of apraxia of speech different from those observed in the dysarthrias?

REFERENCES

1. Bay, E., Principles of classification and their influence on our concepts of aphasia. In De Rueck, A. V., and O'Connor, M., eds., *Disorders of Language*, pp. 122–139. Boston: Little, Brown, 1964.
2. Darley, F. L., Aronson, A. E., and Brown, J. R., Differential diagnostic patterns of dysarthria. *Journal of Speech and Hearing Research*, 1969, *12*:246–269.
3. Darley, F. L., Aronson, A. E., and Brown, J. R., Clusters of deviant speech dimensions in the dysarthrias. *Journal of Speech and Hearing Research*, 1969, *12*:462–496.
4. Darley, F. L., Aronson, A. E., and Brown, J. R., *Motor Speech Disorders*. Philadelphia: Saunders, 1975.
5. De Renzi, E., Pieczuro, A., and Vignolo, L. A., Oral apraxia and aphasia. *Cortex*, 1966, *2*:50–73.
6. Grewel, F., Classification of dysarthrias. *Acta Psychiatrica et Neurologica Scandinavica*, 1957, *32*:325–337.
7. Johns, D. F., and Darley F. L., Phonemic variability in apraxia of speech. *Journal of Speech and Hearing Research*, 1970, *13*:556–583.
8. Schuell, H., Jenkins, J. J., and Jiménez-Pabón, E., *Aphasia in Adults: Diagnosis, Prognosis, and Treatment*. New York: Harper & Row, 1964.
9. Shankweiler, D., and Harris, K. S., An experimental approach to the problems of articulation in aphasia. *Cortex*, 1966, *2*:277–292.
10. Yoss, K. A., and Darley, F. L., Developmental apraxia of speech in children with defective articulation. *Journal of Speech and Hearing Research*, 1974, *17*:399–416.

19

DISORDERS OF ARTICULATION

Frederic L. Darley

Articulation is the aspect of motor speech most frequently involved in disorders of communication. At times we meet a child or adult who presents an articulation disorder in isolation, but more commonly we find that his or her errors in articulation are embedded in a matrix of other communication problems. Sometimes specific features of these articulation difficulties carry differential diagnostic information; more usually we arrive at a decision about the nature of the articulation disorder by observing concomitant aberrations and piecing together related historical information relevant to communication development.

In discerning the significance of an articulation problem, determining its cause or causes, and finally developing a plan for remediation, you will want to make use of various observations described in the appraisal portion of this book. The observations made in evaluating articulation (Chapter 8) are fundamental. How articulation fits into the total speech process can be seen in the overall description of oral communication (Chapter 3). You will need to know whether the articulation problem is part of a larger problem of language development generally, so you will use the measures presented in Chapter 4. In order to determine whether there are important physiological determinants or associations with the articulation problem, you will need to consult the information you have about respiration and phonation (Chapter 6), resonance (Chapter 7), rate and other prosodic features (Chapter 9), and the function of the speech mechanism (Chapter 11). To evaluate the relationship between the articulation problem and problems in auditory sensation or perception, you will use the materials in Chapter 12.

Once you have described the articulation problem of the speaker, you are faced with the task of determining the reasons for it. We will group the possibilities into three main areas: sensory deficits, physiologic limitations, and learning factors.

SENSORY DEFICITS

Hearing Loss

The extent to which articulation is impaired in connection with a hearing loss generally depends upon the degree of hearing loss and the time in the speaker's life when it was acquired. If the speaker had already developed normal speech and language before acquiring a mild or moderate hearing loss, probably little alteration of articulation with the passage of time can be expected. If it is a severe bilateral loss of hearing which is acquired, in time the patient will probably begin to omit final phonemes of words and distort various consonant phonemes, and he may demonstrate some changes in the efficiency with which he monitors the loudness of his voice and his vocal pitch and quality. However, if he has had the benefit of amplification fairly early in the course of the development of the hearing loss, his articulation probably will not be significantly affected.

If the hearing loss exists during the early years when speech and language are developing, impairment of articulation (and language) is much more likely. If the loss is a mild one, the phonemes with low acoustic energy may be impaired; the child may be defective in articulation of the fricative and affricate phonemes, less likely the plosive phonemes, and he may have trouble discriminating between the various fricative and affricate phonemes. Vowels and other consonant phonemes are unlikely to be impaired. If the hearing loss is moderate to severe, there is still greater likelihood that the fricative and affricate phonemes will be distorted. Other consonants—the plosives, semivowels, and nasals —may also be distorted, and even the vowels may be misarticulated.

If the child has no usable hearing, his articulatory repertoire will be extremely limited (22). His speech may consist essentially of poorly differentiated vowels separated from each other with primitive consonantlike sounds. Vowels may be diphthongized, and diphthongs will likely be improperly produced. Some visible phonemes may be more accurately articulated. The fricative and affricate phonemes will probably be so grossly distorted as to be unrecognizable, and consonant clusters will be especially defective. Some phonemes, consonant clusters, and syllables may be omitted. Voiceless phonemes may be voiced. All productions may be hypernasal. Speech will typically be slow and labored, an excessive amount of breath will be exhausted in the production of each phrase, and there will be improper stress, and a lack of inflection or inappropriate inflection.

Oral Anaesthesia

It will be a rare patient who presents an articulation problem attributable to deprivation of sensation in the tongue and mouth. Patients who have facial and oral sensory dysfunction for a variety of reasons, including resection of the trigeminal nerve, ordinarily compensate well and present minor articulatory disturbances if any.

Studies which have used nerve block procedures in order to investigate speech changes with deprivation of oral sensation have reported no substantial change in speech intelligibility. These changes have consisted mostly of distortions and omissions of primarily the fricative and affricate phonemes (*38, 56, 59, 76*). Sometimes fricatives are produced as plosives and bilabials may become labiodentals (*18*). Scott and Ringel (*60*) found little phonemic change during oral anesthesia; their speakers executed basic speech maneuvers including palatal opening and closing, complete vocal tract closures, close vocal tract constrictions, and vocal tract configurations appropriate for vowels. They noted (*61*) that subjects deprived of oral sensation presented articulatory deviations somewhat different from those of a group of dysarthric subjects with which they were compared. Putnam and Ringel (*55*) reported that an experimental subject deprived of labial sensation was able to produce intelligible speech with only minor changes in manner and place of articulation, the disruptive effects becoming more noticeable as the phonetic content of the test words became more complex. In general, noticeable articulatory changes could be described as a loss of refinement in lip movements involving the production of complex consonant clusters, lip rounding, and extent of lip opening relative to normal.

Investigators have considered whether differences in oral tactile discrimination (stereognosis) can account for differences in articulation. Tests of oral sensation-perception have used pairs of small plastic forms placed in a subject's mouth, one at a time, the subject being asked whether the two successive forms are the same or different. Madison and Fucci (*35*) found that in a group of 100 first-grade children the correlation between articulation proficiency and oral tactile discrimination was not statistically significant; children who performed well on the test of oral tactile discrimination did not demonstrate better articulation ability than those who performed poorly.

One may assume that although deprivation of sensory information in the tongue and face may make some contribution to an articulation problem, particularly when associated with motor deficit, a gross articulatory deviation cannot ordinarily be reasonably attributed to sensory deprivation.

PHYSIOLOGIC LIMITATIONS

Palatopharyngeal Incompetence

Children with congenital clefts of lip and palate or of palate only which have undergone primary repair do not necessarily present articulation problems. If the repair has resulted in competent palatopharyngeal closure so that the child can impound adequate intraoral breath pressure, articulation will likely be normal. Pitzner and Morris (53) studied 84 children of the kind described and concluded that children with adequate intraoral breath pressure (indicative of palatopharyngeal competence) showed as a group articulation skills comparable to those of normal children; in that study the only exception to that similarity occurred in the case of fricatives, defects of which might have been caused by special dental problems.

The crucial requirement is for a palatopharyngeal mechanism capable of attaining that degree of closure which makes possible the impounding of a critical amount of intraoral breath pressure. Spriestersbach, Moll, and Morris (71) used an oral manometer to measure nasal leakage in a series of subjects, comparing the breath pressure impounded intraorally with the nostrils occluded with the pressure impounded with nostrils open, the former value being taken to represent maximum since any nasal leak was obviated. (The ratio between these two values is a convenient clinical measure of palatopharyngeal competence: equal values with nostrils open and occluded give a ratio of 1.00, indicating palatopharyngeal competence for this activity; impounding less intraoral breath pressure with the nostrils open than with nostrils occluded yields a ratio of less than 1.00 and indicates nasal escape.) These investigators found that ratios of 0.90 or better usually reflected adequate function for articulation, whereas ratios of 0.89 and lower were associated with significant impairment of articulation skills.

It might be expected that impairment of palatopharyngeal valving which allows even minimal escape of air into the nasal cavities would result in defective articulation since the production of many consonants requires the buildup of substantial intraoral breath pressure and oral impedence of the breath stream. In confirmation of this expectation, Shelton, Brooks, and Youngstrom (62), reporting on a group of 6 patients with palatal inadequacies, 24 patients with surgically repaired cleft palates, and 10 normal subjects, found that gaps between the soft palate and the pharyngeal wall smaller than, as well as larger than, 2.0 mm may have a deleterious effect on articulation.

It is logical to expect that patients who have some demonstrated degree of palatopharyngeal incompetence will have more difficulty with those phonemes which require substantial intraoral breath pressure. Spriestersbach, Darley, and Rouse (70) studied the articulation of 25 children between the ages of 3 and 8, all of whom had congenital clefts of the lip or palate in various stages of repair. The fricatives and affricates were most often defective, the plosives less often defective, the nasals rarely defective; the semivowels and glides, none of which involves a substantial degree of intraoral breath pressure, were defective to variable degrees probably on the basis of developmental immaturity rather than because of any organic deficiency. This would seem to be a reasonable explanation when one compares the data from this study with data from a study by McWilliams (41) of a group of 48 cleft palate adults. The adult subjects demonstrated patterns of difficulty similar to those of the children in the earlier study, demonstrating greater difficulty with fricatives and affricates, much less difficulty with plosives, and minimal difficulty with nasals as well as with semivowels and glides. See Morris (49) for a complete discussion of the causes of articulation impairment in cleft palate.

From a number of studies of the articulation of patients with problems related to the palatopharyngeal mechanism we may derive the following generalizations (9, 41, 46, 68, 70, 71, 77, 78): speakers with palatopharyngeal incompetence have most difficulty in articulating fricatives, affricates, and plosives, that is, the pressure phonemes, and relatively less difficulty with glides, semivowels, and nasals. Voiceless consonants are more frequently misarticulated that their voiced cognates. Although there are some findings to the contrary, patients with cleft of the palate only typically have more articulation difficulties than patients with clefts of lip and palate combined. Patients with clefts of the lip only have no special articulation problems.

A common articulatory characteristic of speakers with palatopharyngeal incompetence is the introduction of glottal articulation, a pulse of air being produced at the level of the glottis as a possible substitute for the impedance of the airstream not achieved within the mouth. Glottal plosives are introduced usually as prevocalic intrusions or substitutions for voiceless consonants, usually for plosives; glottal or pharyngeal fricatives are sometimes substituted for fricatives and affricates (62, 71).

The articulation problems attributable to palatopharyngeal incompetence usually occur in association with a significant degree of hypernasality. In addition, one may frequently note audible nasal emission of air during the production of pressure consonants. These speakers sometimes make facial grimaces in their effort to articulate the phonemes which palatopharyngeal incompetence prevents them from making normally; they may contract the alae of the nares in an attempt to obtain closure at this substitute point.

In this connection it is interesting to note that in a survey of 1061 persons with clefts of lip and palate in various stages of treatment examined at the Lancaster Palate Clinic over a ten-year period, 16.5 percent of the subjects had an articulation defect, 21.5 percent displayed hypernasality, and 27.6 percent presented both an articulation problem and hypernasality (75). This survey reported an incidence of delayed speech of 1.1 percent, a percentage slightly higher than might be expected in a normal population. Others (48, 52, 66, 69) have reported that as a group children with cleft palates are retarded in language development, but this retardation is probably related more to psycho-

social factors than it is to palatopharyngeal incompetence and its consequences. Surveys have indicated that in a group of patients with
palatopharyngeal incompetence the incidence of other communication
disorders is essentially the same as that found in the general population.

Neuromotor Impairment

It is reasonable to expect that patients with a congenital or acquired
impairment of neuromotor function might demonstrate impaired function
of the cranial nerves. If any of the cranial nerves involved in speech
(V, VII, X, XII) is impaired, either centrally or peripherally, we may
expect motor speech in general, including articulation, to be impaired.
The kind and degree of impairment will depend upon the site of the
lesion and the degree to which normal muscle functions are interrupted.
The age at which the central nervous system disorder occurs also is
important in determining the nature of the speech problem and management procedures.

Dysarthria in Cerebral Palsy This group of children with congenital
neuromuscular impairment present a high incidence of involvement of
the speech apparatus. For example, Wolfe (86) reported that of a group of
50 cerebral palsied subjects ranging in age from 5 to 20 years, 43 percent
presented some involvement of the tongue, 59 percent of the lips, 31
percent of the mandible, 57 percent of respiration, 38 percent of the
larynx, and 39 percent of the soft palate. Similarly Palmer (50) in a
group of 100 cerebral palsied children found a wide range of dysfunctions
of the tongue, mandible, and facial muscles. It follows logically that many
cerebral palsied children will have articulatory difficulties, many of them
severe. Wolfe (86) reported that 70 percent of his subjects had inadequate articulation, although not all of the articulation errors were directly
attributable to neuromotor impairment. Achilles (1) found that 43 percent of the cerebral palsied subjects he studied had poor articulation,
45 percent fair articulation. Mecham, Berko, and Berko (42) report that
between 70 and 80 percent of cerebral palsied patients have some type
of articulation problem. In a group of 100 cerebral palsied children with
speech disorders, Palmer (50) reported that 36 percent were speechless,
28 percent presented a severe disorder, 26 percent a moderate disorder.
When Irwin (23) compared the articulatory skills of groups of cerebral
palsied children and mentally retarded children of comparable low I.Q.
(one group, 25–50 I.Q., another 51–80 I.Q.), he found the articulation of
the cerebral palsied children to be significantly poorer than that of the
retarded children.

A number of studies specify the kind of articulation problems we can
expect in cerebral palsy. Both Lencione (33), who studied 129 cerebral
palsied children between the ages of 8 and 14, and Byrne (7), who studied

74 cerebral palsied children between the ages of 2 and 7, found that those consonants requiring complex adjustment of the tongue tip were more frequently in error. For example, Byrne (7) reported the order of difficulty of consonants appearing in the initial position as follows: /θ/ (16.9 percent correct), /r/ (25.1 percent), /ʃ/ (27.8 percent); /s/ (29.5 percent), /dʒ/ (32.2 percent), /z/ (32.7 percent), /l/ (32.8 percent), /tʃ/ (35.5 percent), and /ð/ (36 percent). These investigators found that labial, back of tongue, and simple tongue tip phonemes such as /n/, /t/, /d/, /f/, and /v/ were considerably easier for these children to produce. Byrne found that vowels and diphthongs were produced correctly most of the time. Both Lencione and Byrne found that initial consonants were generally produced correctly more often than consonants in the medial and final positions, a finding also reported by Irwin (24). Irwin (25) found that a group of 96 cerebral palsied children between the ages of 4 and 16 years produced omission and distortion errors primarily, unlike normal subjects, who are more likely to present substitution errors. The studies are in agreement that voiced consonants prove less difficult than their voiceless cognates and that consonant clusters are more difficult than single consonants.

The data are in fairly good agreement that we may expect more articulation problems among cerebral palsied children of the athetoid type than among those of spastic type (7, 10, 24, 33, 86). The intelligibility of the speech of spastic cerebral palsied children is likely to be better than that of the athetoid children.

The articulation problem of the cerebral palsied child is usually one aspect of a comprehensive communication difficulty involving multiple motor speech processes. Many cerebral palsied patients have significant difficulty maintaining adequate breath support for speech. Although restricted vital capacity may not itself constitute a limiting factor for speech, when it is coupled with inadequate valving of the breath stream, speech difficulties are likely to follow (20, 21). Cypreanson (10) found abnormal breathing patterns in 25 cerebral palsied children ranging in age from 8 to 12 years; the better speakers had breathing patterns which approached those of a group of normal subjects more closely than did the breathing patterns of the poorer speakers. Investigators have reported a wide variety of phonatory disorders as well—impaired pitch control, monotonous pitch, breathiness, harshness, hoarseness, inadequate loudness, inadequate control of loudness, and phonation on inhalation (32, 42, 50, 57, 86). There is often significant hypernasality and nasal emission of air. Speech rate is likely to be slow, and stress is likely to be equalized.

Acquired Dysarthria   The adult who as a result of a stroke, neoplasm, infectious process, or trauma suffers impairment of function of the cranial nerves related to speech functions will present a dysarthria which may include defective articulation. The articulation problem will seldom appear in isolation but is usually part of a distinctive pattern of phonatory, resonatory, and prosodic characteristics that provide clues as to the nature of the neurologic impairment and the site of it. One may learn to recognize distinctive patterns of articulatory disorder: (1) the usually consistent distortion and omission errors in articulation resulting from a flaccid paralysis of the speech muscles; (2) the slowly produced articulation characterized by usually consistent distortions and omissions typical of spastic conditions; (3) the often hurried, blurred articulation of the parkinsonian patient producing phonemes in short bursts with inadequate muscle excursion; (4) the irregular articulatory breakdowns resulting from momentary loss of coordination in the ataxic speech which results from cerebellar lesions; (5) the unpredictable alterations of articulation resulting from hyperkinesia of the articulators in movement disorders. The various patterns of articulatory impairment and the clusters of motor speech deviations in which they commonly occur are described in Chapter 17 and are discussed in detail by Darley, Aronson, and Brown (11).

Apraxia of Speech Certain adult patients with lesions of the left cerebral hemisphere have difficulty with the motor programming of phonemes and sequences of them, demonstrating variable difficulty in finding the correct oral postures. This difficulty is identified as apraxia of speech; it is described, as it appears in adults, in Chapter 18, pp. 504–508.

We believe that children may present a developmental form of this disorder. Probably Morley and her associates (47) were the first to use the term apraxia (or dyspraxia) to designate the articulatory behavior of some children. They defined "developmental articulatory dyspraxia" as "the failure or limited ability to control and direct the movements and coordinations of the respiratory, laryngeal and oral muscles for articulation when muscle tone and movement is otherwise adequate." Palmer, Wurth, and Kincheloe (51), Luchsinger and Arnold (34), and Eisenson (13) have described "apraxic" children with persistent articulation problems; scattered uses of the term apraxia throughout the world's literature indicate that people have suspected that some so-called "functional" disorders of articulation in children are actually apraxic in nature.

How does one determine whether a child's articulation problem is the result of apraxia of speech? Yoss and Darley (87) investigated the question and derived a set of criteria which may help differentiate that subset of articulatory defective children whose problem is attributable to a motor-programming deficit. They administered a series of speech and nonspeech oral performance tests to a group of 30 children with moderate to severe articulation problems; the children also were given neurologic examinations, audiometric tests, and psychometric tests. There emerged from the total group a subgroup of children who performed in such manner as to warrant calling them apraxic.

The primary feature which distinguished the apraxic children from the others with articulation problems was their inordinate difficulty in performing certain oral nonspeech tasks volitionally (blowing, licking their lips, puffing out their cheeks, demonstrating a kiss, whistling, coughing, clicking their tongues, etc.). On neurological tests these children also presented more neurologic signs than the other children; they were in some cases identified by the neurologist as being generally dyspraxic, that is, clumsy and awkward. They produced slower oral diadochokinetic rates; when they tried to repeat the series /pʌ—tʌ—kʌ/, they typically produced an incorrect syllable sequence. When asked to repeat polysyllabic words, they often omitted, revised, or added syllables. Analysis of their articulation performance indicated that they made more two- and three-feature errors than the other children with articulation problems, more distortions such as minimal nasalization or voicing errors, and more additions. Especially the older children presented more prosodic errors, such as slowed rate and equalized stress.

Children who present an apraxia of speech typically respond poorly to traditional speech therapy. It is the recalcitrance of their articulation problems to therapy that often calls our attention to them particularly and makes us scrutinize more closely their motor-programming capacities. When these children are studied longitudinally, their clinicians often report that they finally abandoned the usual auditory approach in retraining and resorted to phonetic placement procedures, helping the children make special use of visual, tactile, and kinesthetic cues (88).

Dental Deviations

Can we safely attribute an articulation problem to a speaker's dental condition? Although some clinicians and writers have stated that certain dental conditions "definitely" cause speech defects of given kinds, studies of groups of subjects presenting either abnormal dental conditions or disorders of articulation have failed to demonstrate a one-to-one relationship between any dental condition and any given articulation problem. The conclusion can be drawn, however, that in certain individuals the presence of a dental abnormality may be causally related to an articulation problem. One can also conclude from group data that more severe dental deviations are more likely to cause articulation problems.

In a study of the relationship of speech performance to dental occlusion in 410 university students, Fymbo (17) found that 87 percent of 111 students with defective speech, 62 percent of 129 students with "average" speech, and 35 percent of 100 students with superior speech had a malocclusion. It is impressive that the 35 superior speakers with malocclusion showed no ill effects of the malocclusion. Nevertheless, Fymbo concluded that "severity of the speech defect was found to vary directly with the severity of the dental anomaly." Likewise Fairbanks and Lentner (15), comparing 30 university students with superior and 30 with inferior consonant articulation, found that "marked dental deviations were significantly more numerous among inferior speakers." The conditions that both investigations suggested might be most contributory to defective articulation were anterior openbite (a large interarch distance) and closebite (a small interarch distance), openbite probably being more important as a contributor than closebite.

Probably of greater interest is the relationship between dental conditions and speech in children who are in the process of mastering the phonemes of the language. Of 78 children selected from speech classes receiving therapy because of faulty production of sibilants, Wolf (85) found 74 percent to have malocclusion. In about one-fourth of these cases he "definitely" related the malocclusion to the articulation defect, and in another one-fourth he suggested a secondary or possible relationship. Wolf reported that frontal openbite, protrusion of the upper jaw with openbite, and protrusion of the lower jaw with openbite were all potential causes of articulation problems. In another study of 76 school children aged 8 through 12 with significant openbite, 45 percent were judged to have an interdental lisp sufficiently obvious to warrant speech therapy (45). In still another study Subtelny, Mestre, and Subtelny (73) concluded that some adolescent speakers with an overjet condition may adjust to it in such a way as to produce defective sibilant phonemes. They studied 30 subjects with normal occlusion and speech and 51 subjects with Class II malocclusion (mandibular retrusion associated with protruding incisors), the degree of maxillary dental overjet beyond the mandibular incisors exceeding 6 mm. Thirty-one of the latter subjects had normal articulation, 20 defective articulation. Those with defective articulation protruded the tongue tip beyond the mandibular incisors and tended to approach the lingual surfaces of the protruding maxillary incisors.

Data vary concerning the importance of the completeness and alignment of the incisal edge against which the constricted airstream is directed in the production of sibilant phonemes. Fymbo (17) concluded that "edentulous spaces, particularly those occurring among the upper eight anterior teeth, operated as strong etiologic factors in the production of defective speech" in the college students he studied. He also reported that "spacing of the teeth, due to lack of proximal contact, contributed to the production of defective speech." Wolf (85) also mentions "widely spaced incisors or canines" as a potential cause of sibilant distortion. Snow (67) studied the speech of 498 first-graders to determine the effect of missing or grossly abnormal maxillary incisors upon the articulation of six fricatives (/s/, /z/, /f/, /v/, /θ/, /ð/). Of these children, 314 had abnormal or missing maxillary incisors. She reported that a significantly larger portion of the children with missing or abnormal incisors misarticulated the phonemes than did children with normal dentition. However, most of the children with normal or missing incisors articulated the phonemes correctly and some of the children without dental abnormality misarticulated them. She concluded that "defective incisor teeth usually do not interfere with correct articulation of the single 'dental' sounds studied" but for some children the condition of the maxillary incisors "may be crucial for the development" of the articulation of those phonemes.

In a cephalometric study Weinberg (83) compared 13 children with complete dentition, normal occlusion, and correct production of /s/; 13 children with missing maxillary central incisors, normal molar relationships, and correct /s/; and 13 children with missing maxillary central incisors, normal molar relationships, and defective /s/. The difference between the latter two groups lay in the fact that those with defective /s/ elevated and protruded the tongue tip, whereas those with correct /s/ did not.

We can expect children with congenital clefts of lip and palate to present dental abnormalities which may pose an additional hazard to articulation. A wide variety of dental abnormalities can be expected (5, 27). Following surgical repair of the cleft, one may need to consider carefully whether residual faulty articulation may be related to malocclusion or misalignment of anterior teeth or spaces between the teeth.

Lingual Defects

We have seen that impairment of the innervation of the tongue can lead to various types of articulatory impairment in dysarthria. Anatomic aberrations in tongue size and contour may also be related to articulation problems.

The format of the tongue ranges from essential absence of the tongue or the existence of only a rudimentary form of the tongue in congenital aglossia through various sizes and shapes to the condition of macroglossia, in which the tongue is so large in relationship to the oral cavity that it protrudes from the mouth at rest. Since the tongue plays a crucial role in providing impedance to the breath stream in articulation, it is surprising that the extremes of anatomic variation of the tongue result in no greater articulatory problems than have been observed.

The speech of patients who present aglossia has been described as impaired in articulatory efficiency but intelligible (14, 44). Similarly microglossia due to failure of the tongue to develop normally has been reported to result in multiple articulatory distortions (74). In the patient with macroglossia the tongue is so large in relationship to the mandible, maxilla, or both that it is difficult for it to move with normal speed to the appropriate contact points for precise articulation, most particularly of the tongue tip phonemes.

Drastic reduction in the size of the tongue may be the result of glossectomy or partial glossectomy made necessary by cancer surgery or brought about by accident. The degree of articulatory impairment in this condition will depend in part upon the amount of tongue that has been removed, in part upon the location of the portion that is left, and in large part upon the drive and adaptability of the speaker. It is testimony to the amazing capacity of the human organism to compensate for seemingly insuperable obstacles that most patients with glossectomy continue to speak intelligibly. Patients learn to adjust their rate, produce certain phonemes in atypical ways, and use other parts of the oral speech mechanism to help the tongue compensate for its limitations (2, 6, 16, 19, 29, 31, 36, 64, 65).

LEARNING FACTORS

Mental Retardation

It is a well-documented fact that mentally retarded persons acquire speech and language more slowly than those with normal intelligence and that when speech is acquired, it is likely to be defective (37). The likelihood of there being an articulation problem is increased as the level of mental functioning decreases.

Irwin (26) has reported that the pattern of phoneme production is different in children with low I.Q.'s (7–48) from that found in normal children. The ten mentally retarded children aged 2 through 5 whom he tested over a period of one year used back vowels less frequently than front vowels, demonstrated a ratio of vowels to consonants of 1:1 (adult ratio 1:2, newborn ratio 3:2), and showed a distinctive concentration of labial, postdental, and glottal sounds. Whereas Irwin suggests a different pattern of early articulatory development, other investigators have found that the articulation problems of the retarded are not different in kind from those of individuals not mentally retarded. Karlin and Strazzulla (28) found the following order of decreasing phoneme defectiveness: /s/, /z/, /l/, /r/, /tʃ/, /dʒ/, /ð/, /ʃ/, and /θ/. Bangs (3) reported that a group of 53 institutionalized mentally retarded persons of unspecified ages presented articulatory problems similar to those of nonretarded articulatory defective children except for the greater incidence of omission of phonemes, especially in the final position, and the use of some bizarre substitutions unlike those ordinarily heard among the nonretarded. It should be pointed out that many adults who are judged to be mentally retarded have essentially normal articulation.

There are no reliable data which indicate that individuals who represent specific syndromes of mental retardation present distinctive articulatory patterns. The articulatory problem seen in the mentally retarded constitutes only one aspect of a general speech-language retardation. We can expect to find their articulatory problems associated with reduced recognition and use vocabularies, reduced verbal output, and immature morphologic and syntactic usage.

Specific Language Disability

Children identified as presenting a specific language disability (sometimes designated developmental or congenital aphasia) may present an articulation disorder in connection with other problems in communication. These are children who hear well, but seemingly cannot listen well; it can be determined that they are not mentally retarded, yet intellectually they function inefficiently; they are not emotionally disturbed but some of their behavior may be suggestive of autism. These are children who in the face of seemingly normal or near normal cognitive functions present a markedly disproportionate difficulty in language processing, both input and output. Their problems in communication are evident in the semantic, morphologic, and syntactic aspects of communication and in the phonologic as well.

These children's articulation problems may be attributable to the same kinds of difficulties that account for their language dysfunction. Eisenson (13) has suggested that there may be four conditions, operating singly or in combination, which underlie their difficulty. (1) Their storage system for speech signals may be defective. Although they may be able to imitate phonemes immediately, if there is a brief delay they appear to lose what they have heard and are unable to imitate it. (2) Their discrimination and perception of phonemes in conversation may be impaired. Although they can discriminate between similar phonemes in isolation, when phonemes are blended into words, they may not be able to tell them apart and reproduce them. (3) They may not be able to process auditory signals at the rate at which they receive them. They can't listen fast enough. (4) They cannot keep track of the order in which phonemes arrive, which came first, which came next, and which came last.

To determine whether a child has an articulation problem on the basis of a specific language disability, we must look at his performance on various tests of auditory perception and sequencing and at the kinds of associated language disabilities which he displays. We will be interested in his performance on tests of auditory retention, whether for digits or for word strings. How well can he retain and reproduce sentences of increasing length? How well does he carry out commands which require the processing of more and more bits of information, as in the Token Test (12, 84)? Does he display the variations in morphologic and syntactic form that children of his age usually display, or has he been unable to abstract from the language about him the rules of language structure which most of us learn simply by listening? Can he guess at the identity of words when he hears only fragments of them, as in the Auditory Closure subtest of the Illinois Test of Psycholinguistic Abilities (30)? Can he synthesize a sequence of phonemes into whole nonsense syllables or meaningful words (phonetic fusion or sound blending) (30)? Is his performance on auditory tasks poorer than his performance on comparable visual tasks? Is there a marked discrepancy between his performance on the verbal and performance parts of the Wechsler Intelligence Scale for Children?

When we find evidence of marked auditory processing dysfunction in the face of a normal audiogram, normal or near normal intelligence, and a normal pattern of interpersonal interaction, we may conclude that a child's articulation problem, together with his or her other communication deficits, is attributable to a specific language disability. We will, of course, do well to consider the strong possibility that this articulation problem is not an integral part of his or her specific language disability but is a separate developmental problem which coexists with it. Present diagnostic tools are not adequate to differentiate unequivocally between these two possibilities.

Functional Articulatory Defects

We are left with a group of children whose articulation is defective but for whose problem no cause is evident. These problems have been commonly designated as "functional" articulation problems. Since what we really mean is that these problems are of undetermined origin, the terms "idiopathic" or "developmental" are less misleading.

Clearly these articulatory errors are not haphazard. Several investigators (8, 39, 40, 43, 54, 81, 82) have shown that these children are operating with somewhat different phonologic rules than other children. The rules which a given child uses account for his or her particular set of errors, so there is orderliness and consistency with them.

In Chapter 8 we showed that the acquisition of articulation skills is a gradual process extending over many years. It is a process in which children display marked individual variability for reasons which often we cannot fully specify. "Maturation" is a term that embraces a complex of ways in which children grow, neuromuscularly and perceptually. The norms for phoneme mastery presented in Chapter 8 summarize what we expect the normally maturing child to accomplish, usually by about age 8.

It is evident that some children don't "meet the deadlines" suggested by these norms. They display a "maturational lag" or a "developmental delay" for which we cannot readily account. Yet many of them somehow "catch up," even without help. Van Hattum (79) has pointed out, and offered research data in support, that most people with articulation "problems" develop acceptable speech by adulthood even without therapy. There are abundant data showing that a high percentage of children identified at some age as having an articulation "problem" rather soon progress spontaneously (without speech therapy intervention) to a "nonproblem" status. For example, Van Riper and Erickson (80) found that of 167 beginning first-grade children each of whom "had been judged by a state certified school speech clinician to have functionally defective articulation that was sufficiently deviant to warrant enrollment in a speech therapy program," 47 percent "had spontaneously mastered normal articulation" by the beginning of the third grade, only 53 percent continuing to exhibit articulatory errors. Similar findings have been reported by Barrett and Welsh (4). Sax (58), having observed that apparently "developmental learning of the articulatory process continued for some children beyond the age levels previously reported in developmental studies," followed the articulatory development of 417 children in a four-year longitudinal study. She found that 52 percent of the children improved in articulation during kindergarten; boys continued to improve at a similar rate through the second grade; both boys and girls improved through the third grade, showed a slowing of improvement during the fourth grade, and even in the fifth grade showed some improvement. She concluded that "the development of articulation skills in children is a fluid dynamic progressive process characterized by improvements, regressions, new errors, and stabilization of correct or incorrect consonant sounds."

Here are children, then, who have no obvious physical obstacle to their mastery of articulation skills. Many of them take somewhat longer than average to complete this mastery. Some appear to get stalled along the way, persisting in certain articulatory habits acquired early, seemingly unable to "unlearn" their faulty articulation without special help.

The possibility remains that there are explanatory factors to be discerned if only we had the tools to discern them. Perhaps some of these children have mild forms of the kind of motor-programming difficulty noted in children identified as having a developmental apraxia of speech. Perhaps there are other explanations pertaining to auditory processing or rule learning that at some future time we may be able to specify and designate with distinctive terminology. At the moment the most we can say is that these are children who appear to be normal in most respects relevant to the mastery of phonology but who, nevertheless, have acquired a deviant phonological system in the use of which they persist beyond the time when we would have expected them to replace it with new learning. They remain a large group of articulatory defective children whose challenging problems require creative approaches in diagnosis and therapy.

COMBINATIONS OF FACTORS

Our presentation of factors to consider in differential diagnosis of disorders of articulation may have suggested that a given patient has an articulation problem for any *one* of several reasons—a hearing loss, or a neuromotor impairment, or an anatomic deficiency, or faulty learning. We hasten to remind you that more often than not a given speech deviation has *causes* rather than *a cause*. So it is with articulation problems. There is a strong likelihood that multiple factors underlie a child's defective articulation. To take only one example, if a child has a congenital cleft of the palate, we find that our major diagnostic responsibility is to sort out structural from nonstructural bases for the articulation problem. Can it be related directly and fully to palatopharyngeal incompetence? Can impaired hearing explain part of the child's problem? Do dental deviations play a role? Is there developmental delay due to subnormal intelligence or other learning factors? Are there psychosocial influences complicating the picture further? How have these various potential components interacted in the case of this child?

We may find it impossible to assess definitively the weight of various contributory factors and determine what percentage of the problem is attributable to each of several conceivably relevant variables. Sometimes we may be unable to assign any weight to any of several potential influences; we may end up acknowledging that the behavior is of undetermined origin, a seeming enigma in terms of etiology. But it remains our job to analyze the disorder as completely as we can; to derive if at all possible a rationale for its appearance, its maintenance, and its variability; and consequently to design a program for its amelioration.

ASSIGNMENTS

1. Why do some hard-of-hearing persons have articulation problems? Why not all?
2. Compare and contrast the articulatory impairments observed in sensory deficit and motor deficit of the oral speech mechanism.
3. What degree of palatopharyngeal incompetence can be expected to be reflected in articulatory impairment?
4. Compare and contrast the findings of a study of the articulation of cleft palate children (70) and a study of the articulation of cleft palate adults (41).
5. Why is articulation often defective in children with cleft palates? Contrast the speech problems of patients with cleft palate only and patients with cleft lip only.
6. Why is articulation often defective in cerebral palsied children? Can one generalize and speak of "cerebral palsied speech"?

7. Why is articulation often defective in the dysarthrias? How do we account for different patterns of defective articulation in the various dysarthrias?

8. What articulatory and other behaviors may suggest that a child's articulation problem is apraxic in nature?

9. What dental conditions are particularly likely to be related to articulation problems?

10. Distinguish between the terms "aglossia," "microglossia," and "macroglossia."

11. How does Eisenson (13) account for the existence of articulation problems in children with specific language disability?

12. Discuss the suitability of the term "functional" in the expression "functional articulatory defects." How does Powers rationalize use of the term? See Powers, M. H., Functional disorders of articulation: symptomatology and etiology. In Travis, L. E., ed., *Handbook of Speech Pathology and Audiology*, pp. 837–875. Englewood Cliffs, N.J.: Prentice-Hall, 1971.

REFERENCES

1. Achilles, R., Communicative anomalies of individuals with cerebral palsy: I. Analysis of communicative processes in 151 cases of cerebral palsy. *Cerebral Palsy Review*, 1955, *16*:15–24.

2. Backus, O., Speech rehabilitation following excision of the tip of the tongue. *American Journal of Diseases of Children*, 1940, *60*:368–370.

3. Bangs, J., A critical analysis of the articulatory defects of the feeble-minded. *Journal of Speech Disorders*, 1942, *7*:343–356.

4. Barrett, M. D., and Welsh, J. W., Predictive articulation screening. *Language, Speech, and Hearing Services in Schools*, 1975, *6*:91–95.

5. Bohn, A., *Dental Abnormalities in Harelip and Cleft Palate*. Oslo: Universitelsforloget, Scandinavian University Books, 1963.

6. Brodnitz, F. S., Speech after glossectomy. *Current Problems in Phoniatrics and Logopedics*, 1960, *1*:68–72.

7. Byrne, M. C., Speech and language development of athetoid and spastic children. *Journal of Speech and Hearing Disorders*, 1959, *24*:231–240.

8. Compton, A. J., Generative study of children's phonological disorders. *Journal of Speech and Hearing Disorders*, 1970, *35*:315–339.

9. Counihan, D. T., Articulation skills of adolescents and adults with cleft palates. *Journal of Speech and Hearing Disorders*, 1960, *25*:181–187.

10. Cypreanson, L. E., An investigation of the breathing and speech coordinations and speech intelligibility of normal speaking children and cerebral palsied children with speech defects. Ph.D. dissertation, Syracuse University, 1953.

11. Darley, F. L., Aronson, A. E., and Brown, J. R., *Motor Speech Disorders*. Philadelphia: Saunders, 1975.

12. DeRenzi, E., and Vignolo, L. A., The Token Test: a sensitive test to detect receptive disturbances in aphasia. *Brain*, 1962, *85*:665–678.

13. Eisenson, J., *Aphasia in Children*. New York: Harper & Row, 1972.

14. Eskew, H. A., and Shepard, E., Congenital aglossia. *American Journal of Orthodontics*, 1945, 35:116–119.

15. Fairbanks, G., and Lentner, M. V., A study of minor organic deviations in "functional" disorders of articulation: 4. The teeth and hard palate. *Journal of Speech and Hearing Disorders*, 1951, 16:273–279.

16. Frowine, V. K., and Moser, H., Relationship of dentition to speech. *Journal of the American Dental Association*, 1944, 31:1081–1090.

17. Fymbo, L. H., The relation of malocclusion of the teeth to defects of speech. *Archives of Speech*, 1936, 1:204–216.

18. Gammon, S. A., Smith, P., Daniloff, R., and Kim, C., Articulation and stress/juncture production under oral anesthetization and masking. *Journal of Speech and Hearing Research*, 1971, 14:271–282.

19. Goldstein, M. A., New concepts of the functions of the tongue. *Laryngoscope*, 1940, 50:164–188.

20. Hardy, J. C., A study of pulmonary function in children with cerebral palsy. Ph.D. dissertation, University of Iowa, 1961.

21. Hardy, J. C., Intraoral breath pressure in cerebral palsy. *Journal of Speech and Hearing Disorders*, 1961, 26:309–316.

22. Hudgins, C. V., and Numbers, F., An investigation of the intelligibility of the speech of the deaf. *Genetic Psychology Monographs*, 1942, 25:289–392.

23. Irwin, O. C., Comparison of articulation scores of children with cerebral palsy and mentally retarded children. *Cerebral Palsy Review*, 1961, 22:10–11.

24. Irwin, O. C., Correct status of vowels and consonants in the speech of children with cerebral palsy as measured by an integrated test. *Cerebral Palsy Review*, 1961, 22:21–24.

25. Irwin, O. C., Substitution and omission errors in the speech of children who have cerebral palsy. *Cerebral Palsy Review*, 1956, 17:75.

26. Irwin, O. C., The developmental status of speech sounds of ten feeble-minded children. *Child Development*, 1942, 13:29–39.

27. Jordan, R. E., Kraus, B. S., and Neptune, C. M., Dental abnormalities associated with cleft lip and/or palate. *Cleft Palate Journal*, 1966, 3:22–55.

28. Karlin, I., and Strazzula, M., Speech and language problems of mentally deficient children. *Journal of Speech and Hearing Disorders*, 1952, 17:286–294.

29. Keaster, J., Studies of the anatomy and physiology of the tongue. *Laryngoscope*, 1940, 50:222–258.

30. Kirk, S. A., McCarthy, J. J., and Kirk, W. D., *Illinois Test of Psycholinguistic Abilities*. Rev. ed. Urbana: University of Illinois, 1968.

31. Kremen, A. J., Cancer of the tongue. *Minnesota Medicine*, 1953, 36:828–830.

32. Leith, W. R., and Steer, M. D., Comparison of judged characteristics of athetoids and spastics. *Cerebral Palsy Review*, 1958, 19:15–20.

33. Lencione, R., Speech and language problems in cerebral palsy. In Cruik-

shank, W., ed., *Cerebral Palsy*. 2nd ed. Syracuse, N.Y.: Syracuse University Press, 1966.

34. Luchsinger, R., and Arnold, G. E., *Voice-Speech-Language: Clinical Communicology*. Belmont, Calif.: Wadsworth, 1965.

35. Madison, C. L., and Fucci, D. J., Speech-sound discrimination and tactile-kinesthetic discrimination in reference to speech production. *Perceptual and Motor Skills*, 1971, 33:831–838.

36. Massengill, R., Maxwell, S., and Pickrell, K., An analysis of articulation following partial and total glossectomy. *Journal of Speech and Hearing Disorders*, 1970, 35:170–173.

37. Matthews, J., Communication disorders in the mentally retarded. In Travis, L. E., ed., *Handbook of Speech Pathology and Audiology*, pp. 801–818. Englewood Cliffs, N.J.: Prentice-Hall, 1971.

38. McCroskey, R., Corely, N., and Jackson, G., Some effects of disrupted tactile cues upon the production of consonants. *Southern Speech Journal*, 1959, 25:55–60.

39. McReynolds, L. V., and Bennett, S., Distinctive feature generalization in articulation training. *Journal of Speech and Hearing Disorders*, 1972, 37:462–470.

40. McReynolds, L. V., and Huston, K., A distinctive feature analysis of children's misarticulations. *Journal of Speech and Hearing Disorders*, 1971, 36:155–166.

41. McWilliams, B. J., Articulation problems of a group of cleft palate adults. *Journal of Speech and Hearing Research*, 1958, 1:68–74.

42. Mecham, M., Berko, M., and Berko, F., *Communication Training in Childhood Brain Damage*. Springfield, Ill.: Thomas, 1966.

43. Menyuk, P., The role of distinctive features in children's acquisition of phonology. *Journal of Speech and Hearing Research*, 1968, 11:138–146.

44. Merso, R. M., Speech rehabilitation in congenital aglossia. *Journal of Rehabilitation*, 1967, 33:320–334.

45. Mims, H. A., Kolas, C., and Williams, R., Lisping and persistent thumbsucking among children with open-bite malocclusions. *Journal of Speech and Hearing Disorders*, 1966, 31:176–178.

46. Moll, K. L., Speech characteristics of individuals with cleft lip and palate. In Spriestersbach, D. C., and Sherman, D., eds., *Cleft Palate and Communication*, pp. 61–118. New York: Academic Press, 1968.

47. Morley, M. E., Court, D., and Miller, H., Developmental dysarthria. *British Medical Journal*, 1954, 1:8–10.

48. Morris, H. L., Communication skills of children with cleft lips and palates. *Journal of Speech and Hearing Research*, 1962, 5:79–90.

49. Morris, H. L., Etiological bases for speech problems. In Spriestersbach, D. C., and Sherman, D., eds., *Cleft Palate and Communication*, pp. 119–168. New York: Academic Press, 1968.

50. Palmer, M. F., Speech therapy in cerebral palsy. *Journal of Pediatrics*, 1952, 40:514–524.

51. Palmer, M. F., Wurth, C. W., and Kincheloe, J. W., The incidence of lingual apraxia and agnosia in "functional" disorders of articulation. *Cerebral Palsy Review*, 1964, 25:7–9.

52. Philips, B. J., and Harrison, R. J., Language skills of preschool cleft palate children. *Cleft Palate Journal*, 1969, 6:108–119.

53. Pitzner, J. C., and Morris, H. L., Articulation skills and adequacy of breath pressure ratios of children with cleft palate. *Journal of Speech and Hearing Disorders*, 1966, 31:26–40.

54. Pollack, E., and Rees, N. S., Disorders of articulation: some clinical applications of distinctive feature theory. *Journal of Speech and Hearing Disorders*, 1972, 37:451–461.

55. Putnam, A. H. B., and Ringel, R. L., Some observations of articulation during labial sensory deprivation. *Journal of Speech and Hearing Research*, 1972, 15:529–542.

56. Ringel, R. L., and Steer, M. D., Some effects of tactile and auditory alterations on speech output. *Journal of Speech and Hearing Research*, 1963, 6:369–378.

57. Rutherford, B., A comparative study of loudness, pitch, rate, rhythm, and quality of the speech of children handicapped with cerebral palsy. *Journal of Speech and Hearing Disorders*, 1944, 9:263–271.

58. Sax, M. R., A longitudinal study of articulation change. *Language, Speech, and Hearing Services in Schools*, 1972, 3:41–48.

59. Schliesser, H. F., and Coleman, R., Effectiveness of certain procedures for alteration of auditory and oral tactile sensation for speech. *Perceptual and Motor Skills*, 1968, 26:271–281.

60. Scott, C. M., and Ringel, R. L., Articulation without oral sensory control. *Journal of Speech and Hearing Research*, 1971, 14:804–818.

61. Scott, C. M., and Ringel, R. L., The effects of motor and sensory disruptions on speech: a description of articulation. *Journal of Speech and Hearing Research*, 1971, 14:819–828.

62. Shelton, R. L., Brooks, A. R., and Youngstrom, K. A., Articulation and patterns of palatopharyngeal closure. *Journal of Speech and Hearing Disorders*, 1964, 29:390–408.

63. Sherman, D., Spriestersbach, D. C., and Noll, J. D., Glottal stops in the speech of children with cleft palates. *Journal of Speech and Hearing Disorders*, 1959, 24:37–42.

64. Skelly, M., Donaldson, R. C., Fust, R. S., and Townsend, D. L., Changes in phonatory aspects of glossectomee intelligibility through vocal parameter manipulation. *Journal of Speech and Hearing Disorders*, 1972, 37:379–389.

65. Skelly, M., Spector, D. J., Donaldson, R. C., Brodeur, A., and Paletta, F. X., Compensatory physiologic phonetics for the glossectomee. *Journal of Speech and Hearing Disorders*, 1971, 36:101–114.

66. Smith, R. M., and McWilliams, B. J., Psycholinguistic considerations in the management of children with cleft palate. *Cleft Palate Journal*, 1968, 5:238–249.

67. Snow, K., Articulation proficiency in relation to certain dental abnormalities. *Journal of Speech and Hearing Disorders*, 1961, 26:209–212.

68. Spriestersbach, D. C., and Powers, G. R., Articulation skills, velopharyngeal closure, and oral breath pressure of children with cleft palates. *Journal of Speech and Hearing Research*, 1959, 2:318–325.

69. Spriestersbach, D. C., Darley, F. L., and Morris, H. L., Language skills

in children with cleft palates. *Journal of Speech and Hearing Research,* 1958, *1:*279–285.

70. Spriestersbach, D. C., Darley, F. L., and Rouse, V., Articulation of a group of children with cleft lips and palates. *Journal of Speech and Hearing Disorders,* 1956, *21:*436–445.

71. Spriestersbach, D. C., Moll, K. L., and Morris, H. L., Subject classification and articulation of speakers with cleft palates. *Journal of Speech and Hearing Research,* 1961, *4:*362–372.

72. Subtelny, J. D., and Subtelny, J. D., Intelligibility and associated physiological factors of cleft palate speakers. *Journal of Speech and Hearing Research,* 1959, *2:*353–360.

73. Subtelny, J. D., Mestre, J. C., and Subtelny, J. D., Comparative study of normal and defective articulation of /s/ as related to malocclusion and deglutition. *Journal of Speech and Hearing Disorders,* 1964, *29:*269–285.

74. Sulzmann, J., and Seide, L., Malocclusion with extreme microglossia. *American Journal of Orthodontics,* 1962, *48:*848–857.

75. Takagi, Y., McGlone, R. E., and Millard, R. T., A survey of the speech disorders of individuals with clefts. *Cleft Palate Journal,* 1965, *2:*28–31.

76. Thompson, R. C., The effects of oral sensory disruption upon oral stereognosis and articulation. Paper presented at Forty-fifth Annual Convention of American Speech and Hearing Association, 1969.

77. Van Demark, D. R., Assessment of articulation for children with cleft palate. *Cleft Palate Journal,* 1974, *11:*200–208.

78. Van Demark, D. R., Misarticulations and listener judgments of the speech of individuals with cleft palates. *Cleft Palate Journal,* 1964, *1:*232–245.

79. Van Hattum, R. J., Services of the speech clinician in schools: progress and prospects. *Asha,* 1976, *18:*59–63.

80. Van Riper, C., and Erickson, R., A predictive screening test of articulation. *Journal of Speech and Hearing Disorders,* 1969, *34:*214–219.

81. Waterson, N., Child phonology: a prosodic view. *Journal of Linguistics,* 1971, *7:*179–211.

82. Weber, J. L., Patterning of deviant articulation behavior. *Journal of Speech and Hearing Disorders,* 1970, *35:*135–141.

83. Weinberg, B., A cephalometric study of normal and defective /s/ articulation and variations in incisor dentition. *Journal of Speech and Hearing Research,* 1968, *11:*288–300.

84. Whitaker, H. A., and Noll, J. D., Some linguistic parameters of the Token Test. *Neuropsychologia,* 1972, *10:*395–404.

85. Wolf, I. J., Relation of malocclusion to sigmatism. *American Journal of Diseases of Children,* 1937. *54:*520–528.

86. Wolfe, W., A comprehensive evaluation of fifty cases of cerebral palsy. *Journal of Speech and Hearing Disorders,* 1950, *15:*234–251.

87. Yoss, K. A., and Darley, F. L., Developmental apraxia of speech in children with defective articulation. *Journal of Speech and Hearing Research,* 1974, *17:*399–416.

88. Yoss, K. A., and Darley, F. L., Therapy in developmental apraxia of speech. *Language, Speech, and Hearing Services in Schools,* 1974, *5:*23–31.

20
DIFFERENTIAL DIAGNOSIS OF ORGANIC AND PSYCHOGENIC VOICE DISORDERS

Arnold E. Aronson

Strictly speaking, "voice" refers to phonation, the audible tone produced by vocal cord vibration and resonated by the supraglottic cavities. Nasal and oral resonance, altered by palatopharyngeal closure, will not be discussed. Phonation is produced by periodic opening and closing of the glottis effected by interaction between the exhaled airstream and muscular adduction and tension of the vocal cords. The laryngeal tone is modified by articulation and palatopharyngeal closure. Vocal cord vibration is a necessary component of all vowels, semivowels, and voiced consonants; the cords do not vibrate for production of unvoiced cognates.

Voice is a carrier on which are superimposed the relatively specific, symbolic units of speech. Voice without articulation lacks specificity. Phoneme production is bound by limits which are acoustically well defined; one does not have to stray far in their accuracy of production before we begin to notice deviation from normal. But, what standards are to be applied to voice? What is normal voice? When is it defective? How do we describe it?

In an attempt to isolate the normal and abnormal components of voice, the vocal parameters have been divided into pitch, loudness, and quality, as reviewed in Chapter 6. Pitch, how high or low the voice is, is the psychological perception of the physical quantity, frequency; as it goes up or down, so does pitch. Loudness is the perceptual counterpart of intensity. Quality, the most difficult to characterize, refers to the uniqueness of voice determined by complex overtone structure.

A voice disorder means that the voice is judged abnormal in one or more of these three main dimensions. (1) *Quality*. Examples of voice quality defects are harshness, breathiness, and hoarseness. (2) *Pitch*.

535

Examples of pitch defects are excessively high, excessively low, and monopitch. (3) *Loudness.* Examples of loudness defects are excessive loudness, softness, or monoloudness. An abnormality in any one of these dimensions is called a dysphonia. If there is no voice at all and the patient whispers, the term aphonia is applied. And if the patient neither whispers nor articulates, he or she may be described as mute.

The meaning that an abnormal voice has for the listener depends upon his or her specialty. To a laryngologist, whose chief concern is with the integrity of the airway, an abnormal voice signals organic disease of the larynx. To an internist, an abnormal voice may signify a developing systemic illness which suggests a search for other signs of disease. To a neurologist, an abnormal voice may warn of a lesion in the motor system. Psychiatrists think of voice as it relates to the emotions, use it as a measure of the patient's psychologic state, and may employ it as an indicator of long-term progress in psychotherapy. The speech-language pathologist's interest in voice has to do with its efficiency as an instrument of communication and, when abnormal, the extent to which it interferes with intelligibility, is distracting to the listener, or is disturbing to the speaker. Rehabilitation of the voice to its normal state occupies a large proportion of his or her energies.

Knowledge of the spectrum of illnesses that give rise to abnormal voice can be useful to speech pathologists who work in medical clinics and hospitals. Correlation between certain types of voices and specific disease syndromes can be quite useful to the physician in the diagnosis of illness. Patients may be referred to the speech pathologist with the question: "What is wrong with this patient's voice?" The referring physician is not primarily interested in how the speech clinician would describe the voice in terms of pitch, loudness, and quality, important as this is to the total voice examination, but "With what disease entity do you associate this voice symptom?" A skilled speech pathologist can listen to a patient and say, "That is the voice of myasthenia gravis, . . . this one is of myxedema, . . . that one sounds like bilateral upper motor neuron disease, . . . this one sounds like parkinsonism, . . . or that one sounds like a conversion voice disorder."

Voice disorders can be classified etiologically into the two main groups: organic voice disorders and psychogenic voice disorders.

ORGANIC VOICE DISORDERS

Any interference with muscular adduction, abduction, or tonus of the cords will result in a disturbance of their vibratory characteristics and, consequently, dysphonia or aphonia. Any organic disease that causes an increase in mass of one or both vocal cords or which creates irregularities of their surfaces will result in a disturbance of their vibratory characteristics and, consequently, dysphonia or aphonia.

An organic voice disorder may be defined as any dysphonia or aphonia stemming primarily from structural or neuromuscular pathology of the vocal cords. Alterations in the anatomy of the tissues of the cords themselves or the functioning of the intrinsic or extrinsic laryngeal musculature because of impairment of their innervation are capable of producing such voice changes. Most organic voice disorders can be classified under one of the following etiologic categories: congenital, neoplastic, traumatic, inflammatory, neurologic, and endocrinologic.

Childhood Organic Voice Disorders

Organic voice disorders in infancy and childhood are worthy of study because the parameters of voice quality, loudness, and pitch can be clues to the diagnosis of pediatric laryngologic disorders.

Congenital Laryngeal Anomalies   A condition known as laryngomalacia is a congenital pediatric laryngologic disorder that alerts the listener to its presence by means of inspiratory stridor, described as a high-pitched crow or low-pitched vibratory fluttering, occurring intermittently. The stridor is alleged to be caused by loose or flabby tissue contiguous with the epiglottis and arytenoid cartilages which are seen to flutter back and forth during respiration. The disorder is considered to be temporary and indicative of immaturity of laryngeal development resulting in a less than normally rigid laryngeal framework. The disorder disappears between 18 and 24 months of age (*10*).

Congenital *laryngeal web* is a membrane that covers the anterior two-thirds of the vocal cords and represents an arrest of laryngeal development at approximately the tenth week of fetal life. Most laryngeal webs occur at the level of the vocal cords although some are supraglottic and subglottic. They vary in size. If the web covers most of the glottis, respiration for life support may be threatened. Smaller laryngeal webs are less easily recognized. As a result of obstruction of the airway, stridor on inhalation can occur, and the voice or cry may be weak, hoarse, elevated in pitch, or aphonic. Webs are treated either by dilatation or surgical separation.

Congenital *subglottic stenosis* is an infiltration and thickening of the subglottic areolar tissues that can extend superiorly to involve the inferior surface of the true vocal cords. Because it is a serious threat to an open airway, these children are often candidates for tracheostomy until surgical intervention can be performed when the child is 2 or 3 years of age.

Laryngeal cysts protruding into the glottis from the laryngeal ventricle can obstruct the airway of the newborn resulting in dyspnea and an absent or weakened cry.

Neoplasms   The most common laryngeal neoplasms in children are *papillomas*. These histologically benign lesions originate on the vocal cords as multiple tumors. They can extend superiorly onto the walls of the pharynx and soft palate or inferiorly into the tracheobronchial tree. The onset of papillomas ranges from newborn to elderly. A viral etiology is suspected but not established. The onset and development of the tumors is announced by hoarseness. As the tumors grow, an excessively high pitch develops and, in their more advanced stages of growth, aphonia occurs. Respiratory obstruction, sometimes acute, can occur in advanced papillomas. The therapy of choice is forceps removal which may have to be performed repeatedly as a result of regrowth.

Subglottic hemangioma may occur in infancy and childhood. It is a benign growth of the larynx, not considered to be an actual neoplasm but an extensive vascular malformation (4).

Trauma   Internal trauma to the larynx in children can occur, such as *burns* from the ingestion of caustic solutions, flash burns of the larynx, and intralaryngeal *foreign bodies.* External trauma to the larynx resulting in *fractures* of the laryngeal cartilages result primarily from automobile accidents.

Inflammations   Respiratory and phonatory disorders in children are frequently caused by inflammations of the larynx and surrounding structures resulting from *infections* stemming from such bacteria as streptococcus and staphylococcus.

Neurologic Diseases   *Unilateral and bilateral vocal cord paralyses* in children may be present at birth or acquired in early childhood. They result in breathiness, hoarseness, and stridor. These paralyses are almost always the result of damage to the nucleus ambiguus either unilaterally or bilaterally in the brain stem. They may be associated with such neurologic conditions as cerebral agenesis or they may be congenital failures of development of peripheral nerve nuclei or fibers, or due to trauma. As in adults, left unilateral vocal cord paralyses occur more frequently than right owing to exposure of the recurrent laryngeal nerve to cardiovascular abnormalities, tumors of the mediastinum, or injuries during thoracic and neck surgery.

Voice disorders are associated with more widespread congenital or acquired neurologic diseases in children in which the dysphonia is one of several signs of dysarthria in which respiratory, palatopharyngeal, and articulatory disturbances occur alongside phonatory. The presence or absence, type, and severity of dysphonia in widespread neurologic disease will depend upon location and extent of the lesion. In the so-called "cerebral palsy" syndromes, dysphonia may be a manifestation of spasticity, ataxia, or choreoathetosis. The dysphonias resulting from lesions causing these neurologic conditions are similar to those heard in adults suffering from lesions in the same regions of the nervous system. The specific phonatory characteristics of the dysarthrias will be discussed under adult organic voice disorders.

Adult Organic Voice Disorders

Neurologic   The majority of neurologic diseases which affect the motor speech system cause palatopharyngeal and articulatory defects in addition to phonatory. Only the phonatory manifestations of dysarthria will be given here. A complete discussion of the dysarthrias may be found in Chapter 18.

One exception to the above generalization about neurologic disease affecting multiple systems is the mononeuropathy of unilateral and occasionally bilateral vocal cord paralysis.

A lesion of cranial nerve X, or vagus nerve, at any point along its path to the intrinsic laryngeal musculature will result in *flaccid dysphonia* owing to flaccid paresis or paralysis. The lesion can occur at the nuclear or brain stem level (in which case the paralysis is usually bilateral because of the proximity of both nerve X nuclei); along the nerve itself as it courses to the larynx (more often resulting in unilateral vocal cord paralysis); at the myoneural junction; or within the muscle itself.

Any disease which can damage the brain stem is capable of causing unilateral or bilateral vocal cord paralysis. Vascular disease, such as hemorrhagic infarcts, aneurysms, or thromboembolic occlusions of blood vessels in the medulla are typical examples of vascular causes of tenth nerve damage. Such degenerative diseases or structural anomalies as amyotrophic lateral sclerosis or syringobulbia can have similar effects. Trauma to the brain stem is a common cause of flaccid dysphonia bilaterally. When both vocal cords are flaccid due to brain stem lesions, adductor and abductor paralysis may occur simultaneously resulting in stridor on inhalation and dysphonia which may be characterized as breathy and weak. A reduction in the sharpness of the cough or glottal attack may be a further revelation of the adductor vocal cord weakness.

Infranuclear lesions, that is, lesions affecting cranial nerve X after it has left the brain stem, can result from bony abnormalities of the base of the skull, such as the platybasia of the Arnold-Chiari malformation. Mass lesions in the lateral pharyngeal space may also impinge upon the cranial nerve X resulting in vocal cord paralysis.

Infranuclear lesions of the superior and recurrent laryngeal branches of the vagus nerve in the neck and mediastinum are the most common causes of the more familiar unilateral vocal cord paralysis syndrome. Infranuclear lesions can result from trauma to the nerve during neck and thoracic surgery, neoplasms within the neck and upper thoracic cavity and vascular anomalies, particularly aortic arch aneurysm which can press upon the recurrent laryngeal nerve, particularly the left, which dips more deeply into the thoracic cavity than the right. The left recurrent laryngeal nerve loops around the aortic arch before ascending to reenter the neck to innervate the laryngeal musculature, whereas the right is exposed less to thoracic diseases because it loops under the subclavian artery.

When a lesion of the recurrent laryngeal nerve occurs unilaterally, a combined adductor-abductor paralysis of the vocal cord is the usual result. The vocal cord may be fixed in the paramedian position, that is, abducted from the midline. Because the cord is incapable of adducting to meet the intact cord on the opposite side, a glottal chink remains during phonation resulting in excess air escape resulting in a breathy quality and reduced loudness. Not infrequently, diplophonia can be heard because of unequal rates of vibration of the two cords. Some time after the paralysis has occurred, the intact vocal cord may compensate by overshooting the midline to make contact with the paralyzed cord, in which case the dysphonia becomes less severe.

Bilateral damage to the upper motor neuron (pyramidal) system results in spastic paresis or paralysis causing pseudobulbar or spastic dysphonia, part of the dysarthria that results. The term spastic dysphonia is used here to describe a result of upper neuron disease and should not be confused with the spastic (spasmodic) dysphonia discussed in the section on psychogenic voice disorders. Diseases that cause bilateral upper motor neuron damage are brain stem strokes, tumor, trauma, meningitis, abscess, and amyotrophic lateral sclerosis.

The abnormal muscular action in pseudobulbar dysphonia is hyperadduction of the vocal cords. Instead of the cords failing to aduct fully as in flaccid dysphonia, they overadduct, approximating tightly in the midline, reducing the rate of airflow through the glottis. The ventricular folds often adduct along with the true cords. The dysphonias that result are strained-strangled hoarseness, harshness, excessively low pitch, monopitch, and uncontrolled pitch and loudness changes.

Damage to certain of the nuclei of the basal ganglia results in parkinsonism (hypokinesia) and *hypokinetic dysphonia*. Dysphonia is part of the dysarthria that usually accompanies this disease. Parkinsonism can be familial, due to trauma, infection, or vascular disease. Phonation and often respiration are defective owing to rigidity and reduced amplitude of muscular movements. The dysphonia involves monopitch, monoloudness, hoarseness, harshness, breathiness, excessively low volume, in some excessively low pitch, in others excessively high pitch, and a "hollow" voice quality.

Hyperkinesia refers to three neurologic diseases which are characterized by excessive muscular movements involving many regions of the body. Neurologists often subdivide the hyperkinesias into two types: the quick and the slow.

1. *Chorea* is considered to be a quick hyperkinesia and consists of sudden, jerky movements of the extremities and axial musculature. Relevant to phonation, the laryngeal, thoracic, and abdominal musculature are affected causing choreatic dysphonia. Sydenham's chorea is the childhood type, which is often due to infectious diseases of

the basal ganglia. Huntington's chorea is the adult type, usually heredo-familial. The abnormal muscular action in the choreas is sudden, uncontrolled, jerking of the laryngeal, thoracic, and abdominal musculature. The dysphonia consists of sudden changes in pitch and loudness.

2. *Dystonia* is the slower type of hyperkinesia. Dystonias may be heredo-familial, vascular, or infectious. The abnormal muscular action is slow, uncontrolled changes in tonus of the articulatory, laryngeal, thoracic, and abdominal musculature. Dystonic dysphonia consists of a strained-strangled hoarseness or harshness and slow irregularities in pitch and loudness.

3. *Organic voice tremor,* sometimes called essential tremor, is found in older adults; there may be voice tremor only, tremor of the head and hands only, or both. The disease may be heredo-familial or vascular in origin. The location of the lesion in the nervous system has not been determined. The abnormal muscular action involving phonation is regular tremor of the extrinsic and probably the intrinsic laryngeal musculature having a rate of approximately 4 to 12 cycles per second. Often the larynx can be observed to oscillate synchronously with the voice tremor; this is the major dysphonic characteristic of the disease. However, in severe cases, as the larynx moves upward to the extreme point of its movement during each tremor cycle, the vocal cords adduct tightly, obstructing the airstream momentarily, resulting in intermittent, regular vocal arrests. These arrests of voice strongly resemble those of spastic dysphonia, and vice versa, and the two disorders can be easily confused with one another unless differentiated by careful neurologic examination.

Endocrinologic *Myxedematous dysphonia* occurs in hypothyroidism, in which there is insufficient synthesis of thyroid hormone. An increased amount of hydrophilic mucoprotein ground substance in the skin is responsible for the characteristic puffy appearance around the eyes and dorsa of the hands and feet.

Edematous enlargement of the mucous membranes increases the loading of the vocal cords thereby decreasing their natural frequency of vibration. The acoustic effect of such loading is a dysphonia which most often consists of excessively low pitch and hoarseness.

Acromegalic dysphonia in hyperpituitarism is caused by excessive growth of bone, skin, and connective tissues of the body. There is also a marked increase in the volume of interstitial fluid. An increase in length of the vocal cords as part of the overall excessive growth of body tissues occurs and also an increase in loading of the vocal cords due to the increase in interstitial body fluid. Both of these changes result in a lowering of the natural frequency of the vocal cords which, in turn, causes a dysphonia of excessively low pitch.

Neoplasms   *Growths,* benign and malignant, cause many different kinds of voice changes which have not as yet been correlated with type, size, or location of the growth. The term hoarseness is used generally to refer to these changes, although the varieties of dysphonias that can occur are many.

Some of the benign tumors are papillomas, fibromas, granulomas, lipomas, chondromas, myoblastomas, polyps, and polypoid degeneration of the cords.

The malignant neoplasms of the larynx are squamous cell carcinomas, which are common, and adenocarcinomas, which are rare.

Inflammatory voice disorders can result from an increase in size and mass of the vocal cords due to inflammatory, diphtheritic, and tuberculous laryngitis.

Traumatic dysphonias can occur from contusions and fractures of the larynx due to impact injuries. Patients who have undergone endotracheal anesthesia sometimes develop granuloma of the cords due to the trauma from the endotracheal tube.

The *postsurgical voice disorders* from hemilaryngectomy for cancer of the larynx may be characterized by breathy dysphonia or aphonia.

PSYCHOGENIC VOICE DISORDERS

The term functional, though not a particularly apt one, is more commonly used in the literature than psychogenic to indicate symptoms or signs—pain, loss of sensation, or disorder of muscular control—which do not fit established patterns of disease and for which no organic cause can be found. Eventually, however, functional complaints are found to be of emotional origin, for example, depression, anxiety, or conversion reaction, so that the term functional can be safely thought of as synonymous with psychogenic. A psychogenic voice disorder may be defined as a defect of vocal quality, pitch, or loudness for which no organic disease of the larynx or its neural innervation can be found. Most patients diagnosed as having functional voice disorders are suffering from emotional or personality disorders of which the voice is an external sign.

Three specific etiologic types of functional voice symptoms are (1) vocal abuse, (2) environmental stress, and (3) self-image related. They are found in both children and adults, although the incidence of psychogenic voice disorders is higher in adults.

Childhood Psychogenic Voice Disorders

Vocal Abuse   Vocal abuse means voice usage physically damaging to the vocal cords from sustained or intense speaking, singing, shouting, or screaming, possibly at pitch levels too high or low for the muscular capabilities of the larynx. It is alleged that the vocal cords, under these abusive conditions, strike one another with excess force damaging their surfaces. Two vocal abuse syndromes are recognized—vocal nodule and contact ulcer. Vocal nodule occurs in children and adults, but contact ulcer is almost always an adult disorder.

Vocal Nodule   In children or adults vocal nodule is a small, nodular protuberance on the free margin of the vocal cord about one-third of the distance posterior to the anterior commissure. It may be white or grayish in color, may occur unilaterally or bilaterally and is caused by trauma to the soft, noncartilagenous portions of the vocal cords. As they strike one another a small nodule of hyperkeratotic epithelium with underlying fibrosis forms. In its early stages the nodule is seen as a tiny elevation on the free margin of one vocal cord and later on the other. In some laryngologic circles it is believed that prior to the formation of the nodule a submucous hemorrhage occurs and that the nodule originates from the fibrosis of an organizing hematoma.

People who develop vocal nodule usually abuse their voices at higher than normal pitch levels, alleged to cause the point of greatest trauma to move anteriorly into that region of the cords which contains no cartilagenous undersurface, the friction thereby causing a buildup of epithelial tissue.

Vocal nodule is common among children of both sexes. Nodules result from yelling, screaming, singing, or talking at high pitch and loudness levels, hence the synonyms "screamer's nodules" and "singer's nodules."

The person with developing vocal nodules rarely complains of pain or other physical discomfort. What usually brings him to the physician is the voice change that signals disorder. Depending upon size and number, the dysphonia of vocal nodule involves breathiness, hoarseness, excessively low volume, and excessively low pitch.

The diagnosis of vocal nodule is made by the laryngologist usually on the basis of indirect laryngoscopy. Continued case study by the speech pathologist should stress the following:

In the child, in addition to the question as to whether excess voice use has occurred, one should inquire about a history of tension or conflict in the family. Clinical research studies (5, 9, 11) are now beginning to show a long-suspected presence of family problems in children with vocal nodule; verbal aggressiveness and associated vocal abuse are seen as byproducts of such tensions.

The following case history summaries illustrate the etiologic factors in vocal nodule brought out by the preceding questions:

A 12-year-old boy in the seventh grade is bright, popular, and aggressive. He uses his voice strenuously at home and at school. His father, a child psychiatrist, indicated to us that his son may be using his voice to express his hostilities. He was in direct conflict with his younger sister and under pressure at home to produce good grades. We noted in addition to his breathy, hoarse voice, moments of stutteringlike disfluency in his articulation. He spoke rapidly and urgently.

An 8-year-old girl in the third grade began having a breathy, hoarse voice approximately two weeks after the beginning of the school year. She is described by her mother as aggressive, high-strung, very active, impatient, serious, self-assertive, and competitive. She is short-tempered. She is in constant conflict with her 5-year-old sister.

Environmental Stress   There is no clear separation between the environmental stress associated with the development of vocal nodules and environmental stress causing other types of voice disorders. As we shall see under a discussion of environmentally induced voice disorders in adults, dysphonia, aphonia, and mutism can be the result of interpersonal conflicts. However, these forms of voice disorders rarely occur in children with the possible exception of occasional occurrences of elective aphonia and elective mutism in very young children, usually below the age of 5, in which the voice disorder is consciously employed by the child in order to manipulate adults in his or her environment. Nonspecific hoarseness in children may represent varying degrees of laryngeal tension from external stress even though vocal nodule or other indications of laryngeal irritation are absent. It is reasonable to investigate family and peer relations in all children with dysphonia, with or without vocal nodule.

Self-Image Related

Mutational Falsetto   Also called puberphonia or persistent falsetto, mutational falsetto is a disorder in which the voice represents a psychologic maturational failure on the part of the adolescent to utilize an available anatomically larger phonatory-resonatory apparatus which is capable of producing a vocal tone of lower pitch than his customary preadolescent voice.

At puberty the phonatory-resonatory and respiratory systems increase in size and power. The vocal cords thicken and lengthen in their anteroposterior dimensions, the pharyngeal tract lengthens longitudinally as well as transversally, and vital capacity increases. The net effect of these enlargements on normal voice change is a downward migration of pitch. Although some young men go through a period of "stormy mutation," the majority make the transition without much more trouble than a hoarseness or breathiness or an occasional voice break. The youth who psychologically fails to accept the lowering pitch of his voice is one who is susceptible to a mutational voice disorder.

There have been a few studies to ascertain why some males do not "elect" the lower pitch that nature affords them. Role rejection, or the need to maintain a higher-pitched voice to satisfy the self-image, may spring from a need to remain immature or to perpetuate a more refined or perhaps even feminine self-identification that would be incompatible with a lower pitch.

According to Weiss (10) the abnormal muscular action necessary for the maintenance of the high-pitched voice consists of contraction of the cricothyroid muscle elongating the thyroarytenoid muscle (vocal cords) while at the same time maintaining them at a flaccid state. The larynx is elevated in the neck by action of the thyrohyoid musculature. Exhalation for speech is carried out gently with low infraglottal pressure so as not to cause the vocal cords to vibrate in their entirety; only their medial edges are alleged to vibrate.

The dysphonic effects of these unusual muscular sets consist of excessively high pitch, breathiness, and excessively low volume. Not all patients with mutational falsetto have high pitch; some have progressed downward in pitch but their voices have arrested before reaching the lower levels. This phenomenon is called incomplete mutation. Others show sudden breaks between the high falsetto voice and the lower pitch.

The single most important diagnostic test for mutational falsetto is to have the patient cough sharply, produce an abrupt glottal attack on a vowel, or shout. If the dysphonia is of the falsetto type, a sudden downward shift in pitch and increase in loudness will occur due to the effect of the increased infraglottal air pressure in causing the vocal cords to vibrate fully.

Adult Psychogenic Voice Disorders

Vocal Abuse   Like children, adults are prone to voice disorders from strenuous use of the voice: excess speaking, singing, or shouting characterized by strong force of exhalation, and hyperadduction of the vocal cords. Two vocal abuse syndromes in adults occur: vocal nodule and contact ulcer.

Vocal Nodule   Vocal nodule is found in adults who give histories of vocal abuse at what may be higher than normal pitch levels. In adulthood, females appear to be more prone to the disorder than males. In addition to the mechanical abuse of the vocal cords, it can be shown in adults, as in children, that a high percentage of patients with nodules are under emotional stress and begin to have trouble with their voices at approximately the same time they began having interpersonal or vocational adjustment problems.

The following case histories exemplify adults with vocal nodules:

A 20-year-old male college student and major in music had sung in choirs continuously since high school without ever encountering difficulties with his voice. Shortly after beginning the fall term, he began to notice "vocal fatigue"; after singing for a short period of time his voice would become "weak" and "husky." Laryngoscopic examination revealed bilateral, small vocal nodules. During the social and emotional history he complained of mild but continuous depression beginning during the summer which he believed was related to a stormy relationship with his fiancee and uncertainty over whether he should apply for law school or remain in music.

A 29-year-old attorney's wife began noticing breathy voice about two months before coming to the clinic. She is highly energetic and talks constantly, on the telephone and over coffee. She lives in a large house and finds herself screaming at her young children who are often at some remote corner of the house. She also sings two nights a week in the church choir.

A 21-year-old woman, singing in one of the local nightclubs came to the clinic complaining of a disturbing breathiness and vocal fatigue after singing several numbers during each evening's performance. She was particularly upset by the fact that her voice would suddenly and completely fade out on certain of the higher notes. After visiting the club at which she worked I was astounded to discover that she was singing 30 numbers per evening accompanied by two guitars, drums, and an electric organ, all electronically amplified. The noise level generated by this group was deafening. In a subsequent interview, the patient disclosed that at the time her voice began to lose power and change in quality she had begun competing with the organist as to who was going to perform the loudest during her solo numbers. Obviously she was losing out to his electronically amplified instrument. She was diagnosed as having bilateral vocal nodules, which eventually disappeared following a truce with the organist.

Contact Ulcer Contact ulcer is a small, superficial ulceration of the mucosa covering the vocal cords. The lesion is found on the medial surface of either one or both cords about two-thirds of the way back on the cords going antero-posteriorly. The ulcer, occurring near the tip of the vocal process of the arytenoid cartilage buried beneath the surface of the cord, is caused by the cords forcefully slamming together in this region; the hard undersurface of the cartilage abrades the mucosa of the opposite cord. Inflammation, hyperemia, and granulation tissue form, and a crater develops which may fill with necrotic debris.

Contact ulcer is a disorder which predominantly affects adult males in their forties who are engaged in occupations which require strenuous speaking, for example, teaching, the ministry, law, or saleswork. Such individuals are often smokers and use alcohol to excess. Some give histories of exposure to air pollution, frequent upper respiratory infections, and habits of excessive coughing and throat clearing.

Although many patients with developing contact ulcers do not complain of discomfort, others report pain originating deep in the neck radiating to the lateral neck area, ear, or sternum. Some describe a chronic throat tickle, a nonproductive cough, an urge to clear the throat, a sensation of a lump in the throat, an aching throat, and dryness.

The dysphonia of contact ulcer, as with all voice disorders, varies according to the patient and the severity of the disorder. Typically one hears a low pitched hoarseness and, in some, breathiness.

Following the laryngologist's diagnosis of contact ulcer, usually made by indirect laryngoscopy, the speech pathologist's continued examination concerns the case history. The following questions have been found to be of value both diagnostically and, later, therapeutically.

1. What is the patient's occupation? Is it one of the "talking professions"?
2. How much talking occurs during an average day?
3. Under what conditions does talking occur? Consider environmental noise, air pollution (dust, fumes), distance between speaker and listener, telephone vs. face-to-face conversation, room acoustics.
4. What are the specific conditions under which the patient works with respect to external stresses or pressures to produce?
5. How does the patient feel about his or her work? Is it enjoyed or dreaded? What are the relationships between the patient and other workers? Are there interpersonal conflicts?
6. What is the patient's general energy level? Is the patient tired much of the time? Is he or she putting in abnormally long hours? Have there been concurrent illnesses contributing to depletion of energy reserves?
7. Does the patient use alcohol or tobacco in significant amounts?
8. Does the patient habitually speak at low pitch or high loudness levels because he or she feels this manner of speaking lends authority to the voice?

The following case history summaries illustrate several of the etiologic factors in contact ulcer brought out by the preceding list of questions.

A 57-year-old trial lawyer comes to the clinic with a three-year history of chronic cough and hoarseness. In court he speaks loudly and forcefully, and he is under emotional stress. His medical history indicates an intake of eight to ten glasses of straight whiskey each day. His internist has diagnosed alcoholic gastritis and alcoholism, which the patient refuses to recognize.

A 41-year-old professor of English literature gives a five-year history of hoarseness following his lectures. Recently this has become more severe because of an increase in his teaching load. He describes himself as very conscientious; he overprepares his lectures and approaches them with a mixture of perfectionism, pleasureful anticipation, and anxiety. His style of public speaking is forceful and animated. He admits to using a lower pitch than is comfortable because he feels it is more effective. Toward the end of each lecture he begins to feel fatigue and a tightness in his throat, which is painful at times and radiates up the side of his neck and face and culminates in headaches.

A 48-year-old manager of an automobile plant reports a two-month history of hoarseness accompanying an upper respiratory infection. He has had severe laryngitis for the past six weeks. The patient is an executive in an automobile plant. At the time that his voice symptoms began he had come under much stress caused by manufacturing delays; he found that he had to spend at least six hours every day in the plant talking to personnel over noise levels of 100 decibels. These conversations were often charged with emotion as they had to do with correcting deficiencies and reprimanding employees. In addition, he felt the need to comply with outside speaking responsibilities to civic organizations. He has experienced fatigue during the entire period of his voice disorder and the crisis at the plant. In this patient we have a composite of most of the important etiologic factors in contact ulcer: vocal abuse, emotional stress, upper respiratory infection, and fatigue.

Environmental Stress   If we concede that the emotions of anxiety, anger, or depression stemming from life stress may be minor themes in vocal abuse voice disorders, then we must say that they are major ones in the environmental stress group. Here we are talking about patients who develop a variety of dysphonias or aphonias or become mute primarily as a response to life's problems and interpersonal conflicts. The fact that they reveal their unhappiness and unresolvable conflicts through voice whereas others do so through other organ systems has been of long-standing interest to psychiatrists and psychologists but without adequate explanation as to why people differ in their "selection" of a particular organ system.

These patients gradually or suddenly find themselves without voice or develop a wide range of abnormal voices for purely psychologic or emotional reasons. Vocal abuse is an uncommon finding and they rarely show lesions of the cords, although contact ulcer and vocal nodules sometimes occur as secondary effects.

In the larger psychiatric sense, most of these patients are suffering from conversion reaction, a loss of control over physiologically normal musculature because of emotional reasons. Defined,

Conversion reactions . . . are specific, relatively persistent physical symptoms or syndromes which exist in the absence of sufficiently causative physiological pathology. They constitute an unconscious simulation of illness by the patient who is convinced of their somatic origin; and they enable the patient to remain relatively unaware of conflict, stress, or inadequacies that would otherwise be emotionally disturbing. . . . We find conversion reactions to occur in men as well as women, to be monosymptomatic in some cases and to involve many symptoms in others, to be crude and transparent imitations of illness and sometimes highly precise and accurate simulations (*13*, p. 308).

Loss of sensation, motor "paralyses" of the extremities, atypical gait, loss of vision and hearing, and dysphonias, aphonias, muteness, and even articulatory disturbances have been observed clinically to be based on the mechanism of conversion. If it is difficult to conceive of a disturbing idea, emotion, or conflict communicated through a physical disability, Ziegler and Imboden may help to clarify the concept of conversion in the following quotation:

> We have found it useful to consider the patient with a conversion symptom as someone enacting the role of a person with organic illness, symbolically communicating his distress . . . by means of somatic symptoms. In our conceptual model, this somatic mode of communication is not served to discharge pent-up emotion, but, rather like any other language it is useful as an instrument in negotiating interpersonal transactions. Through the conversion reaction, the fact that the patient is in distress is formulated to himself and communicated to others in . . . terms of physical illness and the patient thereby distracts himself from the more immediate perception of his dysphoric affect. Human beings may communicate their feelings and ideas to themselves . . . and others in a variety of modes such as ordinary consensual language, sign language, dreams, autistic verbal symbols of schizophrenia or autistic somatic symbols of conversion reaction. Conversion may be viewed as operating, in this way, like other psychological processes (*12*, p. 284).

Psychogenic Aphonia Psychogenic, conversion, hysterical, or functional aphonia—terms used interchangeably—refers to patients whose predominant voice symptom is that of aphonia or whispering. In most cases the whispering is rarely pure; careful listening will disclose varying degrees of dysphonia in the background, consisting of high-pitched squeaks and squeals, harshness, and even moments of full voicing which break through the characteristic whisper. Incomplete adduction of the vocal cords is the main reason for the whispering, but in most of these patients there is also pulling upward of the larynx against the hyoid bone. The larynx is rigid and difficult to move from side-to-side manually due to strong muscular contraction.

The acoustic products of these muscular sets are the whispering and transient laryngeal noises already described. The whispering is often harsh, sharp, and piercing, and one's impression is that conversion aphonia is not the passive phenomenon that its inaudibility suggests.

Differential diagnosis between severe organic breathiness due to lower motor neuron disease and conversion aphonia must be made in the course of the laryngologist's examination and often the neurologist's examination. The speech pathologist can add to the diagnostic certainty of one or the other of these two causes by asking the patient to cough sharply. *The conversion aphonic will cough normally* or produce a vowel with abrupt onset because vocal cord adduction strength has not been impaired, whereas the patient with severe neurologic flaccid breathiness will produce a *weak or "mushy" glottal attack* on either coughing or vowel initiation because of adductor muscular weakness. Many conversion aphonics will converse with the examiner using whispered speech, and, while doing so, involuntarily cough sharply with audible voicing. Their lack of insight into the fact that their normal coughing reveals an organically healthy larynx may strike the examiner as odd, but this paradox is completely consistent with the obliviousness that the conversion aphonic has to the realities of his or her disorder.

Rarely does organic disease produce the profound degree of whispering found in conversion aphonia, but not all conversion aphonics are complete whisperers; some have severe breathiness as their main voice symptom, and it is almost impossible to detect the difference between organic and conversion breathiness on the basis of listening alone. Laryngologic and even neurologic examination may be necessary to rule out the many motor unit diseases that are capable of producing breathy voice quality.

Once this has been done and a reasonably secure diagnosis of conversion aphonia made, the speech pathologist can enrich the examination proceedings by enlarging on the psychogenic factors responsible for the disorder. Before suggesting how this might be done, we wish to anticipate a natural question that may arise concerning its propriety. Once the diagnosis of conversion aphonia is made by the laryngologist, shouldn't the patient be sent directly to the psychiatrist for exploration of its causes? This is a logical step and often recommended. In actual clinical practice it can be bad advice. The reason can be found within the very psychodynamics of conversion aphonia; that is, the voice symptom is the patient's way of avoiding conscious awareness of his or her emotional problem. The mechanism of the voice symptom is to shield or distract the patient from the real problem, which is emotional. The effect of this mechanism, clinically, is a patient who presents himself fully believing his voice symptom to be organic. Premature confrontation with the information that his aphonia is due to his emotions and that he needs to see a psychiatrist often results in rejection of this interpretation; either the patient will refuse to see the psychiatrist or he will not cooperate if he does see him. Either the laryngologist or speech pathologist can serve as an intermediary consultant in preparation of the patient for the psychiatric interview. Not immediately identified as specialists who deal with emotional illnesses primarily, they are often more acceptable to the patient and can lead gradually into the idea that the voice disorder is of emotional origin.

One patient in particular comes to mind who illustrated this principle most pointedly.

She was a 50-year-old nun and nursing supervisor who had been diagnosed as having a conversion aphonia. Her voice had just returned to near normalcy after an hour of symptomatic voice therapy. I asked her how she felt now that her voice had returned. "I'm too elated to tell you," she said, and went on to describe what it was like to live with aphonia—how she had to repeat so often, how her voicelessness got on peoples' nerves, and how concerned friends would insist that she do something about her voice. After trying cold steam, ice packs, heat, and massage without benefit, she finally presented herself to the hospital laryngologist. "He took one look at me and said, 'You better report to psychiatry.'" "So I did. He (psychiatrist) talked to me, wanted to know if I had emotional problems and so forth," (and here I could see her anger beginning to mount), "but I *couldn't* give him any reports because I don't have any emotional problems. (She did.) I'm happy in my vocation (she wasn't). I'm happy in doing what I'm doing and I have a good superior . . . and all that stuff!" This climaxed her anger and frustration and she finished by bursting into tears.

In preparation for taking the emotional and social history, we have found it important first to summarize the laryngologist's findings for the patient indicating that from a physical standpoint the larynx was found to be normal. This information is, in itself, therapeutic, for these patients often fear malignant laryngeal disease, and they and their families are relieved to find that their worst fears have failed to materialize.

Following this introduction, the clinician looks for emotional stress or conflict behind the voice disorder. At first the patient's response to the question of emotional causes will range from apathy to strenuous denial. Asked if there were any upsetting emotional problems shortly before or at the time of onset of the aphonia, most will be consciously unable to recall such events.

If the clinician will encourage the patient to talk about any possible problems, however trivial they might seem, what starts out as a discussion of minor irritations or dissatisfactions often blossoms into a revelation of larger, sometimes overwhelming life problems of which the patient was not consciously aware. Although each patient's conflict is different, a common denominator runs through their histories: *a struggle exists within the individual between wanting, but not allowing himself, to express feelings of anger, fear, or remorse verbally. Usually a breakdown in communication with someone close to him has occurred. There is something that the patient is afraid to tell, ashamed to tell, or doesn't know how to tell.*

The following case history summaries illustrate this etiologic principle (*1*).

A 50-year-old nun and nursing supervisor is no longer physically able to carry on with her strenuous nursing duties but is afraid to reveal this condition to her superiors because of her conviction that such a disclosure would signify lack of obedience.

A 26-year-old police officer, unhappy in his work, wishes to return to his old job as a mixer of chemicals in a textile mill but is afraid to tell his parents who had strongly favored his joining the force.

A 63-year-old housewife, highly religious and moralistic, is deeply upset about her married daughter's reading, drinking, and smoking habits but is afraid to express her disapproval for fear that doing so would destroy their relationship.

A 51-year-old wife of a retired army officer cannot cope with her husband's demands that the house be run according to military standards but is afraid to tell him about the aggravation he is causing.

A 39-year-old mother of three young children is having an extramarital affair with an older man at the office where she works. The affair has lost its early romance and intrigue, and now she wishes to break it off. She feels guilty about what she has done and wants to tell her husband about it but cannot bring herself to do so. He is the county sheriff.

Psychogenic Muteness   The most extreme form of conversion communication disorder is muteness. Two variations occur: (1) The patient makes articulatory movements but, unlike the whispering aphonic, fails to accompany these movements with an exhaled airstream. Consequently, no friction noise from the larynx is heard and we would have no idea that the patient was attempting to communicate were it not for the movement of the lips. (2) The patient produces neither articulatory nor exhalatory movements and often resorts to writing notes.

Muteness can occur in psychotic patients, and it is important that a psychiatric consultation be obtained early in the diagnostic workup to determine if indeed severe psychiatric disorder is responsible for their lack of speech. Other mute patients are completely in touch with reality and give histories of dysphonia and aphonia as well as muteness; they are etiologically within the realm of conversion.

Following is a case history of a patient who presented herself as mute. It is given to show the similarity of background to the whispering aphonic and to reinforce the point that conversion voice symptoms are highly variable and interchangeable, even in the patient who presents as mute.

A 44-year-old lady on examination is found to use no respiratory, phonatory, or articulatory activity for communication. She communicates by writing, using a pencil and pad of paper which she carries with her at all times. Psychiatric interview revealed a history of struggle and deprivation almost from birth. She was the youngest of ten, her family being burdened by five other children from her father's former marriage. By the time she was 20, her father then dead and most of the children having left home, she inherited the responsibility of caring for her aging mother and two older sisters. She lived a Cinderella-like existence, doing the household chores and being dominated by her sisters, who rarely allowed her out of the house. It was under these circumstances that, at age 23, she had her first conversion symptom, a "paralysis" of the right arm lasting two weeks. Three years later she became severely depressed and unable to work for several months. Then, at age 27, her mother, ". . . the only person who ever loved me . . ," died. Shortly thereafter she developed a "paralysis" of both legs and became an invalid for one and a half years. Physical therapy effected a "dramatic cure." Her doctors, who knew of her hostile and dependent relationship with her sisters, urged her to get out on her own. Six years later, at age 35, she married a 27-year-old man with a son from a previous marriage. She had made an adjustment to life. However, financial worries and behavior problems in the son arose. She then began to have episodes of *dysphonia* is response to these stresses. During the winter prior to our seeing her she also had episodes of *intermittently phonated-whispered voice.* Nine months before coming to the clinic she lapsed into *complete whispering aphonia* finally giving away to *muteness* and writing of notes.

Muteness can also occur in emotionally disturbed children who come from homes in which they have witnessed or were victims of severe family conflict, rejection, or physical abuse. Elective muteness, a voluntary disorder in children, is recognized. Children on pediatric neurology wards have developed either aphonia or muteness, or both, as anxiety reactions secondary to a sudden apraxia of speech or aphasia stemming from central nervous system diseases. Muteness can occur in severe apraxia of speech, implicating phonation and articulation. It can occur in severe parkinsonism, actually an anarthria. Neurologic diseases affecting other deep brain structures can cause a condition known as akinetic mutism or coma vigil in which the patient appears alert and awake but is unresponsive to commands and does not speak.

Spastic Dysphonia, Intermittent, Adductor   Spastic dysphonia [1] is the acoustic effect of intermittent hyperadduction of the vocal cords. The voice symptoms have been variably described as intermittent partial or complete vocal arrests, strained-strangled voice, hoarseness, harshness, breathiness, excessively high pitch, and excessively low pitch. They have also been described as staccato or stutteringlike, intermittent, jerky,

---

[1] The term spasmodic dysphonia has been suggested as a preferable alternative which could prevent confusion between spastic dysphonia being discussed here and the pseudobulbar dysphonia which is a component of spastic dysarthria (3).

grunting, squeezed, groaning, and effortful. Laughter and phonation at high pitch levels or while singing are often normal.

A given patient with spastic dysphonia can defy some of our best interdisciplinary efforts at establishing an etiologic diagnosis. In some patients the abnormal voice can be traced back to acute emotionally disturbing events. In others it can be linked with chronic emotional stress. In both instances conversion is the mechanism considered to be responsible for the dysphonia. What is disturbing is that in certain of these patients no emotional factors can be found and, because of the presence of scattered neurologic signs, these patients are suspected of having some neurologic disease as responsible for their dysphonia (8). Yet no specific neurologic disease entity or syndrome has been established.

There are, to be sure, definite neurologic syndromes in which spasmodic vocal arrests are present as one of many neurologic signs elsewhere in the body. Although it is unlikely that these diseases would be confused with spastic dysphonia, they might be if the dysphonia were the earliest and only sign of the disease. These syndromes include essential (organic) voice tremor, pseudobulbar palsy, palatopharyngeal myoclonus, spasmodic torticollis, and chorea and dystonia involving the larynx.

Following are pertinent questions that will help identify spastic dysphonia. Comparisons are made with psychogenic aphonia.

1. What was the nature of onset and course of the dysphonia? Rarely do the intermittent arrests of the voice begin suddenly and with full intensity; onset is more often characterized by nonspecific steady hoarseness. As time passes the characteristic intermittency and severity of the spasms become apparent. There is either a gradual worsening of the disorder or the severity remains the same after the initial development of the intermittent spasms. Rarely do patients with spastic dysphonia report spontaneous remissions of their symptoms. Psychogenic aphonic patients experience many such remissions, and this is one of many unexplained differences between the two groups.

2. Was the onset of the voice change associated with any physical illnesses? In conversion aphonia a high percentage of patients began their voice disorder with upper respiratory infections and other physical illnesses involving the head, neck, and chest. Patients with spastic dysphonia as a group give similar histories of cold or flu preceding the development of the hoarseness that ultimately develops into intermittent spasm.

3. Was the onset of the dysphonia associated with a feeling of tightness, lump, or ball in the throat? Tightness, difficulty in swallowing, or general discomfort in the region of the neck and chest are common complaints among patients with both psychogenic aphonia and spastic dysphonia.

4. Has the dysphonia been constant since onset or have there been periods during which the voice has improved, been normal, or worsened? Patients with spastic dysphonia report much less fluctuation in the voice symptoms in comparison with the psychogenically aphonic patient. The typical history is a voice disorder of gradual onset which grows progressively worse with few remissions of symptoms. However, it must be reported that a small number of patients with spastic dysphonia have had episodes of complete aphonia and normal voice after the onset of their voice disorder.

Investigation of the emotional and social factors underlying the dysphonia is carried out in the same manner as that for psychogenic aphonia. We look for life events that have been emotionally upsetting to the patient. In a study by Aronson, Brown, and Litin (2), 18 out of 29 spastic dysphonia patients examined by psychiatrists gave histories and personality characteristics indicative of psychoneurosis. Three common traits emerged: compulsiveness, suppressed anger, and a life history of verbal repression. As a group they were rigid, conscientious, perfectionistic worriers, who showed faulty handling of anger and resentment, tending to keep their anger to themselves, and describing themselves as being "the quiet ones" in their families from childhood on. These personality traits, however, are found in multitudes of people who do not have voice disorders.

When we compared in that same study the histories of psychogenic aphonic with spastic dysphonic patients with respect to the question of emotional events causing the disorder, we had much more difficulty finding distinct precipitating emotional conflicts or trauma that coincided precisely with the onset of spastic dysphonia than we did in patients with aphonia. The spastic group had emotional conflicts to be sure, but they were much less sharply defined in terms of the nature of the conflict and its temporal relationship to the onset of the dysphonia. It is interesting that the psychiatrist in the study just mentioned described the spastic dysphonic as superficially stable and well adjusted in striking contrast to the psychogenically aphonic patient in whom there were obvious evidences of instability. This impression parallels the reports of others concerning the spastic dysphonic's facade of normalcy. Here is a description of a patient reported by Heaver (6, pp. 257–258):

> Psychological examination revealed him to be an anxious, orally dependent, obsessive person, *but did not provide any direct clues to the mechanisms behind his voice loss* (italics mine). Depression was seen only by inference and not by direct evidence . . . *the patient continues to present a remarkably cohesive picture of stabilized adjustment and emotional control* (italics mine). The degree of intactness is in sharp contrast to the amount of disability which his voice loss involves. On the basis of the absence of affect, apart from the depression, the extreme isolation of the symptom and the almost certain functional etiology, it would seem without much doubt that this is a conversion reaction.

Spastic Dysphonia, Constant, Adductor For many years the term ventricular dysphonia has been employed to designate a separate voice disorder entity. It has been characterized as a harsh voice produced by ventricular or false vocal cord hyperadduction. The voice of the patient identified as having ventricular dysphonia is in many ways similar to spastic dysphonia except for the absence of intermittency in the ventricular dysphonic, that is, the spasm is constant. In our experience with patients having constant hyperadduction of the vocal cords which others may have described as ventricular dysphonia, we have found many characteristics similar to those of patients with the intermittent type of spastic dysphonia: they were capable of improved voice at higher pitch levels, laughed normally, could sing, and, etiologically, gave histories of emotional conflict which were undifferentiable from those given by patients having spastic dysphonia. Perhaps the most conclusive behavior that has convinced us of the close relationship between the two groups is that patients with "ventricular dysphonia" who had undergone symptomatic voice therapy improved in the direction of becoming intermittently spastic, and patients with the intermittent spastic dysphonia upon becoming worse had gone from intermittent spastic arrests to the constant type, which, if seen for the first time, would probably have been identified as "ventricular dysphonia."

The abnormal muscular action in the continuous spastic dysphonic is continuous hyperadduction of the false vocal cords alone or both false and true vocal cords, and excessive force on exhalation. The dysphonia consists of continuous strained-strangled hoarseness.

The clinical investigation of the patient with continuous spastic dysphonia or ventricular dysphonia is essentially the same as that for intermittent spastic dysphonia.

Spastic Dysphonia, Abductor Until now we have been talking about laryngospasm in which the direction of vocal cord movement has been medial with hyperadduction in the midline obstructing the exhaled airstream. But there is another type of laryngospasm, less frequently seen, in which the direction of vocal cord movement is away from the midline, that is, abductor spasm. This, then, would be intermittent hyperabduction of the vocal cords as the abnormal muscular action. The effect of intermittent abduction of the vocal cords is to create the dysphonic characteristic of *intermittent moments of breathiness or intermittent whispering*. The listener hears sudden moments of voice loss or breathiness on speech sounds that normally should be phonated.

Thus far, we feel that the abductor type stems from the same dynamics, that is, conversion, as that of the adductor type of spastic dysphonia. Once again, we do not know why patients with conversion voice disorders select their particular voice symptom; the meaning of adductor spasm as opposed to abductor is completely unclear at this time. But the case history backgrounds indicate strong similarities of conflict.

Psychogenic Breathiness, Continuous   At the least dramatic end of the psychogenic voice disorder continuum is the patient with continuously breathy voice quality. The abnormal muscular action is continuous hyperabduction of the vocal cords and the dysphonia is continuous breathiness and excessively low volume.

As we have already mentioned in this chapter, the patient with breathy voice quality presents a medical differential diagnostic problem, as breathiness can be caused by a variety of organic diseases. The patient with psychogenically breathy voice often gives a history similar to that of the psychogenically aphonic patient and, indeed, many patients who ultimately become aphonic begin their disorders with breathy voice quality in varying degrees of severity.

The questioning of the patient during history taking follows the same lines as that for other psychogenic voice disorders and, if the disorder is psychogenic, a history of emotional conflict will usually emerge.

Psychogenic Hoarseness   Another differential diagnostic problem is presented by the patient who is continually hoarse. Hoarseness in mild degrees can be the early dysphonia of either psychogenic aphonia or spastic dysphonia of either adductor or abductor type. Many patients, as we have mentioned before, who develop the intermittent spastic dysphonia begin with nonspecific continuous hoarseness. The abnormal muscular reaction is continuous hyperadduction of the vocal folds and excess force of exhalation. The dysphonia is continuous hoarseness.

Self-Image Related   Certain abnormal voice symptoms are indications of the personality of the individual. In this group the voice disorder is not a transient, fleeting symptom which serves the purpose of extricating the individual from some difficult situation. Rather, the voice has roots at the very core of everyone's personality; it has grown up with one and is as much a part of one as one's way of walking, smiling, or expressing oneself in other unique ways. Many research studies have sought to prove or disprove the statement that the voice reflects the basic personality. Within normal personality limits, apparently voice is not a particularly reliable or valid indicator of specific inner attitudes, traits, or feelings possessed by an individual. However, when personalities begin to nudge the outer limits of normal, voice may quite accurately reflect the developing psychopathology of that individual.

Although the following is not an exhaustive classification of self-image related voice disorders they represent three types of personality related dysphonias that we have seen: (1) mutational falsetto, (2) childlike speech in adults, (3) speech and voice disorders reflecting masculine and feminine tendencies.

Mutational Falsetto   We have discussed this disorder under childhood voice disorders, for it begins during the period of adolescent voice change. However, the disorder will continue into adulthood for an indefinite period of time unless therapeutically changed. The earlier in life training is initiated, the better for the long-term self-image of the person, although individuals in their fifties and sixties have been able to change to the masculine voice without undue difficulty.

Childlike Speech in Adults Occasionally the speech clinician will be confronted by an adult whose entire speech pattern bears a striking resemblance to that of someone much younger and physically smaller. Technically the disorder is not confined to the larynx. The voice may be higher in pitch than normal, reduced in loudness, and accompanied by articulatory postures characterized by smaller than normal mouth openings for consonant and vowel articulation which one speculates facilitates resonation of higher frequencies owing to the artificial creation of a smaller oral cavity. Appropriately immature facial expressions and gestures frequently accompany this type of speech pattern.

Masculine and Feminine Tendencies Voice is often an important component of the self-image of the male with an exaggerated feminine identification and the female with an exaggerated masculine identification. Again, articulation often contributes to this image as well as voice. In the former, the voice is somewhat higher in pitch and articulation more than typically precise for the average male speaker. In the latter, the pitch of the voice is often lowered and the articulation less precise, the total effect pulling the image closer to the masculine range.

The latter two personality-related voice or speech disorders have undergone a minimum of clinical or laboratory investigation and our assertions about them have been based on limited subjective clinical experiences. Moreover, the question arises as to whether the choice of a particular mode of voice and articulation reflecting personality qualifies as a disorder according to our customary definitions of the term or whether they can or should be considered variations along the normal continuum.

ASSIGNMENTS

1. What basic acoustic-psychologic parameters can be employed as a yardstick to determine normalcy or abnormality of voice?
2. What are the fundamental differences between organic and functional voice disorders?
3. What are the three main types of functional voice disorders and how are they different from one another?
4. How do tension, anxiety, and depression affect the laryngeal musculature?
5. Differentiate between contact ulcer and vocal nodule on the basis of location and type of tissue pathology.
6. Give a profile of the person who is most likely to develop contact ulcer.

7. Give a profile of the person who is most likely to develop vocal nodule.
8. Why is there a higher incidence of left unilateral vocal fold paralysis than right?
9. Describe the differences in the sound of the voice among organic voice tremor, unilateral vocal fold paralysis, and myxedema.
10. What is the physical basis for the excessively low pitch of acromegalic dysphonia?
11. What is the meaning of "conversion aphonia" and what is the reason for its occurrence?
12. Describe the voice characteristics of the person with adductor spastic dysphonia.
13. What factors characterize the onset and development of adductor spastic dysphonia?
14. How would you best determine if someone with a high-pitched voice was demonstrating mutational falsetto?
15. If someone came to you before anyone else with a voice disorder, what kinds of medical specialists would you want to examine that person? Why?

REFERENCES

1. Aronson, A. E., *Psychogenic Voice Disorders: An Interdisciplinary Approach to Detection, Diagnosis and Therapy.* Philadelphia: Saunders, 1973.
2. Aronson, A. E., Brown, J. R., and Litin, E. M., Spastic dysphonia: I. Voice, neurologic and psychiatric aspects. *Journal of Speech and Hearing Disorders*, 1968, 33:203–218.
3. Aronson, A. E., Brown, J. R., Litin, E. M., and Pearson, J. S., Spastic dysphonia. II. Comparison with essential (voice) tremor and other neurologic and psychogenic symptoms. *Journal of Speech and Hearing Disorders*, 1968, 33:219–231.
4. Ferguson, C. F., Congenital abnormalities of the infant larynx. *Otolaryngologic Clinics of North America*, June 1970, 3:185–200.
5. Glassel, W. L., A study of personality problems and vocal nodules in children. Paper read at Annual Convention of the American Speech and Hearing Association, San Francisco, November 1972.
6. Heaver, L., Spastic dysphonia: A psychosomatic voice disorder. In Barbara, D. A., ed., *Psychological and Psychiatric Aspects of Speech and Hearing*, pp. 250–263. Springfield, Ill.: Thomas, 1960.
7. Holinger, P. H., Schield, J. A., and Weprin, L., Pediatric laryngology. *Otolaryngologic Clinics of North America*, October 1970, 3:625–637.
8. Robe, E., Brumlik, J., and Moore, P., A study of spastic dysphonia: Neurologic and electroencephalographic abnormalities. *Laryngoscope*, 1960, 70:219–245.
9. Toohill, R. J., The psychosomatic aspects of children with vocal nodules. *Archives of Otolaryngology*, 1975, 101:591–595.

10. Weiss, D. A., The pubertal change of the human voice (mutation). *Folia Phoniatrica*, 1950, *2*:126–159.
11. Wilson, F. B., Emotional stress may cause voice anomalies in kids. *Journal of the American Medical Association*, 1971, *216*:2085.
12. Ziegler, F. J., and Imboden, J. B., Contemporary conversion reactions: II. A conceptual model. *Archives of General Psychiatry*, 1962, *6*:279–287.
13. Ziegler, F. J., Imboden, J. B., and Rodgers, D. A., Contemporary conversion reactions: III. Diagnostic considerations. *Journal of the American Medical Association*, 1963, *186*:307–311.

INDEX

78 79 80 9 8 7 6 5 4 3 2 1